LIPPINCOTT MANUAL
*of* NURSING PRACTICE
Series

# DIAGNOSTIC TESTS

# LIPPINCOTT MANUAL
## *of* NURSING PRACTICE
### Series

# DIAGNOSTIC
# TESTS

◆

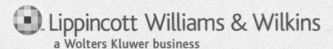

.Lippincott Williams & Wilkins
a Wolters Kluwer business

Philadelphia · Baltimore · New York · London
Buenos Aires · Hong Kong · Sydney · Tokyo

## STAFF

**Executive Publisher**
Judith A. Schilling McCann, RN, MSN

**Editorial Director**
H. Nancy Holmes

**Clinical Director**
Joan M. Robinson, RN, MSN

**Senior Art Director**
Arlene Putterman

**Editorial Project Manager**
Jennifer Lynn Kowalak

**Clinical Project Manager**
Beverly Ann Tscheschlog, RN, BS

**Editor**
Julie Munden

**Clinical Editor**
Maryann Foley, RN, BSN

**Copy Editors**
Kimberly Bilotta (supervisor),
Scotti Cohn, Judith Orioli,
Kelly Pavlovsky, Dona Perkins,
Irene Pontarelli, Lisa Stockslager,
Pamela Wingrod

**Designers**
Debra Moloshok (book design),
Jan Greenberg (project manager)

**Digital Composition Services**
Diane Paluba (manager),
Joyce Rossi Biletz, Donna S. Morris

**Manufacturing**
Patricia K. Dorshaw (director),
Beth J. Welsh

**Editorial Assistants**
Megan L. Aldinger, Karen J. Kirk,
Linda K. Ruhf

**Design Assistant**
Georg Purvis, 4th

**Indexer**
Barbara Hodgson

LMNPDX010206—020307

Library of Congress
Cataloging-in-Publication Data
Diagnostic tests.
     p. ; cm. — (Lippincott manual of nursing practice series)
  Includes bibliographical references and index.
  1. Diagnosis, Laboratory—Handbooks, manuals, etc. 2. Nursing—Handbooks, manuals, etc. I. Lippincott Williams & Wilkins. II. Title. Series.
  [DNLM: 1. Laboratory Techniques and Procedures—Handbooks. 2. Laboratory Techniques and Procedures—Nurses' Instruction. 3. Diagnostic Techniques and Procedures—Handbooks. 4. Diagnostic Techniques and Procedures—Nurses' Instruction. QY 39 D53652 2007]
RT48.5.D528 2007
616.07'5—dc22
ISBN13: 978-1-58255-903-2
ISBN10: 1-58255-903-1 (alk. paper)      2005030525

# CONTENTS

———◆———

# CONTRIBUTORS
# AND CONSULTANTS

◆

**Katrina D. Allen,** RN, MSN, CCRN
*ADN Nursing Faculty*
Faulkner State Community College
Bay Minette, Ala.

**Deborah M. Berry,** RN, MSN
*Clinical Nurse Specialist*
Franklin Square Hospital Center
Baltimore

**Nancy P. Blumenthal,** RN, CRNP, MSN,
CS
*Senior Nurse Practitioner*
Lung Transplant Program
University of Pennsylvania Medical Center
Philadelphia

**Kim D. Cooper,** RN, MSN
*Nursing Department Chair*
Ivy Tech Community College of Indiana
Terre Haute

**Lillian Craig,** RN, MSN, FNP-C
*Family Nurse Practitioner*
Claude (Tex.) Rural Health Clinic
*Instructor*
Oklahoma Panhandle State University
Goodwell

**Colleen Davenport,** RN, MSN
*Med/Surg Nurse*
Wrangell (Alaska) Medical Center

**Louise Diehl-Oplinger,** RN, MSN, CCRN,
APRN-BC
*Advanced Practice Nurse*
CPR for Life & Health Care Consulting, Inc.
Wind Gap, Pa.

**Jennifer E. DiMedio,** RN, MSN, CRNP
*Family Nurse Practitioner*
University of Pennsylvania-West Chester
Family Practice

**Toni Eason,** RN, APRN,BC, MS
*Occupational Health Nurse*
Peace Corps
Washington, D.C.

**Anna L. Easter,** RN, PhD, APRN,BC
*ACNP Orthopedic Surgery*
Central Arkansas Veterans Health Systems
Little Rock

**Nancy A. Emma,** RN, BSN
*OIC,* US Army EMS Programs Office
Academy of Health Sciences
Dept. of Combat Medic Training
Fort Sam Houston, Tex.

**Colleen Fries,** RN, MSN, CRNP, CCRN
*Family Nurse Practitioner*
Newtown (Pa.) Primary Care

**Sharon L.G. Lee,** RN, CCRN, MS, BSN,
FNP-C
*Emergency RN/FNP*
Bryan LGH Medical Center
Lincoln, Nebr.

**Kimberly Hall Oas,** RN, APRN, MSN,
FNP-C
*Faculty*/College of Nursing
Kent (Ohio) State University

**Vanessa G. Southard,** RN, BSN
*Associate Professor*
Darthmouth Medical Center
New Hampshire Community Technical
College
Claremont

**Audrey E. Taleff,** RN, APRN,BC, MSN
*Family Nurse Practitioner*
Waianae (Hawaii) Coast Comprehensive
Health Center

**Dawn M. Zwick,** RN, CRNP, MSN
*Faculty*
Kent (Ohio) State University
*CRNP*
Townhall II Medical Clinic
Kent, Ohio

# ABO blood typing and crossmatching

ABO blood typing classifies blood according to the presence of major antigens A and B on red blood cell (RBC) surfaces and according to serum antibodies anti-A and anti-B. ABO blood typing using forward and reverse methods is required before transfusion to prevent a lethal reaction.

In forward typing, the patient's RBCs are mixed with anti-A serum, then with anti-B serum; the presence or absence of agglutination determines the blood group. In reverse typing, the results of the forward method are verified by mixing the patient's serum with known group A and group B cells. Blood group determination is confirmed when the results of forward and reverse typing match perfectly.

Crossmatching (also known as *compatibility testing*) establishes compatibility or incompatibility of a donor's and a recipient's blood. It's the best antibody detection test available for avoiding lethal transfusion reactions. After the donor's and the recipient's ABO and Rh-factor type are determined, major crossmatching determines compatibility between the donor's RBCs and the recipient's serum. Minor crossmatching determines compatibility between the donor's serum and the recipient's RBCs. Because the antibody-screening test is routinely performed on all blood donors, minor crossmatching is commonly omitted.

Because a complete crossmatch may take from 45 minutes to 2 hours, an incomplete (10-minute) crossmatch may be performed in an emergency such as severe blood loss due to trauma. In an emergency, transfusion can begin with limited amounts of group O packed RBCs while crossmatching is completed. Incomplete typing and crossmatching increase the risk of complications. After crossmatching, compatible units of blood are labeled and a compatibility record is completed.

**Alert** *The most carefully performed crossmatch may not detect all the possible sources of patient-donor incompatibility.*

## PURPOSE

- To establish blood group according to the ABO system
- To check compatibility of donor and recipient blood before transfusion, serving as a final check

## PATIENT PREPARATION

- Tell the patient that ABO blood typing and crossmatching determines his blood group.
- If the patient is scheduled for a transfusion, explain that after his blood group is known, it can be matched with the right donor blood.
- Inform the patient that he need not restrict food and fluids.
- Tell the patient that the test requires a blood sample. Explain who will perform the venipuncture and when.
- Explain to the patient that he may experience slight discomfort from the tourniquet and needle puncture.
- Check the patient's history for recent administration of blood, dextran, or I.V. contrast media.

## PROCEDURE AND POSTTEST CARE

● Perform a venipuncture and collect the sample in a 10-ml tube without additives or EDTA.

● Apply direct pressure to the venipuncture site until bleeding stops.

## PRECAUTIONS

● Label the sample with the patient's name, the health care facility or blood bank number, the date, and the phlebotomist's initials.

● Handle the sample gently to prevent hemolysis and send it to the laboratory immediately with a properly completed laboratory request.

● Follow standard precautions with collection of sample.

● Indicate on the laboratory request the amount and type of blood component needed.

*Alert If more than 72 hours have elapsed since an earlier transfusion, previously crossmatched donor blood must be recrossmatched with a new recipient serum sample to detect newly acquired incompatibilities before transfusion. If the patient is scheduled for surgery and has received blood during the past 3 months, be aware that his blood needs to be crossmatched again if his surgery is rescheduled to detect recently acquired incompatibilities.*

## FINDINGS

In forward typing, if agglutination occurs when the patient's RBCs are mixed with anti-A serum, the A antigen is present and the blood is typed A. If agglutination occurs when the patient's RBCs are mixed with anti-B serum, the B antigen is present and the blood is typed B. If agglutination occurs in both mixes, A and B antigens are present and the blood is typed AB. If it doesn't occur in either mix, no antigens are present and the blood is typed O.

In reverse typing, if agglutination occurs when B cells are mixed with the patient's serum, anti-B is present and the blood is typed A. If agglutination occurs when A cells are mixed, anti-A is present and the blood is typed B. If agglutination occurs when A and B cells are mixed, anti-A and anti-B are present and the blood is typed O. If agglutination doesn't occur when A and B cells are mixed, neither anti-A nor anti-B is present and the blood is typed AB.

With crossmatching, absence of agglutination indicates compatibility between the donor's and the recipient's blood, which means that the transfusion of donor blood can proceed. Note that this doesn't guarantee a safe transfusion.

*Alert Donor blood may be transfused only when ABO compatibility has been confirmed with the recipient's blood. The transfusion of blood containing either A or B antigens to a recipient whose RBCs lack these antigens can cause a potentially fatal reaction.*

## ABNORMAL FINDINGS

A positive crossmatch indicates incompatibility between the donor's blood and the recipient's blood, which means that the donor's blood can't be transfused to the recipient. The sign of a positive crossmatch is agglutination, or clumping, when the donor's RBCs and the recipient's serum are correctly mixed and incubated. Agglutination indicates an undesirable antigen-antibody reaction. The donor's blood must be withheld and the crossmatch continued to determine the cause of the incompatibility and identify the antibody.

## INTERFERING FACTORS

● Recent administration of dextran or I.V. contrast media, causing cellular aggregation resembling antibody-mediated agglutination

● Blood transfusion or pregnancy in the past 3 months (possibility of lingering antibodies)

● Delay of testing for more than 72 hours after sample collection

# ACTH (corticotropin), plasma

The ACTH or corticotropin test measures the plasma levels of corticotropin by radioimmunoassay. Corticotropin stimulates the adrenal cortex to secrete cortisol and, to a lesser degree, androgens and aldosterone. It also induces melanocyte-stimulating activity, increases the uptake of amino acids by muscle cells, promotes lipolysis by fat cells, stimulates pancreatic beta cells to secrete insulin, and possibly contributes to the release of growth hormone. Corticotropin levels vary diurnally, peaking between 6 a.m. and 8 a.m. and ebbing between 6 p.m. and 11 p.m. Through a negative feedback mechanism, plasma cortisol levels control corticotropin secretion—for example, high cortisol levels suppress corticotropin secretion. Emotional and physical stress (pain, surgery, insulin-induced hypoglycemia) stimulate secretion and can override the effects of plasma cortisol levels.

The corticotropin test may be ordered for a patient with signs of adrenal hypofunction (insufficiency) or hyperfunction (Cushing's syndrome). Corticotropin suppression or stimulation testing is usually necessary to confirm diagnosis. The instability and unavailability of corticotropin greatly limit this test's diagnostic significance and reliability.

## PURPOSE

- To facilitate differential diagnosis of primary and secondary adrenal hypofunction
- To aid differential diagnosis of Cushing's syndrome

## PATIENT PREPARATION

- Explain to the patient that the corticotropin test helps determine if his hormonal secretion is normal.
- Advise the patient that he must fast and limit his physical activity for 10 to 12 hours before the test.
- Tell the patient that the test requires a blood sample. Explain who will perform the venipuncture and when.
- Explain to the patient that he may experience slight discomfort from the tourniquet and needle puncture.
- Check the patient's history for medications that may affect the accuracy of test results, as ordered. Withhold these medications for 48 hours or longer before the test. If they must be continued, note this on the laboratory request.
- Arrange with the dietary department to provide a low-carbohydrate diet for 2 days before the test. This requirement may vary, depending on the laboratory.

## PROCEDURE AND POSTTEST CARE

- For a patient with suspected adrenal hypofunction, perform the venipuncture for a baseline level between 6 a.m. and 8 a.m. (peak secretion).
- For a patient with suspected Cushing's syndrome, perform the venipuncture between 6 p.m. and 11 p.m. (low secretion).
- Collect the sample in a plastic EDTA tube (corticotropin may adhere to glass). The tube must be full because excess anticoagulant will affect results.
- Pack the sample in ice and send it to the laboratory immediately, where plasma must be rapidly separated from blood cells at 39.2° F (4° C). The collection technique may vary, depending on the laboratory.
- Apply direct pressure to the venipuncture site until bleeding stops.
- Instruct the patient that he may resume his usual diet, activities, and medications discontinued before the test, as ordered.

## PRECAUTIONS

- Because proteolytic enzymes in plasma degrade corticotropin, a temperature of 39.2° F (4° C) is necessary to retard enzyme activity.
- Immediate transfer of the sample, packed in ice, to the laboratory is essential for reliable test results.

## REFERENCE VALUES

Mayo Medical Laboratories sets baseline values at less than 120 pg/ml (SI, < 26.4 pmol/L at 6 a.m. to 8 a.m.), but these values may vary, depending on the laboratory.

## ABNORMAL FINDINGS

A higher-than-normal corticotropin level may indicate primary adrenal hypofunction (Addison's disease), in which the pituitary gland attempts to compensate for the unresponsiveness of the target organ by releasing excessive corticotropin. The underlying cause of adrenocortical hypofunction may be idiopathic atrophy of the adrenal cortex or partial destruction of the gland by granuloma, neoplasm, amyloidosis, or inflammatory necrosis.

A low-normal corticotropin level suggests secondary adrenal hypofunction resulting from pituitary or hypothalamic dysfunction. The primary determinant may be panhypopituitarism, absence of corticotropin-releasing hormone in the hypothalamus, or chronic blunting of corticotropin levels by long-term corticosteroid therapy.

In suspected Cushing's syndrome, an elevated corticotropin level suggests Cushing's disease, in which pituitary dysfunction (due to adenoma) causes continuous hypersecretion of corticotropin and, consequently, continuously elevated cortisol levels without diurnal variations.

Moderately elevated corticotropin levels suggest pituitary-dependent adrenal hyperplasia and nonadrenal tumors such as oat cell carcinoma of the lung.

A low-normal corticotropin level implies adrenal hyperfunction due to adrenocortical tumor or hyperplasia.

## INTERFERING FACTORS

- Corticosteroids, including cortisone and its analogues (decrease)
- Drugs that increase endogenous cortisol secretion, such as amphetamines, calcium gluconate, estrogens, ethanol, and spironolactone (decrease)
- Lithium carbonate (decreases cortisol levels and may interfere with corticotropin secretion)
- Menstrual cycle and pregnancy
- Radioactive scan performed within 1 week before the test
- Acute stress (including hospitalization and surgery) and depression (increase)

---

# Activated clotting time

---

Activated clotting time, or automated coagulation time, measures whole blood clotting time. It's commonly performed during procedures that require extracorporeal circulation, such as cardiopulmonary bypass, ultrafiltration, hemodialysis, and extracorporeal membrane oxygenation (ECMO), and during invasive procedures, such as cardiac catheterization and percutaneous transluminal coronary angioplasty.

## PURPOSE

- To monitor the effect of heparin
- To monitor the effect of protamine sulfate in heparin neutralization
- To detect severe deficiencies in clotting factors (except factor VII)

## PATIENT PREPARATION

- Explain to the patient that the activated clotting time test is used to monitor the effect of heparin on the blood's ability to coagulate.
- Tell the patient that the test requires a blood sample, which is usually drawn from an existing vascular access site; therefore, no venipuncture will be needed.
- Explain who will perform the test and when, and that it's usually done at the bedside.
- Explain that two blood samples will be drawn. The first one will be discarded so that any heparin in the tubing doesn't interfere with the results.
- If the sample is drawn from a line with a continuous infusion, stop the infusion before drawing the sample.

## PROCEDURE AND POSTTEST CARE

- Withdraw 5 to 10 ml of blood from the line and discard it.
- Withdraw a clean sample of blood into the special tube containing celite provided with the activated clotting time unit.
- Start the activated clotting time unit and wait for the signal to insert the tube.
- Flush the vascular access site according to your facility's policy.

## PRECAUTIONS

- Guard against contamination with heparin if drawn from an access site containing heparin.

## REFERENCE VALUES

In a non-anticoagulated patient, normal activated clotting time is 107 seconds plus or minus 13 seconds (SI, 107 ± 13 s). During cardiopulmonary bypass, heparin is titrated to maintain an activated clotting time between 400 and 600 seconds (SI, 400 to 600 s). During ECMO, heparin is titrated to maintain the activated clotting time between 220 and 260 seconds (SI, 220 to 260 s).

## INTERFERING FACTORS

- Failure to fill the collection tube completely, to use the proper anticoagulant, to adequately mix the sample and the anticoagulant, or to send the sample to the laboratory immediately or place it on ice
- Failure to draw at least 5 ml waste to avoid sample contamination when drawing

the sample from a venous access device that's used for heparin infusion

# Alanine aminotransferase

The alanine aminotransferase (ALT) test is used to measure serum levels of ALT, one of two enzymes that catalyze a reversible amino group transfer reaction in the Krebs cycle. ALT is necessary for tissue energy production. It's found primarily in the liver, with lesser amounts in the kidneys, heart, and skeletal muscles, and is a sensitive indicator of acute hepatocellular disease.

When such damage occurs, ALT is released from the cytoplasm into the bloodstream, typically before jaundice appears, resulting in abnormally high serum levels that may not return to normal for days or weeks. This test measures serum ALT levels using the spectrophotometric method.

## PURPOSE
● To detect and evaluate treatment of acute hepatic disease, especially hepatitis and cirrhosis without jaundice
● To distinguish between myocardial and hepatic tissue damage (used with aspartate aminotransferase)
● To assess the hepatotoxicity of some drugs

## PATIENT PREPARATION
● Explain to the patient that the ALT test is used to assess liver function.
● Tell the patient that the test requires a blood sample. Explain who will perform the venipuncture and when.
● Explain to the patient that he may experience slight discomfort from the tourniquet and needle puncture.
● Inform the patient that he need not restrict food and fluids.
● Notify the laboratory and physician of medications the patient is taking that may affect test results; they may need to be restricted.

## PROCEDURE AND POSTTEST CARE
● Perform a venipuncture and collect the sample in a 4-ml tube without additives.

● Apply direct pressure to the venipuncture site until bleeding stops.
● Instruct the patient that he may resume medications discontinued before the test, as ordered.

## PRECAUTIONS
● Handle the sample gently to prevent hemolysis.
● Know that ALT activity is stable in serum for up to 3 days at room temperature.

## REFERENCE VALUES
Serum ALT levels range from 8 to 50 IU/L (SI, 0.14 to 0.85 µkat/L).

## ABNORMAL FINDINGS
Extremely high ALT levels (up to 50 times normal) suggest viral or severe drug-induced hepatitis or other hepatic disease with extensive necrosis. Moderate to high levels may indicate infectious mononucleosis, chronic hepatitis, intrahepatic cholestasis or cholecystitis, early or improving acute viral hepatitis, or severe hepatic congestion due to heart failure.

Slight to moderate elevations of ALT may appear in any condition that produces acute hepatocellular injury, such as active cirrhosis and drug-induced or alcoholic hepatitis. Marginal elevations occasionally occur in acute myocardial infarction, reflecting secondary hepatic congestion or the release of small amounts of ALT from myocardial tissue.

## INTERFERING FACTORS
● Barbiturates, chlorpromazine (Thorazine), griseofulvin, isoniazid, methyldopa (Aldomet), nitrofurantoin (Macrodantin), para-aminosalicylic acid, phenothiazines, phenytoin (Dilantin), salicylates, tetracycline, and other drugs that cause hepatic injury by competitively interfering with cellular metabolism (false-high)
● Opioid analgesics, such as codeine, meperidine (Demerol), and morphine (possible false-high due to increased intrabiliary pressure)
● Ingestion of lead or exposure to carbon tetrachloride (sharp increase due to direct injury to hepatic cells)

# Aldosterone, plasma and urine

The plasma aldosterone test measures serum aldosterone levels by quantitative analysis and radioimmunoassay. Aldosterone — the principal mineralocorticoid secreted by the zona gomerulosa of the adrenal cortex — regulates ion transport across cell membranes in the renal tubules to promote reabsorption of sodium and chloride in exchange for potassium and hydrogen ions. Consequently, aldosterone helps to maintain blood pressure and volume and to regulate fluid and electrolyte balance.

Aldosterone secretion is controlled primarily by the renin-angiotensin concentration of potassium. Thus, high serum potassium levels elicit secretion of aldosterone through a potent feedback system; similarly, hyponatremia, hypovolemia, and other disorders that provoke the release of renin stimulate aldosterone secretion. The plasma aldosterone test identifies aldosteronism and, when supported by plasma renin levels, distinguishes between the primary and secondary forms of this disorder.

The urine aldosterone test measures urine levels of aldosterone. Urine aldosterone levels, measured through radioimmunoassay, are usually evaluated after measurement of serum electrolyte and renin levels.

## PURPOSE
● To aid in the diagnosis of primary and secondary aldosteronism, adrenal hyperplasia, hypoaldosteronism, and salt-losing syndrome (plasma)
● To aid in the diagnosis of primary and secondary aldosteronism (urine)

## PATIENT PREPARATION
● Explain to the patient that the plasma and urine aldosterone test evaluates hormonal balance.
● Instruct the patient to maintain a normal sodium diet (3 g/day) before the test and to avoid sodium-rich foods, such as bacon, barbecue sauce, corned beef, bouillon cubes or powder, pickles, snack foods (potato chips), and olives. For the plasma test, instruct the patient to maintain a low-carbohydrate, normal-sodium diet for at least 2 weeks or, preferably, for 30 days before the test.
● Withhold drugs that alter fluid, sodium, and potassium balance — especially diuretics, antihypertensives, steroids, hormonal contraceptives, and estrogens — for at least 2 weeks or, preferably, for 30 days before the plasma test, as ordered.
● Withhold all renin inhibitors for 1 week before the plasma test, as ordered. If they must be continued, note this on the laboratory request.
● Tell the patient to avoid licorice for at least 2 weeks before the plasma test because it produces an aldosterone-like effect.
● Tell the patient that the plasma aldosterone test requires a blood sample. Explain who will perform the venipuncture and when.
● Explain to the patient that he may experience slight discomfort from the needle puncture and the tourniquet.
● Advise the patient to avoid strenuous physical exercise and stressful situations during the urine collection period.
● Tell the patient that the urine aldosterone test requires collection of urine during a 24-hour period, and teach him the proper collection technique.
● Notify the laboratory and physician of medications the patient is taking that may affect test results; they may need to be restricted.

## PROCEDURE AND POSTTEST CARE
### Plasma aldosterone
● Perform a venipuncture while the patient is still supine after a night's rest.
● Collect the sample in a 7-ml clot-activator tube and send it to the laboratory immediately.
● Draw another sample 4 hours later, while the patient is standing and after he has been up and about, to evaluate the effect of postural change.
● Collect the second sample in a 7-ml clot-activator tube and send it to the laboratory immediately.
● Apply direct pressure to the venipuncture site until bleeding stops.
● Instruct the patient that he may resume his usual activities, diet, and medications, as ordered.

## Urine aldosterone

- Collect the patient's urine over a 24-hour period, discarding the first specimen and retaining the last. Use a bottle containing a preservative, such as boric acid, to keep the specimen at a pH of 4.0 to 4.5.
- Instruct the patient that he may resume his usual activities, diet, and medications, as ordered.

## PRECAUTIONS

- Handle the blood sample gently to prevent hemolysis.
- Record on the laboratory request whether the patient was supine or standing during the venipuncture.
- If the patient is a premenopausal female, specify the phase of her menstrual cycle on the laboratory slip for plasma aldosterone because aldosterone levels may fluctuate.
- Refrigerate the urine specimen or place it on ice during the collection period.
- Send the plasma or urine specimen to the laboratory as soon as collection is complete.

## REFERENCE VALUES

Laboratory values vary with time of day and posture — upright postures have higher values. In upright individuals, normal values are 7 to 30 ng/dl (SI, 190 to 832 pmol/L). In supine individuals, values are 3 to 16 ng/dl (SI, 80 to 440 pmol/L).

Normally, urine aldosterone levels range from 3 to 19 µg/24 hours (SI, 8 to 51 nmol/d).

## ABNORMAL FINDINGS

Excessive plasma aldosterone levels may indicate primary or secondary disease. Primary aldosteronism (Conn's syndrome) may result from adrenocortical adenoma or carcinoma or from bilateral adrenal hyperplasia. Secondary aldosteronism can result from renovascular hypertension, heart failure, cirrhosis of the liver, nephrotic syndrome, idiopathic cyclic edema, and the third trimester of pregnancy.

Low serum aldosterone levels may indicate primary hypoaldosteronism, salt-losing syndrome, eclampsia, or Addison's disease.

Elevated urine aldosterone levels suggest primary or secondary aldosteronism. The primary form usually arises from an aldosterone-secreting adenoma of the adrenal cortex, but may also result from adrenocortical hyperplasia.

Secondary aldosteronism, the more common form, results from external stimulation of the adrenal cortex such as that produced when the renin-angiotensin system is activated by hypertensive and edematous disorders. Disorders that may result in secondary aldosteronism are malignant hypertension, heart failure, cirrhosis of the liver, nephrotic syndrome, and idiopathic cyclic edema.

Low urine aldosterone levels may result from Addison's disease, salt-losing syndrome, hypokalemia, and toxemia of pregnancy. These levels normally rise during pregnancy, but rapidly decline following parturition.

## INTERFERING FACTORS

- Failure to maintain normal dietary sodium intake as well as excess intake of licorice or glucose
- Failure to avoid strenuous physical exercise and emotional stress before the test (possible increase due to stimulation of adrenocortical secretions)
- Radioactive scan performed within 1 week before the test
- Antihypertensive drugs (possible decrease due to sodium and water retention)
- Diuretics and most steroids (possible increase due to sodium excretion)
- Some corticosteroids such as fludrocortisone (Florinef), which mimic mineralocorticoid activity (possible decrease)

# Alkaline phosphatase

The alkaline phosphatase (ALP) test is used to measure serum levels of ALP, an enzyme that influences bone calcification as well as lipid and metabolite transport. ALP measurements reflect the combined activity of several ALP isoenzymes found in the liver, bones, kidneys, intestinal lining, and placenta. Bone and liver ALP are always present in adult serum, with liver ALP most prominent, except during the third trimester of pregnancy (when the placenta originates about half of all ALP). The intestinal variant of ALP can be a normal component (in less than 10% of normal patterns; almost exclusively in the sera of blood groups B and O), or it can be an abnormal finding associated with hepatic disease.

The ALP test is particularly sensitive to mild biliary obstruction and is a primary indicator of space-occupying hepatic lesions. Although skeletal and hepatic diseases can raise ALP levels, this test is most useful for diagnosing metabolic bone disease. Additional liver function studies are usually required to identify hepatobiliary disorders.

## PURPOSE
● To detect and identify skeletal diseases primarily characterized by marked osteoblastic activity
● To detect focal hepatic lesions causing biliary obstruction, such as a tumor or an abscess
● To assess the patient's response to vitamin D in the treatment of rickets
● To supplement information from other liver function studies and GI enzyme tests

## PATIENT PREPARATION
● Explain to the patient that the ALP test is used to assess liver and bone function.
● Instruct the patient to fast for at least 8 hours before the test because fat intake stimulates intestinal ALP secretion.
● Tell the patient that this test requires a blood sample. Explain who will perform the venipuncture and when.
● Inform the patient that he may experience slight discomfort from the tourniquet and needle puncture.

## PROCEDURE AND POSTTEST CARE
● Perform a venipuncture and collect the sample in a 4-ml clot-activator tube.
● Apply direct pressure to the venipuncture site until bleeding stops.
● Instruct the patient that he may resume his usual diet.

## PRECAUTIONS
● Handle the sample gently to prevent hemolysis.
● Send the sample to the laboratory immediately; ALP activity increases at room temperature because of a rise in pH.

## REFERENCE VALUES
Total ALP levels normally range from 30 to 85 IU/ml (SI, 42 to 128 U/L).

*Age alert  In elderly patients, alkaline phosphatase levels may increase by 8 to* 10 IU/ml possibly due to declining liver function or vitamin D malabsorption and bone demineralization.

## ABNORMAL FINDINGS
Although significant ALP elevations are possible with diseases that affect many organs, they usually indicate skeletal disease or extrahepatic or intrahepatic biliary obstruction causing cholestasis. Many acute hepatic diseases cause ALP elevations before they affect serum bilirubin levels.

Moderate increases in ALP levels may reflect acute biliary obstruction from hepatocellular inflammation in active cirrhosis, mononucleosis, and viral hepatitis. Moderate increases are also seen in osteomalacia and deficiency-induced rickets.

Sharp elevations in ALP levels may indicate complete biliary obstruction by malignant or infectious infiltrations or fibrosis, most common in Paget's disease and, occasionally, in biliary obstruction, extensive bone metastasis, and hyperparathyroidism. Metastatic bone tumors resulting from pancreatic cancer raise ALP levels without a concomitant rise in serum alanine aminotransferase levels.

Isoenzyme fractionation and additional enzyme tests (gamma glutamyl transferase, lactate dehydrogenase, 5'-nucleotidase, and leucine aminopeptidase) are sometimes performed when the cause of ALP elevations is in doubt. Rarely, low levels of serum ALP are associated with hypophosphatasia and protein or magnesium deficiency.

## INTERFERING FACTORS
● Failure to analyze the sample within 4 hours
● Recent ingestion of vitamin D (possible increase due to the effect on osteoblastic activity)
● Recent infusion of albumin prepared from placental venous blood (marked increase)
● Drugs that influence liver function or cause cholestasis, such as barbiturates, chlorpropamide (Diabinese), hormonal contraceptives, isoniazid, methyldopa (Aldomet), phenothiazines, phenytoin (Dilantin), and rifampin (possible mild increase)
● Halothane sensitivity (possible drastic increase)
● Clofibrate (decrease)

- Healing long-bone fractures and the third trimester of pregnancy (possible increase)
- Age and sex (increase in infants, children, adolescents, and individuals over age 45)

# Alpha₁-antitrypsin

A protein produced by the liver, alpha₁-antitrypsin (also known as *AAT* or *alpha₁-AT*) is believed to inhibit the release of protease into body fluids by dying cells and is a major component of alpha₁-globulin. AAT is measured using radioimmunoassay or isoelectric focusing. Congenital absence or deficiency of AAT has been linked to high susceptibility to emphysema in adults and cirrhosis in children.

## PURPOSE
- To screen the patient at high risk for emphysema
- To use as a nonspecific method of detecting inflammation, severe infection, and necrosis
- To test for congenital AAT deficiency

## PATIENT PREPARATION
**Age alert** *Explain to the patient or child's parents that the alpha₁-antitrypsin test is used to diagnose respiratory or liver disease as well as inflammation, infection, or necrosis.*
- Tell the patient that the alpha₁-antitrypsin test requires a blood sample. Explain who will be performing the venipuncture and when.
- Explain to the patient that he may experience slight discomfort from the tourniquet and needle puncture.
- Tell the patient to avoid smoking because irritants in tobacco stimulate leukocytes in the lungs to release protease.
- Tell the patient to avoid hormonal contraceptives and steroids for 24 hours before the test.
- Tell the patient to fast for at least 8 hours before the test.

## PROCEDURE AND POSTTEST CARE
- Perform a venipuncture and collect the sample in a 4-ml tube without additives.
**Age alert** *In a child, puncture the clean area with a sharp needle or lancet, then collect the blood sample in a pipette, a small container, or onto a slide.*
- Apply direct pressure to the venipuncture site until bleeding stops.
- Instruct the patient that he may resume his usual diet and medications discontinued before the test, as ordered.

## PRECAUTIONS
- Handle the sample gently to avoid hemolysis.
- Send the sample to the laboratory promptly.
- If clinically indicated, know that the patient with AAT levels lower than 125 mg/dl (SI, 1.25g/L) should be phenotyped to confirm homozygous and heterozygous deficiencies. (The heterozygous patient doesn't appear to be at increased risk for early emphysema.)

## REFERENCE VALUES
AAT levels vary by age, but the normal range is 110 to 200 mg/dl (SI, 1.1 to 2 g/L).

## ABNORMAL FINDINGS
Decreased AAT levels may occur in early-onset emphysema and cirrhosis, nephrotic syndrome, malnutrition, congenital alpha₁-globulin deficiency and, transiently, in the neonate.

Increased AAT levels can occur in chronic inflammatory disorders, necrosis, pregnancy, acute pulmonary infections, respiratory distress syndrome in infants, hepatitis, systemic lupus erythematosus, and rheumatoid arthritis.

## INTERFERING FACTORS
- Corticosteroids and hormonal contraceptives (possible false-high)
- Smoking or failure to fast for 8 hours before the test (possible false-high)

# Alpha-fetoprotein

Alpha-fetoprotein (AFP) is a glycoprotein produced by fetal tissue and tumors that differentiate from midline embryonic structures. During fetal development, AFP levels in serum and amniotic fluid rise. AFP crosses the placenta and appears in maternal serum.

High maternal serum AFP levels may suggest fetal neural tube defects, such as spina bifida and anencephaly, but positive confirmation requires amniocentesis and ultrasonography. Other congenital anomalies, such as Down syndrome and other chromosomal disorders, may be associated with low maternal serum AFP concentrations.

Elevated AFP levels in the patient who isn't pregnant may occur in cancers such as hepatocellular carcinoma or in certain nonmalignant conditions such as ataxia-telangiectasia. In these conditions, AFP assays are more useful for monitoring the patient's response to therapy than for diagnosis. AFP levels are best determined by enzyme immunoassay on amniotic fluid or serum.

## PURPOSE
- To monitor the effectiveness of therapy in malignant conditions, such as hepatomas and germ cell tumors, and certain nonmalignant conditions such as ataxia-telangiectasia
- To screen for the need for amniocentesis or high-resolution ultrasonography in a pregnant patient

## PATIENT PREPARATION
- Explain that the AFP test helps in monitoring fetal development, screens for a need for further testing, helps detect possible congenital defects in the fetus, and monitors the patient's response to therapy by measuring a specific blood protein, as appropriate.
- Inform the patient that she need not restrict food, fluids, or medications.
- Tell the patient that the test requires a blood sample. Explain who will perform the venipuncture and when.
- Explain to the patient that she may experience slight discomfort from the tourniquet and needle puncture.

## PROCEDURE AND POSTTEST CARE
- Perform a venipuncture and collect the sample in a 7-ml clot-activator tube.
- Record the patient's age, race, weight, and gestational period on the laboratory request.
- Apply direct pressure to the venipuncture site until bleeding stops.

## PRECAUTIONS
- Handle the sample gently to prevent hemolysis.

## REFERENCE VALUES
When testing by immunoassay, AFP values are less than 15 ng/ml (SI, < 15 mg/L) in male patients and nonpregnant female patients. Values in maternal serum normally are less 25 ng/ml (SI, 25 ug/L). At 15 to 18 weeks' gestation, values range from 10 to 150 ng/ml (SI, 10 to 150 ug/L).

## ABNORMAL FINDINGS
Elevated maternal serum AFP levels may suggest neural tube defects or other tube anomalies. Maternal AFP levels rise sharply in the maternal blood of about 90% of women carrying a fetus with anencephaly and in 50% of those carrying a fetus with spina bifida. Definitive diagnosis requires ultrasonography and amniocentesis. High AFP levels may indicate intrauterine death. Sometimes high levels indicate other anomalies, such as duodenal atresia, omphalocele, tetralogy of Fallot, and Turner's syndrome.

Elevated serum AFP levels occur in 70% of nonpregnant patients with hepatocellular carcinoma. Elevated levels are also related to germ cell tumor of gonadal, retroperitoneal, or mediastinal origin. Serum AFP levels rise in ataxia-telangiectasia and sometimes in cancer of the pancreas, stomach, or biliary system and in nonseminiferous testicular tumors. Transient modest elevations can occur in nonneoplastic hepatocellular disease, such as alcoholic cirrhosis and acute or chronic hepatitis. Elevation of AFP levels after remission suggests tumor recurrence.

In hepatocellular carcinoma, a gradual decrease in serum AFP levels indicates a favorable response to therapy. In germ cell tumors, serum AFP levels and serum human chorionic gonadotropin levels should be measured concurrently.

## INTERFERING FACTORS
- Multiple gestations (possible false-positive)

# Alveolar-to-arterial oxygen gradient

Using calculations based on the patient's laboratory values, the alveolar-to-arterial oxygen gradient (A-aDO$_2$) test can help identify the cause of hypoxemia and intrapulmonary shunting by providing an approximation of the partial pressure of oxygenation of the alveoli and arteries. It may help differentiate the cause as ventilated alveoli but no perfusion, unventilated alveoli with perfusion, or collapse of the alveoli and capillaries.

## PURPOSE
● To evaluate the efficiency of gas exchange
● To assess the integrity of the ventilatory control system
● To monitor respiratory therapy

## PATIENT PREPARATION
● Explain to the patient that the A-aDO$_2$ test is used to evaluate how well the lungs are delivering oxygen to the blood and eliminating carbon dioxide.
● Tell the patient that the test requires a blood sample. Explain who will perform the arterial puncture and when.
● Inform the patient that he need not restrict food and fluids.
● Instruct the patient to breathe normally during the test, and warn him that he may experience cramping or throbbing pain at the puncture site.

## PROCEDURE AND POSTTEST CARE
● Perform an arterial puncture or draw blood from an arterial line using a heparinized blood gas syringe.
● Eliminate all air from the sample and place it on ice immediately.
● Apply pressure to the puncture for 3 to 5 minutes or until bleeding has stopped.
● Place a gauze pad over the site and tape it in place, but don't tape the entire circumference.
● Monitor vital signs and observe for signs of circulatory impairment, such as swelling, discoloration, pain, numbness, and tingling in the bandaged arm or leg.

● Watch for bleeding from the puncture site.
● The arterial sample is analyzed for partial pressure of arterial oxygen (PaO$_2$) and partial pressure of arterial carbon dioxide (PaCO$_2$). Also examined are barometric pressure (Pb), water vapor pressure (PH$_2$O), and fraction of inspired oxygen (FIO$_2$) (21% for room air). From these values, the alveolar oxygen tension (PAO$_2$), the arterial-to-oxygen ratio (a/A ratio), and the A-aDO$_2$ are derived by solving these mathematical formulas:

$$PAO_2 = FIO_2 \ (Pb - PH_2O) - 1.25 \ (PaCO_2)$$

$$a/A \ ratio = PaO_2 \ divided \ by \ PAO_2$$

$$A\text{-}aDO_2 = PAO_2 - PaO_2.$$

● Based on the results of the formulas, appropriate interventions to correct patient problems are initiated.

## PRECAUTIONS
● Before sending the sample to the laboratory, note on the laboratory request whether the patient was breathing room air or receiving oxygen therapy when the sample was collected.
● If the patient was receiving oxygen therapy, note the flow rate and method of delivery. If he was on a ventilator, note the FIO$_2$, tidal volume, mode, respiratory rate, and positive end-expiratory pressure.
● Note the patient's core temperature.

## REFERENCE VALUES
Normal values on room air for A-aDO$_2$ at rest is less than 10 mm Hg (SI, < 1.33 kPa) and at maximum exercise is 20 to 30 mm Hg (SI, 2.7 to 4.0 kPa).

## ABNORMAL FINDINGS
● Increased values may be caused by mucus plugs, bronchospasm, or airway collapse (asthma, bronchitis, emphysema). Hypoxemia results in increased A-aDO$_2$ and may be caused by arterial septal defects, pneumothorax, atelectasis, emboli, or edema.

## INTERFERING FACTORS
● Exposing the sample to air (increase or decrease)
● Age and increasing oxygen concentration (increase)

# Ammonia, plasma

The plasma ammonia test measures plasma levels of ammonia, a nonprotein nitrogen compound that helps maintain acid-base balance. In such diseases as cirrhosis of the liver, ammonia can bypass the liver and accumulate in the blood. Plasma ammonia levels may help indicate the severity of hepatocellular damage.

## PURPOSE
● To help monitor the progression of severe hepatic disease and the effectiveness of therapy
● To recognize impending or established hepatic coma

## PATIENT PREPARATION
● Explain to the patient (or family member if patient is comatose) that the plasma ammonia test is used to evaluate liver function.
● Tell the patient that the test requires a blood sample. Explain who will perform the venipuncture and when.
● Explain to the patient that he may experience slight discomfort from the tourniquet and needle puncture.
● Notify the laboratory and physician of medications the patient is taking that may affect test results; they may need to be restricted.

## PROCEDURE AND POSTTEST CARE
● Perform a venipuncture and collect the sample in a 10-ml heparinized tube.
● Apply direct pressure to the venipuncture site until bleeding stops.
● Watch for signs of impending or established hepatic coma if plasma ammonia levels are high.

## PRECAUTIONS
● Notify the laboratory before performing the venipuncture so that preliminary preparations can begin.
● Handle the sample gently to prevent hemolysis.
● Pack the sample in ice and send it to the laboratory immediately.

## REFERENCE VALUES
Plasma ammonia levels in adults usually range from 15 to 45 µg/dl (SI, 11 to 32 µmol/L).

## ABNORMAL FINDINGS
Elevated plasma ammonia levels are common in severe hepatic disease, such as cirrhosis and acute hepatic necrosis, and can lead to hepatic coma. Elevated levels may also occur in Reye's syndrome, severe heart failure, GI hemorrhage, and erythroblastosis fetalis.

## INTERFERING FACTORS
● Acetazolamide (Diamox), ammonium salts, furosemide (Lasix), and thiazides (increase)
● Parenteral nutrition or a portacaval shunt (possible increase)
● Kanamycin (Kantrex), lactulose (Cephulac), and neomycin (Mycifradin) (decrease)
● Smoking, poor venipuncture technique, and exposure to ammonia cleaners in the laboratory (possible increase)

# Amylase, serum

An enzyme that's synthesized primarily in the pancreas and salivary glands and is secreted in the GI tract, amylase (alpha-amylase or AML) helps to digest starch and glycogen in the mouth, stomach, and intestine. In cases of suspected acute pancreatic disease, measurement of serum or urine AML is the most important laboratory test.

## PURPOSE
● To diagnose acute pancreatitis
● To distinguish between acute pancreatitis and other causes of abdominal pain that require immediate surgery
● To evaluate possible pancreatic injury caused by abdominal trauma or surgery

## PATIENT PREPARATION
● Explain to the patient that the serum AML test is used to assess pancreatic function.
● Tell the patient that this test requires a blood sample. Explain who will perform the venipuncture and when.

- Explain to the patient that he may experience slight discomfort from the tourniquet and needle puncture.
- Inform the patient that he need not fast before the test, but must abstain from alcohol.
- Notify the laboratory and physician of medications the patient is taking that may affect test results; they may need to be restricted.

## PROCEDURE AND POSTTEST CARE

- Perform a venipuncture and collect the sample in a 4-ml clot-activator tube.
- Apply direct pressure to the venipuncture site until bleeding stops.
- Instruct the patient that he may resume medications discontinued before the test, as ordered.

## PRECAUTIONS

- If the patient has severe abdominal pain, draw the sample before diagnostic or therapeutic intervention. For accurate results, it's important to obtain an early sample.
- Handle the sample gently to prevent hemolysis.

## REFERENCE VALUES

Normal serum AML levels range from 25 to 85 U/L (SI, 0.39 to 1.45 µkat/L) for adults age 18 and older.

## ABNORMAL FINDINGS

After the onset of acute pancreatitis, AML levels begin to rise within 2 hours, peak within 12 to 48 hours, and return to normal within 3 to 4 days. Determination of urine levels should follow normal serum AML results to rule out pancreatitis.

Moderate serum elevations may accompany obstruction of the common bile duct, pancreatic duct, or ampulla of Vater; pancreatic injury from a perforated peptic ulcer; pancreatic cancer; and acute salivary gland disease. Impaired kidney function may increase serum levels.

Levels may be slightly elevated in a patient who's asymptomatic or responding unusually to therapy. Decreased levels can occur in chronic pancreatitis, pancreatic cancer, cirrhosis, hepatitis, and toxemia of pregnancy.

## UNDERSTANDING MACROAMYLASEMIA

An uncommon, benign condition, macroamylasemia doesn't cause any symptoms, but it occasionally causes elevated serum amylase (AML) levels. This condition occurs when macroamylase — a complex of AML and an immunoglobulin or other protein — is present in a patient's serum.

A patient with macroamylasemia typically has an elevated serum AML level and a normal or slightly decreased urine AML level. This characteristic pattern helps differentiate macroamylasemia from conditions in which serum and urine AML levels rise such as pancreatitis. But it doesn't differentiate macroamylasemia from hyperamylasemia due to impaired renal function, which may raise serum AML levels and lower urine AML levels. Chromatographic, ultracentrifugation, or precipitation tests are necessary to detect macroamylase in serum and definitively confirm macroamylasemia.

## INTERFERING FACTORS

- Ingestion of ethyl alcohol in large amounts (possible false-high)
- Aminosalicylic acid, asparaginase (Elspar), azathioprine (Imuran), corticosteroids, cyproheptadine, hormonal contraceptives, opioid analgesics, rifampin, sulfasalazine (Azulfidine), and thiazide or loop diuretics (possible false-high)
- Recent peripancreatic surgery, perforated ulcer or intestine, abscess, spasm of the sphincter of Oddi or, rarely, macroamylasemia (possible false-high) (see *Understanding macroamylasemia*)

## Amylase, urine

Amylase is a starch-splitting enzyme produced primarily in the pancreas and salivary glands, which is usually secreted into the alimentary tract and absorbed into the blood; small amounts of amylase are also absorbed into the blood directly from these organs.

Following glomerular filtration, amylase is excreted in the urine.

In the presence of adequate renal function, serum and urine levels usually rise in tandem. However, within 2 to 3 days of the onset of acute pancreatitis, serum amylase levels fall to normal, but elevated urine amylase persists for 7 to 10 days. One method for determining urine amylase levels is the dye-coupled starch method.

## PURPOSE

● To diagnose acute pancreatitis when serum amylase levels are normal or borderline
● To aid in the diagnosis of chronic pancreatitis and salivary gland disorders

## PATIENT PREPARATION

● Explain to the patient that the urine amylase test evaluates the function of the pancreas and the salivary glands.
● Inform the patient that he need not restrict food and fluids.
● Tell the patient that the test requires urine collection for 2, 6, 8, or 24 hours, and teach him how to collect a timed specimen.
● Instruct the patient to empty his bladder and then begin timing the collection.
● Notify the laboratory and physician of medications the patient is taking that may affect test results; they may need to be restricted.

## PROCEDURE AND POSTTEST CARE

● Collect the patient's urine over a 2-, 6-, 8-, or 24-hour period.
● A 2-hour test is usually performed because collecting urine for a 2-hour period produces fewer errors than a more diagnostic 24-hour collection.

## PRECAUTIONS

● Cover and refrigerate the specimen during the collection period.
● If the patient is catheterized, keep the collection bag on ice.
● Instruct the patient not to contaminate the specimen with toilet tissue or stool.
● Send the specimen on ice to the laboratory as soon as collection is complete.

## REFERENCE VALUES

Urine amylase is reported in various units of measure; therefore, values differ from laboratory to laboratory. The Mayo Clinic reports normal urinary excretion of 1 to 17 U/hour (SI, 0.017 to 0.29 µkat/h).

## ABNORMAL FINDINGS

Elevated amylase levels occur in acute pancreatitis; obstruction of the pancreatic duct, intestines, or salivary duct; carcinoma of the head of the pancreas; mumps; acute injury of the spleen; renal disease, with impaired absorption; perforated peptic or duodenal ulcers; and gallbladder disease.

Depressed levels occur in pancreatitis, cachexia, alcoholism, cancer of the liver, cirrhosis, hepatitis, and hepatic abscess.

## INTERFERING FACTORS

● Salivary amylase in the urine due to coughing or talking over the sample (possible increase)
● High levels of bacterial contamination of the specimen or blood in the urine
● Bethanechol (Duvoid), codeine, indomethacin (Indocin), meperidine (Demerol), morphine, pentazocine (Talwin), thiazide diuretics, or alcohol within 24 hours of the test (possible increase)
● Fluorides and glucose (possible decrease)

# *Androstenedione*

The androstenedione test helps identify disorders related to altered hormone levels, such as female virilization syndromes and polycystic ovary (Stein-Leventhal) syndrome. Androstenedione is a precursor of cortisol, aldosterone, estrogen, and testosterone. Tumors of the ovaries or adrenal glands can secrete excessive amounts of androstenedione, which then converts to testosterone, resulting in virilizing symptoms, such as hirsutism and sterility.

Increased androstenedione production may induce premature sexual development in children. It may produce renewed ovarian stimulation, endometriosis, bleeding, and polycystic ovaries in postmenopausal females. In obese females, increased levels of estrogen can lead to menstrual irregularities. In males, overproduction of androstenedione may cause feminizing signs such as gynecomastia.

## PURPOSE

● To help determine the cause of gonadal dysfunction, virilizing symptoms, and premature sexual development in males

● To help determine the cause of menstrual or menopausal irregularities, virilizing symptoms, and premature sexual development in females

## PATIENT PREPARATION

● Explain to the patient that the androstenedione test determines the cause of the symptoms.

● Tell the patient that the test requires a blood sample. Explain who will perform the venipuncture and when.

● Explain to the patient that he may experience slight discomfort from the tourniquet and needle puncture.

● Explain to the female patient that the test should be done 1 week before or after her menstrual period and that it may be repeated.

● Withhold steroid and pituitary-based hormones, as ordered. If they must be continued, note this on the laboratory request.

## PROCEDURE AND POSTTEST CARE

● Perform a venipuncture and collect a serum sample in a 7-ml clot-activator tube or collect a plasma sample in a green-top tube. (If a plasma sample is taken, refrigerate it or place it on ice.)

● Label the sample appropriately and send it to the laboratory immediately.

● Apply direct pressure to the venipuncture site until bleeding stops.

● Instruct the patient that he may resume medications discontinued before the test, as ordered.

## PRECAUTIONS

● Handle the sample gently to prevent hemolysis.

● Refrigerate plasma samples or place them on ice.

● Record the patient's age, sex, and (if appropriate) phase of her menstrual cycle on the laboratory request.

## REFERENCE VALUES

Normal values by radioimmunoassay are:
● females — 85 to 275 ng/dl (SI, 3 to 9.6 nmol/L)
● males — 75 to 205 ng/dl (SI, 2.6 to 7.2 nmol/L).

## ABNORMAL FINDINGS

Elevated androstenedione levels are associated with polycystic ovary (Stein-Leventhal) syndrome; Cushing's syndrome; ovarian, testicular, and adrenocortical tumors; ectopic corticotropin-producing tumors; late-onset congenital adrenal hyperplasia; and ovarian stromal hyperplasia. Elevated levels result in increased estrone levels, causing premature sexual development in children; menstrual irregularities in premenopausal women; bleeding, endometriosis, and polycystic ovaries in postmenopausal women; and feminizing signs, such as gynecomastia, in men. Decreased levels occur in hypogonadism.

## INTERFERING FACTORS

● Pituitary hormones and steroids (possible increase)

# *Anion gap*

Total concentrations of cations and anions are usually equal, making serum electrically neutral. Measuring the gap between measured cation and anion levels provides information about the level of anions (including sulfate, phosphate, organic acids, such as ketone bodies and lactic acid, and proteins) that aren't routinely measured in laboratory tests. In metabolic acidosis, measuring the anion gap helps to identify the type of acidosis and possible causes. Further tests are usually needed to determine the specific cause of metabolic acidosis.

## PURPOSE

● To distinguish types of metabolic acidosis

● To monitor renal function and total parenteral nutrition

## PATIENT PREPARATION

● Explain to the patient that the anion gap test is used to determine the cause of acidosis.

● Tell the patient that the test requires a blood sample. Explain who will perform the venipuncture and when.

# Anion Gap and Metabolic Acidosis

Metabolic acidosis with a *normal anion gap* (8 to 14 mEq/L) occurs in conditions characterized by loss of bicarbonate, such as:

♦ hypokalemic acidosis due to renal tubular acidosis, diarrhea, or ureteral diversions

♦ hyperkalemic acidosis due to acidifying agents (for example, ammonium chloride, hydrochloric acid), hydronephrosis, or sickle cell nephropathy.

Metabolic acidosis with an *increased anion gap* (> 14 mEq/L) occurs in conditions characterized by accumulation of organic acids, sulfates, or phosphates, such as:

♦ renal failure

♦ ketoacidosis due to starvation, diabetes mellitus, or alcohol abuse

♦ lactic acidosis

♦ ingestion of toxins, such as salicylates, methanol, ethylene glycol (antifreeze), and paraldehyde.

---

● Explain to the patient that he may experience slight discomfort from the tourniquet and needle puncture.

● Inform the patient that he need not restrict food and fluids.

● Notify the laboratory and physician of medications the patient is taking that may affect test results; they may need to be restricted.

## PROCEDURE AND POSTTEST CARE

● Perform a venipuncture and collect the sample in a 3- or 4-ml clot-activator tube.

● Apply direct pressure to the venipuncture site until bleeding stops.

● Instruct the patient to resume medications discontinued before the test, as ordered.

## PRECAUTIONS

● Handle the sample gently to prevent hemolysis.

## REFERENCE VALUES

Normally, the anion gap ranges from 8 to 14 mEq/L (SI, 8 to 14 mmol/L).

## ABNORMAL FINDINGS

A normal anion gap doesn't rule out metabolic acidosis. It may occur in hyperchloremic acidosis, renal tubular acidosis, and severe bicarbonate-wasting conditions, such as biliary or pancreatic fistulas and poorly functioning ileal loops.

When acidosis results from loss of bicarbonate in the urine or other body fluids, the anion gap remains unchanged. This condition is known as *normal anion gap acidosis*. (See *Anion gap and metabolic acidosis*.)

An increased anion gap indicates an increase in one or more of the unmeasured anions (sulfate; phosphates; organic acids, such as ketone bodies and lactic acid; and proteins). This condition may occur with acidoses that are characterized by excessive organic or inorganic acids, such as lactic acidosis or ketoacidosis.

When acidosis results from an accumulation of metabolic acids — as occurs in lactic acidosis, for example — the anion gap increases (less than 14 mEq/L) with the increase in unmeasured anions. Metabolic acidosis caused by such an accumulation is known as *high anion gap acidosis*.

A decreased anion gap is rare, but may occur with hypermagnesemia and paraproteinemic states, such as multiple myeloma and Waldenström's macroglobulinemia.

## INTERFERING FACTORS

● Chlorpropamide (Diabinese, diuretics, lithium, and vasopressin (Pitressin) (possible decrease due to decreased serum sodium levels)

● Antihypertensives and corticosteroids (possible increase due to increased serum sodium levels)

● Ammonium chloride, acetazolamide (Diamox), dimercaprol (BAL in Oil), ethylene glycol, methyl alcohol, paraldehyde (Paral), and salicylates (possible increase due to decreased serum bicarbonate levels)

● Adrenocorticotropic hormone, cortisone, mercurial or chlorothiazide diuretics, and excessive ingestion of alkali or licorice (possible decrease due to increased serum bicarbonate levels)

- Ammonium chloride, boric acid, cholestyramine, oxyphenbutazone, phenylbutazone, and excessive I.V. infusion of sodium chloride (possible decrease due to increased serum chloride levels)
- Bicarbonates, ethacrynic acid, furosemide, thiazide diuretics, and prolonged I.V. infusion of dextrose 5% in water (possible increase due to decreased serum chloride levels)
- Iodine absorption from wounds packed with povidone-iodine or excessive use of magnesium-containing antacids, especially in patients with renal failure (possible false-low)

# Antegrade pyelography

Antegrade pyelography allows examination of the upper collecting system when ureteral obstruction rules out retrograde ureteropyelography or when cystoscopy is contraindicated. It depends on percutaneous needle puncture for injection of contrast medium into the renal pelvis or calyces.

Renal pressure can be measured during this procedure. Also, urine can be collected for cultures and cytologic studies and for evaluation of renal functional reserve before surgery.

After completing radiographic studies, a nephrostomy tube can be inserted to provide temporary drainage or access for other therapeutic or diagnostic procedures.

## PURPOSE

- To evaluate obstruction of the upper collecting system by stricture, calculus, clot, or tumor
- To evaluate hydronephrosis revealed during excretory urography or ultrasonography and to enable placement of a percutaneous nephrostomy tube
- To evaluate the function of the upper collecting system after ureteral surgery or urinary diversion
- To assess renal functional reserve before surgery

## PATIENT PREPARATION

- Explain to the patient that antegrade pyelography allows radiographic examination of the kidney.
- Tell the patient that he may be required to fast for 6 to 8 hours before the test.
- Tell the patient that he may receive antimicrobial drugs before and after the procedure.
- Tell the patient who will perform the test and where and when it will take place.
- Explain to the patient that a needle will be inserted into the kidney after he's given a sedative and local anesthetic. Explain that urine may be collected from the kidney for testing and that, if necessary, a tube will be left in the kidney for drainage.
- Tell the patient that he may feel mild discomfort during injection of the local anesthetic and contrast medium and that he may also feel transient burning and flushing from the contrast medium.
- Warn the patient that the X-ray machine makes loud, clacking sounds as films are taken.
- Check the patient's history for hypersensitivity reactions to contrast media, iodine, or shellfish. Mark sensitivities clearly on the chart. Also check his history and recent coagulation studies for indications of bleeding disorders.
- Make sure that the patient or a responsible family member has signed an informed consent form.
- Administer a sedative just before the procedure, if needed, and check that pretest blood work, such as kidney function, has been performed, if ordered.

## PROCEDURE AND POSTTEST CARE

- The patient is placed in a prone position on the X-ray table. The skin over the kidney is cleaned with antiseptic solution, and a local anesthetic is injected.
- Previous urographic films or ultrasound recordings are studied for anatomic landmarks. (It's important to determine if the kidney to be studied is in the normal position. If not, the angle of the needle entry must be adjusted during percutaneous puncture.)
- Under guidance of fluoroscopy or ultrasonography, the percutaneous needle is inserted below the 12th rib at the level of the transverse process of the second lumbar vertebra. Aspiration of urine confirms that the

needle has reached the dilated collecting system, which is usually $2^{3}/_{4}$" to $3^{1}/_{8}$" (7 to 8 cm) below the skin surface in adults.

● Flexible tubing is connected to the needle to prevent displacement during the procedure. If intrarenal pressure is to be measured, the manometer is connected to the tubing as soon as it's in place. Urine specimens are then taken, if needed.

● An amount of urine equal to the amount of contrast medium to be injected is withdrawn to prevent overdistention of the collecting system.

● The contrast medium is injected under fluoroscopic guidance. Posteroanterior, oblique, and anteroposterior radiographs are taken. Ureteral peristalsis is observed on the fluoroscope screen to evaluate obstruction.

● A percutaneous nephrostomy tube is inserted if drainage is needed because of increased renal pressure, dilation, or intrarenal reflux. If drainage isn't needed, the catheter is withdrawn and a sterile dressing is applied.

● Check the patient's vital signs every 15 minutes for the first hour, every 30 minutes for the second hour, and then every 2 hours for the next 24 hours.

● Check dressings for bleeding, hematoma, or urine leakage at the puncture site at each vital signs check. For bleeding, apply pressure. For a hematoma, apply warm soaks. Report urine leakage or the patient's failure to void within 8 hours.

● Monitor the patient's fluid intake and urine output for 24 hours. Observe each specimen for hematuria. Report hematuria if it persists after the third voiding.

● Watch for and report signs of sepsis or extravasation of contrast medium (chills, fever, rapid pulse or respirations, and hypotension).

**Alert** *Watch for and report signs that adjacent organs have been punctured, such as pain in the abdomen or flank, or pneumothorax (sudden onset of pleuritic chest pain, dyspnea, tachypnea, decreased breath sounds on the affected side, and tachycardia).*

● If a nephrostomy tube is inserted, check to make sure it's patent and draining well. Irrigate with 5 to 7 ml of sterile saline solution, as ordered, to maintain patency.

● Administer prescribed antibiotics for several days after the procedure and prescribed analgesics.

● If hydronephrosis is present, monitor intake and output, edema, hypertension, flank pain, acid-base status, and glucose level.

## PRECAUTIONS
● Antegrade pyelography is contraindicated in the patient with bleeding disorders and in the pregnant patient unless the benefits outweigh the risks to the fetus.
● Watch for signs of hypersensitivity to the contrast medium.

## NORMAL FINDINGS
After injection of contrast medium, the upper collecting system should fill uniformly and appear normal in size and course. Normal structures should be outlined clearly.

## ABNORMAL FINDINGS
Enlargements of the upper collecting system and parts of the ureteropelvic junction indicate obstruction. Antegrade pyelography shows the degree of dilation, clearly defines obstructions, and demonstrates intrarenal reflux. In hydronephrosis, the ureteropelvic junction shows marked distention. Results of recent surgery or urinary diversion will be obvious; for example, a ureteral stent or a dilated stenotic area will be clearly visualized.

Intrarenal pressure greater than 20 cm $H_2O$ indicates obstruction. Cultures or cytologic studies of urine specimens taken during antegrade pyelography can confirm antegrade pyelonephrosis or malignancy.

## INTERFERING FACTORS
● Recent barium procedures or stool or gas in the bowel (possible poor imaging)
● An obese patient (possible difficulty in needle placement)

# Antibody screening test

Also called the *indirect Coombs' test,* the antibody screening test detects unexpected circulating antibodies in the patient's serum. After incubating the serum with group O red blood cells (RBCs), which are unaffected by anti-A or anti-B antibodies, an antiglobulin (Coombs') serum is added. Agglutination occurs if the patient's serum contains an antibody to one or more antigens on the red cells.

The antibody screening test detects 95% to 99% of the circulating antibodies. After this screening procedure detects them, the antibody identification test can determine the specific identity of the antibodies present.

## PURPOSE

● To detect unexpected circulating antibodies to RBC antigens in the recipient's or donor's serum before transfusion
● To determine the presence of anti-D antibody in maternal blood
● To evaluate the need for $Rh_o(D)$ immune globulin
● To aid in the diagnosis of acquired hemolytic anemia

## PATIENT PREPARATION

● Explain to the prospective blood recipient that the antibody screening test helps evaluate the possibility of a transfusion reaction or to determine if fetal antibodies are in the patient's blood and if treatment is needed, as appropriate.
● If the test is being performed because the patient is anemic, explain to him that it helps identify the specific type of anemia.
● Inform the patient that he need not restrict food and fluids.
● Tell the patient that the test requires a blood sample. Explain who will perform the venipuncture and when.
● Explain to the patient that he may experience slight discomfort from the tourniquet and needle puncture.
● Check the patient's history for recent administration of blood, dextran, or I.V. contrast media.

## PROCEDURE AND POSTTEST CARE

● Perform a venipuncture and collect the sample in two 10-ml tubes. If the antibody screen is positive, antibody identification is performed on the blood.
● Apply direct pressure to the venipuncture site until bleeding stops.

## PRECAUTIONS

● Handle the sample gently to prevent hemolysis.

● Label the sample with the patient's name, the health care facility or blood bank number, the date, and the phlebotomist's initials. Be sure to include on the laboratory request the patient's diagnosis and pregnancy status, history of transfusions, and current drug therapy.
● Send the sample to the laboratory immediately.

## NORMAL FINDINGS

Normally, agglutination doesn't occur, indicating that the patient's serum contains no circulating antibodies other than anti-A or anti-B.

## ABNORMAL FINDINGS

A positive result indicates the presence of unexpected circulating antibodies to RBC antigens. Such a reaction demonstrates donor and recipient incompatibility.

A positive result in a pregnant patient with Rh-negative blood may indicate the presence of antibodies to the Rh factor from an earlier transfusion with incompatible blood or from a previous pregnancy with an Rh-positive fetus.

*Age alert* *A positive result indicates that the fetus may develop hemolytic disease of the neonate. Therefore, repeated testing throughout the patient's pregnancy is necessary to evaluate progressive development of circulating antibody levels.*

## INTERFERING FACTORS

● Previous administration of dextran or I.V. contrast media (causing aggregation resembling agglutination)
● Blood transfusion or pregnancy within the past 3 months (possible presence of antibodies)

# Anti-deoxyribonucleic acid antibodies

About two-thirds of patients with active systemic lupus erythematosus (SLE) have measurable levels of autoantibodies to double-stranded (native) deoxyribonucleic acid (known as *anti-ds-DNA*). These antibodies are rarely detected in patients with other connective tissue diseases.

In autoimmune diseases, such as SLE, native DNA is thought to be the antigen that complexes with antibody and complement, causing local tissue damage where these complexes are deposited. Serum anti-ds-DNA levels are directly related to the extent of renal or vascular damage caused by the disease.

The anti-ds-DNA antibody test measures and differentiates these antibody levels in a serum sample, using radioimmunoassay, agglutination, complement fixation, or immunoelectrophoresis. If anti-ds-DNA antibodies are present, they combine with native DNA and form complexes that are too large to pass through a membrane filter. The test counts these oversized complexes.

## PURPOSE
● To confirm a diagnosis of SLE
● To monitor the patient with SLE for his response to therapy and determine his prognosis

## PATIENT PREPARATION
● Explain to the patient that anti-ds-DNA antibodies test helps diagnose and determine the appropriate therapy for SLE.
● Inform the patient that he need not restrict food and fluids.
● Tell the patient that the test requires a blood sample. Explain who will perform the venipuncture and when.
● Explain to the patient that he may experience slight discomfort from the tourniquet and needle puncture.
● Ask the patient if he has had a recent radioactive test; if so, note this on the laboratory request.

## PROCEDURE AND POSTTEST CARE
● Perform a venipuncture and collect the sample in a 7-ml tube without additives. (Some laboratories may specify a tube with either EDTA or sodium fluoride and potassium oxalate added.)
● Apply direct pressure to the venipuncture site until bleeding stops.

## PRECAUTIONS
● Handle the sample gently to prevent hemolysis.

## REFERENCE VALUES
An anti-ds-DNA antibody level less than 25 IU/ml (SI, < 25 kIU/L) is considered negative for SLE.

## ABNORMAL FINDINGS
Elevated anti-ds-DNA antibody levels may indicate SLE. Values of 25 to 30 IU/ml (SI, 25 to 30 kIU/L) are considered borderline positive. Values of 31 to 200 IU/ml (SI, 31 to 200 kIU/L) are positive, and those greater than 200 IU/ml (SI, > 200 kIU/L) are strongly positive.

Depressed anti-ds-DNA antibody levels may follow immunosuppressive therapy, demonstrating effective treatment of SLE.

## INTERFERING FACTORS
● A radioactive scan performed within 1 week before sample collection

## *Antidiuretic hormone, serum*

Antidiuretic hormone (ADH), also called *vasopressin,* promotes water reabsorption in response to increased osmolality (water deficiency with high concentration of sodium and other solutes). In response to decreased osmolality (water excess), reduced secretion of ADH allows increased excretion of water to maintain fluid balance. Along with aldosterone, ADH helps regulate sodium, potassium, and fluid balance. It also stimulates vascular smooth-muscle contraction, causing an increase in arterial blood pressure.

This relatively rare test, a quantitative analysis of serum ADH levels, may identify diabetes insipidus and other causes of severe homeostatic imbalance. It may be ordered as part of dehydration or hypertonic saline infusion testing, which determines the body's response to states of hyperosmolality.

## PURPOSE
● To aid in the differential diagnosis of pituitary diabetes insipidus, nephrogenic diabetes insipidus (congenital or familial), and syndrome of inappropriate antidiuretic hormone (SIADH)

## PATIENT PREPARATION

• Explain to the patient that the serum ADH test, used to measure hormonal secretion levels, may aid in identifying the cause of his symptoms.
• Instruct the patient to fast and limit physical activity for 10 to 12 hours before the test.
• Tell the patient that the test requires a blood sample. Explain who will perform the venipuncture and when.
• Explain to the patient that he may experience slight discomfort from the tourniquet and needle puncture.
• Withhold medications that may cause SIADH before the test, as ordered. If they must be continued, note this on the laboratory request.
• Make sure the patient is relaxed and recumbent for 30 minutes before the test.

## PROCEDURE AND POSTTEST CARE

• Perform a venipuncture and collect the sample in a plastic collection tube (without additives) or a chilled EDTA tube.
• Immediately send the sample to the laboratory, where serum must be separated from the clot within 10 minutes.
• Perform a serum osmolality test at the same time to help interpret the results.
• Apply direct pressure to the venipuncture site until bleeding stops.
• Instruct the patient that he may resume his usual diet, activities, and medications discontinued before the test, as ordered.

## PRECAUTIONS

• Make sure you use a syringe and collection tube made of plastic because the fragile ADH degrades on contact with glass.

## REFERENCE VALUES

ADH values range from 1 to 5 pg/ml (SI, 1 to 5 mg/L). It may also be evaluated in light of serum osmolality; if serum osmolality is less than 285 mOsm/kg, ADH is normally less than 2 pg/ml (SI, < 2 mg/L); if it's greater than 290 mOsm/kg, ADH may range from 2 to 12 pg/ml (SI, 2 to 12 mg/L).

## ABNORMAL FINDINGS

Absent or below-normal ADH levels indicate pituitary diabetes insipidus, resulting from a neurohypophyseal or hypothalamic tumor, viral infection, metastatic disease, sarcoidosis, tuberculosis, Hand-Schüller-Christian disease, syphilis, neurosurgical procedures, or head trauma.

Normal ADH levels in the presence of signs of diabetes insipidus (such as polydipsia, polyuria, and hypotonic urine) may indicate the nephrogenic form of the disease, marked by renal tubular resistance to ADH; however, levels may rise if the pituitary gland tries to compensate.

Elevated ADH levels may also indicate SIADH, possibly as a result of bronchogenic carcinoma, acute porphyria, hypothyroidism, Addison's disease, cirrhosis of the liver, infectious hepatitis, severe hemorrhage, or circulatory shock.

## INTERFERING FACTORS

• Anesthetics, carbamazepine (Tegretol), chlorothiazide (DIURIL), chlorpropamide (Diabinese), cyclophosphamide (Cytoxan), estrogen, hypnotics, lithium carbonate, morphine, oxytocin, tranquilizers, and vincristine (Oncovin) (increase)
• Stress, pain, and positive-pressure ventilation (increase)
• Alcohol and negative-pressure ventilation (decrease)
• Radioactive scan performed within 1 week before the test

## Antiglobulin test, direct

The direct antiglobulin test (or *direct Coombs' test*) detects immunoglobulins (antibodies) on the surface of red blood cells (RBCs). These immunoglobulins coat RBCs when they become sensitized to an antigen such as the Rh factor.

In this test, antiglobulin (Coombs') serum added to saline-washed RBCs results in agglutination if immunoglobulins or complement is present. This test is "direct" because it requires only one step — the addition of Coombs' serum to washed cells.

## PURPOSE

• To diagnose hemolytic disease of the newborn (HDN)
• To investigate hemolytic transfusion reactions

- To aid in the differential diagnosis of hemolytic anemias, which may be congenital or may result from an autoimmune reaction or use of certain drugs

## PATIENT PREPARATION

*Age alert* *If the patient is a neonate, explain to the parents that the direct antiglobulin test, which requires a blood sample, helps diagnose HDN.*

- If the patient is suspected of having hemolytic anemia, explain that the test determines whether the condition results from an abnormality in the body's immune system, the use of certain drugs, or some unknown cause.
- Inform the adult patient that he need not restrict food and fluids.
- Explain to the patient that he may experience slight discomfort from the tourniquet and needle puncture.
- Withhold medications that may interfere with test results, including quinidine, methyldopa, cephalosporins, sulfonamides, chlorpromazine, diphenylhydantoin, ethosuximide, hydralazine, levodopa, mefenamic acid, melphalan, penicillin, procainamide, rifampin, streptomycin, tetracyclines, and isoniazid, as ordered.

## PROCEDURE AND POSTTEST CARE

- For an adult, perform a venipuncture and collect the sample in two 5-ml EDTA tubes.

*Age alert* *For a neonate, draw 5 ml of umbilical cord blood into a tube with EDTA or additives, as ordered, after the cord is clamped and cut.*

- Apply direct pressure to the venipuncture site until bleeding stops.
- Instruct the patient that he may resume medications discontinued before the test, as ordered.

*Age alert* *Tell the patient or the parents of the neonate with HDN that further tests will be necessary to monitor anemia.*

## PRECAUTIONS

- Handle the sample gently to prevent hemolysis.
- Label the sample with the patient's full name, the health care facility or blood bank number, the date, and the phlebotomist's initials.

- Send the sample to the laboratory immediately.

## NORMAL FINDINGS

A negative test, in which neither antibodies nor complement appears on the RBCs, is normal.

## ABNORMAL FINDINGS

A positive test on umbilical cord blood indicates that maternal antibodies have crossed the placenta and coated fetal RBCs, causing HDN. Transfusion of compatible blood lacking the antigens to these maternal antibodies may be necessary to prevent anemia.

In other patients, a positive test result may indicate hemolytic anemia and help differentiate between autoimmune and secondary hemolytic anemia, which can be drug-induced or associated with an underlying disease. A positive test can also indicate sepsis.

A weakly positive test may suggest a transfusion reaction in which the patient's antibodies react with transfused RBCs containing the corresponding antigen.

## INTERFERING FACTORS

- Cephalosporins, chlorpromazine (Thorazine), ethosuximide (Zarontin), hydralazine (Apresoline), isoniazid, levodopa, mefenamic acid (Ponstel), melphalan (Alkeran), methyldopa (Aldomet), penicillin, procainamide (Procanbid), quinidine, rifampin, streptomycin, sulfonamides, and tetracyclines (positive test results, possibly due to immune hemolysis)

# Anti-insulin antibodies

Some patients with diabetes form antibodies to the insulin they take. These antibodies bind with some of the insulin, making less insulin available for glucose metabolism and necessitating increased insulin dosages. This phenomenon is known as *insulin resistance.*

Performed on the blood of a patient with diabetes who takes insulin, the anti-insulin antibody test detects insulin antibodies. Insulin antibodies are immunoglobulins, called *anti-insulin Ab.* The most common type of anti-insulin Ab is immunoglobulin (Ig) G, but anti-insulin Ab is also found in the other four classes of immunoglobulins — IgA, IgD, IgE, and IgM. IgM may cause insulin resistance, and IgE has been associated with allergic reactions.

## PURPOSE
- To determine insulin allergy
- To confirm insulin resistance
- To determine if hypoglycemia is caused by insulin overuse

## PATIENT PREPARATION
- Explain to the patient that the anti-insulin antibody test is used to determine the most appropriate treatment for his diabetes and to determine if he has insulin resistance or an allergy to insulin.
- Tell the patient that the test requires a blood sample. Explain who will perform the venipuncture and when.
- Explain to the patient that he may experience slight discomfort from the tourniquet and needle puncture.
- Inform the patient that he need not restrict food and fluids.
- Ask the patient if he has had a radioactive test recently; if so, note this on the laboratory request.

## PROCEDURE AND POSTTEST CARE
- Perform a venipuncture and collect the sample in a 7-ml tube without additives.
- Apply direct pressure to the venipuncture site until bleeding stops.

## PRECAUTIONS
- Handle the sample gently to prevent hemolysis.

## NORMAL FINDINGS
There should be less than 3% binding of the patient's serum with labeled beef, human, and pork insulin.

## ABNORMAL FINDINGS
Elevated levels may occur in insulin allergy or resistance and in factitious hypoglycemia.

## INTERFERING FACTORS
- Radioactive test performed within 1 week before the test

# Antimitochondrial antibodies

Usually performed with the test for anti-smooth-muscle antibodies (see page 26), the antimitochondrial antibody test detects antimitochondrial antibodies in serum by indirect immunofluorescence. These autoantibodies are present in several hepatic diseases. Their role in disease pathogenesis is unknown, and there's no evidence that they cause hepatic damage. Most commonly, they're associated with primary biliary cirrhosis and, sometimes, chronic active hepatitis and drug-induced jaundice. Antimitochondrial antibodies are also associated with autoimmune diseases, such as systemic lupus erythematosus, rheumatoid arthritis, pernicious anemia, and idiopathic Addison's disease.

## PURPOSE
- To aid in the diagnosis of primary biliary cirrhosis
- To distinguish between extrahepatic jaundice and biliary cirrhosis

## PATIENT PREPARATION
- Explain to the patient that the antimitochondrial antibody test evaluates liver function.
- Inform the patient that he need not restrict food and fluids.
- Tell the patient that the test requires a blood sample. Explain who will perform the venipuncture and when.
- Explain to the patient that he may experience slight discomfort from the tourniquet and needle puncture.
- Check the patient's medication history for oxyphenisatin use and report it to the laboratory because it may produce antimitochondrial antibodies.

## PROCEDURE AND POSTTEST CARE
- Perform a venipuncture and collect the sample in a 7-ml tube with no additives.
- Because the patient with hepatic disease may bleed excessively, apply pressure to the venipuncture site until bleeding stops.

## INCIDENCE OF SERUM ANTIBODIES IN VARIOUS DISORDERS

This chart shows the percentage of patients with certain disorders who have antimitochondrial or anti-smooth-muscle antibodies in the serum. The presence of these antibodies requires further testing to confirm the diagnosis. (Up to 1% of healthy people also show antimitochondrial antibodies.)

| DISORDER | ANTIMITOCHONDRIAL ANTIBODIES | ANTI-SMOOTH-MUSCLE ANTIBODIES |
|---|---|---|
| Primary biliary cirrhosis | 75% to 95% | 0% to 50%[a] |
| Chronic active hepatitis | 0% to 30% | 50% to 80% |
| Extrahepatic biliary obstruction | 0% to 5% | 0% |
| Cryptogenic cirrhosis | 0% to 25% | 0% to 1% |
| Viral (infectious) hepatitis | 0% | 1% to 2%[b] |
| Drug-induced jaundice | 50% to 80% | |
| Intrinsic asthma | | 20% |
| Rheumatoid arthritis and other collagen diseases | 1% to 2% | |
| Systemic lupus erythematosus | 3% to 5%[c] | 0% |

[a] In chronic disease, values fall at upper end of range.
[b] Much higher incidence occurs with hepatic damage.
[c] Much higher incidence occurs with renal involvement.

## PRECAUTIONS
● Handle the sample gently to prevent hemolysis.
● Send the sample to the laboratory immediately.

## NORMAL FINDINGS
Serum is normally negative for antimitochondrial antibodies. Positive results are titered.

## ABNORMAL FINDINGS
Although antimitochondrial antibodies appear in 79% to 94% of patients with primary biliary cirrhosis, this test alone doesn't confirm the diagnosis. Further tests, such as serum alkaline phosphatase, serum bilirubin, aspartate aminotransferase, alanine aminotransferase and, possibly, liver biopsy or cholangiography, may also be necessary. The autoantibodies also appear in some patients with chronic active hepatitis, drug-induced jaundice, and cryptogenic cirrhosis. (See *Incidence of serum antibodies in various disorders*.) Antimitochondrial antibodies seldom appear in patients with extrahepatic biliary obstruction, and a positive test helps rule out this condition.

## INTERFERING FACTORS
● Confusion of antimitochondrial antibodies with heterophil antibodies, cardiolipin antibodies to syphilis, ribosomal antibodies, and microsomal hepatic or renal autoantibodies

# Antinuclear antibodies

In such conditions as systemic lupus erythematosus (SLE), scleroderma, and certain infections, the body's immune system may perceive portions of its own cell nuclei as foreign and may produce antinuclear antibodies (ANAs). Specific ANAs include antibodies to deoxyribonucleic acid (DNA), nucleoprotein, histones, nuclear ribonucleoprotein, and other nuclear constituents.

Because they don't penetrate living cells, ANAs are harmless, but sometimes form antigen-antibody complexes that cause tissue damage (as in SLE). Because of multiorgan involvement, test results aren't diagnostic and can only partially confirm clinical evidence.

The antinuclear antibody test measures the relative concentration of ANAs in a serum sample through indirect immunofluorescence. Serial dilutions of serum are mixed with either Hep-2 or mouse kidney substrate. If the serum contains ANAs, it forms antigen-antibody complexes with the substrate. After the preparation is mixed with fluorescein-labeled antihuman serum, it's examined under an ultraviolet microscope. If ANAs are present, the complex fluoresces. Titer is taken as the greatest dilution that shows the reaction.

About 99% of patients with SLE exhibit ANAs; a large percentage of these patients do so at high titers. Although this test isn't specific for SLE, it's a useful screening tool. Failure to detect ANAs essentially rules out active SLE.

## PURPOSE
- To screen for SLE
- To monitor the effectiveness of immunosuppressive therapy for SLE

## PATIENT PREPARATION
- Explain to the patient that the antinuclear antibody test evaluates the immune system and that further testing is usually required for diagnosis.
- Inform the patient that the test will be repeated to monitor his response to therapy, if appropriate.
- Inform the patient that he need not restrict food and fluids.
- Tell the patient that the test requires a blood sample. Explain who will perform the venipuncture and when.
- Explain to the patient that he may experience slight discomfort from the tourniquet and needle puncture.
- Check the patient's history for drugs that may affect test results, such as isoniazid and procainamide. Note findings on the laboratory request.

## PROCEDURE AND POSTTEST CARE
- Perform a venipuncture and collect the sample in a 7-ml tube without additives.
- Apply direct pressure to the venipuncture site until bleeding stops.
- Keep a clean, dry bandage over the site for at least 24 hours.
- Because a patient with an autoimmune disease has a compromised immune system, observe the venipuncture site for signs of infection, and report changes to the physician immediately.

## PRECAUTIONS
- Handle the sample gently to prevent hemolysis.
- Send the sample to the laboratory immediately.

## NORMAL FINDINGS
Test results are reported as positive (with pattern and serum titer noted) or negative.

## ABNORMAL FINDINGS
Although the antinuclear antibody test is a sensitive indicator of ANAs, it isn't specific for SLE. Low titers may occur in patients with viral diseases, chronic hepatic disease, collagen vascular disease, and autoimmune diseases and in some healthy adults; the incidence increases with age. The higher the titer, the more specific the test is for SLE (titer typically exceeds 1:256).

The pattern of nuclear fluorescence helps identify the type of immune disease present. A peripheral pattern is almost exclusively associated with SLE because it indicates the presence of anti-DNA antibodies; sometimes anti-DNA antibodies are measured by radioimmunoassay if ANA titers are high or if a peripheral pattern is observed. A homogeneous, or diffuse, pattern is also associated with SLE as well as with related connective tissue disorders; a nucleolar pattern, with scleroderma; and a speckled, irregular pattern, with infectious mononucleosis and mixed connective tissue disorders (for example, SLE and scleroderma).

A single serum sample, especially one collected from a patient with collagen vascular disease, may contain antibodies to several parts of the cell's nucleus. In addition, as serum dilution increases, the fluorescent pattern may change because different antibodies are reactive at different titers.

## INTERFERING FACTORS

- Most commonly isoniazid, hydralazine (Apresoline), and procainamide (Procanbid), but also para-aminosalicylic acid, chlorpromazine (Thorazine), phenytoin (Dilantin), griseofulvin, ethosuximide (Zarontin), gold salts, methyldopa (Aldomet), hormonal contraceptives, penicillin, propylthiouracil, streptomycin, sulfonamides, tetracyclines, quinidine, and primidone (Mysoline), (possible production of a syndrome resembling SLE)

---

# Anti-smooth-muscle antibodies

---

Using indirect immunofluorescence, the anti-smooth-muscle antibodies test measures the relative concentration of anti-smooth-muscle antibodies in serum; it's usually performed with the test for antimitochondrial antibodies (see page 23). The serum sample is exposed to a thin section of smooth muscle and incubated; then a fluorescent-labeled antiglobulin is added. This antiglobulin binds only to antibodies that have complexed with smooth muscle and appears fluorescent when viewed through the microscope under ultraviolet light.

Anti-smooth-muscle antibodies appear in several hepatic diseases, especially chronic active hepatitis and, less commonly, primary biliary cirrhosis. Although anti-smooth-muscle antibodies are usually associated with hepatic diseases, their etiologic role is unknown, and there's no evidence that they cause hepatic damage.

## PURPOSE

- To aid in the diagnosis of active chronic hepatitis and primary biliary cirrhosis

## PATIENT PREPARATION

- Explain to the patient that the anti-smooth-muscle antibody test helps evaluate liver function.
- Inform the patient that he need not restrict food and fluids.
- Tell the patient that the test requires a blood sample. Explain who will perform the venipuncture and when.
- Explain to the patient that he may experience slight discomfort from the tourniquet and needle puncture.

## PROCEDURE AND POSTTEST CARE

- Perform a venipuncture and collect the sample in a 7-ml tube without additives.
- Because the patient with hepatic disease may bleed excessively, apply direct pressure to the venipuncture site until bleeding stops.

## PRECAUTIONS

- Handle the sample gently to prevent hemolysis.
- Send the sample to the laboratory immediately.

## REFERENCE VALUES

A normal titer of anti-smooth-muscle antibodies is negative. Positive results are titered.

## ABNORMAL FINDINGS

The test for anti-smooth-muscle antibodies isn't specific; these antibodies appear in many patients with chronic active hepatitis and in fewer patients with primary biliary cirrhosis.

Anti-smooth-muscle antibodies may also be present in patients with infectious mononucleosis, acute viral hepatitis, a malignant tumor of the liver, and intrinsic asthma (see *Incidence of serum antibodies in various disorders,* page 24).

## INTERFERING FACTORS

- None significant

# Antistreptolysin-O test

The antistreptolysin-O (known as ASO) test measures the relative serum concentrations of the antibody to streptolysin-O. A serum sample is diluted with a commercial preparation of streptolysin-O and incubated. After the addition of human red blood cells, the tube is reincubated and examined visually. Failure of hemolysis to develop indicates recent streptococcal infection. The end point is read in Todd units, the reciprocal of the highest dilution (titer) that inhibits hemolysis.

## PURPOSE
● To confirm recent or ongoing streptococcal infection
● To help diagnose rheumatic fever and poststreptococcal glomerulonephritis in the presence of clinical symptoms (See *Test for anti-DNase B*, for information about another method of diagnosing these two diseases.)
● To distinguish between rheumatic fever and rheumatoid arthritis when joint pains are present

## PATIENT PREPARATION
● Explain to the patient that the ASO test detects an immunologic response to certain bacteria (streptococci).
● Inform the patient that he need not restrict food and fluids (although a fasting sample is preferred).
● Tell the patient that the test requires a blood sample. Explain who will perform the venipuncture and when.
● Explain to the patient that he may experience slight discomfort from the tourniquet and needle puncture.
● If the test is to be repeated at regular intervals to identify active and inactive states of rheumatic fever or to confirm acute glomerulonephritis, tell the patient that measuring changes in antibody levels helps determine the effectiveness of therapy.
● Check the patient's history for drugs that may suppress the streptococcal antibody responses. If such drugs must be continued, note this on the laboratory request.

---

## TEST FOR ANTI-DNASE B

The antideoxyribonuclease B (anti-DNase B) test, a process similar to the antistreptolysin-O (ASO) test, detects antibodies to DNase B, a potent antigen produced by all group A streptococci.

For adults, normal anti-DNase B titer is less than 85 Todd units/ml; for school-age children, it's less than 170 Todd units/ml; and for preschoolers, it's less than 80 Todd units/ml.

Elevated anti-DNase B titers appear in 80% of patients with acute rheumatic fever, in 75% of those with poststreptococcal glomerulonephritis (following streptococcal pharyngitis), and in 60% of those with glomerulonephritis (following group A streptococcal pyoderma). This patient group reflects a much higher percentage than those with ASO titer elevations (25%), making the test for anti-DNase B especially valuable in detecting a reaction to group A streptococcal pyoderma.

Other streptococcal antigens are of limited diagnostic value, or their use is controversial.

---

## PROCEDURE AND POSTTEST CARE
● Perform a venipuncture and collect the sample in a 7-ml tube without additives.
● Apply direct pressure to the venipuncture site until bleeding stops.

## PRECAUTIONS
● Handle the sample gently to prevent hemolysis.

## REFERENCE VALUES
★ *Age alert* *Even healthy people have some detectable ASO titers from previous minor streptococcal infections. Normal ASO titers range as follows:*
● *school-age children: 170 Todd units/ml*
● *preschoolers and adults: 85 Todd units/ml.*

## ABNORMAL FINDINGS
High ASO titers usually occur only after prolonged or recurrent infections. Generally, a

titer higher than 166 Todd units/ml is considered a definite elevation. A low titer is good evidence of the absence of active rheumatic fever. A higher titer doesn't necessarily mean that rheumatic fever or glomerulonephritis is present; however, it does indicate the presence of a streptococcal infection.

Serial titers, determined at 10- to 14-day intervals, provide more reliable information than does a single titer. An increase in titer 2 to 5 weeks after the acute infection, which peaks 4 to 6 weeks after the initial increase, confirms poststreptococcal disease.

## INTERFERING FACTORS
● Streptococcal skin infections, seldom producing abnormal ASO titers even with poststreptococcal disease (probable false-negative)
● Antibiotic or corticosteroid therapy (possible suppression of the streptococcal antibody response)

---

# Antithyroid antibodies

---

In autoimmune disorders — such as Hashimoto's thyroiditis and Graves' disease (hyperthyroidism) — thyroglobulin, the major colloidal storage compound, is released into the blood. Because thyroxine usually separates from thyroglobulin before its release into the blood, thyroglobulin doesn't normally enter the circulation. When it does, antithyroglobulin antibodies are formed to attack this foreign substance; the ensuing autoimmune response damages the thyroid gland. The serum of a patient whose autoimmune system produces antithyroglobulin antibodies usually contains antimicrosomal antibodies, which react with the microsomes of the thyroid epithelial cells.

The tanned red cell hemagglutination test detects antithyroglobulin and antimicrosomal antibodies. Another laboratory technique, indirect immunofluorescence, can detect antimicrosomal antibodies.

## PURPOSE
● To detect circulating antithyroglobulin antibodies when clinical evidence indicates Hashimoto's thyroiditis, Graves' disease, or other thyroid diseases

## PATIENT PREPARATION
● Explain to the patient that the antithyroid antibody test evaluates thyroid function.
● Inform the patient that he need not restrict food and fluids.
● Tell the patient that the test requires a blood sample. Explain who will perform the venipuncture and when.
● Explain to the patient that he may experience slight discomfort from the tourniquet and needle puncture.

## PROCEDURE AND POSTTEST CARE
● Perform a venipuncture and collect the sample in a 7-ml tube without additives.
● Apply direct pressure to the venipuncture site until bleeding stops.

## PRECAUTIONS
● Handle the sample gently to prevent hemolysis.
● Send the sample to the laboratory immediately.

## REFERENCE VALUES
The normal titer is less than 1:100 for antithyroglobulin and antimicrosomal antibodies.

## ABNORMAL FINDINGS
The presence of antithyroglobulin or antimicrosomal antibodies in serum can indicate subclinical autoimmune thyroid disease, Graves' disease, or idiopathic myxedema. Titers of 1:400 or greater strongly suggest Hashimoto's thyroiditis.

Antithyroglobulin antibodies may also occur in some patients with other autoimmune disorders, such as systemic lupus erythematosus, rheumatoid arthritis, and autoimmune hemolytic anemia.

## INTERFERING FACTORS
● None significant

# Arginine test

The arginine test, also known as the *human growth hormone (hGH) stimulation test,* measures hGH levels after I.V. administration of arginine, an amino acid that normally stimulates hGH secretion. It's commonly used to identify pituitary dysfunction in infants and children with growth retardation and to confirm hGH deficiency. This test may be performed concomitantly with an insulin tolerance test or after administration of other hGH stimulants, such as glucagon, vasopressin, and levodopa.

## PURPOSE
- To aid diagnosis of pituitary tumors
- To confirm hGH deficiency in infants and children with low baseline levels

## PATIENT PREPARATION
- Explain to the patient, or his parents if the patient is a child, that the arginine test identifies hGH deficiency.
- Instruct the patient to fast and limit physical activity for 10 to 12 hours before the test.
- Explain to the patient that this test requires I.V. infusion of a drug and collection of several blood samples. Tell him that the test takes at least 2 hours to perform.
- Withhold all steroid medications, including pituitary-based hormones, as ordered. If they must be continued, record this on the laboratory request.
- Tell the patient to lie down and relax for at least 90 minutes before the test.

## PROCEDURE AND POSTTEST CARE
- Between 6 a.m. and 8 a.m., perform a venipuncture and collect 6 ml of blood (basal sample) in a clot-activator tube.
- Use an indwelling venous catheter to avoid repeated venipunctures. Start I.V. infusion of arginine (0.5 g/kg of body weight) in normal saline solution, and continue for 30 minutes.
- Discontinue the I.V. infusion, and then draw a total of three 6-ml samples at 30-minute intervals. Collect each sample in a clot-activator tube, and label it appropriately.

- Apply direct pressure to the venipuncture site until bleeding stops.
- Instruct the patient that he may resume his usual diet, activities, and medications discontinued before the test, as ordered.

## PRECAUTIONS
- Collect each sample at the scheduled time, and specify the collection time on the laboratory request.
- Send each sample to the laboratory immediately because hGH has a half-life of only 20 to 25 minutes.
- Handle the samples gently to prevent hemolysis.

## REFERENCE VALUES
Arginine should raise hGH levels to more than 10 ng/ml (SI, > 10 µg/L) in males, more than 15 ng/ml (SI, >15 µg/L) in females, and more than 48 ng/ml (SI, > 48 µg/L) in children. Such an increase may appear in the first sample collected 30 minutes after arginine infusion is discontinued or in the samples collected 60 and 90 minutes afterward.

## ABNORMAL FINDINGS
Levels that are elevated during fasting or that rise during sleep help to rule out hGH deficiency. Failure of hGH levels to rise after arginine infusion indicates decreased anterior pituitary hGH reserve. In children, this deficiency causes dwarfism; in adults, it can indicate panhypopituitarism. When hGH levels fail to reach 10 ng/ml, retesting is required at the same time of day as the original test.

## INTERFERING FACTORS
- Radioactive scan performed within 1 week before the test

# Arterial blood gas analysis

Arterial blood gas (ABG) analysis is used to measure the partial pressure of arterial oxygen ($PaO_2$), the partial pressure of arterial carbon dioxide ($PaCO_2$), and the pH of an arterial sample. Oxygen content ($O_2CT$), arterial oxygen saturation ($SaO_2$), and bicarbonate ($HCO_3^-$) values are also measured.

A blood sample for ABG analysis may be drawn by percutaneous arterial puncture or from an arterial line.

The $PaO_2$ indicates how much oxygen the lungs are delivering to the blood. The $PaCO_2$ indicates how efficiently the lungs eliminate carbon dioxide. The pH indicates the acid-base level of the blood, or the hydrogen ion (H+) concentration. Acidity indicates H+ excess; alkalinity, H+ deficit. (See *Balancing pH*.) $O_2CT$, $SaO_2$, and $HCO_3^-$ values also aid diagnosis.

## PURPOSE

- To evaluate the efficiency of pulmonary gas exchange
- To assess the integrity of the ventilatory control system
- To determine the acid-base level of the blood
- To monitor respiratory therapy

## PATIENT PREPARATION

- Explain to the patient that ABG analysis is used to evaluate how well the lungs are delivering oxygen to blood and eliminating carbon dioxide.
- Tell the patient that the test requires a blood sample. Explain who will perform the arterial puncture and when, and which site — radial, brachial, or femoral artery — has been selected for the puncture.
- Inform the patient that he need not restrict food and fluids.
- Instruct the patient to breathe normally during the test, and warn him that he may experience a brief cramping or throbbing pain at the puncture site.

## PROCEDURE AND POSTTEST CARE

- Perform an arterial puncture or draw blood from an arterial line. Use a heparinized blood gas syringe to draw the sample. Eliminate air from the sample, place it on ice immediately, and transport it for analysis.
- After applying pressure to the puncture site for 3 to 5 minutes and when bleeding has stopped, tape a gauze pad firmly over it. (If the puncture site is on the arm, don't tape the entire circumference; this may restrict circulation.)
- If the patient is receiving anticoagulants or has a coagulopathy, apply pressure to the puncture site longer than 5 minutes if necessary.

- Monitor vital signs and observe for signs of circulatory impairment, such as swelling, discoloration, pain, numbness, and tingling in the bandaged arm or leg.
- Watch for bleeding from the puncture site.

## PRECAUTIONS

- Wait at least 20 minutes before drawing arterial blood when starting, changing, or discontinuing oxygen therapy; after initiating or changing settings of mechanical ventilation; or after extubation.
- Before sending the sample to the laboratory, note on the laboratory request whether the patient was breathing room air or receiving oxygen therapy when the sample was collected.
- If the patient was receiving oxygen therapy, note the flow rate and method of delivery. If he's on a ventilator, note the fraction of inspired oxygen, tidal volume mode, respiratory rate, and positive-end expiratory pressure.
- Note the patient's core temperature.

## REFERENCE VALUES

Normal ABG values fall within these ranges:
- $PaO_2$ — 80 to 100 mm Hg (SI, 10.6 to 13.3 kPa)
- $PaCO_2$ — 35 to 45 mm Hg (SI, 4.7 to 5.3 kPa)
- pH — 7.35 to 7.45 (SI, 7.35 to 7.45)
- $O_2CT$ — 15% to 23% (SI, 0.15 to 0.23)
- $SaO_2$ — 94% to 100% (SI, 0.94 to 1)
- $HCO_3^-$ — 22 to 25 mEq/L (SI, 22 to 25 mmol/L).

## ABNORMAL FINDINGS

Low $PaO_2$, $O_2CT$, and $SaO_2$ levels and a high $PaCO_2$ may result from conditions that impair respiratory function, such as respiratory muscle weakness or paralysis, respiratory center inhibition (from head injury, brain tumor, or drug abuse), and airway obstruction (possibly from mucus plugs or a tumor). Similarly, low readings may result from bronchiole obstruction caused by asthma or emphysema, from an abnormal ventilation-perfusion ratio due to partially blocked alveoli or pulmonary capillaries, or from alveoli that are damaged or filled with fluid because of disease, hemorrhage, or near-drowning.

When inspired air contains insufficient oxygen, $PaO_2$, $O_2CT$, and $SaO_2$ decrease, but

# BALANCING pH

To measure the acidity or alkalinity of a solution, chemists use a pH scale of 1 to 15 that measures hydrogen ion concentrations. As hydrogen ions and acidity increase, pH falls below 7.0, which is neutral. Conversely, when hydrogen ions decrease, pH and alkalinity increase. Acid-base balance, or homeostasis of hydrogen ions, is necessary if the body's enzyme systems are to work properly.

The slightest change in ionic hydrogen concentration alters the rate of cellular chemical reactions; a sufficiently severe change can be fatal. To maintain a normal blood pH — generally between 7.35 and 7.45 — the body relies on three mechanisms.

## BUFFERS

Chemically composed of two substances, buffers prevent radical pH changes by replacing strong acids added to a solution (such as blood) with weaker ones. For example, strong acids capable of yielding many hydrogen ions are replaced by weaker ones that yield fewer hydrogen ions. Because of the principal buffer coupling of bicarbonate and carbonic acid — normally in a ratio of 20:1 — the plasma acid-base level rarely fluctuates. Increased bicarbonate, however, indicates alkalosis, whereas decreased bicarbonate points to acidosis. Increased carbonic acid indicates acidosis, and decreased carbonic acid indicates alkalosis.

## RESPIRATION

Respiration is important in maintaining blood pH. The lungs convert carbonic acid to carbon dioxide and water. With every expiration, carbon dioxide and water leave the body, decreasing the carbonic acid content of the blood. Consequently, fewer hydrogen ions are formed, and blood pH increases. When the blood's hydrogen ion or carbonic acid content increases, neurons in the respiratory center stimulate respiration.

Hyperventilation eliminates carbon dioxide and hence carbonic acid from the body, reduces hydrogen ion formation, and increases pH. Conversely, increased blood pH from alkalosis — decreased hydrogen ion concentration — causes hypoventilation, which restores blood pH to its normal level by retaining carbon dioxide and thus increasing hydrogen ion formation.

## URINARY EXCRETION

The third factor in acid-base balance is urine excretion. Because the kidneys excrete varying amounts of acids and bases, they control urine pH, which in turn affects blood pH. For example, when blood pH is decreased, the distal and collecting tubules remove excessive hydrogen ions (carbonic acid forms in the tubular cells and dissociates into hydrogen and bicarbonate) and displaces them in urine, thereby eliminating hydrogen from the body. In exchange, basic ions in the urine — usually sodium — diffuse into the tubular cells, where they combine with bicarbonate. This sodium bicarbonate is then reabsorbed in the blood, resulting in decreased urine pH and, more importantly, increased blood pH.

---

$PaCO_2$ may be normal. Such findings are common in pneumothorax, impaired diffusion between alveoli and blood (due to interstitial fibrosis, for example), or an arteriovenous shunt that permits blood to bypass the lungs.

Low $O_2CT$ — with normal $PaO_2$, $SaO_2$ and, possibly, $PaCO_2$ values — may result from severe anemia, decreased blood volume, and reduced hemoglobin oxygen-carrying capacity.

In addition to clarifying blood oxygen disorders, ABG values can give considerable information about acid-base disorders. (See *Acid-base disorders,* page 32.)

## INTERFERING FACTORS

- Exposing the sample to air (increase or decrease in $PaO_2$ and $PaCO_2$)
- Venous blood in the sample (possible decrease in $PaO_2$ and increase in $PaCO_2$)
- $HCO_3^-$, ethacrynic acid, hydrocortisone, metolazone, prednisone, and thiazides (possible increase in $PaCO_2$)
- Acetazolamide (Diamox), nitrofurantoin (Macrodantin), and tetracycline (possible decrease in $PaCO_2$)
- Fever (possible false-high $PaO_2$ and $PaCO_2$)

# ACID-BASE DISORDERS

| DISORDERS AND ABG FINDINGS | POSSIBLE CAUSES | SIGNS AND SYMPTOMS |
|---|---|---|
| **RESPIRATORY ACIDOSIS (EXCESS $CO_2$ RETENTION)** | | |
| pH < 7.35 (SI, < 7.35)<br>$HCO_3^-$ > 26 mEq/L<br>(SI, > 26 mmol/L) (if compensating)<br>$Paco_2$ > 45 mm Hg (SI, > 5.3 kPa) | ◆ Central nervous system depression from drugs, injury, or disease<br>◆ Asphyxia<br>◆ Hypoventilation due to pulmonary, cardiac, musculoskeletal, or neuromuscular disease<br>◆ Obesity<br>◆ Postoperative pain<br>◆ Abdominal distention | Diaphoresis, headache, tachycardia, confusion, restlessness, apprehension |
| **RESPIRATORY ALKALOSIS (EXCESS $CO_2$ EXCRETION)** | | |
| pH > 7.45 (SI, > 7.45)<br>$HCO_3^-$ < 22 mEq/L<br>(SI, < 22 mmol/L) (if compensating)<br>$Paco_2$ < 35 mm Hg (SI, < 4.7 kPa) | ◆ Hyperventilation due to anxiety, pain, or improper ventilator settings<br>◆ Respiratory stimulation caused by drugs, disease, hypoxia, fever, or high room temperature<br>◆ Gram-negative bacteremia<br>◆ Compensation for metabolic acidosis (chronic renal failure) | Rapid, deep breathing; paresthesia; lightheadedness; twitching; anxiety; fear |
| **METABOLIC ACIDOSIS ($HCO_3^-$ LOSS, ACID RETENTION)** | | |
| pH < 7.35 (SI, < 7.35)<br>$HCO_3^-$ < 22 mEq/L<br>(SI, < 22 mmol/L)<br>$Paco_2$ < 35 mm Hg (SI, < 4.7 kPa) (if compensating) | ◆ $HCO_3^-$ depletion due to renal disease, diarrhea, or small-bowel fistulas<br>◆ Excessive production of organic acids due to hepatic disease; endocrine disorders, including diabetes mellitus, hypoxia, shock, and drug intoxication<br>◆ Inadequate excretion of acids due to renal disease | Rapid, deep breathing; fruity breath; fatigue; headache; lethargy; drowsiness; nausea; vomiting; coma (if severe) |
| **METABOLIC ALKALOSIS ($HCO_3^-$ RETENTION, ACID LOSS)** | | |
| pH > 7.45 (SI, > 7.45)<br>$HCO_3^-$ > 26 mEq/L<br>(SI, > 26 mmol/L)<br>$Paco_2$ > 45 mm Hg (SI, > 5.3 kPa) | ◆ Loss of hydrochloric acid from prolonged vomiting or gastric suctioning<br>◆ Loss of potassium due to increased renal excretion (as in diuretic therapy) or steroid overdose<br>◆ Excessive alkali ingestion<br>◆ Compensation for chronic respiratory acidosis | Slow, shallow breathing; hypertonic muscles; restlessness; twitching; confusion; irritability; apathy; tetany; seizures; coma (if severe) |

# Arterial-to-alveolar oxygen ratio

Using calculations based on the patient's laboratory values, the arterial-to-alveolar oxygen ratio (a/A ratio) test can help identify the cause of hypoxemia and intrapulmonary shunting by providing an approximation of the partial pressure of oxygenation of the alveoli and arteries. It may help differentiate the cause as ventilated alveoli but no perfusion, unventilated alveoli with perfusion, or collapse of the alveoli and capillaries.

## PURPOSE
- To evaluate the efficiency of gas exchange
- To assess the integrity of the ventilatory control system
- To monitor respiratory therapy

## PATIENT PREPARATION
- Explain to the patient that the a/A ratio test is used to evaluate how well the lungs are delivering oxygen to the blood and eliminating carbon dioxide.
- Tell the patient that the test requires a blood sample. Explain who will perform the arterial puncture and when.
- Inform the patient that he need not restrict food and fluids.
- Instruct the patient to breathe normally during the test, and warn him that he may experience cramping or throbbing pain at the puncture site.

## PROCEDURE AND POSTTEST CARE
- Perform an arterial puncture or draw blood from an arterial line using a heparinized blood gas syringe.
- Eliminate all air from the sample and place it on ice immediately.
- Apply pressure to the puncture for 3 to 5 minutes or until bleeding stops.
- Place a gauze pad over the site and tape it in place, but don't tape the entire circumference.
- Monitor vital signs and observe for signs of circulatory impairment, such as swelling, discoloration, pain, numbness, and tingling in the bandaged arm or leg.

- Watch for bleeding from the puncture site.
- The arterial sample is analyzed for partial pressure of arterial oxygen ($PaO_2$) and partial pressure of arterial carbon dioxide ($PaCO_2$). Also examined are barometric pressure ($Pb$), water vapor pressure ($PH_2O$), and fractional concentration of inspired oxygen ($FIO_2$) (21% for room air). From these values, the alveolar oxygen tension ($PAO_2$), the a/A ratio, and the alveolar-to-arterial oxygen gradient ($A\text{-}aDO_2$) are derived by solving these mathematical formulas:

$$PaO_2 = FIO_2 \ (Pb - PH_2O) - 1.25 \ (PaCO_2)$$

$$\text{a/A ratio} = PaO_2 \div PAO_2$$

$$A\text{-}aDO_2 = PAO_2 - PaO_2$$

- Based on the results of the formulas, appropriate interventions to correct patient problems are initiated.

## PRECAUTIONS
- Before sending the sample to the laboratory, note on the laboratory request whether the patient was breathing room air or receiving oxygen therapy when the sample was collected.
- If the patient was receiving oxygen therapy, note the flow rate and method of delivery. If he was on a ventilator, note the $FIO_2$, tidal volume, mode, respiratory rate, and positive end-expiratory pressure.
- Note the patient's rectal temperature.

## REFERENCE VALUES
A normal a/A ratio is 75%.

## ABNORMAL FINDINGS
Increased values may be caused by mucus plugs, bronchospasm, or airway collapse (asthma, bronchitis, emphysema). Hypoxemia results in increased $A\text{-}aDO_2$ and may be caused by arterial septal defects, pneumothorax, atelectasis, emboli, or edema.

## INTERFERING FACTORS
- Exposing the sample to air (increase or decrease)
- Age and increasing oxygen concentration (increase)

# Arthrography

Arthrography allows radiographic examination of a joint after injection of a radiopaque dye, air, or both (double-contrast arthrogram) to outline soft-tissue structures and the contour of the joint. The joint is put through its range of motion while a series of radiographs are taken.

Indications for arthrography include persistent unexplained joint discomfort or pain. Complications may include persistent joint crepitus and allergic reactions to the contrast dye. Magnetic resonance imaging of the joint may be used in place of this test.

## PURPOSE
● To identify acute or chronic tears or other abnormalities of the joint capsule or supporting ligaments of the knee, shoulder, ankle, hips, or wrist
● To detect internal joint derangements
● To locate synovial cysts

## PATIENT PREPARATION
● Describe arthrography to the patient and answer any questions he may have. Explain that this test permits examination of a joint.
● Inform the patient that he need not restrict food and fluids.
● Tell the patient who will perform the procedure and where it will take place.
● Explain that the fluoroscope allows the physician to track the contrast medium as it fills the joint space.
● Inform the patient that standard X-ray films will also be taken after diffusion of the contrast medium.
● Tell the patient that, although the joint area will be anesthetized, he may experience a tingling sensation or pressure in the joint when the contrast medium is injected.
● Instruct the patient to remain as still as possible during the procedure, except when following instructions to change position.
● Stress to the patient the importance of his cooperation in assuming various positions because films must be taken as quickly as possible to ensure optimum quality.
● Check the patient's history to determine if he's hypersensitive to local anesthetics, iodine, seafood, or dyes used for other diagnostic tests.

## PROCEDURE AND POSTTEST CARE
### Knee arthrography
● The knee is cleaned with an antiseptic solution and the area around the puncture site is anesthetized. (It isn't usually necessary to anesthetize the joint space itself.)
● A 2″ needle is then inserted into the joint space between the patella and femoral condyle and fluid is aspirated. The aspirated fluid is usually sent to the laboratory for analysis.
● While the needle is still in place, the aspirating syringe is removed and replaced with a syringe containing dye.
● If fluoroscopic examination demonstrates correct placement of the needle, the dye is injected into the joint space.
● After the needle is removed, the site is rubbed with a sterile sponge and the wound may be sealed with collodion.
● The patient is asked to walk a few steps or to move his knee through a range of motion to distribute the dye in the joint space. A film series is quickly taken with the knee held in various positions.
● If the films are clean and demonstrate proper dye placement, the knee is bandaged, typically with an elastic bandage.
● Tell the patient to keep the bandage in place for several days and teach him how to rewrap it.

### Shoulder arthrography
● The skin is prepared and a local anesthetic is injected subcutaneously just in front of the acromioclavicular joint.
● Additional anesthetic is injected directly onto the head of the humerus.
● The short lumbar puncture needle is inserted until the point is embedded in the joint cartilage.
● The stylet is removed, a syringe of contrast medium is attached and, using fluoroscopic guidance, about 1 ml of dye is injected into the joint space, as the needle is withdrawn slightly.
● If fluoroscopic examination demonstrates correct needle placement, the rest of the dye is injected while the needle is slowly withdrawn and the site is wiped with a sterile sponge.
● A film series is taken quickly to achieve maximum contrast.

# COMPARING NORMAL AND ABNORMAL ARTHROGRAMS

The arthrogram on the left (below) shows a normal medial meniscus. The view on the right shows a torn medial meniscus.

**Normal arthrogram of knee**

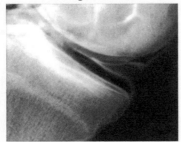

**Abnormal arthrogram of knee**

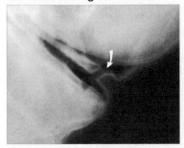

The arthrogram on the left (below) shows a normal shoulder. The arthrogram on the right shows a shoulder with a ruptured rotator cuff. Contrast medium has collected in the subacromial bursa (indicated by the arrows).

**Normal arthrogram of shoulder**

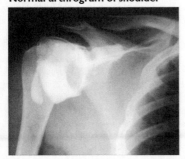

**Abnormal arthrogram of shoulder**

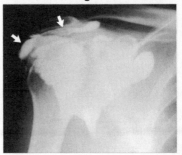

## Both types

● Tell the patient to rest the joint for at least 12 hours.

● Inform the patient that he may experience some swelling or discomfort or may hear crepitant noises in the joint after the test, but that these symptoms usually disappear after 1 or 2 days; tell him to report persistent symptoms.

● Advise the patient to apply ice to the joint if swelling occurs and to take a mild analgesic for pain.

● Instruct the patient to report signs of infection at the needle insertion site, such as warmth, redness, swelling, or foul-smelling drainage.

## PRECAUTIONS

● Know that arthrography is contraindicated during pregnancy and in the patient with active arthritis, joint infection, or previous sensitivity to radiopaque media.

## NORMAL FINDINGS

A normal knee arthrogram shows a characteristic wedge-shaped shadow, pointed toward the interior of the joint, which indicates a normal medial meniscus. A normal shoulder arthrogram shows the bicipital tendon sheath, redundant inferior joint capsule, and subscapular bursa intact. (See *Comparing normal and abnormal arthrograms*.)

## ABNORMAL FINDINGS

Arthrography accurately detects medial meniscal tears and lacerations in 90% to 95% of cases. Because the entire joint lining is opacified, arthrography can demonstrate extra-meniscal lesions, such as osteochondritis dissecans, chondromalacia patellae, osteochondral fractures, cartilaginous abnormalities, synovial abnormalities, tears of the cruciate ligaments, and disruption of the joint capsule and collateral ligaments.

Arthrography can reveal shoulder abnormalities, such as adhesive capsulitis, bicipital tenosynovitis or rupture, and rotator cuff tears. It can also evaluate damage from recurrent dislocations.

## INTERFERING FACTORS

● Dilution of the contrast medium due to incomplete aspiration of joint effusion (possible poor imaging)
● Improper injection technique (possible displacement of contrast medium)

## *Arthroscopy*

Arthroscopy is the visual examination of the interior of a joint (most commonly a major joint, such as a shoulder, hip, or knee) with a specially designed fiber-optic endoscope that's inserted through a cannula in the joint cavity. It usually follows and confirms a diagnosis made through physical examination, radiography, and arthrography.

Arthroscopy may be performed under local anesthesia, but it's usually performed under a spinal or general anesthesia, particularly when surgery is anticipated. A camera may be attached to the arthroscope to photograph areas for later study. (See *Arthroscopy of the knee*.)

Complications associated with arthroscopy are rare and may include infection, hemarthrosis, swelling, thrombophlebitis, and joint injury.

## PURPOSE

● To detect and diagnose meniscal, patellar, condylar, extrasynovial, and synovial diseases
● To monitor disease progression
● To perform joint surgery

● To monitor the effectiveness of therapy

## PATIENT PREPARATION

● Explain to the patient that arthroscopy is used to examine the interior of the joint, to evaluate joint disease, or to monitor his response to therapy, as appropriate.
● Describe the procedure to the patient and answer his questions.
● If surgery or another treatment is anticipated, explain that this may be accomplished during arthroscopy.
● Instruct the patient to fast after midnight before the procedure.
● Tell the patient who will perform the procedure and when and where it will be done.
● If local anesthesia is to be used, tell the patient that he may experience slight discomfort from the injection of the local anesthetic and the pressure of the tourniquet on his leg. The patient will also feel a thumping sensation as the cannula is inserted in the joint capsule.
● Make sure that the patient or a responsible family member has signed an informed consent form.
● Check the patient's history for hypersensitivity to the anesthetic.
● Be aware that the surgical site is prepared by shaving the area 5″ (12.7 cm) above and below the joint and a sedative is administered, as ordered. The patient is positioned and draped according to facility policy.

## PROCEDURE AND POSTTEST CARE

● Arthroscopic techniques vary depending on the surgeon and the type of arthroscope used.
● The patient's leg is elevated and wrapped with an elastic bandage to drain as much blood from the leg as possible, or a mixture of lidocaine with epinephrine and normal saline is instilled into the patient's knee to distend the knee and help reduce bleeding.
● The local anesthetic is administered, a small incision is made, and a cannula is passed through the incision and positioned in the joint cavity.
● The arthroscope is then inserted, and the knee structures are visually examined and photographed for further study.
● After visual examination, a synovial biopsy or appropriate surgery is performed as indicated.

# ARTHROSCOPY OF THE KNEE

With the patient's knee flexed about 40 degrees, the arthroscope is introduced into the joint. The examiner flexes, extends, and rotates the knee to view the joint space. Counterclockwise from the top right, these illustrations show a normal patellofemoral joint with smooth joint surfaces; the articular surface of the patella showing chondromalacia; and a tear in the anterior cruciate ligament.

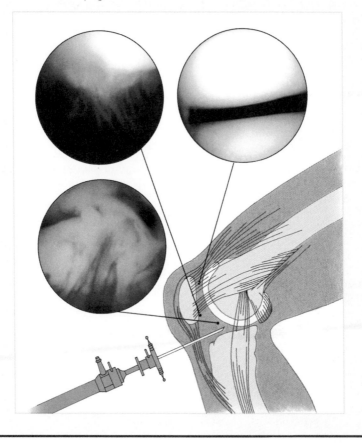

● When the examination is completed, the arthroscope is removed, the joint is irrigated, the cannula is removed, and an adhesive strip and compression dressing are applied over the incision site.

● Watch the patient for fever, swelling, increased pain, and localized inflammation at the incision site. If the patient reports discomfort, provide an analgesic, as ordered.

● Monitor the patient's circulation and sensation in his leg.

● Advise the patient to elevate the leg and apply ice for the first 24 hours.

● Instruct the patient to report fever, bleeding, drainage, or increased swelling or pain in the joint.

● Advise the patient to bear only partial weight, using crutches, a walker, or a cane for 48 hours.

● If an immobilizer is ordered, teach the patient how to apply it.

- Tell the patient that showering is permitted after 48 hours, but a tub bath should be avoided until after the postoperative visit.
- Tell the patient that he may resume his usual diet, as ordered.

## PRECAUTIONS
- Know that arthroscopy is contraindicated in a patient with fibrous ankylosis with flexion of less than 50 degrees.
- Know that arthroscopy is contraindicated when a patient with local skin or wound infections has a risk of subsequent joint involvement.

## NORMAL FINDINGS
The knee is a typical diarthrodial joint surrounded by muscles, ligaments, cartilage, and tendons and lined with a synovial membrane. In children, the menisci are smooth and opaque, with their thick outer edges attached to the joint capsule and their inner edges lying snugly against the condylar surfaces, unattached. Articular cartilage appears smooth and white; ligaments and tendons appear cablelike and silvery. The synovium is smooth and marked by a fine vascular network. Degenerative changes begin during adolescence.

## ABNORMAL FINDINGS
Arthroscopic examination can reveal meniscal disease, such as a torn medial or lateral meniscus or other meniscal injuries; patellar disease, such as chondromalacia, dislocation, subluxation, parapatellar synovitis or fracture; condylar disease, such as degenerative articular cartilage, osteochondritis dissecans, and loose bodies; extrasynovial disease, such as torn anterior cruciate or tibial collateral ligaments, Baker's cyst, and ganglionic cyst; and synovial disease, such as synovitis, rheumatoid and degenerative arthritis, and foreign bodies associated with gout, pseudogout, and osteochondromatosis.

Depending on test findings, appropriate treatment or surgery can follow arthroscopy. If arthroscopic surgery can't be performed, arthrotomy is the procedure of choice.

## INTERFERING FACTORS
- None significant

# Aspartate aminotransferase

Aspartate aminotransferase (AST) is one of two enzymes that catalyze the conversion of the nitrogenous portion of an amino acid to an amino acid residue. It's essential to energy production in the Krebs cycle. AST is found in the cytoplasm and mitochondria of many cells, primarily in the liver, heart, skeletal muscles, kidneys, pancreas, and red blood cells. It's released into serum in proportion to cellular damage.

Although a high correlation exists between myocardial infarction (MI) and elevated AST levels, this test is sometimes considered superfluous for diagnosing an MI because of its relatively low organ specificity; it doesn't allow differentiation between acute MI and the effects of hepatic congestion due to heart failure.

## PURPOSE
- To aid detection and differential diagnosis of acute hepatic disease
- To monitor patient progress and prognosis in cardiac and hepatic diseases
- To aid diagnosis of an MI in correlation with creatine kinase and lactate dehydrogenase levels

## PATIENT PREPARATION
- Explain to the patient that the AST test is used to assess heart and liver function.
- Inform the patient that the test usually requires three venipunctures (one on admission and one each day for the next 2 days).
- Tell the patient that he need not restrict food and fluids.
- Explain to the patient that he may experience slight discomfort from the tourniquet and needle puncture.
- Notify the laboratory and physician of medications the patient is taking that may affect test results; they may need to be restricted.

## PROCEDURE AND POSTTEST CARE
- Perform a venipuncture and collect the sample in a 4-ml clot-activator tube.
- Apply direct pressure to the venipuncture site until bleeding stops.

- Instruct the patient that he may resume medications discontinued before the test, as ordered.

## PRECAUTIONS
- To avoid missing peak AST levels, draw serum samples at the same time each day.
- Handle the sample gently to prevent hemolysis.
- Send the sample to the laboratory immediately.

## REFERENCE VALUES
AST levels range from 8 to 46 U/L (SI, 0.14 to 0.78 µkat/L) in males and from 7 to 34 U/L (SI, 0.12 to 0.5 µkat/L) in females.

*Age alert  Normal values are typically higher ranging from 47 to 150 U/L (SI, 0.78 to 2.5 µkat/L) in neonates and from 9 to 80 U/L (SI, 0.15 to 1.3 µkat/L) in children.*

## ABNORMAL FINDINGS
AST levels fluctuate in response to the extent of cellular necrosis, being transiently and minimally increased early in the disease process and extremely increased during the most acute phase. Depending on when the initial sample is drawn, AST levels may increase, indicating increasing disease severity and tissue damage, or decrease, indicating disease resolution and tissue repair.

Maximum elevations (more than 20 times normal) may indicate acute viral hepatitis, severe skeletal muscle trauma, extensive surgery, drug-induced hepatic injury, or severe passive liver congestion.

High levels (10 to 20 times normal) may indicate a severe MI, severe infectious mononucleosis, or alcoholic cirrhosis. High levels also occur during the prodromal or resolving stages of conditions that cause maximum elevations.

Moderate to high levels (5 to 10 times normal) may indicate dermatomyositis, Duchenne's muscular dystrophy, or chronic hepatitis. Moderate to high levels also occur during prodromal and resolving stages of diseases that cause high elevations.

Low to moderate levels (2 to 5 times normal) occur at some time during the preceding conditions or diseases or may indicate hemolytic anemia, metastatic hepatic tumors, acute pancreatitis, pulmonary emboli, delirium tremens, or fatty liver. AST levels rise slightly after the first few days of biliary duct obstruction.

## INTERFERING FACTORS
- Antitubercular agents, chlorpropamide (Diabinese), dicumarol, erythromycin, methyldopa (Aldomet), opioids, pyridoxine, and sulfonamides; large doses of acetaminophen (Tylenol), salicylates, or vitamin A; and many other drugs known to affect the liver (increase)
- Strenuous exercise and muscle trauma due to I.M. injections (increase)

# Atrial natriuretic peptides, plasma

Atrial natriuretic peptides (ANP), also known as *plasma atrial natriuretic factor* or *atriopeptins,* is a radioimmunoassay that measures the plasma level of ANP. An extremely potent natriuretic agent and vasodilator, ANP rapidly produces diuresis and increases the glomerular filtration rate. ANP's role in regulating extracellular fluid volume, blood pressure, and sodium metabolism appears critical. It promotes sodium excretion, inhibits the renin-angiotensin system's effect on aldosterone secretion, and decreases atrial pressure by decreasing venous return, thereby reducing blood pressure and volume.

The patient with overt heart failure has highly elevated plasma levels of ANP. The patient with cardiovascular disease and elevated cardiac filling pressure but without heart failure also has markedly elevated ANP levels. ANP may provide a marker for early asymptomatic left ventricular dysfunction and increased cardiac volume.

## PURPOSE
- To confirm heart failure
- To identify asymptomatic cardiac volume overload

## PATIENT PREPARATION
- As appropriate, explain the purpose of the plasma ANP test to the patient.
- Inform the patient that he must fast for 12 hours before the test.
- Tell the patient that the test requires a blood sample. Explain who will perform the venipuncture and when.
- Explain to the patient that he may experience slight discomfort from the tourniquet and needle puncture.

- Explain that the test results will be available within 4 days.
- Check the patient's history for medications that can influence test results.
- Withhold beta-adrenergic blockers, calcium antagonists, diuretics, vasodilators, and cardiac glycosides for 24 hours before collection, as ordered.

## PROCEDURE AND POSTTEST CARE
- Perform a venipuncture and collect the sample in a prechilled potassium-EDTA tube.
- After chilled centrifugation, the EDTA plasma should be promptly frozen and sent to the laboratory.
- Apply direct pressure to the venipuncture site until bleeding stops.
- Instruct the patient that he may resume his usual diet and medications discontinued before the test, as ordered.

## PRECAUTIONS
- Handle the sample gently to prevent hemolysis.

## REFERENCE VALUES
Normal ANP levels range from 20 to 77 pg/ml.

## ABNORMAL FINDINGS
- Markedly elevated levels of ANP occur in the patient with frank heart failure and significantly elevated cardiac filling pressure.
- Cardiovascular drugs, including beta-adrenergic blockers, calcium antagonists, diuretics, vasodilators, and cardiac glycosides

## INTERFERING FACTORS
- Cardiovascular drugs including beta-adrenergic blockers, calcium antagonists, cardiac glycosides, diuretics, and vasodilators

---

# Auditory evoked potentials (brain stem evoked-response testing)

---

Auditory brain stem evoked-response (ABR, also called *brain stem auditory evoked-response*) testing is the most common form of auditory evoked potentials testing. In ABR testing, electrodes are attached to the surface of the patient's scalp, following cleaning and mild abrasion of the electrode sites. EEG activity, including the auditory evoked potential present in response to a signal, is amplified, filtered, digitized, and subjected to time-domain signal averaging to separate the response from the background EEG. The resulting traces are analyzed to determine if a response is present, and the characteristics of that response are noted. Various peaks are associated with the ABR (the most prominent are labeled I, III, and V). They occur at predictable times after signal presentation in the patient with normal hearing and normal neural synchronization.

The stimulus characteristics depend upon the type of evoked potential and its use. In threshold estimation and hearing screening, the signal may be tonal or may be a very short duration square wave, or click. The click contains energy throughout the frequency spectrum, but the evoked response generally comes from the high-frequency region of the cochlea.

Various forms of auditory evoked responses can be used to evaluate the function of the auditory pathways in a child or adult suspected of having auditory processing deficits.

Electrocochleography (ECoG or ECochG) can be used in the differential diagnosis of Ménière's disease (endolymphatic hydrops), although its diagnostic sensitivity and specificity is considered by some to be lacking, particularly in the early stages of the disease.

## PURPOSE
- To screen neonatal hearing
- To estimate or confirm the extent of hearing loss in infants and toddlers
- To estimate threshold in other difficult-to-test patients, such as those with developmental disabilities and those suspected of nonorganic hearing loss
- To evaluate cranial nerve (CN) VIII and lower brain stem auditory synchronization, which is abnormal with lesions of this area and with auditory dyssynchronization (auditory neuropathy)

## PATIENT PREPARATION
- Cerumen removal is required before referring the patient for this form of testing, which is conducted by an audiologist, and

sometimes at a neurology facility. Clean ear canals are particularly important when referring for ECoG.

> **Age alert** *Depending on the age of the child, sedation may be required. Sedated ABR testing can only be conducted at health care facilities. In other facilities, sleep deprivation of the child may be required to ensure that the patient sleeps during testing.*

● The patient should be advised to dress comfortably and be aware that although the test is painless, electrodes will be applied to the skin and will require 1 to 1½ hours to complete.

## PROCEDURE AND POSTTEST CARE

● Electrodes are connected to a physiologic amplifier that allows the minute voltages coming from the auditory system to be amplified enough to allow them to be read by the signal-averaging computer. The waveforms are displayed as the amplitude of the response across the time after the presentation of the signals.

● Threshold estimation is typically conducted by an audiologist. In this testing, he varies the intensity of the signal until the threshold of the response is obtained. The response threshold is typically slightly suprathreshold, but threshold estimation is possible if the patient has normal neural synchrony.

● In neurodiagnostic testing for CN VIII and auditory brain stem response, click signals are presented at intensities that are clearly audible and should elicit good synchronization of CN VIII. Typically, the click signals are presented at different presentation rates. More rapid presentations may reveal auditory pathology more readily. A click stimulus is presented at a supra-threshold level. The time at which wave V occurs in each ear, the time difference between the evoked waves I and V in each ear, and the time difference between both of these measures is used to indicate the probability of retrocochlear pathology. Assessment of central auditory processing ability typically involves assessing brain stem potentials and one or more of the potentials generated by the neural structures superior to the brain stem.

● ECoG also involves the presentation of relatively intense signals. The recording electrodes are placed in the ear canal of the patient or on the tympanic membrane. Rarely, a physician places the electrode through the tympanic membrane and rests it on the promontory of the middle ear. The cochlear potentials and CN VIII response are recorded.

● If the patient required sedation, he must be medically supervised until he completely recovers.

## PRECAUTIONS

● Know that accurate test results require passive patient cooperation.

● Know that rarely, skin abrasion for electrode placement causes irritation and minor allergic reactions.

● Be aware that ECoG using tympanic membrane electrodes requires skill on the part of the audiologist to place the electrode in contact with the tympanic membrane without creating patient discomfort.

## NORMAL FINDINGS

ABR wave latencies (time of the waveform occurrence after stimulus presentation) occur at predictable times for the patient with normal hearing or with cochlear loss for the patient who's hearing signals that are sufficiently above hearing threshold. The latency between wave I and V are approximately 4 ms (no longer than about 4.4 ms). The interaural latency difference of wave V and the I-V interaural latency differences are small, generally less than 0.3 or 0.4 ms. (See *Auditory brain evoked response,* page 42.)

The threshold of the ABR is typically about 10 to 20 dB nHL for click or high-frequency stimuli, and 20 or 30 dB nHL for lower-frequency stimuli.

ECoG reveals an amplitude ratio of the summating potential and action potential that's within normal limits for the type of electrode used.

## ABNORMAL FINDINGS

Cochlear loss increases the threshold of the ABR response, but doesn't typically alter the wave V latency for stimuli that are well above the threshold. The time between waves I and V is unaffected or shortens with cochlear loss; however, establishing wave I may be more difficult. Prolongation of the I-V interpeak latency is an indicator of CN VIII or lower brain stem pathology. This condition requires confirmation with imaging studies. Asymmetry of the I-V interpeak in-

# AUDITORY BRAIN EVOKED RESPONSE

These graphs are an example of an auditory brain stem evoked response elicited by 100 ms click stimuli. The patient's auditory neural activity is recorded using surface electrodes. The peaks on the graphs represent activity from cranial nerve VIII and brain stem structures. Traces are repeated for accuracy at each intensity. The morphology and time between labeled peaks is evaluated when assessing the patient's neural integrity. Additionally, the symmetry of left and right ear responses are evaluated (not illustrated). When used to estimate the hearing threshold, the stimuli's intensity is decreased. A prolonged wave V occurs. The lowest intensity eliciting an evoked potential is assumed to be slightly supra-threshold.

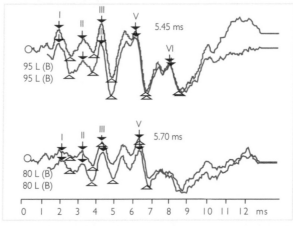

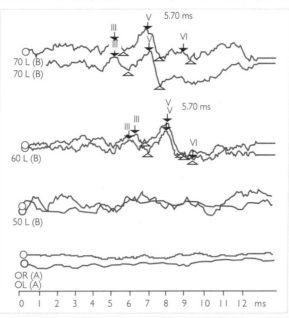

terval between ears is also a strong sign of a retrocochlear disorder. Asymmetry of absolute latency of wave V, abnormal prolongation of V with an increase in the stimulus repetition rate, poor replicability or morphology, and atypical amplitude ratios of waves I to V fail to rule out a retrocochlear abnormality.

A normal supra-threshold response — for example, an ABR to a 80 dB nHL click — doesn't indicate normal hearing. Assessment of the threshold of the ABR must be conducted. The threshold of the ABR is slightly above the expected actual hearing threshold. The audiologist interprets the findings in terms of probable hearing loss type and degree. While ABR testing is subject to some level of imprecision, amplification shouldn't be delayed because of incomplete test results. Amplification should be provided using conservative gain levels and protection against high output levels that can damage hearing. Careful audiologic follow-up is required. The goals of neonatal hearing screening programs are to identify hearing problems in children at birth and provide amplification by age 6 months.

ECoG that indicates abnormally large summating potential amplitude, compared to action potential amplitude, is a positive indicator of Ménière's disease.

## INTERFERING FACTORS

- Hearing loss developed after birth, for instance from such congenital diseases as maternal cytomegalovirus infection and some genetic hearing losses or progressive hearing loss
- Patient movement leading to inaccurate results: if the young child isn't asleep or if the older child or adult is restless
- Threshold testing with click stimuli, possibly creating false-negative results with normal hearing occurring due to a region of residual hearing
- Some uncertainty of ABR threshold estimation
- Auditory dyssynchronization, possibly eliminating an ABR even though cochlear function may be normal (The use of otoacoustic emissions testing in conjunction with ABR testing is recommended.)
- Lack of use of age-specific norms (Neonates and infants have longer latency responses than adults.)

- Asymptomatic Ménière's disease, leading to high false-negative results via ECoG (Normal ECoG findings don't rule out Ménière's disease.)

## *Bacterial meningitis antigen*

The bacterial meningitis antigen test can detect specific antigens of *Streptococcus pneumoniae, Neisseria meningitidis,* and *Haemophilus influenzae* type B, the principal etiologic agents in meningitis. It can be performed on samples of serum, cerebrospinal fluid (CSF), urine, pleural fluid, and joint fluid, but CSF and urine are preferred.

### PURPOSE
● To identify the etiologic agent in meningitis
● To aid in the diagnosis of bacterial meningitis when the Gram stain smear and culture are negative

### PATIENT PREPARATION
● Explain the purpose of the bacterial meningitis antigen test to the patient, as appropriate.
● Inform the patient that this test requires a specimen of urine or CSF. Explain who will perform the procedure and when.
● If a CSF specimen is required, describe how it will be obtained.
● Explain to the patient that he may experience discomfort from the needle puncture.
● Advise the patient that a headache is the most common complication of lumbar puncture, but that his cooperation during the test minimizes such an effect.
● Make sure the patient or a family member has signed an informed consent form.

### PROCEDURE AND POSTTEST CARE
● Collect a 10-ml urine specimen or a 1-ml CSF specimen in a sterile container.

### PRECAUTIONS
● Maintain specimen sterility during collection.
● Wear gloves when obtaining or handling the specimen.
● Make sure the cap is tightly fastened on the specimen container.
● Place the specimen on a refrigerated coolant and send it to the laboratory immediately.

### NORMAL FINDINGS
Normally, results are negative for bacterial antigens.

### ABNORMAL FINDINGS
Positive results identify the specific bacterial antigen including *S. pneumoniae, N. meningitidis, H. influenzae* type B, or group B streptococci.

### INTERFERING FACTORS
● Previous antimicrobial therapy

## *Barium enema*

Also called *lower GI examination,* barium enema is the radiographic examination of the large intestine after rectal instillation of barium sulfate (single-contrast technique) or barium sulfate and air (double-contrast technique). It's indicated in patients with histories of altered bowel habits, lower abdominal pain, or the passage of blood, mucus, or pus in the stool. It may also be indicated after colostomy or ileostomy; in these patients, barium (or barium and air) is instilled through the stoma. Complications include perforation of the colon, water intoxication, barium granulomas and, rarely, intraperitoneal and extraperitoneal extravasation of barium and barium embolism.

The single-contrast technique provides a profile view of the large intestine; the double-contrast technique provides profile and frontal views. The latter technique best detects small intraluminal tumors (especially polyps), the early mucosal changes of inflammatory disease, and subtle intestinal bleeding caused by ulcerated polyps or the shallow ulcerations of inflammatory disease.

Although barium enema clearly outlines most of the large intestine, proctosigmoidoscopy provides the best view of the rectosigmoid region. Barium enema should precede the barium swallow and upper GI and small-bowel series because barium ingested in the latter procedure may take several days to pass through the GI tract and thus may interfere with subsequent X-ray studies.

## PURPOSE

- To aid in the diagnosis of colorectal cancer and inflammatory disease
- To detect polyps, diverticula, and structural changes in the large intestine

## PATIENT PREPARATION

- Explain to the patient that the barium enema test permits examination of the large intestine through X-rays taken after a barium enema.
- Describe the test, including who will perform it and when and where it will take place.
- Because residual fecal material in the colon obscures normal anatomy on X-rays, instruct the patient to carefully follow the prescribed bowel preparation, which may include diet, laxatives, or an enema. However, in certain conditions, such as ulcerative colitis and active GI bleeding, their use may be prohibited.
- Stress that accurate test results depend on the patient's cooperation with prescribed dietary restrictions and bowel preparation. A common bowel preparation technique includes restricted intake of dairy products and maintenance of a liquid diet for 24 hours before the test. The patient is encouraged to drink five 8-oz glasses of water or clear liquids 12 to 24 hours before the test. Administer a bowel preparation supplied by the radiography department. (A GoLYTELY preparation isn't recommended because it leaves the bowel too wet for the barium to coat the walls of the bowel.)

- Advise the patient to administer prescribed enemas until return is clear.
- Tell the patient not to eat breakfast before the procedure; if the test is scheduled for late afternoon (or delayed), he may have clear liquids.
- Tell the patient that he'll be placed on a tilting X-ray table and adequately draped. Assure him that he'll be secured to the table and will be assisted to various positions.
- Tell the patient that he may experience cramping pains or the urge to defecate as the barium or air is introduced into the intestine. Instruct him to breathe deeply and slowly through his mouth to ease discomfort.
- Tell the patient to keep his anal sphincter tightly contracted against the rectal tube; this holds the tube in position and helps prevent leakage of barium. Stress the importance of retaining the barium enema; if the intestinal walls aren't adequately coated with barium, test results may be inaccurate.
- Assure the patient that the barium enema is fairly easy to retain because of its cool temperature.

## PROCEDURE AND POSTTEST CARE

- After the patient is in a supine position on a tilting X-ray table, spot films of the abdomen are taken.
- The patient is assisted to Sims' position, and a well-lubricated rectal tube is inserted through the anus. If the patient has anal sphincter atony or severe mental or physical debilitation, a rectal tube with a retaining balloon may be inserted.
- The barium is administered slowly and the filling process is monitored fluoroscopically. To aid filling, the table may be tilted or the patient assisted to supine, prone, and lateral decubitus positions.
- As barium flow is observed, spot films are taken of significant findings. When the

intestine is filled with barium, overhead films of the abdomen are taken. The rectal tube is withdrawn, and the patient is escorted to the toilet or provided with a bedpan and is instructed to expel as much barium as possible.

- After evacuation, an additional overhead film is taken to record the mucosal pattern of the intestine and to evaluate the efficiency of colonic emptying.
- A double-contrast barium enema may directly follow this examination or may be performed separately. If it's performed immediately, a thin film of barium remains in the patient's intestine, coating the mucosa, and air is carefully injected to distend the bowel lumen.
- When the double-contrast technique is performed separately, a colloidal barium suspension is instilled, filling the patient's intestine to either the splenic flexure or the middle of the transverse colon. The suspension is then aspirated and air is forcefully injected into the intestine. If the intestine is filled to the lower descending colon, air is forcefully injected without previous aspiration of the suspension.
- The patient is then assisted to erect, prone, supine, and lateral decubitus positions in sequence. Barium filling is monitored fluoroscopically, and spot films are taken of significant findings. After the required films are taken, the patient is escorted to the toilet or provided with a bedpan.
- Make sure further studies haven't been ordered before allowing the patient food and fluids. Encourage extra fluid intake because bowel preparation and the test itself can cause dehydration.
- Encourage rest because this test and the bowel preparation that precedes it is usually exhausting.
- Because barium retention after this test can cause intestinal obstruction or fecal impaction, administer a mild cathartic or an enema. Tell the patient his stool will be light colored for 24 to 72 hours. Record and describe any stool passed by the patient in the health care facility.

## PRECAUTIONS

- Know that barium enema is contraindicated in the patient with tachycardia, fulminant ulcerative colitis associated with systemic toxicity and megacolon, toxic megacolon, or suspected perforation.

- Know that this test should be performed cautiously in the patient with obstruction, acute inflammatory conditions (such as ulcerative colitis and diverticulitis), acute vascular insufficiency of the bowel, acute fulminant bloody diarrhea, and suspected pneumatosis cystoides intestinalis.
- Be aware that barium enema is contraindicated in the pregnant patient because of radiation's possible teratogenic effects.

## NORMAL FINDINGS

In the single-contrast enema, the intestine is uniformly filled with barium, and colonic haustral markings are clearly apparent. The intestinal walls collapse as the barium is expelled, and the mucosa has a regular, feathery appearance on the postevacuation film. In the double-contrast enema, the intestines uniformly distend with air and have a thin layer of barium, providing excellent detail of the mucosal pattern. As the patient is assisted to various positions, the barium collects on the dependent walls of the intestine by the force of gravity.

## ABNORMAL FINDINGS

Although most colonic cancers occur in the rectosigmoid region and are best detected by proctosigmoidoscopy, X-rays may reveal adenocarcinoma and, rarely, sarcomas occurring higher in the intestine. Carcinoma usually appears as a localized filling defect, with a sharp transition between the normal and necrotic mucosa. If it's circumferential, it will have an "apple core" appearance. These characteristics help distinguish carcinoma from the more diffuse lesions of inflammatory disease, but endoscopic biopsy may be necessary to confirm the diagnosis.

X-ray studies demonstrate and define the extent of inflammatory disease, such as diverticulitis, ulcerative colitis, and granulomatous colitis. Ulcerative colitis usually originates in the anal region and ascends through the intestine; granulomatous colitis usually originates in the cecum and terminal ileum and then descends through the intestine. However, biopsy may be necessary to confirm diagnosis.

Barium X-rays may also reveal saccular adenomatous polyps, broad-based villous polyps, structural changes in the intestine (such as intussusception, telescoping of the bowel, sigmoid volvulus [360-degree turn or greater], and sigmoid torsion [up to a 180-

degree turn]), gastroenteritis, irritable colon, vascular injury due to arterial occlusion, and selected cases of acute appendicitis.

## INTERFERING FACTORS
● Inadequate bowel preparation (possible poor imaging)
● Retention of barium from previous studies (possible poor imaging)
● The patient's inability to retain barium

# Basal gastric secretion test

The basal gastric secretion test measures basal secretion during fasting by aspirating stomach contents through a nasogastric (NG) tube. It's indicated in the patient with obscure epigastric pain, anorexia, and weight loss. Because external factors — such as the sight or odor of food — and psychological stress stimulate gastric secretion, accurate testing requires that the patient be relaxed and isolated from all sources of sensory stimulation. Although abnormal basal secretion test results can suggest various gastric and duodenal disorders, a complete evaluation of secretions requires the gastric acid stimulation test.

## PURPOSE
● To determine gastric output while the patient is fasting

## PATIENT PREPARATION
● Explain to the patient that the basal gastric secretion test measures the stomach's secretion of acid.
● Instruct the patient to restrict food for 12 hours and fluids and smoking for 8 hours before the test.
● Tell the patient who will perform the test and that the procedure takes approximately $1^1/_4$ hours (or $2^1/_4$ hours, if followed by the gastric acid stimulation test).
● Inform the patient that the test requires insertion of a tube through the nose and into the stomach, that he may initially experience discomfort, and that he may cough or gag.
● Notify the laboratory and physician of medications the patient is taking that may affect test results; they may need to be restrict-

ed. If these drugs must be continued, note this on the laboratory request.
● Check the patient's pulse rate and blood pressure just before the test. Then encourage him to relax.

## PROCEDURE AND POSTTEST CARE
● Insert the NG tube after seating the patient comfortably.
● Attach a 20-ml syringe to it and aspirate the stomach contents.
● To ensure complete emptying of the stomach, ask the patient to assume three positions in sequence — supine and right and left lateral decubitus — while stomach contents are aspirated.
● Label the specimen container residual contents.
● Connect the NG tube to the suction machine. Aspirate gastric contents by continuous low suction for 1 hour. Aspiration can also be performed manually with a syringe.
● Collect a specimen every 15 minutes, but discard the first two; this eliminates the specimens that could be affected by the stress of the intubation.
● Record the color and odor of each specimen and note the presence of food, mucus, bile, or blood.
● Label these specimens basal contents, and number them 1 through 4.
● Measure secretion volume and acid concentration.
● If the NG tube is to be left in place, clamp it or attach it to low intermittent suction, as ordered.
● Watch for complications, such as nausea, vomiting, and abdominal distention or pain, following removal of the NG tube.
● If the patient complains of a sore throat, provide soothing lozenges.
● Instruct the patient that he may resume his usual diet and medications, as ordered, unless the gastric acid stimulation test will also be performed.

## PRECAUTIONS
● Know that the basal gastric secretion test is contraindicated in the patient with a condition that prohibits NG intubation.
*Alert* During insertion, make sure that the NG tube enters the esophagus and not the trachea; remove it immediately if the patient develops cyanosis or paroxysmal coughing.

- Monitor the patient's vital signs during intubation and observe him carefully for arrhythmias.
- To prevent contamination of the specimens with saliva, instruct the patient to expectorate excess saliva.
- Send the specimens to the laboratory immediately after the collection is completed.

## REFERENCE VALUES

Normally, basal secretion ranges from 1 to 5 mEq/hour in males and from 0.2 to 3.3 mEq/hour in females.

## ABNORMAL FINDINGS

Abnormal basal secretion findings are non-specific and must be considered with the results of the gastric acid stimulation test. Elevated secretion may suggest a duodenal or jejunal ulcer (after partial gastrectomy); markedly elevated secretion suggests Zollinger-Ellison syndrome. Depressed secretion may indicate gastric carcinoma or a benign gastric ulcer. Absence of secretion may indicate pernicious anemia.

## INTERFERING FACTORS

- Failure to observe pretest restrictions (increase)
- Psychological stress (possible increase)
- Adrenergic blockers, adrenocorticosteroids, alcohol, cholinergics, and reserpine (possible increase)
- Antacids, anticholinergics, histamine-2 blockers, and proton pump inhibitors (possible decrease)

## Bence Jones protein

Bence Jones proteins are abnormal light-chain immunoglobulins of low molecular weight that are derived from the clone of a single plasma cell. This globulin appears in the urine of 50% to 80% of patients with multiple myeloma and in most patients with Waldenström's macroglobulinemia.

Screening tests, such as thermal coagulation and Bradshaw's test, can detect Bence Jones proteins, but urine immunoelectrophoresis is usually the method of choice for quantitative studies. Serum immunoelectrophoresis, which is sometimes used, is less sensitive than other tests. Nevertheless, urine and serum studies are usually used when multiple myeloma is suspected.

## PURPOSE

- To confirm the presence of multiple myeloma in the patient with characteristic clinical signs, such as bone pain (especially in the back and the thorax) and persistent anemia and fatigue

## PATIENT PREPARATION

- Tell the patient that the Bence Jones protein test can detect an abnormal protein in the urine.
- Tell the patient that the test requires an early-morning urine specimen; teach him how to collect a specimen.

## PROCEDURE AND POSTTEST CARE

- Collect an early-morning, midstream clean-catch urine specimen of at least 50 ml.

## PRECAUTIONS

- Instruct the patient not to contaminate the urine specimen with toilet tissue or stool.
- Send the specimen to the laboratory immediately after collection, or refrigerate it if transport is delayed. A refrigerated specimen must be analyzed within 24 hours, or it should be discarded.

## NORMAL FINDINGS

Normal urine should contain no Bence Jones proteins.

## ABNORMAL FINDINGS

The presence of Bence Jones proteins in urine suggests multiple myeloma or Waldenström's macroglobulinemia. Very low levels in the absence of other symptoms may result from benign monoclonal gammopathy. However, clinical evidence figures prominently in the diagnosis of multiple myeloma.

## INTERFERING FACTORS

- Connective tissue disease, renal insufficiency, and certain cancers (possible false-positive)
- Contamination of the specimen with menstrual blood, prostatic secretions, or semen (possible false-positive)
- Failure to properly store the specimen during the collection period or to send the sample to the laboratory immediately after

the collection is completed (possible false-positive from protein deterioration)

# *Bilirubin*

The bilirubin test is used to measure serum levels of bilirubin, the predominant pigment in bile. Bilirubin is the major product of hemoglobin catabolism. Serum bilirubin measurements are especially significant in neonates because elevated unconjugated bilirubin can accumulate in the brain, causing irreparable damage.

## PURPOSE
- To evaluate liver function
- To aid in the differential diagnosis of jaundice and monitor its progress
- To aid in the diagnosis of biliary obstruction and hemolytic anemia
- To determine whether a neonate requires an exchange transfusion or phototherapy because of dangerously high unconjugated bilirubin levels

## PATIENT PREPARATION
- Explain to the patient that the bilirubin test is used to evaluate liver function and the condition of red blood cells.
- Tell the patient that the test requires a blood sample. Explain who will perform the venipuncture and when.

*Age alert* *If the patient is an infant, tell the parents that a small amount of blood will be drawn from his heel. Tell them who will be performing the heelstick and when.*

- Explain to the patient that he may experience slight discomfort from the tourniquet and needle puncture.
- Inform the adult patient that he need not restrict fluids, but should fast for at least 4 hours before the test.

*Age alert* *Fasting isn't necessary for the neonate.*

## PROCEDURE AND POSTTEST CARE
- If the patient is an adult, perform a venipuncture and collect the sample in a 3- or 4-ml clot-activator tube.

*Age alert* *If the patient is an infant, perform a heelstick and fill the microcapillary tube to the designated level with blood.*

- Apply direct pressure to the venipuncture site until bleeding stops.

## PRECAUTIONS
- Protect the sample from strong sunlight and ultraviolet light.
- Handle the sample gently and send it to the laboratory immediately.

## REFERENCE VALUES
In adults, normal indirect serum bilirubin levels are 1.1 mg/dl (SI, 19 µmol/L), and direct serum bilirubin levels are less than 0.5 mg/dl (SI, < 6.8 µmol/L).

*Age alert* *In neonates, total serum bilirubin levels are 2 to 12 mg/dl (SI, 34 to 205 µmol/L).*

## ABNORMAL FINDINGS
Elevated indirect serum bilirubin levels usually indicate hepatic damage. High levels of indirect bilirubin are also likely in severe hemolytic anemia. If hemolysis continues, direct and indirect bilirubin levels may rise. Other causes of elevated indirect bilirubin levels include congenital enzyme deficiencies such as Gilbert syndrome.

Elevated direct serum bilirubin levels usually indicate biliary obstruction. If obstruction continues, direct and indirect bilirubin levels may rise. In severe chronic hepatic damage, direct bilirubin concentrations may return to normal or near normal levels, but indirect bilirubin levels remain elevated.

In neonates, total bilirubin levels of 15 mg/dl (SI, 257 µmol/L) or more indicate the need for an exchange transfusion.

## INTERFERING FACTORS
- Exposure of the sample to direct sunlight or ultraviolet light (possible decrease)
- Hemolytic agents, hepatotoxic drugs, methyldopa (Aldomet), and rifampin (possible increase)
- Barbiturates and sulfonamides (possible decrease)

# *Bioterrorism infectious agents testing*

Numerous agents can be used to treat the effects of bioterrorism. The most common infections associated with bioterrorism include botulism; anthrax; hemorrhagic fever, Hantaan virus, Ebola virus, and yellow fever infections; plague; smallpox; and tularemia. Various specimen collection methods may be used to diagnose an infection with a bioterroristic agent depending on the causative agent and site of entry. (See *Understanding bioterrorism infectious agents*.) These methods include cultures of blood, sputum, urine, emesis or gastric aspirate, stool, lymph node aspirate, or scrapings from lesions. Regardless of the method used, suspected cases of infection must be reported to local, state, and federal health departments.

## PURPOSE
- To isolate and identify the causative organism

## PATIENT PREPARATION
- Explain to the patient that the bioterrorism infectious agents test is used to help identify the organism causing his signs and symptoms.
- Describe the method and procedure to be used to obtain the specimen, such as blood, stool, or sputum.
- Tell the patient when the specimen will be collected and who will be collecting it.
- Tell the patient how many samples will need to be collected.
- Inform the patient that he not need restrict food or fluids.
- If botulism is suspected, inform the patient that an electromyogram may be done to identify the cause of acute flaccid paralysis.

## PROCEDURE AND POSTTEST CARE
- Obtain the specimens as ordered based on the suspicion of infectious agent.
- Place blood samples on ice; refrigerate all specimens for botulinum toxin testing.

*Alert* *If stool is being cultured for botulism testing and the patient is constipated, administer an enema using sterile water as the solution to ensure that an adequate sample is obtained.*
- Send the specimen to the laboratory for a "mouse" assay to evaluate for botulinum toxin.
- Collect vesicular fluid from a previously unopened lesion on at least one culture swab when testing for cutaneous anthrax and smallpox.

- Obtain three blood cultures along with specimens of gastric aspirate, stool, or food, if GI anthrax is suspected.
- When obtaining specimens for tularemia, have the patient provide a forced deep cough for a sputum specimen; obtain a lesional specimen from the leading edge of the lesion.
- Send any food that's being tested (for botulism) in its original container.
- Send each specimen to the laboratory immediately.

## PRECAUTIONS
- Adhere to standard precautions during collection of all specimens.
- Institute airborne precautions and use negative pressure rooms for patients with suspected infection of hemorrhagic fever, Hantaan virus, Ebola virus, and yellow fever.
- Clean contaminated surfaces and spills with appropriate solution such as a hypochlorite bleach solution.
- Make sure that specimens being examined for smallpox are performed in a Biosafety laboratory (level 4); specimens for other infections are performed in a Biosafety laboratory (level 2).

## NORMAL FINDINGS
Cultures are negative for the suspected organism. If an electromyogram was done for a patient suspected of botulism, the response to repetitive nerve stimulation reveals no increase.

## ABNORMAL FINDINGS
Evidence of growth of the causative organism indicates infection. In addition, for smallpox, Guarnieri's bodies are present in the lesion scrapings and brick-shaped virions are noted when the specimen is viewed by an electron microscope.

## INTERFERING FACTORS
- Use of saline solution in an enema to collect a stool specimen in a patient with botulism
- Use of anticholinesterase agents by the patient being tested for botulism

## UNDERSTANDING BIOTERRORISM INFECTIOUS AGENTS

| INFECTIOUS AGENT | MODE OF TRANSMISSION | MODE OF ENTRY | SPECIMEN FOR TESTING |
|---|---|---|---|
| *Clostridium botulinum* (spore-forming obligate anaerobe causing botulism) | ◆ Soil<br>◆ Undercooked food not kept warm | ◆ Mucosal surface (GI tract, lung)<br>◆ Wound | ◆ Blood, stool, gastric aspirate, emesis<br>◆ Suspected contaminated food substance |
| *Bacillus anthracis* (spore-forming, gram-positive bacillus causing anthrax) | ◆ Undercooked meat from infected animals<br>◆ Inhalation of animal products such as the animal's wool<br>◆ Intentional release of spores | ◆ Skin<br>◆ Inhalation<br>◆ GI tract | ◆ Blood, sputum, or stool<br>◆ Fluid from lesion |
| Viruses for hemorrhagic fever and yellow fever (including Hantaan virus, Ebola virus) | ◆ Bite of infected animal, rodent, or insect | ◆ Skin | ◆ Blood, sputum, tissue, or urine |
| *Yersinia pestis* (causing plague) | ◆ Infected flea bite | ◆ Skin | ◆ Blood, sputum, or lymph node aspirate |
| Variola virus (causing smallpox) | ◆ Airborne via coughing<br>◆ Direct contact<br>◆ Contaminated clothing or bedding | ◆ Lungs | ◆ Fluid from lesion |
| *Francisella tularensis* (intracellular parasite causing tularemia) | ◆ Infected animals, such as mice, squirrels, or rabbits<br>◆ Contaminated water, soil, or vegetation | ◆ Skin, mucous membranes<br>◆ Lungs<br>◆ GI tract | ◆ Respiratory secretions and blood<br>◆ Lymph node biopsy<br>◆ Lesion scrapings |

## *Bladder cancer markers*

Tumor markers are substances produced and secreted by tumor cells to help determine tumor activity. They can be found in the serum or urine of the patient with cancer. Specific tests are ordered depending on the type of cancer. For bladder cancer, two specific markers in the urine have been identified: BTA and NMP22.

BTA is a protein-related substance produced by bladder cancer cells. NMP22 is a protein of the nuclear matrix that's excreted in the urine when the nucleus of the bladder cancer cells becomes disrupted. In the patient without bladder cancer, these elements are absent or present in only very minimal amounts. However, in the patient with bladder cancer, these elements are elevated.

Bladder cancer markers are helpful in monitoring the patient diagnosed with bladder cancer to evaluate for recurrence after surgical resection. Often these tests are done in conjunction with a cystoscopy. In addition, NMP22 also may be used to screen for individuals who may be at highest risk for recurrence as well as screening for individuals who are at risk for developing bladder cancer.

## PURPOSE

- To monitor and detect bladder cancer recurrence
- To identify individuals at risk for bladder cancer

## PATIENT PREPARATION

- Explain the purpose of the bladder cancer marker test and how it may be helpful in monitoring the patient's disorder, as appropriate.
- Inform the patient that the procedure involves obtaining a urine specimen.
- Tell the patient that he need not restrict food or fluids.

## PROCEDURE AND POSTTEST CARE

- Obtain a random voided urine specimen before noon.

## PRECAUTIONS

- Send the specimen to the laboratory immediately.
- Refrigerate the specimen if there will be a delay in transport.

## REFERENCE VALUES

Normal values for bladder cancer markers are: BTA less than 14 units/ml and NMP22 less than 10 units/ml.

## ABNORMAL FINDINGS

Elevations of BTA and NMP22 indicate bladder cancer.

## INTERFERING FACTORS

- Failure to stabilize urine immediately after collection
- Recent urologic surgery, urinary tract infection, or urinary calculi (increase in BTA levels)
- Presence of cancer of the ureters or renal pelvis (increase in both markers)

# Bleeding time

Bleeding time is used to measure the duration of bleeding after a measured skin incision. Bleeding time may be measured by one of two methods: Ivy or Duke. The template method is the most commonly

used and the most accurate because the incision size is standardized. Bleeding time depends on the elasticity of the blood vessel wall and on the number and functional capacity of platelets.

Although the bleeding time test is usually performed on the patient with a personal or family history of bleeding disorders, it's also useful—along with a platelet count—for preoperative screening. The test isn't usually recommended for the patient with a platelet count of less than 75,000/µl (SI, 75 × 10⁹/L).

## PURPOSE

- To assess overall hemostatic function (platelet response to injury and functional capacity of vasoconstriction)
- To detect congenital and acquired platelet function disorders

## PATIENT PREPARATION

- Explain to the patient that the bleeding time test is used to measure the time required to form a clot and stop bleeding.
- Tell the patient who will be performing the test and when it will take place.
- Inform the patient that he need not restrict food and fluids.
- Inform the patient that he may feel some discomfort from the incisions, the antiseptic, and the tightness of the blood pressure cuff. Also inform the patient that depending on the method used, incisions or punctures may leave tiny scars that should be barely visible when healed.
- Notify the laboratory and physician of medications the patient is taking that may affect test results; they may need to be restricted.

## PROCEDURE AND POSTTEST CARE
### Ivy method

- After applying the pressure cuff and preparing the test site, make three small punctures with a disposable lancet.
- Start the stopwatch immediately.
- Taking care not to touch the punctures, blot each site with filter paper every 30 seconds until the bleeding stops.
- Average the bleeding time of the three punctures and record the result.

## Duke method

● Drape the patient's shoulder with a towel.
● Clean the earlobe and let the skin air-dry.
● Make a puncture wound 2 to 4 mm deep on the earlobe with a disposable lancet.
● Start the stopwatch.
● Being careful not to touch the ear, blot the site with filter paper every 30 seconds until bleeding stops.
● Record bleeding time.

## Both methods

● In a patient with a bleeding tendency (hemophilia), maintain a pressure bandage over the incision for 24 to 48 hours to prevent further bleeding. Check the test area frequently; keep the edges of the cuts aligned to minimize scarring.
● In other patients, a piece of gauze held in place by an adhesive bandage is sufficient.
● Instruct the patient that he may resume medications discontinued before the test, as ordered.

## PRECAUTIONS

● Be sure to maintain a cuff pressure of 40 mm Hg throughout the test.
  **Alert** *If the bleeding doesn't diminish after 15 minutes, discontinue the test.*
● Apply direct pressure to the test site until bleeding stops.

## REFERENCE VALUES

The normal range of bleeding time is from 3 to 6 minutes in the Ivy method and from 1 to 3 minutes (SI, 1 to 3 min) in the Duke method.

## ABNORMAL FINDINGS

Prolonged bleeding time may indicate the presence of disorders associated with thrombocytopenia, such as Hodgkin's disease, acute leukemia, disseminated intravascular coagulation, hemolytic disease of the newborn, Schönlein-Henoch purpura, severe hepatic disease (cirrhosis, for example), or severe deficiency of factors I, II, V, VII, VIII, IX, and XI. Prolonged bleeding time in a patient with a normal platelet count suggests a platelet function disorder (thrombasthenia, thrombocytopathia) and requires further investigation with clot retraction, prothrombin consumption, and platelet aggregation tests.

## INTERFERING FACTORS

● Anticoagulants, antineoplastics, aspirin and aspirin compounds, nonsteroidal anti-inflammatory drugs, sulfonamides, thiazide diuretics, vitamin E supplementation, and some nonnarcotic analgesics (prolonged bleeding time)

## *Blood culture*

A blood culture is performed to isolate and aid in the identification of the pathogens in bacteremia (bacterial invasion of the bloodstream) and septicemia (systemic spread of such infection). It requires inoculating a culture medium with a blood sample and incubating it.

Blood culture can identify about 67% of pathogens within 24 hours and up to 90% within 72 hours.

Bacteria from local tissue infection usually invade the bloodstream through the lymphatic system by way of the thoracic duct. (See *The lymphatic system,* page 54.) Occasionally, they enter the bloodstream directly through infusion lines, thrombophlebitis, or bacterial endocarditis from prosthetic heart valve replacements.

Bacteremia may be transient, intermittent, or continuous. The timing of specimen collection for blood cultures varies; it usually depends on the type of bacteremia (intermittent or continuous) suspected and whether drug therapy needs to be started regardless of test results.

## PURPOSE

● To confirm bacteremia
● To identify the causative organism in bacteremia and septicemia

## PATIENT PREPARATION

● Explain to the patient that the blood culture procedure is used to help identify the organism causing his symptoms.
● Inform the patient that he need not restrict food and fluids.
● Tell the patient how many samples the test will require and who will perform the venipunctures and when.

# THE LYMPHATIC SYSTEM

The lymphatic system—a network of capillary and venous channels—returns excess interstitial fluids and proteins to the blood. Materials flowing through these channels pass into the thoracic and right lymph ducts. The thoracic duct, the larger of the two, drains the lymphatic vessels from all but the upper right quadrant. This lymphatic drainage (commonly called *lymph*, the tissue fluid absorbed in the lymphatic vessels) then flows into the junction of the left internal jugular and left subclavian veins. The right lymph duct drains interstitial fluid from the upper right quadrant into the right subclavian vein.

Bacteria from local tissue infection usually enter the bloodstream through this system. When functioning properly, however, the lymphatic system provides a strong defense against bacteria and viruses. Before lymph reenters the bloodstream, afferent lymphatic vessels transport it to lymph nodes or glands—clusters of lymphatic tissues throughout the body—where numerous lymphocytes destroy microorganisms and foreign particles.

If the lymphatic system fails to destroy harmful particles before they enter the bloodstream, white blood cells (WBCs) in the spleen, liver, and bone marrow act as another defense mechanism. As blood circulates through the body, it flows into the spleen, where it's filtered. There, residing lymphocytes ingest abnormal or foreign cells while normal cells pass through. Bacteria that accompany digested food particles into the portal vein—which supplies the liver—are ingested by reticulum cells. Likewise, WBCs formed in the bone marrow protect the body from invading bacteria.

Macrophages constitute still another defense system. These WBCs in the tissues, lymph nodes, and red bone marrow are usually immobile, but they migrate to inflamed areas, where they ingest and destroy infective particles.

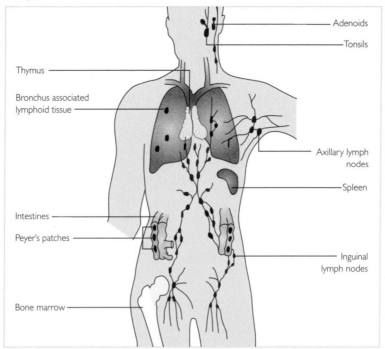

Illustration from Timby, B.K., and Smith, N.E., *Essentials of Nursing: Care of Adults and Children*. Philadelphia: Lippincott Williams & Wilkins, 2005.

- Explain to the patient that he may experience slight discomfort from the tourniquet and needle punctures.

## PROCEDURE AND POSTTEST CARE
- Put on gloves.
- Clean the venipuncture site with an alcohol swab and then with an iodine swab, working in a circular motion from the site outward.
- Wait at least 1 minute for the patient's skin to dry, and remove the residual iodine with an alcohol swab or remove the iodine after venipuncture.
- Apply the tourniquet.
- Perform a venipuncture; draw 10 to 20 ml of blood for an adult or 2 to 6 ml for a child.
- Clean the diaphragm tops of the culture bottles with alcohol or iodine (or other antiseptic agent as per facility policy), and change the needle on the syringe.
- If broth is used, add blood to each bottle until a 1:5 or 1:10 dilution is obtained. For example, add 10 ml of blood to a 100-ml bottle. (The size of the bottle varies, depending on facility procedure.)
- If a special resin is used, add blood to the resin in the bottles and invert them gently to mix.
- If you're using the lysis-centrifugation technique (Isolator), draw the blood directly into a special collection and processing tube.
- Indicate the tentative diagnosis on the laboratory request, and note current or recent antimicrobial therapy.
- Apply direct pressure to the venipuncture site until bleeding stops.

## PRECAUTIONS
- Wear gloves when performing the procedure and handling samples.
- Send each sample to the laboratory immediately after collection.
- Don't draw blood from an existing I.V. catheter. Use a vein below an I.V. catheter or in the opposite arm.
- Know that whenever possible, blood cultures should be collected before administering antimicrobial agents.

## NORMAL FINDINGS
Normally, blood cultures are negative for pathogens.

## ABNORMAL FINDINGS
Positive blood cultures don't necessarily confirm pathologic septicemia. Mild, transient bacteremia may occur during the course of many infectious diseases or may complicate other disorders. Persistent, continuous, or recurrent bacteremia reliably confirms the presence of serious infection. To detect most causative agents, blood cultures are ideally drawn on 2 consecutive days.

Isolation of most organisms takes about 72 hours; negative cultures are held for 1 or more weeks before being reported negative.

Common blood pathogens include *Streptococcus pneumoniae* and other *Streptococcus* species, *Haemophilus influenzae, Staphylococcus aureus, Pseudomonas aeruginosa,* Bacteroides, *Brucella, Enterobacteriaceae,* coliform bacilli, and *Candida albicans.* Although 2% to 3% of cultured blood samples are contaminated by skin bacteria, such as *Staphylococcus epidermidis,* diphtheroids, and *Propionibacterium,* these organisms may be clinically significant when isolated from multiple cultures or from immunocompromised patients. Debilitated or immunocompromised patients may have isolates of *C. albicans.* In patients with human immunodeficiency virus infection, *Mycobacterium tuberculosis* and *M. avium* complex may be isolated as well as other *Mycobacterium* species on a less frequent basis.

## INTERFERING FACTORS
- Previous or current antimicrobial therapy on the laboratory request (possible false-negative)
- Removal of culture bottle caps at the bedside (possible prevention of anaerobic growth)
- Use of the incorrect bottle and media (possible prevention of aerobic growth)

# Blood urea nitrogen

The blood urea nitrogen (BUN) test is used to measure the nitrogen fraction of urea, the chief end product of protein metabolism. Formed in the liver from ammonia and excreted by the kidneys, urea constitutes 40% to 50% of the blood's nonprotein nitrogen. BUN level reflects protein intake and renal excretory capacity, but is a less reliable indicator of uremia than the serum creatinine level.

## PURPOSE
- To evaluate kidney function and aid in the diagnosis of renal disease
- To aid in the assessment of hydration

## PATIENT PREPARATION
- Tell the patient that the BUN test is used to evaluate kidney function.
- Inform the patient that he need not restrict food and fluids, but should avoid a diet high in meat.
- Tell the patient that the test requires a blood sample. Explain who will perform the venipuncture and when.
- Explain to the patient that he may experience slight discomfort from the tourniquet and needle puncture.
- Notify the laboratory and physician of medications the patient is taking that may affect test results; they may need to be restricted.

## PROCEDURE AND POSTTEST CARE
- Perform a venipuncture and collect the sample in a 3- to 4-ml clot-activator tube.
- Apply direct pressure to the venipuncture site until bleeding stops.
- Inform the patient that he may resume his usual medications discontinued before the test, as ordered.

## PRECAUTIONS
- Handle the sample gently to prevent hemolysis.

## REFERENCE VALUES
BUN values normally range from 8 to 20 mg/dl (SI, 2.9 to 7.5 mmol/L).

*Age alert* *In elderly patients, BUN will show slightly higher values, possibly to 69 mg/dl (SI, 25.8 mmol/L).*

## ABNORMAL FINDINGS
Elevated BUN levels occur in renal disease, reduced renal blood flow (due to dehydration, for example), urinary tract obstruction, and increased protein catabolism (such as with burns).

Low BUN levels occur in severe hepatic damage, malnutrition, and overhydration.

## INTERFERING FACTORS
- Chloramphenicol and tetracyclines (possible decrease)
- Anabolic steroids, aminoglycosides, and amphotericin B (possible increase)

# *Bone biopsy*

Bone biopsy is the removal of a piece or a core of bone for histologic examination. It's performed either by using a special drill needle under local anesthesia or by surgical excision under general anesthesia.

Bone biopsy is indicated in patients with bone pain and tenderness after bone scan, computed tomography scan, X-ray, or arteriography reveals a mass or deformity. Excision provides a larger specimen than does drill biopsy and permits immediate surgical treatment if quick histologic analysis of the specimen reveals cancer.

Possible complications include bone fracture, damage to surrounding tissue, infection (osteomyelitis) and, possibly, contamination of normal tissue with tumor cells.

## PURPOSE
- To distinguish between benign and malignant bone tumors

## PATIENT PREPARATION
- Describe the bone biopsy procedure to the patient, and answer his questions.
- Explain that this procedure permits microscopic examination of a bone specimen.
- If the patient is to have a drill biopsy, he need not restrict food and fluids; if he's to have open biopsy, he must fast overnight before the procedure.
- Tell the patient who will perform the biopsy and when and where it will be done.
- Tell the patient that he'll receive a local anesthetic but will still experience discomfort and pressure when the biopsy needle enters the bone.
- Explain that a special bone drill forces the needle into the bone; if possible, show him a photograph of the drill. Stress the importance of his cooperation during the biopsy.
- Make sure the patient or a responsible family member has signed an informed consent form.

- Check the patient's history for hypersensitivity to the local anesthetic.

## PROCEDURE AND POSTTEST CARE
### Drill biopsy
- The patient is properly positioned, and the biopsy site is shaved and prepared.
- After the local anesthetic is injected, a small incision (usually about 3 mm) is made and the biopsy needle is pushed with a pointed trocar into the bone, and then it's rotated about 180 degrees.
- When the bone core is obtained, the trocar is withdrawn and the specimen is placed in a properly labeled bottle containing 10% formalin solution. Then pressure is applied to the site with a sterile gauze pad.
- When bleeding stops, apply a topical antiseptic (povidone-iodine ointment) and an adhesive bandage or other sterile covering to close the wound and prevent infection.

### Open biopsy
- The patient is anesthetized, and the biopsy site is shaved, cleaned with surgical soap, and disinfected with an iodine wash and alcohol.
- An incision is made, and a piece of bone is removed and sent to the histology laboratory immediately for analysis. Further surgery can then be performed, depending on findings.

### Both procedures
- Check the patient's vital signs and the dressing at the biopsy site. Determine how much drainage is expected and report excessive drainage.
- If the patient experiences pain, administer an analgesic.
- *Alert* For several days after the biopsy, watch for and report indications of bone infection including fever, headache, pain on movement, and redness or abscess near the biopsy site. Notify the physician if any of these signs or symptoms develop.
- Advise the patient that he may resume his usual diet.

### PRECAUTIONS
- Know that the bone biopsy should be performed cautiously in the patient with coagulopathy to reduce the risk of bleeding.

- Send the specimen to the laboratory immediately.

## NORMAL FINDINGS
Normal bone tissue consists of fibers of collagen, osteocytes, and osteoblasts. It may be compact or cancellous. Compact bone has dense, concentric layers of mineral deposits, or lamellae. Cancellous bone has widely spaced lamellae, with osteocytes and red and yellow marrow between them.

## ABNORMAL FINDINGS
Histologic examination of a bone specimen can reveal benign or malignant tumors. Benign tumors, generally well circumscribed and nonmetastasizing, include osteoid osteoma, osteoblastoma, osteochondroma, unicameral bone cyst, benign giant-cell tumor, and fibroma. Malignant tumors, which spread irregularly and rapidly, most commonly include multiple myeloma and osteosarcoma; the most lethal is Ewing's sarcoma.

Most malignant tumors spread to the bone through the blood and lymphatic system from the breasts, lungs, prostate, thyroid, or kidneys.

## INTERFERING FACTORS
- Failure to obtain a representative bone specimen
- Failure to use the proper fixative

# *Bone densitometry*

Bone densitometry assesses bone mass quantitatively. This noninvasive technique, also known as *dual energy X-ray absorptiometry (DEXA)*, uses an X-ray tube to measure bone mineral density, but exposes the patient to only minimal radiation. The images detected are computer-analyzed to determine bone mineral status. The computer calculates the size and thickness of the bone as well as its volumetric density to determine its potential resistance to mechanical stress. It may be performed in the radiology department of a health care facility, a physician's office, or a clinic.

## PURPOSE
- To determine bone mineral density

- To identify the risk of osteoporosis
- To evaluate clinical response to therapy for reducing the rate of bone loss

## PATIENT PREPARATION

- Reassure the patient that the bone densitometry test is painless and that the exposure to radiation is minimal.
- Tell the patient that the test will take from 10 minutes to 1 hour, depending on the areas to be scanned.
- Tell the patient who will perform the test and when and where it will take place.

## PROCEDURE AND POSTTEST CARE

- Instruct the patient to remove all metallic objects from the area to be scanned.
- Know that the patient is positioned on a table under the scanning device, with the radiation source below and the detector above. The detector measures the bone's radiation absorption and produces a digital readout.

## PRECAUTIONS

- Bone densitometry is contraindicated during pregnancy.

## NORMAL FINDINGS

Computer-analyzed results of the bone densitometry scan are within normal limits for the patient's age, sex, and height. The patient's rate of bone loss can be treated over time.

## ABNORMAL FINDINGS

The value and reliability of bone densitometry as a predictor of fractures are under investigation. Controversy exists regarding the scanning site and whether bone loss occurs as a general phenomenon or occurs first in the spine. Also, large-scale studies are being conducted to establish an "at-risk" level of bone density to help predict fractures.

## INTERFERING FACTORS

- Osteoarthritis (possible decrease)
- Fat tissue (poor visualization)
- Fractures
- Size of region to be scanned

# Bone marrow aspiration and biopsy

Bone marrow, the soft tissue contained in the medullary canals of the long bone and in the interstices of cancellous bone, may be removed by aspiration or needle biopsy under local anesthesia. The histologic and hematologic examination of bone marrow provides reliable diagnostic information about blood disorders.

Marrow may be removed by aspiration or needle biopsy under local anesthesia. In aspiration biopsy, a fluid specimen in which pustulae of marrow are suspended is removed from the bone marrow. In needle biopsy, a core of marrow cells (not fluid) is removed. These methods are typically used concurrently to obtain the best possible marrow specimens. Red marrow, which constitutes about 50% of an adult's marrow, actively produces stem cells that ultimately evolve into red blood cells, white blood cells, and platelets. Yellow marrow contains fat cells and connective tissue and is inactive, but it can become active in response to the body's needs.

Bleeding and infection may result from bone marrow biopsy at any site, but the most serious complications occur at the sternum. Such complications are rare but include puncture of the heart and major vessels, causing severe hemorrhage, and puncture of the mediastinum, causing mediastinitis or pneumomediastinum. (See *Common sites of bone marrow aspiration and biopsy,* pages 60 and 61.)

## PURPOSE

- To diagnose thrombocytopenia, leukemias, and granulomas as well as aplastic, hypoplastic, and pernicious anemias
- To diagnose primary and metastatic tumors
- To determine the cause of infection
- To aid in the staging of disease such as Hodgkin's disease
- To evaluate the effectiveness of chemotherapy and monitor myelosuppression

## PATIENT PREPARATION

- Explain to the patient that the bone marrow aspiration and biopsy procedure permits microscopic examination of a bone marrow specimen.

- Describe the procedure to the patient, and answer his questions.
- Inform the patient that he need not restrict food and fluids.
- Tell the patient who will perform the biopsy and when and where it will be done.
- Inform the patient that more than one bone marrow specimen may be required and that a blood sample will be collected before biopsy for laboratory testing.
- Make sure the patient or a responsible family member has signed an informed consent form.
- Check the patient's history for hypersensitivity to the local anesthetic.
- Tell the patient which bone — the sternum, anterior or posterior iliac crest, vertebral spinous process, rib, or tibia — will be the biopsy site.
- Inform the patient that he'll receive a local anesthetic but will feel pressure on insertion of the biopsy needle and a brief, pulling pain on removal of the marrow. Administer a mild sedative 1 hour before the test.
- Preparation for children requires additional steps. (See *Preparing a child for bone marrow biopsy*.)

## PROCEDURE AND POSTTEST CARE

- After positioning the patient, instruct him to remain as still as possible.
- Offer emotional support during the biopsy by talking quietly to the patient, describing what's being done, and answering questions.

## Aspiration biopsy

- After the skin over the biopsy site is prepared and the area is draped, the local anesthetic is injected. With a twisting motion, the marrow aspiration needle is inserted through the skin, the subcutaneous tissue, and the cortex of the bone.
- The stylet is removed from the needle, and a 10- to 20-ml syringe is attached. The examiner aspirates 0.2 to 0.5 ml of marrow and then withdraws the needle.
- Apply pressure to the site for 5 minutes, while the marrow slides are being prepared. (If the patient has thrombocytopenia, apply pressure to the site for 10 to 15 minutes.)

---

### PREPARING A CHILD FOR BONE MARROW BIOPSY

To prepare a child for a bone marrow biopsy, give him his own biopsy kit: a syringe without a needle, cotton balls, and adhesive bandages. Act out the procedure by using a doll or a stuffed animal as a model. This will help you gain the child's confidence and answer any questions he may have. Be sure to prepare him by describing the kinds of pressure and discomfort he will feel during the procedure.

Before the biopsy, explain the equipment on the tray to the child. Encourage the parents to get involved by helping you hold the child still and reassuring him. Tell the child that he'll feel some pain when the health care provider aspirates the bone marrow and that it's okay to cry or yell if he wants to, but the pain will go away quickly.

---

- The biopsy site is cleaned again, and a sterile adhesive bandage is applied.
- If an adequate marrow specimen isn't obtained on the first attempt, the needle may be repositioned within the marrow cavity or removed and reinserted in another site within the anesthetized area. If the second attempt fails, a needle biopsy may be needed.

## Needle biopsy

- After preparing the biopsy site and draping the area, the examiner marks the skin at the site with an indelible pencil or marking pen.
- A local anesthetic is then injected intradermally, subcutaneously, and at the bone's surface.
- The biopsy needle is inserted into the periosteum, and the needle guard is set as indicated. The needle is advanced with a steady boring motion until the outer needle passes through the bone's cortex.
- The inner needle with trephine tip is inserted into the outer needle. By alternately rotating the inner needle clockwise and counterclockwise, the examiner directs the needle into the marrow cavity and then removes a tissue plug.

# COMMON SITES OF BONE MARROW ASPIRATION AND BIOPSY

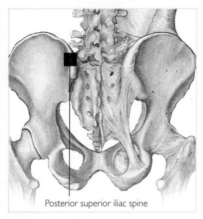

Posterior superior iliac spine

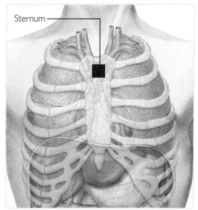

Sternum

The *posterior superior iliac spine* is usually the preferred site for bone marrow aspiration and biopsy because no vital organs or vessels are located nearby. With the patient in a lateral position with one leg flexed, the health care provider inserts the needle several centimeters lateral to the iliosacral junction, entering the bone plane crest with the needle directed downward and toward the anterior inferior spine, or entering a few centimeters below the crest at a right angle to the surface of the bone.

The *sternum* involves the greatest risk but is commonly used for marrow aspiration because it's near the surface, the cortical bone is thin, and the marrow cavity contains numerous cells and relatively little fat or supporting bone. For this procedure, the patient is supine on a firm bed or examining table with a small pillow beneath the shoulders to elevate the chest and lower the head. The health care provider secures the needle guard 3 to 4 mm from the tip of the needle to avoid accidental puncture of the heart or a major vessel. Then he inserts the needle at the midline of the sternum at the second intercostal space.

---

● The needle assembly is withdrawn, and the marrow is expelled into a labeled bottle containing Zenker's acetic acid solution.

● After the biopsy site is cleaned, a sterile adhesive bandage or a pressure dressing is applied.

## Both procedures

● Check the biopsy site for bleeding and inflammation.

● Observe the patient for signs and symptoms of hemorrhage and infection, such as rapid pulse rate, low blood pressure, and fever.

## PRECAUTIONS

● Know that bone marrow biopsy is contraindicated in the patient with a severe bleeding disorder.

● Send the tissue specimen or slides to the laboratory immediately.

## NORMAL FINDINGS

Yellow marrow contains fat cells and connective tissue; red marrow contains hematopoietic cells, fat cells, and connective tissue. In addition, special stains that are used to detect hematologic disorders produce these normal findings: The iron stain, which is used to measure hemosiderin (storage iron), has a +2 level; the Sudan black B (SBB)

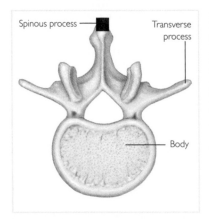

Spinous process — Transverse process

Body

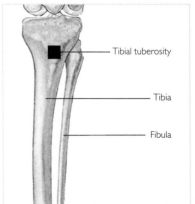

Tibial tuberosity

Tibia

Fibula

The *spinous process* is the preferred site if multiple punctures are necessary, marrow is absent at other sites, or the patient objects to sternal puncture. For this procedure, the patient sits on the edge of the bed, leaning over the bedside stand; or, if he's uncooperative, he may be placed in the prone position with restraints. The health care provider selects the spinous process of the third or fourth lumbar vertebra and inserts the needle at the crest or slightly to one side, advancing the needle in the direction of the bone plane.

The *tibia* is the site of choice for infants under age 1. The infant is placed in a prone position on a bed or examining table with a sandbag beneath the leg. The foot is taped to the surface of the table, or an assistant holds the leg stationary by placing a hand under it. The health care provider inserts the needle about ⅜″ (1 cm) below the tibial tuberosity and slightly toward the medial side, being careful to angle the needle point toward the foot to avoid epiphyseal injury.

Illustrations from Anatomical Chart Company. *Atlas of Human Anatomy*. Springhouse, 2001.

fat stain, which shows granulocytes, is negative; and the periodic acid–Schiff (PAS) stain, which is used to detect glycogen reactions, is negative.

## ABNORMAL FINDINGS

Histologic examination of a bone marrow specimen can be used to detect myelofibrosis, granulomas, lymphoma, and cancer. Hematologic analysis, including the differential count and myeloid-erythroid ratio, can implicate a wide range of disorders. (See *Bone marrow: Normal values and implications of abnormal findings,* pages 62 and 63.)

In an iron stain, decreased hemosiderin levels may indicate a true iron deficiency. Increased levels may accompany other types of anemias and blood disorders. A positive SBB stain can differentiate acute granulocytic leukemia from acute lymphocytic leukemia (SBB-negative) or may indicate granulation in myeloblasts. A positive PAS stain may indicate acute or chronic lymphocytic leukemia, amyloidosis, thalassemia, lymphomas, infectious mononucleosis, iron deficiency anemia, or sideroblastic anemia.

## INTERFERING FACTORS
- Failure to obtain a representative specimen
- Failure to use a fixative for histologic analysis

# BONE MARROW: NORMAL VALUES AND IMPLICATIONS OF ABNORMAL FINDINGS

| CELL TYPES | NORMAL MEAN VALUES | | | CLINICAL IMPLICATIONS |
| --- | --- | --- | --- | --- |
| | Adults | Children | Infants | |
| *Normoblasts, total* | 25.6% | 23.1% | 8% | *Elevated values*: polycythemia vera |
| Pronormoblasts | 0.2% to 1.3% | 0.5% | 0.1% | *Depressed values*: vitamin B$_{12}$ or folic acid deficiency; hypoplastic or aplastic anemia |
| Basophilic | 0.5% to 2.4% | 1.7% | 0.34% | |
| Polychromatic | 17.9% to 29.2% | 18.2% | 6.9% | |
| Orthochromatic | 0.4% to 4.6% | 2.7% | 0.54% | |
| *Neutrophils, total* | 56.5% | 57.1% | 32.4% | *Elevated values*: acute myeloblastic or chronic myeloid leukemia |
| Myeloblasts | 0.2% to 1.5% | 1.2% | 0.62% | *Depressed values*: lymphoblastic, lymphatic, or monocytic leukemia; aplastic anemia |
| Promyelocytes | 2.1% to 4.1% | 1.4% | 0.76% | |
| Myelocytes | 8.2% to 15.7% | 18.3% | 2.5% | |
| Metamyelocytes | 9.6% to 24.6% | 23.3% | 11.3% | |
| Bands | 9.5% to 15.3% | 0 | 14.1% | |
| Segmented | 6% to 12% | 12.9% | 3.6% | |
| *Eosinophils* | 3.1% | 3.6% | 2.6% | *Elevated values*: bone marrow carcinoma, lymphadenoma, myeloid leukemia, eosinophilic leukemia, pernicious anemia (in relapse) |
| *Plasma cells* | 1.3% | 0.4% | 0.02% | *Elevated values*: myeloma, collagen disease, infection, antigen sensitivity, malignancy |
| *Basophils* | 0.01% | 0.06% | 0.07% | *Elevated values*: no relation between basophil count and symptoms *Depressed values*: no relation between basophil count and symptoms |
| *Lymphocytes* | 16.2% | 16.2% | 49% | *Elevated values*: B- and T-cell chronic lymphocytic leukemia, other lymphatic leukemias, lymphoma, mononucleosis, aplastic anemia, macroglobulinemia |
| *Plasma cells* | 1.3% | 0.4% | 0.02% | *Elevated values*: myeloma, collagen disease, infection, antigen sensitivity, malignancy |

## BONE MARROW: NORMAL VALUES AND IMPLICATIONS OF ABNORMAL FINDINGS *(continued)*

| CELL TYPES | NORMAL MEAN VALUES | | | CLINICAL IMPLICATIONS |
| --- | --- | --- | --- | --- |
| | Adults | Children | Infants | |
| Megakaryocytes | 0.1% | 0.1% | 0.05% | *Elevated values:* advanced age, chronic myeloid leukemia, polycythemia vera, megakaryocytic myelosis, infection, idiopathic thrombocytopenic purpura, thrombocytopenia<br>*Depressed values:* pernicious anemia |
| Myeloiderythroid ratio | 2:1 to 4:1 | 2.9:1 | 4.4:1 | *Elevated values:* myeloid leukemia, infection, leukemoid reactions, depressed hematopoiesis<br>*Depressed values:* agranulocytosis, hematopoiesis after hemorrhage or hemolysis, iron deficiency anemia, polycythemia vera |

# Bone scan

A bone scan involves imaging the skeleton by a scanning camera after I.V. injection of a radioactive tracer compound. The tracer of choice, radioactive technetium diphosphonate, collects in bone tissue in increased concentrations at sites of abnormal metabolism. When scanned, these sites appear as hot spots that are typically detectable months before an X-ray can reveal a lesion. To promote early detection of lesions, this test may be performed with a gallium scan.

## PURPOSE
● To detect or to rule out malignant bone lesions when radiographic findings are normal but cancer is confirmed or suspected
● To detect occult bone trauma due to pathologic fractures
● To monitor degenerative bone disorders
● To detect infection
● To evaluate unexplained bone pain
● To stage cancer

## PATIENT PREPARATION
● Describe the bone scan procedure to the patient. Explain that this test may detect skeletal abnormalities sooner than is possible with ordinary X-rays.
● Tell the patient who will perform the test, where it will take place, and that he may have to assume various positions on a scanner table. Emphasize that he must keep still for the scan.
● Assure the patient that the scan itself is painless and that the isotope, although radioactive, emits less radiation than a standard X-ray machine.
● Make sure that the patient or a responsible family member has signed an informed consent form, if required.
● If a bone scan is ordered to diagnose cancer, evaluate the patient's emotional state and offer support.
● Administer prescribed analgesics.
● After the patient receives an I.V. injection of the tracer and imaging agent, encourage him to increase his intake of fluids for the next 1 to 3 hours to facilitate renal clearance of the circulating free tracer.

# COMPARING NORMAL AND ABNORMAL BONE SCANS

The scans below compare a normal bone scan with an abnormal scan. The scan on the left is normal because the isotope is distributed evenly throughout the skeletal tissue. The scan on the right is abnormal because the isotope has accumulated in multiple metastases in the ribs and spine.

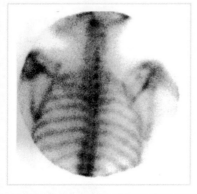 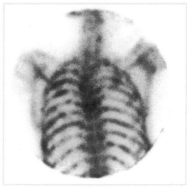

## PROCEDURE AND POSTTEST CARE

- Be aware that the patient receives an I.V. injection of tracer and imaging agent. Encourage increased fluids for the next 1 to 3 hours to facilitate renal clearance.
- Instruct the patient to void immediately before the procedure (otherwise, a urinary catheter may be inserted to empty the bladder), and then position him on the scanner table.
- As the scanner head moves back and forth over the patient's body, know that it detects low-level radiation emitted by the skeleton and translates this into a film, paper chart, or both to produce two-dimensional pictures of the area scanned.
- If appropriate, assist with repositioning the patient several times during the test to obtain adequate views. (The scanner takes as many views as needed to cover the specified area.)

*Age alert* Anticipate the need to administer sedation to the child who can't hold still for the scan.

- Check the injection site for redness or swelling.
- Don't schedule other radionuclide tests for 24 to 48 hours.

- Instruct the patient to drink lots of fluids and to empty his bladder frequently for the next 24 to 48 hours.
- Provide analgesics for pain resulting from positioning on the scanning table, as needed.

## PRECAUTIONS

- To avoid exposing the fetus or infant to radiation, be aware that a bone scan is contraindicated during pregnancy or lactation.
- Know that allergic reactions to radionuclides may occur.

## NORMAL FINDINGS

The tracer concentrates in bone tissue at sites of new bone formation or increased metabolism. The epiphyses of growing bone are normal sites of high concentration, or hot spots.

## ABNORMAL FINDINGS

Although a bone scan demonstrates hot spots that identify sites of bone formation, it doesn't distinguish between normal and abnormal bone formation. But scan results can identify all types of bone malignancy, infection, fracture, and other disorders if viewed in light of the patient's medical and surgical history, X-rays, and other laboratory tests.

(See *Comparing normal and abnormal bone scans*.)

## INTERFERING FACTORS
- Distended bladder (possible obscuring of pelvic detail)
- Improper injection technique (possible seepage of tracer into muscle tissue, creating false hot spots)
- Antihypertensives (invalidate test results)

# Breast biopsy

## BRCA TESTING

Genetic researchers have located two genes, BRCA1 and BRCA2, that are linked to certain forms of breast cancer. BRCA testing can detect the presence of BRCA gene mutations, which may increase an individual's susceptibility to some breast cancers.

The BRCA test, performed on a blood sample, is available for a woman with a family history of breast cancer.

Breast biopsy is performed to confirm or rule out breast cancer after clinical examination, mammography, or thermography has identified a mass. Fine-needle or needle biopsy is usually done on a mass that has been identified by ultrasonography as being fluid-filled. Both methods have limited diagnostic value because of the small and perhaps unrepresentative specimens they provide. Open biopsy provides complete tissue system, which can be sectioned to allow more accurate evaluation. Local anesthesia can usually be given to outpatients for these three techniques. Stereotactic breast biopsy immobilizes the breast and allows the computer to calculate the exact location of the mass based on X-rays from two angles.

An excisional biopsy may be done under general anesthesia. If sufficient tissue is obtained and the mass is found to be a malignant tumor, specimens are sent for estrogen and progesterone receptor assays to assist in determining future therapy and the prognosis.

Because breast cancer remains the most prevalent cancer in women, genetic researchers are continually working to identify women at risk. (See *BRCA testing*.)

## PURPOSE
- To differentiate between benign and malignant breast tumors

## PATIENT PREPARATION
- Describe the procedure to the patient, and explain that the breast biopsy procedure permits microscopic examination of a breast tissue specimen. Offer her emotional support, and assure her that breast masses don't always indicate cancer.
- If the patient is to receive a local anesthetic, tell her that she need not restrict food, fluids, and medication.
- If the patient is to receive a general anesthetic, advise her to fast from midnight before the procedure until after the biopsy.
- Tell the patient who will perform the biopsy and when and where it will be done.
- Explain that pretest studies, such as blood tests, urine tests, and chest X-rays, may be required.
- Make sure the patient or a responsible family member has signed an informed consent form.
- Check the patient's history for hypersensitivity to anesthetics.

## PROCEDURE AND POSTTEST CARE
### Needle biopsy
- Instruct the patient to undress to the waist, and guide her to a sitting or recumbent position with her hands at her sides, reminding her to remain still.
- The biopsy site is prepared, a local anesthetic is administered, and the syringe (luer-lock syringe for aspiration, Vim-Silverman needle for tissue specimen) is introduced into the lesion.
- Fluid aspirated from the breast is expelled into a properly labeled, heparinized tub; the tissue specimen is placed in a labeled specimen bottle containing normal saline solution or formalin.
- With fine-needle aspiration, a slide is made for cytology and viewed immediately under a microscope.

Pressure is exerted on the biopsy site and, after bleeding stops, an adhesive bandage is applied. Because breast fluid aspiration isn't considered diagnostically accurate, some physicians aspirate fluid only from cysts. If such fluid is clear yellow and the mass disappears, the aspiration procedure is diagnostic and therapeutic, and the aspirate is discarded. If aspiration yields no fluid or if the lesion recurs two or three times, an open biopsy is then considered appropriate.

## Open biopsy

- After the patient receives a general or local anesthetic, an incision is made in the breast to expose the mass.
- The examiner may then incise a portion of tissue or excise the entire mass. If the mass is smaller than $3/4''$ (2 cm) in diameter and appears benign, it's usually excised; if it's larger or appears malignant, a specimen is usually incised before the mass is excised. Incisional biopsy generally provides an adequate specimen for histologic analysis.
- The specimen is placed in a properly labeled specimen bottle containing 10% formalin solution. Tissue that appears malignant is sent for frozen section and receptor assays. Receptor assay specimens must not be placed in the formalin solution.
- The wound is sutured, and an adhesive bandage applied.

## All procedures

- If the patient has received a general or local anesthetic, check the patient's vital signs, and provide medication for pain. If she has received a general anesthetic, check her vital signs every 15 minutes for 1 hour, every 30 minutes for 2 hours, every hour for the next 4 hours, and then every 4 hours.
- Administer an analgesic, as ordered. An ice bag may provide comfort. Instruct the patient to wear a support bra at all times until healing is complete.
- Watch for and report bleeding, tenderness, and redness at the biopsy site.
- Provide emotional support to the patient who's awaiting diagnosis.

## PRECAUTIONS

- Know that open breast biopsy is contraindicated in the patient with a condition that precludes surgery.
- Send the specimen to the laboratory immediately.

## NORMAL FINDINGS

Normally, breast tissue consists of cellular and noncellular connective tissue, fat lobules, and various lactiferous ducts. It's pink, more fatty than fibrous, and shows no abnormal development of cells or tissue elements.

## ABNORMAL FINDINGS

Abnormal breast tissue may exhibit a wide range of malignant or benign pathology. Breast tumors are common in women and account for 32% of female cancers; such tumors are rare in men (0.2% of male cancers). Benign tumors include fibrocystic disease, adenofibroma, intraductal papilloma, mammary fat necrosis, and plasma cell mastitis (mammary duct ectasia). Malignant tumors include adenocarcinoma, cystosarcoma, intraductal carcinoma, infiltrating carcinoma, inflammatory carcinoma, medullary or circumscribed carcinoma, colloid carcinoma, lobular carcinoma, sarcoma, and Paget's disease.

The receptor assays evaluate tumors for estrogen and progesterone protein and assign a positive or negative value to the estrogen and progesterone receptors. This positive or negative value assists in the prognosis and treatment of breast cancer.

## INTERFERING FACTORS

- Failure to obtain an adequate tissue specimen
- Failure to place the specimen in the proper solution

# Bronchoscopy

Bronchoscopy allows direct visualization of the larynx, trachea, and bronchi through a flexible fiber-optic bronchoscope or a rigid metal bronchoscope. A more recent approach is the use of virtual bronchoscopy. (See *Virtual bronchoscopy.*)

Although a flexible fiber-optic bronchoscope allows a wider view and is used more commonly, the rigid metal bronchoscope is required to remove foreign objects, excise endobronchial lesions, and control massive hemoptysis. A brush, biopsy forceps, or catheter may be passed through the bron-

# VIRTUAL BRONCHOSCOPY

Using a computer and data from a spiral computed tomography (CT) scan, physicians can now examine the respiratory tract noninvasively with virtual bronchoscopy. Although still in its early stages, researchers believe that this test can enhance screening, diagnosis, preoperative planning, surgical technique, and postoperative follow-up.

Unlike its counterpart — conventional bronchoscopy — virtual bronchoscopy is noninvasive, doesn't require sedation, and provides images for examination beyond the segmental bronchi, thus allowing for possible diagnosis of areas that may be stenosed, obstructed, or compressed from an external source. The images obtained from the CT scan include views of the airways and lung parenchyma. Anatomic structures and abnormalities can be precisely identified and, there-fore, can be helpful in locating potential biopsy sites to be obtained with conventional bronchoscopy and provide simulation for planning the optimal surgical approach.

Virtual bronchoscopy does have disadvantages. This technique doesn't allow for specimen collection or actual biopsies to be obtained from tissue sources. It also can't demonstrate details of the mucosal surface, such as color or texture. Moreover, if an area contains viscous secretions, such as mucus or blood, visualization becomes difficult.

More research on this technique is needed. However, researchers believe that virtual bronchoscopy may play a major role in the screening and early detection of certain cancers, thus allowing for treatment at an earlier, possibly curable stage.

---

choscope to obtain specimens for cytologic examination.

## PURPOSE
- To visually examine a tumor, an obstruction, secretions, bleeding, or a foreign body in the tracheobronchial tree
- To help diagnose bronchogenic carcinoma, tuberculosis, interstitial pulmonary disease, and fungal or parasitic pulmonary infection by obtaining a specimen for bacteriologic and cytologic examination
- To remove foreign bodies, malignant or benign tumors, mucus plugs, and excessive secretions from the tracheobronchial tree

## PATIENT PREPARATION
- Explain to the patient that bronchoscopy is used to examine the lower airways.
- Describe the procedure, and instruct the patient to fast for 6 to 12 hours before the test.
- Tell the patient who will perform the test, when and where it will be done, and that the room will be darkened.
- Tell the patient that a chest X-ray and blood studies will be performed before the bronchoscopy and afterward, if appropriate.
- Advise the patient that he may receive an I.V. sedative to help him relax.
- If the procedure isn't being performed under general anesthesia, inform the patient that a local anesthetic will be sprayed into his nose and mouth to suppress the gag reflex. Warn him that the spray has an unpleasant taste and that he may experience discomfort during the procedure.
- Reassure the patient that his airway won't be blocked during the procedure and that oxygen will be administered through the bronchoscope.
- Make sure that the patient or a responsible family member has signed an informed consent form.
- Check the patient's history for hypersensitivity to the anesthetic.
- Obtain the patient's baseline vital signs.
- Administer the preoperative sedative.
- Have the patient remove his dentures, if appropriate, before he receives a sedative.

## PROCEDURE AND POSTTEST CARE
- Place the patient in the supine position or have him sit upright in a chair.
- Tell the patient to remain relaxed with his arms at his sides and to breathe through his nose.
- Provide supplemental oxygen by nasal cannula, if necessary.
- After the local anesthetic is sprayed into the patient's throat and it takes effect, assist as appropriate as a bronchoscope is introduced through the patient's mouth or nose.

When the scope is just above the vocal cords, about 3 to 4 ml of 2% to 4% lidocaine is flushed through the inner channel of the scope to the vocal cords to anesthetize deeper areas. The physician inspects the anatomic structure of the trachea and bronchi, observes the color of the mucosal lining, and notes masses or inflamed areas.

● As indicated, provide biopsy forceps that may be used to remove a tissue specimen from a suspect area, a bronchial brush to obtain cells from the surface of a lesion, and a suction apparatus to remove foreign bodies or mucus plugs. Bronchoalveolar lavage may be performed to diagnose the infectious causes of infiltrates in an immunocompromised patient or to remove thickened secretions.

● After collection, place the specimens in their respective, properly labeled containers in accordance with laboratory and pathology guidelines and send them to the laboratory at once.

● Be aware that bronchoscopy may require fluoroscopic guidance for distal evaluation of lesions for a transbronchial biopsy in alveolar areas.

● Check the patient's vital signs per facility policy, or at least every 15 minutes until the patient is stable and then every 30 minutes for 4 hours, every hour for the next 4 hours, and then every 4 hours for 24 hours. Immediately notify the physician of adverse reactions to the anesthetic or sedative.

● Place the conscious patient in semi-Fowler's position; place the unconscious patient on his side with his head slightly elevated to prevent aspiration.

● Provide an emesis basin and instruct the patient to spit out saliva rather than swallow it. Observe sputum for blood and report excessive bleeding immediately.

● Tell the patient who has had a biopsy to refrain from clearing his throat and coughing, which may dislodge the clot at the biopsy site and cause hemorrhaging.

● If biopsies are taken, obtain a postprocedure chest X-ray as ordered.

● Immediately report subcutaneous crepitus around the patient's face and neck because this may indicate tracheal or bronchial perforation.

✦ **Alert** *Watch for, listen for, and immediately report symptoms of respiratory difficulty resulting from laryngeal edema or laryngospasm,* such as laryngeal stridor and dyspnea. Observe for signs and symptoms of hypoxemia, pneumothorax, bronchospasm, and bleeding.

● Restrict food and fluids to avoid aspiration until the gag reflex returns (usually in 1 to 2 hours). The patient may then resume his usual diet, beginning with sips of clear liquid or ice chips.

● Reassure the patient that hoarseness, loss of voice, and sore throat are temporary. Provide lozenges or a soothing liquid gargle to ease discomfort when his gag reflex returns.

## PRECAUTIONS

● Know that a patient with respiratory failure who can't breathe adequately by himself should be placed on a ventilator before bronchoscopy.

● Send the specimens to the laboratory immediately.

## NORMAL FINDINGS

The trachea normally consists of smooth muscle containing C-shaped rings of cartilage at regular intervals, and it's lined with ciliated mucosa. The bronchi appear structurally similar to the trachea; the right bronchus is slightly larger and more vertical than the left. Smaller segmental bronchi branch off the main bronchi.

## ABNORMAL FINDINGS

Bronchial wall abnormalities include inflammation, swelling, protruding cartilage, ulceration, enlargement of the mucous gland orifices or submucosal lymph nodes, and tumors. Endotracheal abnormalities include stenosis, compression, ectasia (dilation of tubular vessel), irregular bronchial branching, and abnormal bifurcation due to diverticulum.

Abnormal substances in the trachea or bronchi include blood, secretions, calculi, and foreign bodies.

Results of tissue and cell studies may indicate interstitial pulmonary disease, cancer, tuberculosis, or other pulmonary infections. Correlation of radiographic, bronchoscopic, histopathologic, and cytologic findings with clinical signs and symptoms is essential.

## INTERFERING FACTORS

● Failure to place specimens in the appropriate containers

# B-type natriuretic peptide assay

B-type natriuretic peptide (BNP) is a neuro-hormone produced predominantly by the heart ventricle. BNP is released from the heart in response to blood volume expansion or pressure overload.

Plasma BNP increases with the severity of heart failure. Studies have demonstrated that the heart is the major source of circulating BNP. It's an excellent hormonal marker of ventricular systolic and diastolic dysfunction.

## PURPOSE
- To aid in the diagnosis and severity of heart failure

## PATIENT PREPARATION
- Explain to the patient that the BNP assay is used to identify the presence and severity of heart failure.
- Tell the patient that the assay requires a blood sample. Explain who will perform the venipuncture and when.
- Explain to the patient that he may experience slight discomfort from the tourniquet and needle puncture.
- Inform the patient that he need not restrict food and fluids.

## PROCEDURE AND POSTTEST CARE
- Perform a venipuncture and collect the sample in a 3.5-ml EDTA tube.
- Apply direct pressure to the venipuncture site until bleeding stops.

## PRECAUTIONS
- Handle the sample gently to prevent hemolysis.

## REFERENCE VALUES
The normal value is less than 100 pg/ml (SI, < 100 ng/L).

## ABNORMAL FINDINGS
Blood concentrations greater than 100 pg/ml are an accurate predictor of heart failure. The level of BNP in the blood is related to the severity of heart failure. The higher the level, the worse the symptoms of heart failure. (See *Linking BNP levels to heart failure symptom severity*.)

## INTERFERING FACTORS
- None significant

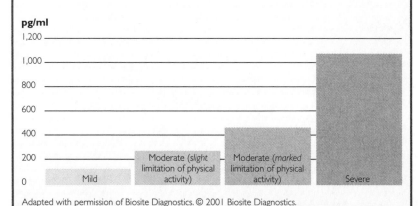

## LINKING BNP LEVELS TO HEART FAILURE SYMPTOM SEVERITY

This chart shows the level of B-type natriuretic peptide (BNP) levels and its correlation with symptoms of heart failure. The higher the level of BNP, the more severe the symptoms.

pg/ml

Mild — Moderate (*slight* limitation of physical activity) — Moderate (*marked* limitation of physical activity) — Severe

Adapted with permission of Biosite Diagnostics. © 2001 Biosite Diagnostics.

# Calcitonin, plasma

The plasma calcitonin test is a radioimmunoassay that measures plasma levels of calcitonin (thyrocalcitonin). The exact role of calcitonin in normal human physiology hasn't been fully defined. However, calcitonin is known to act as an antagonist to parathyroid hormone and to lower serum calcium levels.

The usual clinical indication for this test is suspected medullary carcinoma of the thyroid, which causes hypersecretion of calcitonin (without associated hypocalcemia). Equivocal results require provocative testing with I.V. pentagastrin or calcium to rule out disease.

## PURPOSE
● To aid diagnosis of thyroid medullary carcinoma and ectopic calcitonin-producing tumors (rare)

## PATIENT PREPARATION
● Explain to the patient that the plasma calcitonin test helps evaluate thyroid function.
● Instruct the patient to fast overnight because food may interfere with calcium homeostasis and, subsequently, calcitonin levels.
● Tell the patient that the test requires a blood sample. Explain who will perform the venipuncture and when.
● Explain to the patient that he may experience slight discomfort from the tourniquet and needle puncture.
● Tell him that the laboratory requires several days to complete the analysis.

## PROCEDURE AND POSTTEST CARE
● Perform a venipuncture and collect the sample in a 7-ml heparinized tube.
● Apply direct pressure to the venipuncture site until bleeding stops.
● If a hematoma develops at the venipuncture site, apply pressure.
● Instruct the patient that he may resume his usual diet.

## PRECAUTIONS
● Handle the sample gently to prevent hemolysis.
● Send the sample to the laboratory immediately.

## REFERENCE VALUES
Serum calcitonin levels (basal) normally are 40 pg/ml (SI, 40 ng/L) for males and 20 pg/ml (SI, 20 ng/L) for females.

Reference values after 4-hour calcium infusion are:
● males — 190 pg/ml (SI, 190 ng/L)
● females — 130 pg/ml (SI, 130 ng/L).

Values after testing with pentagastrin infusion are:
● males — 110 pg/ml (SI, 110 ng/L)
● females — 30 pg/ml (SI, 30 ng/L).

## ABNORMAL FINDINGS
Elevated serum calcitonin levels in the absence of hypocalcemia usually indicate medullary carcinoma of the thyroid. Transmitted as an autosomal dominant trait, thyroid medullary carcinoma may occur as part of multiple endocrine neoplasia. Occasionally, increased calcitonin levels may be due to

ectopic calcitonin production by oat cell carcinoma of the lung or by breast carcinoma.

## INTERFERING FACTORS
- Ingestion of food or fluids before the test

# Calcium, serum; calcium and phosphates, urine

About 99% of the body's calcium is found in the teeth. Approximately 1% of total calcium in the body circulates in the blood. Of this, about 50% is bound to plasma proteins and 40% is ionized, or free. Evaluation of serum calcium levels measures the total amount of calcium in the blood, and ionized calcium measures the fraction of serum calcium that's in the ionized form.

Urine calcium and phosphates test measures the urine levels of calcium and phosphates, elements essential for bone formation and resorption. Urine calcium and phosphate levels generally parallel serum levels.

Normally absorbed in the upper intestine and excreted in stool and urine, calcium and phosphates help maintain tissue and fluid pH, electrolyte balance in cells and extracellular fluids, and permeability of cell membranes. Calcium promotes enzymatic processes, aids blood coagulation, and lowers neuromuscular irritability; phosphates aid carbohydrate metabolism.

## PURPOSE
- To evaluate endocrine function, calcium metabolism and excretion, and acid-base balance
- To guide therapy in patients with renal failure, renal transplant, endocrine disorders, malignancies, cardiac disease, and skeletal disorders
- To monitor treatment of calcium or phosphate deficiency (urine testing)

## PATIENT PREPARATION
### Serum calcium
- Explain to the patient that the serum calcium test is used to determine blood calcium levels.

- Tell the patient that the test requires a blood sample. Explain who will perform the venipuncture and when.
- Explain to the patient that he may experience slight discomfort from the tourniquet and needle puncture.
- Inform the patient that he need not restrict food and fluids.

### Urine calcium and phosphates
- Explain that the urine calcium and phosphates test measures the amount of calcium and phosphates in the urine.
- Encourage the patient to be as active as possible before the test.
- Tell the patient that the test requires urine collection over a 24-hour period. If the patient is to collect the specimen, teach him the proper technique.
- Provide a diet that contains about 130 mg of calcium/24 hours for 3 days before the test or provide a copy of the diet for the patient to follow at home. Check the laboratory for parameters related to dietary instructions.
- Notify the laboratory and physician of medications the patient is taking that may affect test results; they may need to be restricted.

## PROCEDURE AND POSTTEST CARE
### Serum calcium
- Perform a venipuncture (without a tourniquet if possible) and collect the sample in a 3- or 4-ml clot-activator tube.
- Apply direct pressure to the venipuncture site until bleeding stops.
- If a hematoma develops at the venipuncture site, apply pressure.

### Urine calcium and phosphates
- Collect the patient's urine over a 24-hour period, discarding the first specimen and retaining the last.
- Observe the patient with low urine calcium levels for tetany.
- Inform the patient that he may resume his usual diet, activities, and medications, as ordered.

## PRECAUTIONS
- Handle the serum sample carefully to prevent hemolysis.

## DISORDERS THAT AFFECT URINE CALCIUM AND URINE PHOSPHATE LEVELS

| DISORDER | URINE CALCIUM LEVEL | URINE PHOSPHATE LEVEL |
|---|---|---|
| Hyperparathyroidism | Elevated | Elevated |
| Vitamin D intoxication | Elevated | Suppressed |
| Metastatic carcinoma | Elevated | Normal |
| Sarcoidosis | Elevated | Suppressed |
| Renal tubular acidosis | Elevated | Elevated |
| Multiple myeloma | Elevated or normal | Elevated or normal |
| Paget's disease | Normal | Normal |
| Milk-alkali syndrome | Suppressed or normal | Suppressed or normal |
| Hypoparathyroidism | Suppressed | Suppressed |
| Acute nephrosis | Suppressed | Suppressed or normal |
| Chronic nephrosis | Suppressed | Suppressed |
| Acute nephritis | Suppressed | Suppressed |
| Renal insufficiency | Suppressed | Suppressed |
| Osteomalacia | Suppressed | Suppressed |
| Steatorrhea | Suppressed | Suppressed |

- Tell the patient not to contaminate the urine specimen with toilet tissue or stool.

## REFERENCE VALUES

Normally, total serum calcium levels range from 8.2 to 10.2 mg/dl (SI, 2.05 to 2.54 mmol/L) in adults. Ionized calcium levels are 4.65 to 5.28 mg/dl (SI, 1.1 to 1.25 mmol/L).

**Age alert** *In children, total calcium levels range from 8.6 to 11.2 mg/dl (SI, 2.15 to 2.79 mmol/L).*

Normal urine values depend on dietary intake. For a normal diet, urine calcium levels for a 24-hour period range from 100 to 300 mg/24 hours (SI, 2.5 to 7.5 mmol/d). Normal excretion of phosphate is less than 1,000 mg/24 hours.

## ABNORMAL FINDINGS

Abnormally high serum calcium levels (hypercalcemia) may occur in hyperparathyroidism and parathyroid tumors, Paget's disease of the bone, multiple myeloma, metastatic carcinoma, multiple fractures, and prolonged immobilization. Elevated levels may also result from inadequate excretion of calcium, such as adrenal insufficiency and renal disease; from excessive calcium ingestion; and from overuse of antacids such as calcium carbonate.

**Alert** *Observe the patient with hypercalcemia for deep bone pain, flank pain due to renal calculi, and muscle hypotonicity. Hypercalcemic crisis begins with nausea, vomiting, and dehydration, leading to stupor and coma, and can end in cardiac arrest.*

Low serum calcium levels (hypocalcemia) may result from hypoparathyroidism, total parathyroidectomy, and malabsorption. Decreased serum calcium levels may also occur with Cushing's syndrome, renal failure, acute pancreatitis, peritonitis, malnutrition with hypoalbuminemia, and blood transfusions (due to citrate).

In the patient with hypocalcemia, be alert for circumoral and peripheral numbness and tingling, muscle twitching, Chvostek's sign (facial muscle spasm), tetany, muscle cramping, Trousseau's sign (carpopedal spasm), seizures, arrhythmias, laryngeal spasm, decreased cardiac output, prolonged bleeding time, fractures, and a prolonged Q interval.

Many disorders may affect urine calcium and phosphorus levels. (See *Disorders that affect urine calcium and urine phosphate levels*.)

## INTERFERING FACTORS
### Serum calcium
● Venous stasis due to prolonged tourniquet application (possible false-high)
● Excessive ingestion of vitamin D or its derivatives (dihydrotachysterol, calcitrol) or use of androgens, asparaginase, calciferol-activated calcium salts, progestins-estrogens, thiazide diuretics, and thyroid hormones (increase)
● Acetazolamide, anticonvulsants, chronic laxative use, cisplatin, corticosteroids, hormonal contraceptives, magnesium salts, plicamycin, and excessive transfusions of citrated blood (possible increase or decrease)

### Urine calcium and phosphates
● Parathyroid hormones (increase phosphates excretion and decrease calcium excretion)
● Estrogen-containing medications, lithium carbonate, and thiazide diuretics (decreases calcium excretion)
● Prolonged inactivity and ingestion of antacids, anticonvulsants, calcitonin, corticosteroids, and sodium phosphate (increases calcium excretion)
● Vitamin D (increases phosphate absorption and excretion)

# Candida *antibodies*

Commonly present in the body, *Candida albicans* is a saprophytic yeast that can become pathogenic when the environment favors proliferation or the host's defenses have been significantly weakened.

Candidiasis is usually limited to the skin and mucous membranes, but may cause life-threatening systemic infection. Susceptibility to candidiasis is associated with antibacterial, antimetabolic, and corticosteroid therapy as well as with immunologic defects, pregnancy, obesity, diabetes, and debilitating diseases. Oral candidiasis is common and benign in children; in adults, it may be an early indication of acquired immunodeficiency syndrome.

Diagnosis of candidiasis is usually made by culture or histologic study. When such diagnosis can't be made, identifying *Candida* antibodies may be helpful in diagnosing systemic candidiasis. Be aware that serologic testing to detect antibodies in candidiasis isn't reliable, and investigators continue to disagree about its usefulness.

## PURPOSE
● To aid in the diagnosis of candidiasis when culture or histologic study can't confirm the diagnosis

## PATIENT PREPARATION
● Explain the purpose of the *Candida* antibodies test to the patient, as appropriate.
● Inform the patient that he need not restrict food and fluids.
● Tell the patient that the test requires a blood sample. Explain who will perform the venipuncture and when.
● Explain to the patient that he may experience slight discomfort from the tourniquet and needle puncture.

## PROCEDURE AND POSTTEST CARE
● Perform a venipuncture and collect the sample in a 5-ml sterile collection tube without additives.
● Apply direct pressure to the venipuncture site until bleeding stops.
● If a hematoma develops at the venipuncture site, apply pressure.

## PRECAUTIONS

- Handle the sample gently to prevent hemolysis.
- Send the sample to the laboratory immediately.
- Note recent antimicrobial therapy on the laboratory request form.
- Because the patient's immune system may be compromised, keep the venipuncture site clean and dry.

## NORMAL FINDINGS

A normal test result is negative for *Candida* antibodies.

## ABNORMAL FINDINGS

A positive test for *C. albicans* antibodies is common in patients with disseminated candidiasis. However, this test yields a significant percentage of false-positive results.

## INTERFERING FACTORS

- None significant

# Carcinoembryonic antigen

Carcinoembryonic antigen (CEA) is a protein normally found in embryonic entodermal epithelium and fetal GI tissue. Production of CEA stops before birth, but it may begin again later if a neoplasm develops. Because CEA levels are also raised by biliary obstruction, alcoholic hepatitis, chronic heavy smoking, and other conditions, this test can't be used as a general indicator of cancer. The measurement of enzyme CEA levels by immunoassay is useful for staging and monitoring treatment of certain cancers. (See *Using CEA to monitor cancer treatment*.)

## PURPOSE

- To monitor the effectiveness of cancer therapy
- To assist in preoperative staging of colorectal cancers, assess the adequacy of surgical resection, and test for the recurrence of colorectal cancers

## PATIENT PREPARATION

- Explain to the patient that the CEA test detects and measures a special protein that isn't normally present in adults.

- Inform the patient that the test will be repeated to monitor the effectiveness of therapy, if appropriate.
- Inform the patient that he need not restrict food, fluids, or medications.
- Tell the patient that the test requires a blood sample. Explain who will perform the venipuncture and when.
- Explain to the patient that he may experience slight discomfort from the tourniquet and needle puncture.

## PROCEDURE AND POSTTEST CARE

- Perform a venipuncture and collect the sample in a 7-ml tube without additives.
- Apply direct pressure to the venipuncture site until bleeding stops.
- If a hematoma develops at the venipuncture site, apply pressure.

## PRECAUTIONS

- Handle the sample gently to prevent hemolysis.
- Send the sample to the laboratory immediately.

## REFERENCE VALUES

Normal serum CEA values are less than 5 ng/ml (SI, < 5 mg/L).

## ABNORMAL FINDINGS

Persistent elevation of CEA levels suggests residual or recurrent tumor. If levels exceed normal before surgical resection, chemotherapy, or radiation therapy, their return to normal within 6 weeks suggests successful treatment.

High CEA levels are characteristic in various malignant conditions, particularly entodermally derived neoplasms of the GI organs and lungs, and in certain nonmalignant conditions, such as benign hepatic disease, hepatic cirrhosis, alcoholic pancreatitis, inflammatory bowel disease, and renal failure.

Elevated CEA concentrations may occur in nonendodermal carcinomas, such as breast and ovarian cancers.

## INTERFERING FACTORS

- Chronic cigarette smoking (possible increase)

# Using CEA to monitor
## Cancer Treatment

Because many patients in the early stages of colorectal cancer have normal or low levels of carcinoembryonic antigen (CEA), the CEA test doesn't screen successfully for early malignancy. It's a good tool, however, for monitoring response to cancer therapy.

After a patient's serum CEA level has dropped following surgery, chemotherapy, or other treatment, an increase suggests recurrence of cancer or diminished effectiveness of treatment.

Both charts below illustrate CEA levels in patients during and after treatment for colorectal cancer. In the left chart, initial results show the usual dramatic drop in response to treatment; the subsequent rise in CEA indicates a diminishing response to chemotherapy. In the right chart, the progressive rise in CEA signals a recurrence of cancer 8 months before clinical symptoms or radiologic evidence.

**CEA levels**

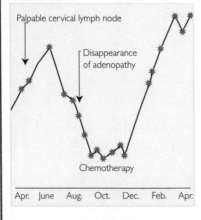

**CEA levels**

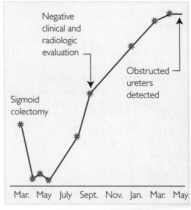

---

## Cardiac blood pool imaging

Cardiac blood pool imaging evaluates regional and global ventricular performance after I.V. injection of human serum albumin or red blood cells (RBCs) tagged with the isotope technetium 99m ($^{99m}$Tc) pertechnetate. In first-pass imaging, a scintillation camera records the radioactivity emitted by the isotope in its initial pass through the left ventricle. Higher counts of radioactivity occur during diastole because there's more blood in the ventricle; lower counts occur during systole as the blood is ejected. The portion of isotope ejected during each heartbeat can then be calculated to determine the ejection fraction; the presence and size of intracardiac shunts can also be determined.

Gated cardiac blood pool imaging, performed after first-pass imaging or as a separate test, has several forms; however, most forms use signals from an electrocardiogram (ECG) to trigger the scintillation camera. In two-frame gated imaging, the camera records left ventricular end-systole and end-diastole for 500 to 1,000 cardiac cycles; superimposition of these gated images allows assessment of left ventricular contraction to find areas of hypokinesia or akinesia.

In multiple-gated acquisition (MUGA) scanning, the camera records 14 to 64 points of a single cardiac cycle, yielding sequential images that can be studied like motion picture films to evaluate regional wall motion and determine the ejection fraction and other indices of cardiac function. In the stress MUGA test, the same test is performed at rest and after exercise to detect changes in ejection fraction and cardiac output. In the nitroglycerin MUGA test, the scintillation camera records points in the cardiac cycle after sublingual nitroglycerin administration to assess its effect on ventricular function.

Cardiac blood pool imaging is more accurate and involves less risk to the patient than does left ventriculography in assessing cardiac function.

## PURPOSE
- To evaluate left ventricular function
- To detect aneurysms of the left ventricle and other motion abnormalities of the myocardial wall (areas of akinesia or dyskinesia)
- To detect intracardiac shunting

## PATIENT PREPARATION
- Explain to the patient that cardiac blood pooling imaging permits assessment of the heart's left ventricle.
- Describe the test, including who will perform it, where it will take place, and its expected duration.
- Tell the patient that he need not restrict food and fluids.
- Explain to the patient that he'll receive an I.V. injection of a radioactive tracer and that a detector positioned above his chest will record the circulation of this tracer through the heart.
- Reassure the patient that the tracer poses no radiation hazard and rarely produces adverse effects.
- Inform the patient that he may experience slight discomfort from the needle puncture, but that the imaging itself is painless.
- Instruct the patient to remain silent and motionless during imaging, unless otherwise instructed.
- Make sure that the patient or a responsible family member has signed an informed consent form.

## PROCEDURE AND POSTTEST CARE
- The patient is placed in a supine position beneath the detector of a scintillation camera, and 15 to 20 millicuries of albumin or RBCs tagged with $^{99m}$Tc pertechnetate are injected I.V.
- For the next minute, the scintillation camera records the first pass of the isotope through the heart so that the aortic and mitral valves can be located.
- Then, using an ECG, the camera is gated for selected 60-msec intervals, representing end-systole and end-diastole, and 500 to 1,000 cardiac cycles are recorded on X-ray or Polaroid film.
- To observe septal and posterior wall motion, the patient may be assisted to modified left anterior oblique position or he may be assisted to a right anterior oblique position and given 0.4 mg of nitroglycerin sublingually. The scintillation camera then records additional gated images to evaluate abnormal contraction in the left ventricle.
- The patient may be asked to exercise as the scintillation camera records gated images.

*Age alert* *If the patient is elderly or physically compromised, assist him to a sitting position and make sure he isn't dizzy. Then provide assistance to get him off the examination table.*

## PRECAUTIONS
- Be aware that cardiac blood pool imaging is contraindicated during pregnancy.

## NORMAL FINDINGS
Normally, the left ventricle contracts symmetrically, and the isotope appears evenly distributed in the scans. Normal ejection fraction is 55% to 65%.

## ABNORMAL FINDINGS
The patient with coronary artery disease usually has asymmetrical blood distribution to the myocardium, which produces segmental abnormalities of ventricular wall motion; such abnormalities may also result from preexisting conditions such as myocarditis. In contrast, the patient with a cardiomyopathy shows globally reduced ejection fractions. In the patient with a left-to-right shunt, the recirculating radioisotope prolongs the downslope of the curve of scintigraphic data; early arrival of activity in the left ventricle or aorta signifies a right-to-left shunt.

## INTERFERING FACTORS
- None significant

# Cardiac catheterization

Cardiac catheterization involves passing a catheter into the right or left side of the heart. Catheterization can determine blood pressure and blood flow in the chambers of the heart, permit blood sample collection, and record films of the heart's ventricles (contrast ventriculography) or arteries (coronary arteriography or angiography).

In catheterization of the left side of the heart, a catheter is inserted into an artery in the antecubital fossa or into the radial or femoral artery through a puncture or cutdown procedure. Guided by fluoroscopy, the catheter is advanced retrograde through the aorta into the coronary artery orifices and left ventricle. Then a contrast medium is injected into the ventricle, permitting radiographic visualization of the ventricle and coronary arteries and filming (cineangiography) of heart activity.

Catheterization of the left side of the heart assesses the patency of the coronary arteries, mitral and aortic valve function, and left ventricular function. It aids in the diagnosis of left ventricular enlargement, aortic stenosis and insufficiency, aortic root enlargement, mitral insufficiency, aneurysm, and intracardiac shunt.

In catheterization of the right side of the heart, the catheter is inserted into an antecubital vein or the femoral vein and is advanced through the inferior vena cava or right atrium into the right side of the heart and the pulmonary artery. Catheterization of the right side of the heart assesses tricuspid and pulmonic valve function and pulmonary artery pressures.

## PURPOSE

● To evaluate valvular insufficiency or stenosis, septal defects, congenital anomalies, myocardial function and blood supply, and cardiac wall motion

## PATIENT PREPARATION

● Explain to the patient that cardiac catheterization evaluates the function of the heart and its vessels.
● Instruct the patient to restrict food and fluids for at least 6 hours before the test, but to continue his prescribed drug regimen unless directed otherwise.
● Describe the test, including who will perform it and where it will take place.
● Make sure that the patient or a responsible family member has signed an informed consent form.
● Inform the patient that he may receive a mild sedative, but will remain conscious during the procedure. He'll lie on a padded table as the camera rotates so that his heart can be examined from different angles.
● Tell the patient that the catheterization team will wear gloves, masks, and gowns to protect him from infection.
● Inform the patient that he'll have an I.V. needle inserted in his arm to administer medication. Assure him that the electrocardiography (ECG) electrodes attached to his chest during the procedure will cause no discomfort.
● Tell the patient that the catheter will be inserted into an artery or a vein in his arm or leg; if the skin above the vessel is hairy, it will be shaved and cleaned with an antiseptic.
● Explain to the patient that he'll experience a slight stinging sensation when a local anesthetic is injected to numb the incision site for catheter insertion and that he may experience pressure as the catheter moves along the blood vessel. Assure him that these sensations are normal.
● Inform the patient that injection of a contrast medium through the catheter may produce a hot, flushing sensation or nausea that quickly passes; instruct him to follow directions to cough or breathe deeply.
● Explain to the patient that he'll be given medication if he experiences chest pain during the procedure and that he may also receive nitroglycerin periodically to dilate coronary vessels and aid visualization. Reassure him that complications, such as a myocardial infarction or thromboembolism, are rare.
● Check the patient's history for hypersensitivity to shellfish, iodine, or the contrast media used in other diagnostic tests; notify the physician of any hypersensitivities.
● Discontinue any anticoagulant therapy, as ordered, to reduce the risk of complications from venous bleeding.
● Just before the procedure, tell the patient to void and put on a gown.

## PROCEDURE AND POSTTEST CARE

- The patient is placed in the supine position on a tilt-top table and secured by restraints. ECG leads are applied for continuous monitoring, and an I.V. line, if not already in place, is started with dextrose 5% in water or normal saline solution at a keep-vein-open rate.
- After a local anesthetic is injected at the catheterization site, a small incision or percutaneous puncture is made into the artery or vein, and the catheter is passed through the needle into the vessel; the catheter is guided to the cardiac chambers or coronary arteries using fluoroscopy.
- When the catheter is in place, the contrast medium is injected through it to visualize the cardiac vessels and structures.
- The patient may be asked to cough or breathe deeply. Coughing helps counteract nausea or light-headedness caused by the contrast medium and can correct arrhythmias produced by its depressant effect on the myocardium; deep breathing can ease catheter placement into the pulmonary artery or the wedge position and moves the diaphragm downward, making the heart easier to visualize.
- During the procedure, the patient may be given nitroglycerin to eliminate catheter-induced spasm or to measure its effect on the coronary arteries.
- Monitor the patient's heart rate and rhythm, respiratory and pulse rates, and blood pressure frequently during the procedure.
- After completion of the procedure, the catheter is removed and pressure should be applied to the incision site for about 30 minutes either manually or with a mechanical compression device. An adhesive bandage or clear occlusive dressing should be applied to protect the site and permit visualization for detection of bleeding or hematoma formation.
- Monitor the patient's vital signs every 15 minutes for 2 hours after the procedure, every 30 minutes for the next 2 hours, and then every hour for 2 hours. If no hematoma or other problems arise, begin checking every 4 hours. If vital signs are unstable, check every 5 minutes and notify the physician.

- Observe the insertion site for a hematoma or blood loss. Additional compression may be necessary to control bleeding.
- Check the patient's color, skin temperature, and peripheral pulse below the puncture site. The brachial approach is associated with a higher incidence of vasospasm (characterized by cool fingers and hands and weak pulses on the affected side); this condition usually resolves within 24 hours.
- Enforce bed rest for 8 hours. If the femoral route was used for catheter insertion, keep the patient's leg extended for 6 to 8 hours; if the antecubital fossa was used, keep the patient's arm extended for at least 3 hours.
- If medications were withheld before the test, check with the physician about resuming their administration.
- Administer prescribed analgesics.
- Make sure a posttest ECG is scheduled to check for possible myocardial damage.

## PRECAUTIONS

- Know that coagulopathy, impaired renal function, and debilitation usually contraindicate catheterization of both sides of the heart. Unless a temporary pacemaker is inserted to counteract induced ventricular asystole, left bundle-branch block contraindicates catheterization of the right side of the heart.
- If the patient has valvular heart disease, be aware that prophylactic antimicrobial therapy may be indicated to guard against subacute bacterial endocarditis.

## NORMAL FINDINGS

Cardiac catheterization should reveal no abnormalities of heart chamber size or configuration, wall motion or thickness, direction of blood flow, or valve motion; the coronary arteries should have a smooth and regular outline and vessels should be patent.

Cardiac catheterization provides information on pressures in the heart's chambers and vessels. Higher pressures than normal are clinically significant; lower pressures, except in shock, usually aren't significant. (See *Normal pressure curves*. See also *Upper limits of normal pressures in cardiac chambers and great vessels in recumbent adults,* page 80.)

## ABNORMAL FINDINGS

Common abnormalities confirmable by cardiac catheterization include coronary artery

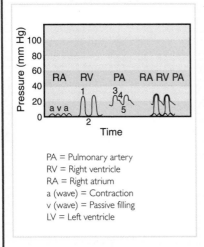
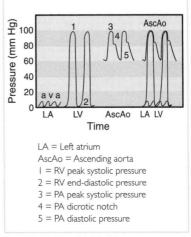
disease (CAD), myocardial incompetence, valvular heart disease, and septal defects.

In CAD, catheterization shows constriction of the lumen of the coronary arteries. Constriction greater than 70% is especially significant, particularly in proximal lesions. Narrowing of the left main coronary artery and occlusion or narrowing high in the left anterior descending artery are commonly indications for revascularization surgery. (This lesion responds best to coronary artery bypass grafting.)

Impaired wall motion can indicate myocardial incompetence from CAD, aneurysm, cardiomyopathy, or congenital anomalies. Comparing the size of the left ventricle in systole and diastole helps assess the efficiency of cardiac muscle contraction, segmental wall motion, chamber size, and ejection fraction. An ejection fraction under 35% generally increases the risk of complications and decreases the probability of successful surgery.

Valvular heart disease is indicated by a gradient, or difference in pressures, above and below a heart valve. For example, systolic pressure measurements on both sides of a stenotic aortic valve show a gradient across the valve. The higher the gradient, the greater the degree of stenosis. If left ventricular systolic pressure measures 200 mm Hg and aortic systolic pressure measures 120 mm Hg, the gradient across the valve is 80 mm Hg. Because these pressures should normally be equal during systole, when the aortic valve is open, a gradient of this magnitude indicates the need for corrective surgery. Incompetent valves can be visualized during ventriculography by watching retrograde flow of the contrast medium across the valve during systole.

Septal defects (atrial and ventricular) can be confirmed by measuring blood oxygen content in both sides of the heart. Elevated blood oxygen levels on the right side indicate

## UPPER LIMITS OF NORMAL PRESSURES IN CARDIAC CHAMBERS AND GREAT VESSELS IN RECUMBENT ADULTS

This chart details the upper limits of normal pressures within the cardiac chambers and great vessels in recumbent adults. Higher-than-normal pressures usually are clinically significant.

| CHAMBER OR VESSEL | PRESSURE (MM HG) |
| --- | --- |
| Right atrium | 6 (mean) |
| Right ventricle | 30/6* |
| Pulmonary artery | 30/12* (mean, 18) |
| Left atrium | 12 (mean) |
| Left ventricle | 140/12* |
| Ascending aorta | 140/90* (mean, 105) |
| Pulmonary artery wedge | Almost identical (±1 to 2 mm Hg) to left atrial mean pressure |

* Peak systolic and end-diastolic

a left-to-right atrial or ventricular shunt; decreased oxygen levels on the left side indicate a right-to-left shunt.

Cardiac output can be measured by analyzing blood oxygen levels in the cardiac chambers. This analysis may be accomplished by drawing blood from cardiac chambers or by injecting contrast medium into the venous circulation and measuring its concentration as it moves past a thermodilution catheter.

### INTERFERING FACTORS
● Equipment malfunction and poor technique
● Patient anxiety (increase in heart rate and cardiac chamber pressures)

## Cardiac magnetic resonance imaging

A great asset in the diagnosis of cardiac disorders, cardiac magnetic resonance imaging (MRI) has the ability to "see through" bone and to delineate fluid-filled soft tissue in great detail as well as produce images of organs and vessels in motion.

In this noninvasive procedure, the patient is placed in a magnetic field, into which a radiofrequency beam is introduced. Resulting energy changes are measured and used by the MRI computer to generate images on a monitor. Cross-sectional images of the anatomy are viewed in multiple planes and recorded for the permanent record.

### PURPOSE
● To identify anatomic sequelae related to myocardial infarction, such as formation of ventricular aneurysm, ventricular wall thinning, and mural thrombus
● To detect and evaluate cardiomyopathy
● To detect and evaluate pericardial disease
● To identify paracardiac or intracardiac masses
● To detect congenital heart disease, such as atrial or ventricular septal defects, and the degree of malposition of the great vessel
● To identify vascular disease, such as thoracic aneurysm and thoracic dissection
● To assess the structure of the pulmonary vasculature

## PATIENT PREPARATION

- Explain to the patient that cardiac MRI assesses the heart's function and structure.
- Tell the patient who will perform the test and where it will take place.
- Inform the patient that he'll be positioned on a narrow bed, which slides into a large cylinder that houses the MRI magnets. Tell him that the scanner will make clicking, whirring, and thumping noises as it moves inside its housing and that he may receive earplugs.
- Explain to the patient who's claustrophobic or anxious about the test's duration that he'll receive a mild sedative to reduce his anxiety or he may need to be scanned in an open MRI scanner, which may take longer, but is less confining.
- Explain to the patient the need to lie flat.
- Reassure the patient that he'll be able to communicate with the technician at all times and that the procedure will be stopped if he feels claustrophobic.
- Immediately before the test, have the patient remove all metal objects. Double-check to make sure that he doesn't have a pacemaker or any surgically implanted joints, pins, clips, valves, or pumps containing metal that could be attracted to the strong MRI magnet. If he does, he won't be able to undergo the test.
- Make sure that the patient or a responsible family member has signed an informed consent form.
- Administer the prescribed sedative.

## PROCEDURE AND POSTTEST CARE

- At the scanner room door, check the patient one last time for metal objects.
- The patient is placed supine on a narrow, padded, nonmetallic bed that slides to the desired position inside the scanner. Radiofrequency waves are directed at his chest. The resulting images are displayed on a monitor and recorded on film or magnetic tape for permanent storage.
- The radiologist may vary the waves and use the computer to manipulate and enhance the images.
- Remind the patient to remain still throughout the procedure.
- Assess how the patient responds to the enclosed environment. Provide reassurance, if necessary.

**Alert** *If the patient is sedated, monitor his hemodynamic, cardiac, respiratory, and mental status until the effects of the sedative have worn off.*

## PRECAUTIONS

- Be aware that the claustrophobic patient may experience anxiety. Be sure to monitor the cardiac patient for signs of ischemia (chest pressure, shortness of breath, or changes in hemodynamic status).
- Know that MRI can't be performed on the patient with a pacemaker or an intracranial aneurysm clip.
- If the patient is unstable, make sure an I.V. line with no metal components is in place and that all equipment is compatible with MRI imaging. If necessary, monitor the patient's oxygen saturation, cardiac rhythm, and respiratory status during the test.
- Know that an anesthesiologist may be needed to monitor a heavily sedated patient.
- Keep in mind that a nurse or radiology technician should maintain verbal contact with the conscious patient.

## NORMAL FINDINGS

MRI should reveal no anatomic or structural dysfunctions in cardiovascular tissue.

## ABNORMAL FINDINGS

MRI can detect cardiomyopathy and pericardial disease. It can also detect atrial or ventricular septal defects or other congenital defects. MRI is useful for identifying paracardiac or intracardiac masses. In addition, it can evaluate the extent of pericardial or vascular disease.

## INTERFERING FACTORS

- The patient's inability to remain still during the procedure

## *Cardiac positron emission tomography*

Cardiac positron emission tomography (PET) scanning combines elements of computed tomography scanning and conventional radionuclide imaging. Like radionuclide imaging, cardiac PET scans measure emissions of injected radioisotopes and convert these values to tomographic images. PET uses radioisotopes of biologically important elements — oxygen, nitrogen, carbon, and fluorine — which emit particles called *positrons*. During positron emissions, gamma rays are detected by the PET scanner and reconstructed to form an image. One distinct advantage of PET scans is that positron emitters can be chemically "tagged" to biologically active molecules, such as carbon monoxide, neurotransmitters, hormones, and metabolites (particularly glucose), enabling study of their uptake and distribution in tissue.

## PURPOSE

- To detect coronary artery disease
- To evaluate myocardial metabolism and contractility
- To distinguish viable from infarcted cardiac tissue, especially during the early stages of myocardial infarction

## PATIENT PREPARATION

- If cardiac PET is ordered to assess myocardial contractility, explain to the patient that the test distinguishes viable tissue from tissue injured by infarction and may also help the physician assess mitochondrial impairment associated with ischemia or evaluate coronary artery obstruction.
- Describe the test to the patient, including who will perform it and where it will take place. Also take the time to describe the equipment.
- Tell the patient that the test is painless, unless an I.V. infusion is planned, in which case he may experience slight discomfort from the tourniquet and needle puncture.
- If fasting is ordered, describe food and fluid restrictions to the patient.
- Explain to the patient that he'll be given a radioactive substance, either by injection or I.V. infusion, and that a highly specialized camera will detect the radioactive decay of this substance and send these data to a computer, which converts the data to an image.
- Tell the patient that he'll undergo an attenuation scan for about 30 minutes. Then he'll receive the appropriate positron emitter and undergo PET scanning.

*Age alert* *Because the radioisotope may be harmful to a fetus, the female patient of child-bearing age should be screened carefully before undergoing cardiac PET.*

## PROCEDURE AND POSTTEST CARE

- The patient is placed in a supine position with his arms above his head.
- An attenuation scan, lasting about 30 minutes, is performed.
- The appropriate positron emitter is administered and scanning is completed.
- An additional positron emitter may be given if comparative studies are needed.
- Instruct the patient to move slowly after the procedure to avoid postural hypotension.
- Encourage increased oral fluid intake to flush the radioisotope from the bladder.

## PRECAUTIONS

- Stress to the patient the importance of remaining still during the study.

## NORMAL FINDINGS

Normally, no areas of ischemic tissue are present. If the patient receives two tracers, the flow and distribution should match, indicating normal tissue.

## ABNORMAL FINDINGS

Reduced blood flow with increased glucose use, indicates ischemia. Reduced blood flow with decreased glucose use, indicates necrotic, scarred tissue.

## INTERFERING FACTORS

- Patient's inability to maintain proper positioning

# Cardiac radiography

Among the most frequently used tests for evaluating cardiac disease and its effects on the pulmonary vasculature, cardiac radiography provides images of the thorax, mediastinum, heart, and lungs. In a routine evaluation, posteroanterior and left lateral views are taken. The posteroanterior view is preferable to the anteroposterior view because it places the heart slightly closer to the plane of the film, providing a sharper, less distorted image. Cardiac radiography may be performed on a bedridden patient using portable equipment, but such equipment can provide only anteroposterior views.

## PURPOSE
- To help detect cardiac disease and abnormalities that change the size, shape, or appearance of the heart and lungs
- To ensure correct positioning of pulmonary artery and cardiac catheters and of pacemaker wires

## PATIENT PREPARATION
- Explain to the patient that cardiac radiography reveals the size and shape of the heart. Tell him who will perform the test and where it will take place. Reassure him that the test uses little radiation and is harmless.
- Instruct the patient to remove jewelry, other metallic objects, and clothing above his waist and to put on a gown that has ties instead of metal snaps.

## PROCEDURE AND POSTTEST CARE
### Posteroanterior view
- The patient stands erect about 6' (2 m) from the X-ray machine with his back to the machine and his chin resting on top of the film cassette holder.
- The holder is adjusted to slightly hyperextend the patient's neck. The patient places his hands on his hips, with his shoulders touching the holder, and centers his chest against it.
- The patient is asked to take a deep breath and hold it during the X-ray film exposure.

### Left lateral view
- The patient is positioned with his arms extended over his head and his left torso flush against the cassette and centered.
- The patient is asked to take a deep breath and hold it during the X-ray film exposure.

### Anteroposterior view (bedridden patient)
- The head of the bed is elevated as much as possible.
- The patient is assisted to an upright position to reduce visceral pressure on the diaphragm and other thoracic structures.
- The film cassette is centered under the patient's back. Although the distance between the patient and the X-ray machine may vary a little, the path between the two should be clear.
- The patient is instructed to take a deep breath and hold it during the X-ray film exposure.

## PRECAUTIONS
- Be aware that cardiac radiography is usually contraindicated during the first trimester of pregnancy. If it's performed during pregnancy, a lead shield or apron should cover the patient's abdomen and pelvic area during the X-ray exposure.
- When testing an ambulatory patient, make sure the radiographic order stipulates a posteroanterior view and not an anteroposterior view. Include on the order any pertinent findings from previous cardiac radiographs as well as the indication for this test.
- When testing a bedridden patient, make sure anyone else in the room is protected from X-rays by a lead shield, a room divider, or sufficient distance.

## NORMAL FINDINGS
Normally, in the posteroanterior view, the thoracic cage appears at least twice as wide as the heart. However, in the anteroposterior view, relative heart size and position may look different, and the cardiac silhouette and vascular markings may increase.

If cardiac radiography is performed to evaluate the position of cardiac catheters and pacemakers, the films should confirm accurate placement.

## ABNORMAL FINDINGS
Cardiac X-ray films must be evaluated based on the patient's history, physical examination, electrocardiography results, and results of previous radiographic tests for cardiac abnormalities.

An abnormal cardiac silhouette usually reflects left or right ventricular or left atrial enlargement, or even a multichamber enlargement. In left ventricular enlargement, the posteroanterior view shows the border of the left side of the heart to be rounded and convex, with lateral extension of the lower left border; the lateral view shows posterior bulging of the left ventricle. In right ventricular enlargement, the posteroanterior view shows secondary prominence of the pulmonary artery segment at the border of the left side of the heart; the lateral view shows anterior bulging in the region of the right ventricular outflow tract.

In left atrial enlargement, the posteroanterior view shows double density of the enlarged left atrium, straightening of the border of the left side of the heart, elevation of the left mainstem bronchus and, rarely, lateral extension of the border of the right side of the heart superior to the right ventricle; the lateral view shows a posterior bulge at the level of the left atrium.

In the posteroanterior view, dilation of pulmonary venous shadows in the superior lateral aspect of the hilus and vascular shadows horizontally and inferiorly along the margin of the right side of the heart may be the first signs of pulmonary vascular congestion. Chronic pulmonary venous hypertension produces an "antler" pattern, caused by dilated superior pulmonary veins and normal or constricted inferior pulmonary veins. Acute alveolar edema may produce a "butterfly" appearance, with increased densities in central lung fields; interstitial pulmonary edema, a cloudy or "cotton-puff" appearance.

## INTERFERING FACTORS
● Patient's inability to maintain inspiration or to remain motionless
● The patient's chest off-center on the film cassette (may hinder viewing of costophrenic angle on X-ray)
● Thoracic deformity such as scoliosis (possible misleading results)
● Underexposure or overexposure of films

# Cardiolipin antibodies

The cardiolipin antibodies test measures serum concentrations of immunoglobulin (Ig) G and IgM antibodies in relation to the phospholipid cardiolipin. These antibodies appear in some patients with lupus erythematosus (LE) whose serum also contains a coagulation inhibitor (lupus anticoagulant). They also appear in some patients who don't fulfill all the diagnostic criteria for LE, but who experience recurrent episodes of spontaneous thrombosis, fetal loss, or thrombocytopenia. Serum concentrations of cardiolipin antibodies are measured by enzyme-linked immunosorbent assay.

## PURPOSE
● To aid in the diagnosis of cardiolipin antibody syndrome in the patient with or without LE who experiences recurrent episodes

of spontaneous thrombosis, fetal loss, or thrombocytopenia

## PATIENT PREPARATION
● Tell the patient that the cardiolipin antibodies test helps diagnose cardiolipin antibody syndrome and LE.
● Inform the patient that he need not restrict food and fluids.
● Tell the patient that the test requires a blood sample. Explain who will perform the venipuncture and when.
● Explain to the patient that he may experience slight discomfort from the tourniquet and needle puncture.

## PROCEDURE AND POSTTEST CARE
● Perform a venipuncture and collect the sample in a 5-ml tube without additives.
● Apply direct pressure to the venipuncture site until bleeding stops.
● If a hematoma develops at the venipuncture site, apply pressure.

## PRECAUTIONS
● Handle the sample gently to prevent hemolysis.
● Send the sample to the laboratory immediately.

## REFERENCE VALUES
Cardiolipin antibody results are reported as negative or positive. A positive result is titered.

## ABNORMAL FINDINGS
A positive result along with a history of recurrent spontaneous thrombosis, fetal loss, or thrombocytopenia suggests cardiolipin antibody syndrome. Treatment may involve anticoagulant or platelet inhibitor therapy.

## INTERFERING FACTORS
● None significant

# Catecholamines, plasma

The plasma catecholamines test, a quantitative (total or fractionated) analysis of plasma catecholamines, has clinical importance in the patient with hypertension and signs of adrenal medullary tumor as well as in the patient with a neural tumor that affects endocrine function. Elevated plasma catecholamine levels necessitate supportive confirmation by urinalysis.

Major catecholamines include the hormones epinephrine, norepinephrine, and dopamine. When secreted into the bloodstream, catecholamines produced in the adrenal medulla prepare the body for the fight-or-flight response. They increase heart rate and contractility, constrict blood vessels and redistribute circulating blood toward the skeletal and coronary muscles, mobilize carbohydrate and lipid reserves, and sharpen alertness. Excessive catecholamine secretion by tumors causes hypertension, weight loss, episodic sweating, headache, palpitations, and anxiety.

Plasma levels commonly fluctuate in response to temperature, stress, postural change, diet, smoking, anoxia, volume depletion, renal failure, obesity, and many drugs.

## PURPOSE
- To rule out pheochromocytoma (adrenal medullary or extra-adrenal) in the patient with hypertension
- To help identify neuroblastoma, ganglioneuroblastoma, and ganglioneuroma
- To distinguish between adrenal medullary tumors and other catecholamine-producing tumors through fractional analysis (Urinalysis for catecholamine degradation products is recommended to support the diagnosis.)
- To aid diagnosis of autonomic nervous system dysfunction such as idiopathic orthostatic hypotension

## PATIENT PREPARATION
- Explain to the patient that the plasma catecholamines test helps determine if hypertension or other symptoms are related to improper hormonal secretion.
- As ordered, instruct the patient to refrain from using self-prescribed medications, especially cold and allergy remedies that may contain sympathomimetics, for 2 weeks before the test.
- Tell the patient to exclude amine-rich foods and beverages, such as bananas, avocados, cheese, coffee, tea, cocoa, beer, and Chianti, from his diet for 48 hours; to maintain vitamin C intake, which is necessary for formation of catecholamines; to abstain from smoking for 24 hours; and to fast for 10 to 12 hours before the test.
- Tell the patient that the test requires one or two blood samples. Explain who will perform the venipuncture and when.
- Explain to the patient that he may experience slight discomfort from the tourniquet and needle puncture.
- If the patient is in your facility, withhold medications that affect catecholamine levels, such as amphetamines, phenothiazines (chlorpromazine), sympathomimetics, and tricyclic antidepressants, as ordered.
- Insert an intermittent venous access device (heparin lock) 24 hours before the test because the stress of the venipuncture itself may significantly raise catecholamine levels.
- Make sure the patient is relaxed and recumbent for 45 to 60 minutes before the test.
- If necessary, provide blankets to keep the patient warm; low temperatures stimulate catecholamine secretion.

## PROCEDURE AND POSTTEST CARE
- Perform a venipuncture between 6 a.m. and 8 a.m.
- Collect the sample in a 10-ml chilled EDTA tube (sodium metabisulfite solution), which can be obtained from the laboratory on request.
- If a second sample is requested, have the patient stand for 10 minutes and draw the sample into another tube exactly like the first.
- If a heparin lock is used, it may be necessary to discard the first 1 or 2 ml of blood. Check with the laboratory for the preferred procedure.
- Apply direct pressure to the venipuncture site until bleeding stops.
- If a hematoma develops at the venipuncture site, apply pressure.
- Instruct the patient that he may resume his usual diet and medications discontinued before the test, as ordered.

## PRECAUTIONS
- After collecting each sample, roll the tube slowly between your palms to distribute the EDTA without agitating the blood.

- Pack the tube in crushed ice to minimize deactivation of catecholamines and send it to the laboratory immediately.
- Indicate on the laboratory request whether the patient was supine or standing during the venipuncture and the time the sample was drawn.

## REFERENCE VALUES

In fractional analysis, catecholamine levels range as follows:
- supine — epinephrine, undetectable to 110 pg/ml (SI, undetectable to 600 pmol/L); norepinephrine, 70 to 750 pg/ml (SI, 413 to 4,432 pmol/L)
- standing — epinephrine, undetectable to 140 pg/ml (SI, undetectable to 764 pmol/L); norepinephrine, 200 to 1,700 pg/ml (SI, 1,182 to 10,047 pmol/L).

## ABNORMAL FINDINGS

High catecholamine levels may indicate pheochromocytoma, neuroblastoma, ganglioneuroblastoma, or ganglioneuroma. Elevations are possible, but don't directly confirm thyroid disorders, hypoglycemia, and cardiac disease. Electroconvulsive therapy, shock resulting from hemorrhage, endotoxins, and anaphylaxis also raise catecholamine levels.

In the patient with normal or low baseline catecholamine levels, failure to show an increase in the sample taken after standing suggests autonomic nervous system dysfunction.

Fractional analysis helps identify the cause of elevated catecholamine levels. For example, adrenal medullary tumors secrete epinephrine, whereas ganglioneuromas, ganglioblastomas, and neuroblastomas secrete norepinephrine.

## INTERFERING FACTORS

- Amphetamines, decongestants, epinephrine, levodopa, phenothiazines, sympathomimetics, and tricyclic antidepressants (increase)
- Reserpine (decrease)
- Radioactive scan performed within 1 week before the test

# Catecholamines, urine

The test for urine catecholamines uses spectrophotofluorimetry to measure urine levels of the major catecholamines — epinephrine, norepinephrine, and dopamine. Epinephrine is secreted by the adrenal medulla; dopamine, by the central nervous system; and norepinephrine, by both. Catecholamines help regulate metabolism and prepare the body for the fight-or-flight response to stress. Certain tumors can also secrete catecholamines.

A 24-hour urine specimen is preferred because catecholamine secretion fluctuates diurnally and in response to pain, heat, cold, emotional stress, physical exercise, hypoglycemia, injury, hemorrhage, asphyxia, and drugs. However, a random specimen may be useful for evaluating catecholamine levels after a hypertensive episode.

For a complete diagnostic workup of catecholamine secretion, urine levels of catecholamine metabolites are also measured. These metabolites — metanephrine, normetanephrine, homovanillic acid (HVA), and vanillylmandelic acid (VMA) — normally appear in the urine in greater quantities than do catecholamines.

## PURPOSE

- To aid in the diagnosis of pheochromocytoma in a patient with unexplained hypertension
- To aid in the diagnosis of neuroblastoma, ganglioneuroma, and dysautonomia

## PATIENT PREPARATION

- Explain to the patient that the urine catecholamine test evaluates adrenal function.
- Inform the patient that he should avoid amine-rich foods and beverages, such as chocolate, coffee, bananas, avocados, cheese, tea, cocoa, beer, and Chianti, for 7 hours before the test and should avoid stressful situations and excessive physical activity during the collection period.
- Tell the patient that the test requires either the collection of urine over 24 hours or a random specimen, and explain the collection procedure.
- Notify the laboratory and physician of medications the patient is taking that

may affect test results; they may need to be restricted.

## PROCEDURE AND POSTTEST CARE
● Collect the patient's urine over a 24-hour period. Use a bottle containing a preservative to keep the specimen acidified to a pH of 3.0 or less. (If a random specimen is ordered, collect it immediately after a hypertensive episode.)
● Instruct the patient that he may resume his usual activities, diet, and medications, as ordered.

## PRECAUTIONS
● Refrigerate a 24-hour specimen or place it on ice during the collection period.
● Send the specimen to the laboratory as soon as the collection is complete.

## REFERENCE VALUES
Values for catecholamine fractionalization range as follows:
● epinephrine — 0 to 20 µg/24 hours (SI, 0 to 109 nmol/24 hours)
● norepinephrine — 15 to 80 µg/24 hours (SI, 89 to 473 nmol/24 hours)
● dopamine — 65 to 400 µg/24 hours (SI, 425 to 2,610 nmol/24 hours).

## ABNORMAL FINDINGS
In a patient with undiagnosed hypertension, elevated urine catecholamine levels following a hypertensive episode usually indicate a pheochromocytoma. If tests indicate a pheochromocytoma, the patient may also be tested for multiple endocrine neoplasia. With the exception of HVA — a dopamine metabolite — catecholamine metabolites may also be elevated. Abnormally high HVA levels rule out a pheochromocytoma because this tumor mainly secretes epinephrine, whose primary metabolite is VMA, not HVA.

Elevated catecholamine levels, without marked hypertension, may be due to a neuroblastoma or a ganglioneuroma, although HVA levels reflect these conditions more accurately. Elevated levels are also seen in severe systemic situations (burns, peritonitis, shock, and septicemia), cor pulmonale, manic depressive disorders, or depressive neurosis. Myasthenia gravis and progressive muscular dystrophy commonly cause urine catecholamine levels to rise above normal, but this test is rarely performed to diagnose these disorders. Consistently low-normal catecholamine levels may indicate dysautonomia marked by orthostatic hypotension.

## INTERFERING FACTORS
● Excessive physical exercise or emotional stress (increase)
● Aminophylline, B-complex vitamins, caffeine, chloral hydrate, insulin, isoproterenol, levodopa, nitroglycerin, methyldopa, monoamine oxidase inhibitors, quinidine, quinine, sympathomimetics, tetracycline, and tricyclic antidepressants (possible increase)
● Clonidine, contrast media containing iodine, guanethidine, and reserpine (possible decrease)
● Erythromycin, methenamine compounds, and phenothiazines (possible increase or decrease)

# *Celiac and mesenteric arteriography*

Celiac and mesenteric arteriography involves the radiographic examination of the abdominal vasculature after intra-arterial injection of a contrast medium through a catheter. Most commonly, the catheter is passed through the femoral artery into the aorta and then, using fluoroscopy, is positioned in the celiac, superior mesenteric, or inferior mesenteric artery. Injection of a contrast medium into one or more of these arteries provides a map of abdominal vasculature; injection into specific arterial branches, called *superselective angiography,* permits detailed visualization of a particular area. As the contrast medium flows through the abdominal vasculature, serial radiographs outline abdominal vessels in the arterial, capillary, and venous phases of perfusion.

Celiac and mesenteric arteriography is indicated when endoscopy can't locate the source of GI bleeding or when barium studies, ultrasonography, and nuclear medicine or computed tomography scanning prove inconclusive in evaluating neoplasms. It's also used to evaluate cirrhosis and portal hypertension (especially when a portacaval shunt is being considered); to evaluate vascular damage, particularly in the spleen and liver, after abdominal trauma; and to detect vascular abnormalities.

Because arteriography can demonstrate the portal vein even when portal venous flow is reversed, it's used more often than splenoportography.

Complications associated with this test include hemorrhage, venous and intracardiac thrombosis, cardiac arrhythmia, and emboli caused by dislodging atherosclerotic plaques.

## PURPOSE
- To locate the source of GI bleeding
- To help distinguish between benign and malignant neoplasms
- To evaluate cirrhosis and portal hypertension
- To evaluate vascular damage after abdominal trauma
- To detect vascular abnormalities

## PATIENT PREPARATION
- Explain to the patient that celiac and mesenteric arteriography permits examination of the abdominal blood vessels after injection of a contrast medium.
- Instruct the patient to fast for 8 hours before the test.
- Tell the patient that he'll receive I.V. conscious sedation and a local anesthetic and that he may feel a brief, stinging sensation as the anesthetic is injected. He may also feel pressure when the femoral artery is palpated, but the local anesthetic will minimize the pain when the needle is introduced into the artery.
- Tell the patient that he may feel a transient burning as the contrast medium is injected.
- Tell the patient that the X-ray equipment makes a loud, clacking sound as the films are taken.
- Instruct the patient to lie still during the test to avoid blurring the films and inform him that restraints may be used to help him remain still.
- Warn the patient that he may feel some temporary stiffness after the test from lying still on the hard X-ray table.
- Tell the patient who will perform the test, where it will take place, and that it takes 30 minutes to 3 hours, depending on the number of vessels studied.

- Make sure that the patient or a responsible family member has signed an informed consent form.
- Check the patient's history for hypersensitivity to iodine, shellfish, or the contrast medium.
- Make sure blood studies (hemoglobin and hematocrit levels; clotting, prothrombin, and partial thromboplastin times; and platelet count) have been completed.
- Just before the procedure, instruct the patient to put on a gown and to remove jewelry and other objects that might obscure anatomic detail on X-ray films.
- Tell the patient to void, and then record his baseline vital signs.
- Administer a sedative if prescribed.

## PROCEDURE AND POSTTEST CARE
- After the patient is placed in a supine position on the X-ray table, an I.V. infusion is started to maintain hydration and to permit emergency administration of medication. The patient is attached to a heart monitor and pulse oximeter and his blood pressure is monitored according to your facility's policy.
- Spot films of the patient's abdomen are taken, and the peripheral pulses are palpated and marked.
- The puncture site is cleaned with soap and water; the area is shaved, cleaned with povidone-iodine preparation, and surrounded by sterile drapes.
- The local anesthetic is injected and the femoral artery is located by palpation. The needle is gently inserted until a pulsing blood flow is obtained.
- A guide wire is passed through the needle into the aorta, and then the needle is removed, leaving the guide wire in place.
- The catheter is inserted over the guide wire and then withdrawn to inject the contrast medium to check for catheter placement. The guide wire is again inserted into the selected artery for fluoroscopic guidance.
- When the wire is in position, the catheter is advanced over it into the artery. The wire is then removed and placement verified by hand injection of contrast medium.
- The automatic injector is then attached to the catheter. As the contrast medium is injected, a series of films is taken in rapid sequence.

- After injecting into one or more major arteries, superselective catheterization may be performed. Using fluoroscopy, the catheter is repositioned in a specific branch of a major artery, contrast medium is injected, and rapid-sequence films are taken. If necessary, several specific branches may be catheterized.
- If an occlusion is detected, balloon angioplasty is performed.
- After filming, the catheter is withdrawn and firm pressure is applied to the puncture site for about 15 minutes.
- Observe the puncture site for hematoma formation and check peripheral pulses.
- Inform the patient that he'll be on bed rest for 4 to 6 hours and that he must keep the leg with the puncture site straight. Don't raise the bed more than 30 degrees. He'll be able to logroll and may use the unaffected leg to reposition himself to use the bedpan.
- Monitor the patient's vital signs until stable and check peripheral pulses. Note the color and temperature of the leg that was used for the test.
- Check the puncture site for bleeding and hematoma. If bleeding develops, apply pressure to the site. If a hematoma develops, apply warm soaks.
- Confirm whether the patient can resume his usual diet. If the patient isn't receiving I.V. infusions, encourage intake of fluids to speed excretion of the contrast medium.

## PRECAUTIONS
- Know that celiac and mesenteric arteriography should be performed cautiously in the patient with coagulopathy.
- **Alert** *Be aware that most reactions to the contrast medium occur within 30 minutes. Watch the patient carefully for cardiovascular shock or arrest, flushing, laryngeal stridor, or urticaria.*
- Know that this test is contraindicated in the pregnant patient because of radiation's possible teratogenic effects.

## NORMAL FINDINGS
X-rays show the three phases of perfusion — arterial, capillary, and venous. The arteries normally taper regularly, becoming gradually smaller with subsequent divisions. The contrast medium then spreads evenly within the sinusoids. The portal vein appears 10 to 20 seconds after the injection as the contrast medium empties from the spleen into the splenic vein or from the intestine into the superior mesenteric vein and further into the portal vein.

## ABNORMAL FINDINGS
GI hemorrhage appears on the angiogram as the extravasation of contrast medium from the damaged vessels. Upper GI hemorrhage can result from such conditions as Mallory-Weiss syndrome, a gastric or peptic ulcer, hemorrhagic gastritis, and an eroded hiatal hernia. Esophageal hemorrhage rarely appears on the angiogram because the contrast medium usually fails to fill the esophageal vein. Lower GI hemorrhage can result from such conditions as bleeding diverticula, carcinoma, and angiodysplasia.

Abdominal neoplasms — carcinoid tumors, adenomas, leiomyomas, angiomas, and adenocarcinomas — can disrupt the normal vasculature in several ways. Neoplasms can invade or encase nearby arteries and veins, distorting their regular channel-like appearance and, in late stages, displacing them. Vessels within the neoplasm, known as *neovasculature,* appear as abnormal vascular areas. Areas of necrosis appear as puddles of contrast medium. Contrast medium may also remain in the neoplasm longer during capillary perfusion, producing a tumor blush or stain on the angiogram. Arteriovenous shunting may also be present, depending on the size and location of the tumor. Because these characteristics aren't uniformly present in all neoplasms, combinations of these characteristics can usually distinguish between benign and malignant neoplasms.

In early or mild cirrhosis, portal venous flow to the liver remains relatively unaffected, and the hepatic artery and its branches appear normal. As this disease progresses, portal venous flow diminishes, the hepatic artery and its branches become dilated and tortuous, and collateral veins develop. In advanced cirrhosis, portal venous flow reverses. However, the portal vein still appears on the X-ray film, which may also show thrombi.

Abdominal trauma commonly causes splenic injury; less commonly, hepatic injury. Splenic rupture usually displaces intrasplenic arterial branches, causing the contrast medium to leak from splenic arteries into the splenic pulp. When rupture occurs without subcapsular hematoma, the spleen usually maintains its normal size. However, in subcapsular hematoma, the spleen enlarges to displace the splenic artery and vein; the subcapsular hematoma itself appears as a large, avascular mass that stretches intrasplenic arteries and compresses the splenic pulp away from the capsule.

Hepatic injury causes similar vascular distortion such as displacement of the common hepatic artery and extrahepatic branches. Intrahepatic and subcapsular hematomas displace and stretch intrahepatic arteries. As the hepatic vascular supply is disrupted, an arteriovenous fistula may develop between the hepatic artery and portal vein.

Various abnormalities affecting the diameter and course of an artery may appear on the angiogram. Atherosclerotic plaques or atheromas — lipid deposits on the intima — narrow the arterial lumen and may even occlude it, resulting in collateral formation. Other identifiable vascular abnormalities include aneurysms, thrombi, and emboli.

## INTERFERING FACTORS
● The patient's inability to remain still during the procedure
● Barium, gas, or stool from a previous procedure (possible poor imaging)
● Presence of an atherosclerotic lesion in the vessel to be cannulated (prevents the entry and passage of catheter)

# Cerebral angiography

Cerebral angiography involves injecting a contrast medium to allow radiographic examination of the cerebral vasculature. Possible injection sites include the femoral, carotid, and brachial arteries. Because it allows visualization of four vessels (the carotid and the vertebral arteries), the femoral artery is used most commonly.

Usually, this test is performed on patients with suspected abnormality of the cerebral vasculature; abnormalities may be suggested by intracranial computed tomography, lumbar puncture, magnetic resonance imaging, or magnetic resonance angiography.

## PURPOSE
● To detect cerebrovascular abnormalities, such as aneurysm or arteriovenous malformation (AVM), thrombosis, narrowing, or occlusion
● To study vascular displacement caused by tumor, hematoma, edema, herniation, vasospasm, increased intracranial pressure (ICP), or hydrocephalus
● To locate clips applied to blood vessels during surgery and to evaluate the postoperative status of affected vessels

## PATIENT PREPARATION
● Explain to the patient that cerebral angiography shows blood circulation in the brain.
● Describe the test, including who will administer it and where it will take place.
● Tell the patient to fast for 8 to 10 hours before the test.
● Make sure that any pretest blood work results are on the chart to determine bleeding tendency or kidney function.
● Explain to the patient that he'll wear a gown and that he must remove all jewelry, dentures, hairpins, and other metallic objects in the radiographic field.
● If ordered, administer a sedative and an anticholinergic drug 30 to 45 minutes before the test.
● Make sure the patient voids before leaving his room.
● Tell the patient that he'll be positioned on an X-ray table with his head immobilized and that he should remain still.
● Explain that a local anesthetic will be administered (some patients — especially children — receive a general anesthetic).
● Explain to the patient that he'll feel a transient burning sensation as the medium is injected; a warm, flushed feeling; a transient headache; a salty or metallic taste in his mouth; or nausea and vomiting after the dye is injected.
● Make sure that the patient or a responsible family member has signed an informed consent form, if required.

*Alert* Check the patient's history for hypersensitivity to iodine, iodine-containing substances (such as shellfish), or other contrast media. Note any hypersensitivities on his chart and report them as appropriate.

## PROCEDURE AND POSTTEST CARE

● Have the patient recline on an X-ray table and instruct him to lie still with his arms at his sides.

● Shave the injection site (femoral, carotid, or brachial artery) and clean it with alcohol and povidone-iodine.

● A local anesthetic is injected. Then the artery is punctured with the appropriate needle and catheterized.

● In the femoral artery approach, a catheter is threaded to the aortic arch.

● In the brachial artery approach (least common), a blood pressure cuff is placed distal to the puncture site and inflated before injection to prevent the contrast medium from flowing into the forearm and hand.

● After X-rays or fluoroscopy verifies placement of the needle or catheter, the contrast medium is injected. Observe the patient for an adverse reaction, such as hives, flushing, or laryngeal stridor.

● An initial series of lateral and anteroposterior X-rays is taken, developed, and reviewed. Depending on the results, more contrast medium may be injected and another series taken.

● During the test, maintain arterial catheter patency by continuous or periodic flushing. Monitor the patient's vital and neurologic signs.

● When a satisfactory series of X-rays is obtained, the needle (or catheter) is withdrawn. Apply firm pressure to the puncture site for 15 minutes.

● After the test, observe the patient for bleeding, check distal pulses, and apply a pressure bandage.

● Typically, the patient will be on bed rest for 6 to 8 hours. Administer prescribed pain medications and monitor his vital signs and neurologic status for 6 hours. The patient is usually discharged the same day.

● Observe the puncture site for signs of extravasation (redness, swelling) and apply an ice bag to ease the patient's discomfort and minimize swelling. If bleeding occurs, apply firm pressure to the puncture site and inform the physician.

⚕ *Alert  If the femoral approach was used, keep the patient's affected leg straight for 6 hours or longer and routinely check pulses distal to the site (dorsalis pedis, popliteal). Monitor the leg for temperature, color, and sensation. Thrombosis or hematoma can occlude blood flow; extravasation*

*can also impede blood flow by exerting pressure on the artery.*

● Monitor the patient for disorientation and weakness or numbness in the extremities (signs of thrombosis or hematoma) and for arterial spasms, which may produce symptoms of transient ischemic attacks.

● If the brachial approach was used, immobilize the affected arm for 6 hours or longer and routinely check the radial pulse.

● Place a sign near the patient's bed warning personnel not to take blood.

● Observe the patient's arm and hand for changes in color, temperature, or sensation. If they become pale, cool, or numb, report these changes at once.

● After the test, tell the patient he may resume his usual diet. Encourage him to drink fluids to help him pass the contrast medium.

## PRECAUTIONS

● Know that cerebral angiography is contraindicated in the patient with hepatic, renal, or thyroid disease.

● Be aware that this test is also contraindicated in the patient with a hypersensitivity to iodine or contrast media.

● If the patient has been receiving aspirin or other anticoagulants such as warfarin daily, take extra care when compressing the puncture site. Anticoagulants may need to be discontinued for 3 days before testing.

⚕ *Alert  Monitor the catheter puncture site frequently and closely for hemorrhage or hematoma formation. If either occurs, notify the physician immediately.*

## NORMAL FINDINGS

During the arterial phase of perfusion, the contrast medium fills and opacifies superficial and deep arteries and arterioles; it opacifies superficial and deep veins during the venous phase. The finding of apparently normal (symmetrical) cerebral vasculature must be correlated with the patient's history and clinical status.

## ABNORMAL FINDINGS

Changes in the caliber of vessel lumina suggest vascular disease, possibly due to spasms, plaques, fistulas, AVM, or arteriosclerosis. Diminished blood flow to vessels may be related to increased ICP. (See *Comparing normal and abnormal cerebral angiograms,* page 92.)

## COMPARING NORMAL AND ABNORMAL CEREBRAL ANGIOGRAMS

The angiograms below show the differences between normal and abnormal cerebral vasculature. The cerebral angiogram on the left is normal. The cerebral angiogram on the right shows occluded blood vessels caused by a large arteriovenous malformation.

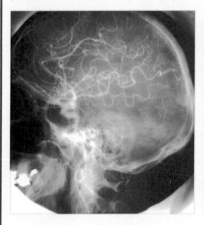 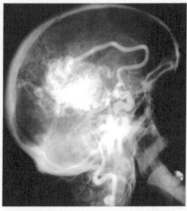

Vessel displacement may reflect the presence and size of a tumor, areas of edema, or obstruction of the cerebrospinal fluid pathway. Cerebral angiography may also show circulation within a tumor, usually giving precise information on its position and nature. Meningeal blood supply originating in the external carotid artery may indicate an extracerebral tumor, but usually designates a meningioma. Such a tumor may arise outside the brain substance, but it may still be within the cerebral hemisphere.

### INTERFERING FACTORS
● Head movement during the test (possible poor imaging)
● Metal objects in X-ray field (possible poor imaging)

# Cerebrospinal fluid analysis

Cerebrospinal fluid (CSF), a clear substance that circulates in the subarachnoid space, has many vital functions. It protects the brain and spinal cord from injury and transports products of neurosecretion, cellular biosynthesis, and cellular metabolism through the central nervous system (CNS).

For qualitative analysis, CSF is most commonly obtained by lumbar puncture (usually between the third and fourth lumbar vertebrae) and, rarely, by cisternal or ventricular puncture. A CSF specimen may also be obtained during other neurologic tests such as myelography.

### PURPOSE
● To measure CSF pressure as an aid in detecting an obstruction of CSF circulation
● To aid in the diagnosis of viral or bacterial meningitis, subarachnoid or intracranial hemorrhage, tumors, and brain abscesses
● To aid in the diagnosis of neurosyphilis and chronic CNS infections
● To check for Alzheimer's disease

### PATIENT PREPARATION
● Describe the procedure to the patient and explain that CSF analysis analyzes the fluid around the spinal cord.

- Inform the patient that he need not restrict food and fluids.
- Tell the patient who will perform the procedure and where it will take place.
- Advise the patient that a headache is the most common adverse effect of a lumbar puncture, but reassure him that his cooperation during the test helps minimize this effect.
- Make sure that the patient or a responsible family member has signed an informed consent form.
- If the patient is unusually anxious, assess and report his vital signs.

## PROCEDURE AND POSTTEST CARE

- Position the patient on his side at the edge of the bed with his knees drawn up to his abdomen and his chin on his chest. Provide pillows to support the spine on a horizontal plane. This position allows full flexion of the spine and easy access to the lumbar subarachnoid space. Help him maintain this position by placing one arm around his knees and the other arm around his neck.
- If the sitting position is preferred, have the patient sit up and bend his chest and head toward his knees. Help him maintain this position throughout the procedure.
- After the skin is prepared for injection, the area is draped. Warn the patient that he'll probably experience a transient burning sensation when the local anesthetic is injected.
- Tell the patient that when the spinal needle is inserted, he may feel slight local pain as the needle transverses the dura mater.
- Ask the patient to report pain or sensations that differ from or continue after this expected discomfort because such sensations may indicate irritation or puncture of a nerve root, requiring needle repositioning.
- Instruct the patient to remain still and breathe normally; movement and hyperventilation can alter pressure readings or cause injury.
- The anesthetic is injected, and the spinal needle is inserted in the midline, between the spinous processes of the vertebrae (usually between the third and fourth lumbar vertebra). At this point, initial (or opening) CSF pressure is measured and a specimen is obtained.
- After the specimen is collected, label the containers in the order in which they were filled and find out if specific instructions are required for the laboratory.
- Next, a final pressure reading is taken, and the needle is removed.
- Clean the puncture site with a local antiseptic, such as povidone-iodine solution, and apply a small adhesive bandage.
- Check whether the patient must lie flat or if the head of his bed may be slightly elevated. In most cases, you'll be instructed to keep the patient lying flat for 8 hours after lumbar puncture. Some physicians, however, allow a 30-degree elevation at the head of the bed. Remind the patient that although he must not raise his head, he can turn from side to side.
- Encourage the patient to drink fluids. Provide a flexible straw.
- Check the puncture site for redness, swelling, and drainage every hour for the first 4 hours, and then every 4 hours for the first 24 hours.
- If CSF pressure is elevated, assess the patient's neurologic status every 15 minutes for 4 hours. If he's stable, assess him every hour for 2 hours and then every 4 hours or according to the pretest schedule.

**Alert** *Watch the patient for complications of lumbar puncture, such as reaction to the anesthetic, meningitis, bleeding into the spinal canal, cerebellar tonsillar herniation, and medullary compression. Signs of meningitis include fever, neck rigidity, and irritability; signs of herniation include decreased level of consciousness, changes in pupil size and equality, altered vital signs (including widened pulse pressure, decreased pulse rate, and irregular respirations), and respiratory failure.*

## PRECAUTIONS

- Be aware that infection at the puncture site contraindicates removal of CSF; in a patient with increased intracranial pressure, CSF should be removed with extreme caution because the rapid reduction in pressure that follows withdrawal of fluid can cause cerebellar tonsillar herniation and medullary compression.
- During the procedure, observe closely for adverse reactions, such as elevated pulse rate, pallor, or clammy skin. Report any significant changes immediately.
- Record the collection time on the test request form. Send the form and labeled specimens to the laboratory immediately after collection.

# FINDINGS IN CEREBROSPINAL FLUID ANALYSIS

| Test | Normal | Abnormality | Implications |
|------|--------|-------------|--------------|
| Pressure | 50 to 180 mm $H_2O$ | Increase | Increased intracranial pressure |
| | | Decrease | Spinal subarachnoid obstruction above puncture site |
| Appearance | Clear, colorless | Cloudy | Infection |
| | | Xanthochromic or bloody | Subarachnoid, intracerebral, or intra-ventricular hemorrhage; spinal cord obstruction; traumatic tap (usually noted only in initial specimen) |
| | | Brown, orange, or yellow | Elevated protein levels, red blood cell (RBC) breakdown (blood present for at least 3 days) |
| Protein | 15 to 50 mg/dl (SI, 0.15 to 0.5 q/L) | Marked increase | Tumors, trauma, hemorrhage, diabetes mellitus, polyneuritis, blood in cerebrospinal fluid (CSF) |
| | | Marked decrease | Rapid CSF production |
| Gamma globulin | 3% to 12% of total protein | Increase | Demyelinating disease, neurosyphilis, Guillain-Barré syndrome |
| Glucose | 50 to 80 mg/dl (SI, 2.8 to 4.4 mmol/L) | Increase | Systemic hyperglycemia |
| | | Decrease | Systemic hypoglycemia, bacterial or fungal infection, meningitis, mumps, postsubarachnoid hemorrhage |
| Cell count | 0 to 5 white blood cells | Increase | Active disease: meningitis, acute infection, onset of chronic illness, tumor, abscess, infarction, demyelinating disease |
| | No RBCs | RBCs | Hemorrhage or traumatic lumbar puncture |
| Venereal Disease Research Laboratories, test for syphilis, and other serologic tests | Nonreactive | Positive | Neurosyphilis |
| Chloride | 118 to 130 mEq/L (SI, 118 to 130 mmol/L) | Decrease | Infected meninges |
| Gram stain | No organisms | Gram-positive or gram-negative organisms | Bacterial meningitis |

## FINDINGS

For a summary of normal and abnormal findings in CSF analysis, see *Findings in cerebrospinal fluid analysis.*

Normally, the CSF pressure is recorded and the appearance of the specimen is checked. Three tubes are collected routinely and are sent to the laboratory for protein, sugar, and cell analysis as well as for serologic testing such as the Venereal Disease Research Laboratory test for neurosyphilis. A separate specimen is also sent to the laboratory for culture and sensitivity testing. Electrolyte analysis and Gram stain may be ordered as supplementary tests. CSF electrolyte levels are of special interest in the patient with abnormal serum electrolyte levels or CSF infection and in the patient receiving hyperosmolar agents.

## INTERFERING FACTORS

- Patient position and activity (possible increase or decrease in CSF pressure)
- Crying, coughing, or straining (possible increase in CSF pressure)
- Delay between collection time and laboratory testing (possible invalidation of test results, especially cell counts)

## *Cervical punch biopsy*

Cervical punch biopsy or cervical biopsy is the excision by sharp forceps of a tissue specimen from the cervix for histologic examination. Generally, multiple biopsies are done to obtain specimens from all areas with abnormal tissue or from the squamocolumnar junction and other sites around the cervical circumference. The biopsy site is selected by direct visualization of the cervix with a colposcope or by Schiller's test, which stains normal squamous epithelium a dark mahogany, but fails to color abnormal tissue. Other biopsies are done to detect other gynecological disorders. The biopsy is performed when the cervix is least vascular, usually 1 week after menses.

## PURPOSE

- To evaluate suspicious cervical lesions
- To diagnose cervical cancer

## PATIENT PREPARATION

- Describe the procedure to the patient, and explain that it provides a cervical tissue specimen for microscopic study.
- Tell the patient who will perform the biopsy and where it will be done.
- Tell the patient that she may experience mild discomfort during and after the biopsy.
- Advise the outpatient to have someone accompany her home after the biopsy.
- Make sure the patient or a responsible family member has signed an informed consent form.
- Ask the patient to void just before the biopsy.

## PROCEDURE AND POSTTEST CARE

- Place the patient in the lithotomy position, and tell her to relax as the unlubricated speculum is inserted.
- For direct visualization, the colposcope is inserted through the speculum, the biopsy site is located, and the cervix is cleaned with a swab soaked in 3% acetic acid solution. The biopsy forceps are then inserted through the speculum or the colposcope, and tissue is removed from any lesion or from selected sites, starting from the posterior lip to avoid obscuring other sites with blood. Each specimen is immediately put in 10% formalin solution in a labeled bottle. To control bleeding after biopsy, the cervix is swabbed with 5% silver nitrate solution (cautery or sutures may be used instead). If bleeding persists, the examiner may insert a tampon.
- For Schiller's test, an applicator stick saturated with iodine solution is inserted through the speculum. This stains the cervix to identify lesions for biopsy.
- Record the patient's and physician's names and the biopsy sites on the laboratory request.
- Instruct the patient to avoid strenuous exercise for 24 hours after the biopsy. Encourage the outpatient to rest briefly before leaving the office.
- If a tampon was inserted after the biopsy, tell the patient to leave it in place for 8 to 24 hours. Inform her that some bleeding may occur, but tell her to report heavy bleeding (heavier than menses). Warn the patient to avoid using additional tampons, which can irritate the cervix and provoke bleeding.
- Tell the patient to avoid douching and intercourse for 2 weeks, or as directed, if

she has undergone such treatments as cryotherapy or laser treatment during the procedure.
● Tell the patient that a foul-smelling, gray-green vaginal discharge is normal for several days after the biopsy and may persist for 3 weeks.

## PRECAUTIONS
● Send the specimens to the laboratory immediately.

## NORMAL FINDINGS
Normal cervical tissue is composed of columnar and squamous epithelial cells, loose connective tissue, and smooth-muscle fibers with no dysplasia or abnormal cell growth.

## ABNORMAL FINDINGS
Histologic examination of a cervical tissue specimen is used to identify abnormal cells and to differentiate the tissue as intraepithelial neoplasia or invasive cancer. If the cause of an abnormal Papanicolaou test isn't demonstrated by cervical biopsy or if the specimen shows advanced dysplasia or carcinoma in situ, a cone biopsy is performed under general anesthesia to obtain a larger tissue specimen and to allow a more accurate evaluation of dysplasia.

## INTERFERING FACTORS
● Nonrepresentative specimens obtained

## Chest radiography

In chest radiography, X-rays or electromagnetic waves penetrate the chest and cause an image to form on specially sensitized film. Air appears radiolucent, whereas normal tissue, bone, and abnormalities — such as infiltrates, foreign bodies, fluids, and tumors — appear as densities on the film. A chest X-ray is most useful when compared with previous films to detect changes. (See *Selected clinical implications of chest X-ray films.*)

## PURPOSE
● To detect cardiopulmonary disorders, such as emphysema, pneumonia, atelectasis, pneumothorax, pulmonary bullae, pleurisy, cardiomegaly, heart failure, and tumors
● To detect mediastinal abnormalities, such as tumors, and cardiac disease such as heart failure
● To determine the correct placement of pulmonary catheters, endotracheal tubes, and other chest tubes
● To determine the location and size of lesions or foreign bodies
● To help assess pulmonary status
● To evaluate the patient's response to interventions

## PATIENT PREPARATION
● Explain to the patient that chest radiography assesses chest anatomy.
● Tell the patient that he need not restrict food and fluids.
● Describe the test, including who will perform it and when it will take place.
● Provide a gown without snaps, and instruct the patient to remove jewelry and other metallic objects that may be in the X-ray field.
● Explain to the patient that he'll be asked to take a deep breath and to hold it momentarily while the film is being taken to provide a clearer view of pulmonary structures.

## PROCEDURE AND POSTTEST CARE
● If a stationary X-ray machine is used, the patient stands or sits in front of the machine so films can be taken of the posteroanterior and left lateral views.
● If a portable X-ray machine is used at the patient's bedside, the patient is moved to the top of the bed, if his tolerance permits. Nipple markers are placed on the patient's areolae to identify nipples, which may have a distinct density and otherwise appear as nodules. The head of the bed is elevated for maximum upright positioning. The patient must take a deep breath and hold it for several seconds.
● Place cardiac monitoring lead wires, I.V. tubing from central lines, pulmonary artery catheter lines, and safety pins as far from the X-ray field as possible.

## PRECAUTIONS
● Know that chest radiography is usually contraindicated during the first trimester of pregnancy; however, when radiography is absolutely necessary, a lead apron placed

# SELECTED CLINICAL IMPLICATIONS OF CHEST X-RAY FILMS

| NORMAL ANATOMIC LOCATION AND APPEARANCE | POSSIBLE ABNORMALITY | IMPLICATIONS |
|---|---|---|
| **TRACHEA** | | |
| Visible midline in the anterior mediastinal cavity; translucent tubelike appearance | ◆ Deviation from midline | ◆ Tension pneumothorax, atelectasis, pleural effusion, consolidation, mediastinal nodes or, in children, enlarged thymus |
| | ◆ Narrowing with hourglass appearance and deviation to one side | ◆ Substernal thyroid or stenosis secondary to trauma |
| **HEART** | | |
| Visible in the anterior left mediastinal cavity; solid appearance due to blood contents; edges may be clear in contrast with surrounding air density of the lung | ◆ Shift<br>◆ Hypertrophy<br>◆ Cardiac borders obscured by stringy densities ("shaggy heart") | ◆ Atelectasis, pneumothorax<br>◆ Cor pulmonale, heart failure<br>◆ Cystic fibrosis |
| **AORTIC KNOB** | | |
| Visible as water density; formed by the arch of the aorta | ◆ Solid densities, possibly indicating calcifications<br>◆ Tortuous shape | ◆ Atherosclerosis<br><br>◆ Atherosclerosis |
| **MEDIASTINUM (MEDIASTINAL SHADOW)** | | |
| Visible as the space between the lungs; shadowy appearance that widens at the hilum of the lungs | ◆ Deviation to nondiseased side; deviation to diseased side by traction<br>◆ Gross widening | ◆ Pleural effusion or tumor, fibrosis or collapsed lung<br><br>◆ Neoplasms of esophagus, bronchi, lungs, thyroid, thymus, peripheral nerves, lymphoid tissue; aortic aneurysm; mediastinitis; cor pulmonale |
| **RIBS** | | |
| Visible as thoracic cage | ◆ Break or misalignment<br>◆ Widening of intercostal spaces | ◆ Fractured sternum or ribs<br>◆ Emphysema |
| **SPINE** | | |
| Visible midline in the posterior chest; straight bony structure | ◆ Spinal curvature<br>◆ Break or misalignment | ◆ Scoliosis, kyphosis |

*(continued)*

| NORMAL ANATOMIC LOCATION AND APPEARANCE | POSSIBLE ABNORMALITY | IMPLICATIONS |
|---|---|---|
| **CLAVICLES** | | |
| Visible in upper thorax; intact and equidistant in properly centered X-ray films | ◆ Break or misalignment | ◆ Fractures |
| **HILA (LUNG ROOTS)** | | |
| Visible above the heart, where pulmonary vessels, bronchi, and lymph nodes join the lungs; appear as small, white, bilateral densities | ◆ Shift to one side<br>◆ Accentuated shadows | ◆ Atelectasis<br>◆ Pneumothorax, emphysema, pulmonary abscess, tumor, enlarged lymph nodes |
| **MAINSTEM BRONCHUS** | | |
| Visible; part of the hila with translucent tubelike appearance | ◆ Spherical or oval density | ◆ Bronchogenic cyst |
| **BRONCHI** | | |
| Usually not visible | ◆ Visible | ◆ Bronchial pneumonia |
| **LUNG FIELDS** | | |
| Usually not visible throughout, except for the blood vessels | ◆ Visible<br>◆ Irregular | ◆ Atelectasis<br>◆ Resolving pneumonia, infiltrates, silicosis, fibrosis, neoplasm |
| **HEMIDIAPHRAGM** | | |
| Rounded, visible; right side 3/8" to 3/4" (1 to 2 cm) | ◆ Elevation of diaphragm (difference in elevation can be measured on inspiration and expiration to detect movement)<br>◆ Flattening of diaphragm<br>◆ Unilateral elevation of either side<br>◆ Unilateral elevation of left side only | ◆ Active tuberculosis, pneumonia, pleurisy, acute bronchitis, active disease of the abdominal viscera, bilateral phrenic nerve involvement, atelectasis<br>◆ Asthma, emphysema<br>◆ Possible unilateral phrenic nerve paresis<br>◆ Perforated ulcer (rare), gas distention of stomach or splenic flexure of colon, free air in abdomen |

over the patient's abdomen can shield the fetus.

● If the patient is intubated, check that no tubes have been dislodged during positioning.

● To avoid exposure to radiation, leave the room or the immediate area while the films are being taken. If you must stay in the area, wear a lead-lined apron or protective clothing.

## FINDINGS

For an overview of normal and abnormal chest radiography findings, see *Selected clinical* implications of chest X-ray films. For an accurate diagnosis, radiography findings must be correlated with the results of additional radiologic and pulmonary tests as well as physical assessment findings. For example, pulmonary hyperinflation with a low diaphragm and generalized increased radiolucency may suggest emphysema, but may also occur in a healthy person.

## INTERFERING FACTORS
● Portable chest X-rays (possibly lower-quality image than stationary X-rays)
● Portable chest X-rays taken in the anteroposterior position (may show larger cardiac shadowing than do other X-rays due to shorter distance between beam and anterior structures)
● Patient in a supine position (hides fluid levels that are visible in decubitus views)
● Patient's inability to take a full inspiration
● Underexposure or overexposure of films
● Incorrect view of the area (For example, lateral film views reveal infiltrates [pneumonia, atelectasis] that may not be seen in anteroposterior views or posteroanterior views because of heart obstruction.)
● Extrathoracic structures, such as breast implants or body piercings (may be radiopaque and obscure anatomical area of interest)

---

# Chlamydia trachomatis *culture*

---

The most common sexually transmitted disease in the United States, chlamydia is caused by the organism *Chlamydia trachomatis*. Identification of this parasite requires cultivation in the laboratory. After incubation, Chlamydia-infected cells can be detected by fluorescein isothiocyanate-conjugated monoclonal antibodies or by iodine stain.

Detection in cell cultures of *C. psittaci* and *C. pneumoniae* requires specific technical manipulations and reagents; deoxyribonucleic acid detection may also be performed in women who may be susceptible to the infections, whether they have symptoms or not.

Culture is the detection method of choice, but rapid noncultural (antigen detection) procedures are also available.

## PURPOSE
● To confirm infections caused by *C. trachomatis*

## PATIENT PREPARATION
● Explain the purpose of the *C. trachomatis* culture test to the patient.
● Describe the procedure for collecting a specimen for culture.
● If the specimen will be collected from the patient's genital tract, instruct him not to urinate for 3 to 4 hours before the specimen is taken.
● Tell the female patient not to douche for 24 hours before the test.
● Tell the male patient that he may experience some burning and pressure as the culture is taken, but that the discomfort will subside after a few minutes.

## PROCEDURE AND POSTTEST CARE
● Obtain a specimen of the epithelial cells from the infected site. In adults, these sites may include the eye, urethra (rather than from the purulent exudate that may be present), endocervix, and rectum.
● Obtain a urethral specimen by inserting a cotton-tipped applicator ¾″ ( to 2″ (2 to 5 cm) into the urethra.
● To collect a specimen from the endocervix, use a microbiologic transport swab or cytobrush.
● Extract the specimen into 2SP transport medium.
● Specimens collected from the throat, eye, or nasopharynx and aspirates from infants should be extracted into 2SP transport medium. The specimens are sent to the laboratory at 39.2° F (4° C).
● If the anticipated time between specimen collection and inoculation into cell culture is more than 24 hours, freeze the 2SP transport medium and send it to the laboratory with dry ice.

🔬 **Alert**  *In the patient suspected of being sexually abused, be sure to process the specimen by culture rather than by antigen detection methods.*
● Advise the patient to avoid all sexual contact until after test results are available.
● If the culture confirms infection, provide counseling for the patient about treatment of sexual partners.

## PRECAUTIONS

- Place the male patient in the supine position to prevent him from falling if vasovagal syncope occurs when the cotton swab or wire loop is introduced into the urethra. Observe for profound hypotension, bradycardia, pallor, and sweating.
- Wear gloves when performing the procedures and handling the specimens.
- Collect a urethral specimen at least 1 hour after the patient has voided to prevent loss of urethral secretions.
- After collecting the specimens, carefully dispose of gloves, swabs, and speculum to prevent staff exposure.

## NORMAL FINDINGS

Normally, no *C. trachomatis* appears in the culture.

## ABNORMAL FINDINGS

A positive culture confirms *C. trachomatis* infection.

## INTERFERING FACTORS

- Use of an antimicrobial drug within a few days before specimen collection (possible inability to recover *C. trachomatis*)
- In males, voiding within 1 hour of specimen collection; in females, douching within 24 hours of specimen collection (fewer organisms available for culture)
- Contamination of the specimen due to fecal material in a rectal culture
- Menses

# Chloride, serum

The serum chloride test is used to measure serum levels of chloride, the major extracellular fluid (ECF) anion. Chloride helps maintain osmotic pressure of blood and, therefore, helps regulate blood volume and arterial pressure. Chloride levels also affect acid-base balance. Chloride is absorbed from the intestines and excreted primarily by the kidneys.

## PURPOSE

- To detect acid-base imbalance (acidosis or alkalosis) and to aid evaluation of fluid status and extracellular cation-anion balance

## PATIENT PREPARATION

- Explain to the patient that the serum chloride test is used to evaluate the chloride content of blood.
- Tell the patient that the test requires a blood sample. Explain who will perform the venipuncture and when.
- Explain to the patient that he may experience slight discomfort from the tourniquet and needle puncture.
- Inform the patient that he need not restrict food and fluids.
- Notify the laboratory and physician of medications the patient is taking that may affect test results; they may need to be restricted.

## PROCEDURE AND POSTTEST CARE

- Perform a venipuncture and collect the sample in a 3- or 4-ml clot-activator tube.
- Apply direct pressure to the venipuncture site until bleeding stops.
- If a hematoma develops at the venipuncture site, apply pressure.
- Instruct the patient to resume any medications discontinued before the test, as ordered.

## PRECAUTIONS

- Handle the sample gently to prevent hemolysis.

## REFERENCE VALUES

Normally, serum chloride levels range from 100 to 108 mEq/L (SI, 100 to 108 mmol/L) in adults.

## ABNORMAL FINDINGS

Chloride levels are inversely related to bicarbonate levels, reflecting acid-base balance. Excessive loss of gastric juices or other secretions containing chloride may cause hypochloremic metabolic alkalosis; excessive chloride retention or ingestion may lead to hyperchloremic metabolic acidosis.

An increase in chloride levels may be evident in severe dehydration, complete renal shutdown, head injury (producing neurogenic hyperventilation), and primary aldosteronism.

Decreased levels of chloride may result from low sodium and potassium levels due to prolonged vomiting, gastric suctioning, intestinal fistula, chronic renal failure, and Addison's disease. Heart failure or edema resulting in excess ECF can cause dilutional hypochloremia.

**Alert** *Observe the patient with hypochloremia for hypertonicity of muscles, tetany, depressed respirations, and decreased blood pressure with dehydration. In the patient with hyperchloremia, be alert for signs of developing stupor, rapid deep breathing, and weakness, which may lead to coma.*

## INTERFERING FACTORS

- Use of acetazolamide, ammonium chloride, androgens, boric acid, cholestyramine, estrogens, excessive I.V. infusion of sodium chloride, nonsteroidal anti-inflammatory agents, oxyphenbutazone, and phenylbutazone (possible increase)
- Use of bicarbonates, ethacrynic acid, furosemide, laxatives, or thiazide diuretics, and prolonged I.V. infusion of dextrose 5% in water (decrease)

# Chromosome analysis

Chromosome analysis studies the relationship between the microscopic appearance of chromosomes and an individual's phenotype — the expression of the genes in physical, biochemical, or physiologic traits.

Ideally, chromosomes are studied during metaphase, the middle phase of mitosis, when new cell poles appear. During metaphase, colchicine (a cell poison) is added to arrest cell division. Cells are harvested, stained, and then examined under a microscope. These cells are then photographed to record the karyotype — the systematic arrangement of chromosomes in groupings according to size and shape.

Only rapidly dividing cells, such as bone marrow or neoplastic cells, permit direct, immediate study. In other cells, mitosis is stimulated by the addition of phytohemagglutinin. Indications for the test determine the specimen required (blood, bone marrow, amniotic fluid, skin, or placental tissue) and the specific analytic procedure. Umbilical cord sampling may also be used to perform chromosome analysis.

## PURPOSE

- To identify chromosomal abnormalities, such as hypoploidy or hyperploidy, as the underlying cause of malformation, maldevelopment, or disease

## PATIENT PREPARATION

- Explain to the patient or his parents, if appropriate, the purpose of the chromosome analysis.
- Tell the patient who will perform the test and what kind of specimen will be required.
- Inform the patient when results will be available, according to the specimen required.

## PROCEDURE AND POSTTEST CARE

- Collect a blood sample (in a 5- to 10-ml heparinized tube), a tissue specimen, 1 ml of bone marrow, or at least 20 ml of amniotic fluid.
- Provide appropriate posttest care, depending on the procedure used to collect the specimen.
- Explain the test results and their implications to the patient or his parents, if he's a child, with a chromosomal abnormality.
- Recommend appropriate genetic or other counseling and follow-up care, if necessary, such as an infant stimulation program for a patient with Down syndrome.

## PRECAUTIONS

- Keep all specimens sterile, especially those requiring a tissue culture.
- To facilitate interpretation of test results, send the specimen to the laboratory immediately after collection, with a brief patient history and the indication for the test.
- Refrigerate the specimen if transport is delayed, but never freeze it.

**Alert** *Before a skin biopsy, make sure the povidone-iodine solution is thoroughly removed with alcohol. This solution could prevent cell growth.*

## NORMAL FINDINGS

The normal cell contains 46 chromosomes: 22 pairs of nonsex chromosomes (autosomes) and 1 pair of sex chromosomes (Y for the male-determining chromosome, X for the female-determining chromosome). On a karyotype, chromosomes are arranged according to size and the location of their primary constrictions, or centromeres.

The centromere may be medial (metacentric), slightly to one end of the chromosome (submetacentric), or entirely to one end

## CHROMOSOME ANALYSIS FINDINGS

| SPECIMEN AND INDICATION | RESULT | IMPLICATIONS |
|---|---|---|
| **BLOOD** | | |
| To evaluate abnormal appearance or development, suggesting chromosomal irregularity | ◆ Abnormal chromosome number (aneuploidy) or arrangement | ◆ Identifies specific chromosomal abnormality |
| To evaluate couples with a history of miscarriages or to identify balanced translocation carriers having unbalanced offspring | ◆ Normal chromosomes<br><br>◆ Parental balanced translocation carrier | ◆ Miscarriage unrelated to parental chromosomal abnormality<br>◆ Increased risk of repeated abortion or unbalanced offspring requiring amniocentesis in future pregnancies |
| To detect chromosomal rearrangements in rare genetic diseases predisposing the patient to malignant neoplasms | ◆ Chromosomal rearrangements, gaps, and breaks | ◆ Occurs in Bloom's syndrome, Fanconi's syndrome, telangiectasia; patient predisposed to malignant neoplasms |
| **BLOOD OR BONE MARROW** | | |
| To identify Philadelphia chromosome and confirm chronic myelogenous leukemia | ◆ Translocation of chromosome 22q (long arm) to another chromosome (often chromosome 9)<br>◆ Aneuploidy (usually due to abnormalities in chromosomes 8 and 12)<br>◆ Trisomy 21 | ◆ Aids in the diagnosis of chronic myelogenous leukemia<br><br>◆ Occurs in acute myelogenous leukemia<br><br>◆ Occasionally occurs in chronic lymphocytic leukemia cells |
| **SKIN** | | |
| To evaluate abnormal appearance or development, suggesting chromosomal irregularity | ◆ All chromosomal abnormalities possible | ◆ Same as chromosomal abnormality in blood; rarely, mosaic individual has normal blood but abnormal skin chromosomes |
| **AMNIOTIC FLUID** | | |
| To evaluate the developing fetus with possible chromosomal abnormality | ◆ All chromosomal abnormalities possible | ◆ Same as chromosomal abnormality in blood or fetus |

(acrocentric). The largest chromosomes are displayed first; the others are arranged in order of decreasing size, with the two sex chromosomes traditionally placed last. By convention, the centromere is always placed at the top in a karyotype. Thus, if the two pairs of chromosomal arms are of unequal length, the arm above the centromere will be shorter. The letter "p" designates the short arm; the letter "q", the long arm.

Special stains identify individual chromosomes and locate and enumerate particular

CHROMOSOME ANALYSIS FINDINGS *(continued)*

| SPECIMEN AND INDICATION | RESULT | IMPLICATIONS |
|---|---|---|
| **PLACENTAL TISSUE** | | |
| To evaluate products of conception after a miscarriage to determine if the abnormality is fetal or placental in origin | ◆ All chromosomal abnormalities possible | ◆ More than 50% of aborted tissue is chromosomally abnormal |
| **TUMOR TISSUE** | | |
| For research purposes only | ◆ Many chromosomal abnormalities possible | ◆ Although malignant tumors aren't associated with specific chromosomal aberrations, most are aneuploid, usually hyperploid |

portions of chromosomes. Trypsin, alkali, heat denaturation, and Giemsa stain are used for visible light microscopy; quinacrine stain, for ultraviolet microscopy. These techniques produce nonuniform staining of each chromosome in a repetitive, banded pattern. The mechanism of chromosome banding is unknown, but seems related to primary deoxyribonucleic acid sequence and protein composition of the chromosome.

## ABNORMAL FINDINGS

Chromosomal abnormalities may be numerical or structural. Implications of chromosome analysis results depend on the specimen and indications for the test. (See *Chromosome analysis findings.*) Any numerical deviation from the norm of 46 chromosomes is called *aneuploidy.* Less than 46 chromosomes is called *hypoploidy;* more than 46, *hyperploidy.* Special designations exist for whole multiples of the haploid number 23: diploidy for the normal somatic number of 46, triploidy for 69, tetraploidy for 92, and so forth.

When the deviation occurs within a single pair of chromosomes, the suffix "-somy" is used, as in trisomy for the presence of three chromosomes instead of the usual pair or monosomy for the presence of only one chromosome.

Aneuploidy most commonly follows failure of the chromosomal pair to separate

(nondisjunction) during anaphase, the mitotic stage that follows metaphase. It may also result from anaphase lag, in which one of the normally separated chromosomes fails to move to a pole and is left out of the daughter cells.

If nondisjunction or anaphase lag occurs during meiosis, the cells of the zygote will all be the same. Errors in mitotic division after zygote formation will produce more than one cell line (mosaicism).

Structural chromosomal abnormalities result from chromosome breakage. Intrachromosomal rearrangement occurs within a single chromosome in these forms:
● deletion — loss of an end (terminal) or middle (interstitial) portion of a chromosome
● inversion — end-to-end reversal of a chromosome segment, which may be pericentric inversion (including the centromere) or paracentric inversion (occurring in only one arm of the chromosome)
● ring chromosome formation — breakage of both ends of a chromosome and reunion of the ends
● isochromosome formation — abnormal splitting of the centromere in a transverse rather than a longitudinal plane.

Interchromosomal rearrangements (of more than one chromosome, usually two) also occur. The most common rearrangement is translocation, or exchange, of genetic material between two chromosomes. Translocations may be balanced, in which the cell neither loses nor gains genetic material; unbalanced, in which a piece of genetic material is gained or lost from each cell; reciprocal (in children), in which two chromosomes exchange material; or Robertsonian, in which two chromosomes join to form one combined chromosome with little or no loss of material.

## INTERFERING FACTORS

● Chemotherapy (possible abnormal results due to chromosome breaks)

● Contamination of tissue with bacteria, fungus, or a virus (possible inhibition of culture growth)

● Inclusion of maternal cells in a specimen obtained by amniocentesis, with subsequent culturing (possible false results)

# Cold agglutinins

Cold agglutinins are antibodies, usually of the immunoglobulin M type, that cause red blood cells (RBCs) to aggregate at low temperatures. They may occur in small amounts in healthy people. Transient elevations of these antibodies develop during certain infectious diseases, notably primary atypical pneumonia. This test reliably detects such pneumonia within 1 to 2 weeks after its onset.

Patients with high cold agglutinin titers, such as those with primary atypical pneumonia, may develop acute transient hemolytic anemia after repeated exposure to cold; patients with persistently high titers may develop chronic hemolytic anemia.

## PURPOSE

● To help confirm primary atypical pneumonia

● To provide additional diagnostic evidence for cold agglutinin disease associated with many viral infections and lymphoreticular cancer

● To detect cold agglutinins in the patient with suspected cold agglutinin disease

## PATIENT PREPARATION

● Explain to the patient that the cold agglutinins test detects antibodies in the blood

that attack RBCs after exposure to low temperatures.

● Tell the patient that the test will be repeated to monitor his response to therapy, if appropriate.

● Tell the patient that he need not restrict food and fluids.

● Tell the patient that the test requires a blood sample. Explain who will perform the venipuncture and when.

● Explain to the patient that he may experience slight discomfort from the tourniquet and needle puncture.

● If the patient is receiving antimicrobial drugs, note this on the laboratory request because the use of such drugs may interfere with the development of cold agglutinins.

## PROCEDURE AND POSTTEST CARE

● Perform a venipuncture and collect the sample in a 7-ml tube without additives that has been prewarmed to 98.6° F (37° C).

● If cold agglutinin disease is suspected, keep the patient warm. If he's exposed to low temperatures, agglutination may occur within peripheral vessels, possibly leading to frostbite, anemia, Raynaud's phenomenon and, rarely, focal gangrene.

✷ *Alert  Watch for signs of vascular abnormalities, such as mottled skin, purpura, jaundice, pallor, pain or swelling of extremities, and cramping of fingers and toes. Hemoglobinuria may result from severe intravascular hemolysis on exposure to severe cold.*

● Apply direct pressure to the venipuncture site until bleeding stops.

● If a hematoma develops at the venipuncture site, apply pressure.

## PRECAUTIONS

● Handle the sample gently to prevent hemolysis.

● Send the sample to the laboratory immediately.

✷ *Alert  Don't refrigerate the sample; cold agglutinins will coat the RBCs, leaving none in the serum for testing.*

## REFERENCE VALUES

Cold agglutinin screening results are reported as negative or positive. A positive result, indicating the presence of cold agglutinin, is titered. A normal titer is less than 1:64.

## ABNORMAL FINDINGS

High titers may occur as primary phenomena or secondary to infections or lymphoreticular cancer. They may be present in infectious mononucleosis, cytomegalovirus infection, hemolytic anemia, multiple myeloma, scleroderma, malaria, cirrhosis of the liver, congenital syphilis, peripheral vascular disease, pulmonary embolism, trypanosomiasis, tonsillitis, staphylococcemia, scarlatina, influenza and, occasionally, pregnancy.

Chronically elevated titers are most commonly associated with pneumonia and lymphoreticular cancer; an acute transient elevation typically accompanies many viral infections.

In primary atypical pneumonia, cold agglutinins appear in serum in one-half to two-thirds of all patients during the first week of acute infection, even before antimycoplasmal antibodies can be detected by complement fixation or metabolic inhibition tests. Thus, titers usually become positive at 7 days, peak above 1:32 in 4 weeks, and disappear rapidly after 6 weeks. When sequential titers verify this pattern and clinical evidence of pneumonia exists, the diagnosis is confirmed.

Extremely high titers (greater than 1:2,000) can occur with idiopathic cold agglutinin disease that precedes lymphoma development. Patients with titers this high are susceptible to intravascular agglutination, which causes significant clinical problems.

## INTERFERING FACTORS

- Refrigeration of the sample before serum is separated from RBCs (possible false-low titer)
- Antimicrobial drugs

## *Colonoscopy*

Colonoscopy uses a flexible fiber-optic video endoscope to permit visual examination of the lining of the large intestine. It's indicated for patients with a history of constipation or diarrhea, persistent rectal bleeding, and lower abdominal pain when the results of proctosigmoidoscopy and a barium enema test are negative or inconclusive.

## PURPOSE

- To detect or evaluate inflammatory and ulcerative bowel disease
- To locate the origin of lower GI bleeding
- To aid in the diagnosis of colonic strictures and benign or malignant lesions
- To evaluate the colon postoperatively for recurrence of polyps and malignant lesions

## PATIENT PREPARATION

- Check the patient's medical history for allergies, medications, and information pertinent to the current complaint.
- Tell the patient that colonoscopy permits examination of the lining of the large intestine.
- Instruct the patient to maintain a clear-liquid diet for 24 to 48 hours before the test and to take nothing by mouth after midnight the night before.
- Describe the procedure and tell the patient who will perform it and where it will take place.
- Explain that the large intestine must be thoroughly cleaned to be clearly visible. Instruct the patient to take a laxative, as ordered, or 1 gallon of GoLYTELY solution in the evening (drinking the chilled solutions at 8 oz [236.6 ml] every 10 minutes until the entire gallon is consumed).
- If fecal results aren't clear, the patient will receive a laxative, suppository, or tap water enema.

*Alert* Don't administer a soapsuds enema because this irritates the mucosa and stimulates mucus secretions that may hinder the examination.

- Inform the patient that an I.V. line will be started before the procedure and that a sedative will be administered just before the procedure. Advise him to arrange for someone to drive him home if he receives sedation.
- Assure the patient that the colonoscope is well lubricated to ease its insertion, that it initially feels cool, and that he may feel an urge to defecate when it's inserted and advanced.
- Explain to the patient that air may be introduced through the colonoscope to distend the intestinal wall and to facilitate viewing the lining and advancing the instrument. Tell him that flatus normally escapes around the instrument because of air insufflation and that he shouldn't attempt to control it.

# VIRTUAL COLONOSCOPY

Virtual colonoscopy combines computed tomography (CT) scanning and X-ray images with sophisticated image processing computers to generate three-dimensional (3-D) images of the patient's colon. These images are interpreted by a skilled radiologist to recreate and evaluate the colon's inner surface. Although this procedure isn't as accurate as a routine colonoscopy, it's less invasive and is useful in screening the patient with small polyps. The colon must be free from residue and fecal material. Bowel preparation consists of following a clear-liquid diet for 24 hours before the procedure; also, the patient performs GoLYTELY bowel preparation the evening before and takes a rectal suppository on the morning of the test.

Before performing the CT scan, a thin, red rectal tube is placed, and air is introduced into the colon to distend the bowel. This insertion may produce mild cramping. The CT scan is done with the patient in the supine position and again while prone. The scans are then shipped over a network to a 3-D image processing computer, and a radiologist evaluates the images obtained. If polyps are identified, a colonoscopy may be scheduled to remove them.

---

- Tell the patient that suction may be used to remove blood or liquid stool that obscure vision, but that this won't cause discomfort.
- Make sure that the patient or a responsible family member has signed an informed consent form.

## PROCEDURE AND POSTTEST CARE

- Place the patient on his left side with his knees flexed and drape him.
- Obtain the patient's baseline vital signs. Be prepared to monitor vital signs throughout the procedure. If the patient has known cardiac disease, continuous electrocardiographic monitoring should be instituted. Continuous or periodic pulse oximetry is advisable, particularly in the high-risk patient with possible respiratory depression secondary to sedation.
- Instruct the patient to breathe deeply and slowly through his mouth as the physician palpates the mucosa of the anus and rectum and inserts the lubricated colonoscope through the patient's anus into the sigmoid colon under direct vision.
- Insufflate a small amount of air to locate the bowel lumen and then advance the scope through the rectum.
- When the instrument reaches the descending sigmoid junction, assist the patient to a supine position to aid the scope advance, if necessary. After passing the splenic flexure, the scope is advanced through the transverse colon, through the hepatic flexure, and into the ascending colon and cecum.
- Abdominal palpation or fluoroscopy may be used to help guide the colonoscope through the large intestine.
- Suction may be used to remove blood and secretions that obscure vision.
- Biopsy forceps or a cytology brush may be passed through the colonoscope to obtain specimens for histologic or cytologic examination; an electrocautery snare may be used to remove polyps.
- If the examiner removes a tissue specimen, immediately place it in a specimen bottle containing 10% formalin; immediately place cytology smears in a Coplin jar containing 95% ethyl alcohol. Send specimens to the laboratory immediately. Specimens should be collected in accordance with laboratory and pathology guidelines.
- Observe the patient closely for signs of bowel perforation. Report such signs immediately.
- Check the patient's vital signs and document them according to your facility's policy.
- After the patient has recovered from sedation, he may resume his usual diet unless the physician orders otherwise.
- Provide privacy while the patient rests after the procedure; tell him that he may pass large amounts of flatus after insufflation.
- If a polyp has been removed, inform the patient that his stool may contain some blood, but excessive bleeding should be reported immediately.

# Abnormal colonoscopy

These two views, taken with a fiber-optic colonscope, show ulcerative colitis (left) and diverticulosis (right).

**Fiber-optic colonoscope**

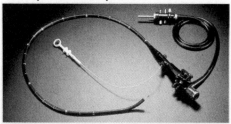

**Ulcerative colitis**

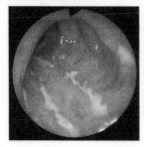

**Diverticulosis**

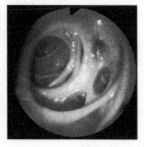

Photos from *Stedman's Medical Dictionary*, 27e. Philadelphia: Lippincott Williams & Wilkins, 2004.

## PRECAUTIONS

- Although it's usually a safe procedure, be aware that colonoscopy can cause perforation of the large intestine, excessive bleeding, and retroperitoneal emphysema.
- Know that this procedure is contraindicated in the pregnant woman near term, the patient who has had a recent acute myocardial infarction or abdominal surgery, and one with ischemic bowel disease, acute diverticulitis, peritonitis, fulminant granulomatous colitis, perforated viscus, or fulminant ulcerative colitis. For these cases or for screening purposes, a virtual colonoscopy may be an option to help visualize polyps early before they become concerns. (See *Virtual colonoscopy*.)

> **Alert** *Watch the patient closely for adverse effects of the sedative. Have available emergency resuscitation equipment and an opioid antagonist, such as naloxone, for I.V. use if necessary.*

- If a polyp is removed but not retrieved during the examination, give enemas and strain stools to retrieve it if the physician requests it.

## NORMAL FINDINGS

Normally, the mucosa of the large intestine beyond the sigmoid colon appears light pink-orange and is marked by semilunar folds and deep tubular pits. Blood vessels are visible beneath the intestinal mucosa, which glistens from mucus secretions.

## ABNORMAL FINDINGS

Visual examination of the large intestine, coupled with histologic and cytologic test results, may indicate proctitis, granulomatous or ulcerative colitis, Crohn's disease, and malignant or benign lesions. Diverticular disease or the site of lower GI bleeding can be detected through colonoscopy alone. (See *Abnormal colonoscopy*.)

## INTERFERING FACTORS

- Fixation of the sigmoid colon due to inflammatory bowel disease, surgery, or radiation therapy (may hinder passage of the colonoscope)
- Blood from acute colonic hemorrhage (hinders visualization)
- Insufficient bowel preparation or barium retained in the intestine from previous diagnostic studies (makes accurate visual examination impossible)

# Colposcopy

In colposcopy, the cervix and vagina are visually examined by an instrument containing a magnifying lens and a light (colposcope). This test is primarily used to evaluate abnormal cytology or grossly suspicious lesions and to examine the cervix and vagina after a positive Papanicolaou (Pap) test.

During the examination, a biopsy may be performed and photographs taken of suspicious lesions with the colposcope and its attachments. Risks of biopsy include bleeding (especially during pregnancy) and infection.

## PURPOSE

- To help confirm cervical intraepithelial neoplasia or invasive carcinoma after a positive Pap test
- To evaluate vaginal or cervical lesions
- To monitor conservatively treated cervical intraepithelial neoplasia
- To monitor the patient whose mother received diethylstilbestrol during pregnancy

## PATIENT PREPARATION

- Explain to the patient that the colposcopy magnifies the image of the vagina and cervix, providing more information than does a routine vaginal examination.
- Inform the patient that she need not restrict food and fluids.
- Tell the patient who will perform the examination, where it will be done, and that it's safe and painless.
- Tell the patient that a biopsy may be performed during colposcopy and that this procedure may cause minimal but easily controlled bleeding and mild cramping.

- Make sure that the patient or a responsible family member has signed an informed consent form.

## PROCEDURE AND POSTTEST CARE

- The examiner puts on gloves. With the patient in the lithotomy position, the examiner inserts the speculum and, if indicated, performs a Pap test. Help the patient relax during insertion by telling her to breathe through her mouth and concentrate on relaxing her abdominal muscles.
- The cervix is gently swabbed with acetic acid solution to remove mucus.
- After the cervix and vagina are examined, biopsy is performed on areas that appear abnormal.
- Bleeding is stopped by applying pressure, hemostatic solutions, or by cautery.
- After a biopsy, instruct the patient to abstain from intercourse and to avoid inserting anything in her vagina (including a tampon) until healing of the biopsy site is confirmed (in approximately 10 days).

## NORMAL FINDINGS

Surface contour of the cervical vessels should be smooth and pink; columnar epithelium appears grapelike. Different tissue types are sharply demarcated.

## ABNORMAL FINDINGS

Abnormal colposcopy findings include white epithelium (leukoplakia) or punctate and mosaic patterns, which may indicate underlying cervical intraepithelial neoplasia; keratinization in the transformation zone, which may indicate cervical intraepithelial neoplasia or invasive carcinoma; and atypical vessels, which may indicate invasive carcinoma.

Other abnormalities visible on colposcopic examination include inflammatory changes (usually from infection), atrophic changes (usually from aging or, less commonly, the use of hormonal contraceptives), erosion (probably from increased pathogenicity of vaginal flora due to changes in vaginal pH), and papilloma and condyloma (possibly from viruses).

Histologic study of the biopsy specimen confirms colposcopic findings. If the examination and biopsy results are inconsistent with the Pap test and biopsy of the squamocolumnar junction results, conization of the cervix for biopsy may be indicated.

## INTERFERING FACTORS

- Presence of menstrual blood or foreign materials in the cervix, such as creams and medications (possible obstruction to visualization)

# Complement assays

*Complement* is a collective term for a system of at least 20 serum proteins designed to destroy foreign cells and help remove foreign materials. The system may be triggered by contact with antigen-antibody complexes or by clotting factor XIIa. A cascade of events follows, resulting in the formation of a complex that ruptures cell membranes.

Complement components are numerically designated as C1 through C9, with C1 having three subcomponents: C1q, C1r, and C1s. These components constitute 3% to 4% of total serum globulins and play a key role in antibody-mediated immune reactions.

Complement can function as a defense by promoting the removal of infectious agents or as a threat by triggering destructive reactions in host tissues. Therefore, complement deficiency can increase susceptibility to infection and can predispose a person to other diseases. Complement assays are thus indicated in patients with known or suspected immunomediated disease or a repeatedly abnormal response to infection.

Normally, complement is present in serum in an inactive state until "fixed," or activated, in the classic pathway by binding to an antibody-coated surface. In the classic pathway, a specific antibody identifies and coats an antigen that enters the body. C1 then recognizes and binds with this specific antibody, activating the complement cascade (a series of enzymatic reactions involving all complement components) and producing a coordinated inflammatory response, which usually results in cell lysis or some other damaging outcome.

In the alternate pathway, substances, such as polysaccharides, bacterial endotoxins, and aggregated immunoglobulins, react with properdin and factors B, D, H, and I, producing an enzyme that activates C3. In turn, C3 activates the remainder of the complement cascade.

In both pathways, specific inhibitors regulate the sequential activation of complement components. The C1 esterase inhibitor, the most commonly studied inhibitor, regulates the classic pathway; the C3b inhibitor can regulate either pathway because C3 is a pivotal component of both.

Various laboratory methods are used to evaluate and measure total complement and its components; hemolytic assay, laser nephelometry, and radial immunodiffusion are the most common.

Although complement assays provide valuable information about the patient's immune system, the results must be considered in light of serum immunoglobulin and autoantibody tests for a definitive diagnosis of immunomediated disease or an abnormal response to infection.

## PURPOSE

- To help detect immunomediated disease and genetic complement deficiency
- To monitor the effectiveness of therapy

## PATIENT PREPARATION

- Explain to the patient that the complement assay test measures a group of proteins that fight infection.
- Inform the patient that he need not restrict food and fluids.
- Tell the patient that the test requires a blood sample. Explain who will perform the venipuncture and when.
- Explain to the patient that he may experience slight discomfort from the tourniquet and needle puncture.
- If the patient is scheduled for C1q assay, check his history for recent heparin therapy. Report such therapy to the laboratory.

## PROCEDURE AND POSTTEST CARE

- Perform a venipuncture and collect the sample in a 7-ml tube without additives.
- Because many patients with complement defects have a compromised immune system, keep the venipuncture site clean and dry.
- Apply direct pressure to the venipuncture site until bleeding stops.
- If a hematoma develops at the venipuncture site, apply pressure.

## PRECAUTIONS

* Handle the sample gently to prevent hemolysis.
* Send the sample to the laboratory immediately because complement is heat labile and deteriorates rapidly.

## REFERENCE VALUES

Normal values for complement range as follows:

* total complement—25 to 110 U/ml (SI, 0.25 to 1.1 g/L)
* C3—70 to 150 mg/dl (SI, 0.7 to 1.5 g/L)
* C4—15 to 45 mg/dl (SI, 0.15 to 0.45 g/L).

## ABNORMAL FINDINGS

Complement abnormalities may be genetic or acquired; acquired abnormalities, however, are most common. Depressed total complement levels (which are clinically more significant than are elevations) may result from excessive formation of antigen-antibody complexes, insufficient complement synthesis, inhibitor formation, or increased complement catabolism and are characteristic in such conditions as systemic lupus erythematosus (SLE), acute poststreptococcal glomerulonephritis, and acute serum sickness. Low levels may also occur in some patients with advanced cirrhosis of the liver, multiple myeloma, hypogammaglobulinemia, or rapidly rejecting allografts.

Elevated total complement may occur in obstructive jaundice, thyroiditis, acute rheumatic fever, rheumatoid arthritis, acute myocardial infarction, ulcerative colitis, and diabetes.

C1 esterase inhibitor deficiency is characteristic in hereditary angioedema, the most common genetic abnormality associated with complement; C3 deficiency is characteristic in recurrent pyogenic infection and disease activation in SLE; C4 deficiency is characteristic in SLE and rheumatoid arthritis. C4 is increased in autoimmune hemolytic anemia.

## INTERFERING FACTORS

* Recent heparin therapy

# Computed tomography of the liver and biliary tract

In computed tomography (CT) of the liver and biliary tract, multiple X-rays pass through the upper abdomen and are measured while detectors record differences in tissue attenuation. A computer reconstructs these data as a two-dimensional image on a monitor. CT scanning accurately distinguishes the biliary tract and the liver if the ducts are large. Use of I.V. contrast media during CT scanning can accentuate different densities.

Although CT scanning and ultrasonography detect biliary tract and liver disease equally well, the latter technique is performed more commonly. CT scanning is more expensive than ultrasonography and requires exposure to moderate amounts of radiation. However, it's the test of choice in patients who are obese and in those with livers positioned high under the rib cage because bone and excessive fat hinder ultrasound transmission.

## PURPOSE

* To distinguish between obstructive and nonobstructive jaundice
* To detect intrahepatic tumors and abscesses, subphrenic and subhepatic abscesses, cysts, and hematomas

## PATIENT PREPARATION

* Explain to the patient that CT scanning helps detect biliary tract and liver disease.
* Tell the patient that he'll be given a contrast medium to drink and then he should fast until after the examination. If contrast isn't ordered, fasting isn't necessary.
* Explain to the patient who will perform the test and where it will take place.
* Inform the patient that he'll be placed on an adjustable table, which is positioned inside a scanning gantry. Assure him that the test will be painless.
* Tell the patient that he'll be asked to remain still during the test and to hold his breath when instructed. Stress the importance of remaining still during the test because movement can cause artifact, thereby prolonging the test and limiting its accuracy.

- If I.V. contrast medium is being used, inform the patient that he may experience transient discomfort from the needle puncture and a localized feeling of warmth on injection as well as a salty or metallic taste. Tell him to immediately report nausea, vomiting, dizziness, headache, and hives.
- Check the patient's history for hypersensitivity to iodine, seafood, or the contrast media used in other diagnostic tests.
- If a contrast medium has been ordered, give the patient the oral contrast medium supplied by the radiology department.
- Make sure that the patient or a responsible family member has signed an informed consent form.

## PROCEDURE AND POSTTEST CARE
- The patient is placed in a supine position on an X-ray table, and the table is positioned within the opening of the scanning gantry.
- A series of transverse X-ray films is taken and recorded on magnetic tape. This information is reconstructed by a computer and appears as images on a television screen.
- These images are studied, and selected ones are photographed. When the first series of films is completed, the images are reviewed.
- Contrast enhancement may be performed. After the contrast medium is injected, a second series of films is taken, and the patient is carefully observed for an allergic reaction.

## PRECAUTIONS
- Be aware that CT scanning of the biliary tract and liver is usually contraindicated during pregnancy.
- Know that use of an I.V. contrast medium is contraindicated in the patient with hypersensitivity to iodine or with severe renal or hepatic disease.

## NORMAL FINDINGS
Normally, the liver has a uniform density that's slightly greater than that of the pancreas, kidneys, and spleen. Linear and circular areas of slightly lower density, representing hepatic vascular structures, may interrupt this uniform appearance. The portal vein is usually visible; the hepatic artery usually isn't. I.V. contrast medium enhances the isodensity of vascular structures and liver parenchyma.

Typically, intrahepatic biliary radicles aren't visible, but the common hepatic and bile ducts may be visible as low-density structures. Because bile has the same density as water, use of an I.V. contrast medium improves demarcation of the biliary tract by enhancing the surrounding parenchyma and vascular structures.

Like the biliary ducts, the gallbladder is visible as a round or elliptic low-density structure. A contracted gallbladder may be impossible to visualize.

## ABNORMAL FINDINGS
Most focal hepatic defects appear less dense than do the normal parenchyma, and CT scans can detect small lesions. Use of rapid-sequence scanning with an I.V. contrast medium helps distinguish between the two because the normal parenchyma shows greater enhancement than focal defects.

Primary and metastatic neoplasms may appear as well-circumscribed or poorly-defined areas of slightly lower density than the normal parenchyma. However, some lesions have the same density as the liver parenchyma and may be undetectable. Neoplasms that are especially large may distort the liver's contour. Hepatic abscesses appear as relatively low-density, homogeneous areas, usually with well-defined borders. Hepatic cysts appear as sharply defined round or oval structures and have a density lower than do abscesses and neoplasms.

The density of a hepatic hematoma varies with its age. A recent clot is as dense as or slightly denser than the normal parenchyma; a resolving clot is somewhat less dense than the normal parenchyma. Intrahepatic hematomas vary in shape; subcapsular hematomas are usually crescent-shaped and compress the liver away from the capsule.

When distinguishing between obstructive and nonobstructive jaundice, biliary duct dilation indicates the former and an absence of dilation indicates the latter. Dilated intrahepatic bile ducts appear as low-density linear and circular branching structures. Dilation of the common hepatic duct, common bile duct, and gallbladder may also be apparent, depending on the site and severity of obstruction. Use of an I.V. contrast medium helps detect biliary dilation, especially when the ducts are only slightly dilated.

Usually, CT scanning can identify the cause of obstruction — for example, calculi or pancreatic carcinoma. However, if the site of obstruction must be located before surgery, percutaneous transhepatic cholangiography or endoscopic retrograde cholangiopancreatography (less common) may be performed as well.

## INTERFERING FACTORS
● Presence of oral or I.V. contrast media, including barium, in the bile duct from earlier tests (possible poor imaging)

# Computed tomography of the pancreas

In computed tomography (CT) of the pancreas, multiple X-rays penetrate the upper abdomen while a detector records the differences in tissue attenuation, which is then displayed as an image on a television screen. A series of cross-sectional views can provide a detailed look at the pancreas. CT scanning accurately distinguishes the pancreas and surrounding organs and vessels if enough fat is present between the structures. Use of an I.V. or oral contrast medium can further accentuate differences in tissue density.

CT scanning is replacing ultrasonography as the test of choice for examining the pancreas. Although ultrasonography costs less and involves less risk for the patient, it's also less accurate. In retroperitoneal disorders, specifically when pancreatitis is suspected, CT scanning goes beyond ultrasonography by showing the general swelling that accompanies acute inflammation of the gland. In chronic cases, CT scanning easily detects calcium deposits commonly missed by simple radiography, particularly in obese patients.

## PURPOSE
● To detect pancreatic carcinoma or pseudocysts
● To detect or evaluate pancreatitis
● To distinguish between pancreatic disorders and disorders of the retroperitoneum

## PATIENT PREPARATION
● Explain to the patient that CT scanning helps detect disorders of the pancreas.
● Instruct the patient to fast after administration of the oral contrast medium.

● Describe the test, including who will perform it and where it will take place.
● Tell the patient that he'll be placed on an adjustable table that's positioned inside a scanning gantry. Assure him that the procedure is painless.
● Explain to the patient that he'll need to remain still during the test and periodically hold his breath.
● Inform the patient that he may be given an I.V. contrast medium, an oral contrast medium, or both to enhance visualization of the pancreas. Describe possible adverse reactions to the medium, such as nausea, flushing, dizziness, and sweating, and tell him to report these symptoms.
● Check the patient's history for recent barium studies and for hypersensitivity to iodine, seafood, or contrast media used in previous tests.
● Make sure that the patient or a responsible family member has signed an informed consent form.
● Administer the oral contrast medium.

## PROCEDURE AND POSTTEST CARE
● Help the patient into the supine position on the X-ray table and position the table within the opening of the scanning gantry.
● A series of transverse X-rays is taken and recorded on magnetic tape. The varying tissue absorption is calculated by a computer, and the information is reconstructed as images on a television screen. These images are studied, and selected ones are photographed.
● After the first series of films is completed, the images are reviewed. Then contrast enhancement may be ordered. After the contrast medium is administered, another series of films is taken, and the patient is observed for an allergic reaction, such as itching, hypotension, hypertension, diaphoresis, or dyspnea.
● After the procedure, tell the patient he may resume his usual diet.
● Observe for a delayed allergic reaction to the contrast dye, such as urticaria, headache, and vomiting.

## PRECAUTIONS
● Know that CT scanning of the pancreas is contraindicated in the pregnant patient.
● If a contrast medium is used, be aware that the test is contraindicated in the patient

# NORMAL CT SCAN OF THE PANCREAS

This normal pancreatic computed tomography (CT) scan shows the pancreas opacified by contrast medium.

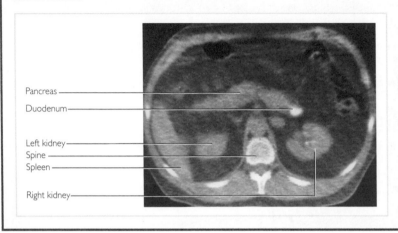

Pancreas
Duodenum

Left kidney
Spine
Spleen

Right kidney

with a history of hypersensitivity to iodine or severe renal or hepatic disease.

## NORMAL FINDINGS

Usually, the pancreatic parenchyma displays a uniform density, especially when an I.V. contrast medium is used. The gland normally thickens from tail to head and has a smooth surface. A contrast medium administered orally opacifies the adjacent stomach and duodenum and helps outline the pancreas, particularly in the patient with little peripancreatic fat, such as a child or a thin adult. (See *Normal CT scan of the pancreas*.)

## ABNORMAL FINDINGS

Because the tissue density of pancreatic carcinoma resembles that of the normal parenchyma, changes in pancreatic size and shape help demonstrate carcinoma and pseudocysts. Usually, carcinoma first appears as a localized swelling of the head, body, or tail of the pancreas and may spread to obliterate the fat plane, dilate the main pancreatic duct and common bile duct by obstructing them, and produce low-density focal lesions in the liver from metastasis. Use of an I.V. contrast medium helps detect metastases by opacifying the pancreatic and hepatic parenchyma.

Adenocarcinoma and islet cell tumors are the most common carcinomas of the pancreas. Cystadenomas and cystadenocarcinomas, usually multilocular, occur most frequently in the body and tail of the pancreas and appear as low-density focal lesions marked by internal septa. Contrast medium administered by mouth helps distinguish between bowel loops and tumors in the tail of the pancreas.

Acute pancreatitis, either edematous (interstitial) or necrotizing (hemorrhagic), produces diffuse enlargement of the pancreas. In acute edematous pancreatitis, parenchyma density is uniformly decreased. In acute necrotizing pancreatitis, the density is nonuniform because of the presence of necrosis and hemorrhage. The areas of tissue necrosis have diminished density. In acute pancreatitis, inflammation typically spreads into the peripancreatic fat, causes stranding in the mesenteric fat, and blurs the gland margin.

Abscesses, phlegmons, and pseudocysts may occur as complications of acute pancreatitis. Abscesses, either within or outside the pancreas, appear as low-density areas and are most readily detected when they contain gas. Pseudocysts, which may be unilocal or multilocal, appear as sharply circumscribed, low-density areas that may contain debris.

Ascites and pleural effusion may also be apparent in acute pancreatitis.

In chronic pancreatitis, the pancreas may appear normal, enlarged (localized or generalized), or atrophic, depending on disease severity. Duct calcification and dilation of the main pancreatic duct are characteristic. Pseudocysts, obliteration of the fat plane, and secondary complications, such as biliary obstruction, may occur.

## INTERFERING FACTORS

● Barium or other contrast media in the GI tract from earlier tests (possible poor imaging)

● Excessive peristalsis or excessive patient movement

# Computed tomography of the spine

Much more versatile than conventional radiography, spinal computed tomography (CT) provides detailed high-resolution images in the cross-sectional, longitudinal, sagittal, and lateral planes. Multiple X-ray beams from a computerized body scanner are directed at the spine from different angles; these pass through the body and strike radiation detectors, producing electrical impulses. A computer then converts these impulses into digital information, which is displayed as a three-dimensional image on a monitor. Storage of the digital information allows electronic recreation and manipulation of the image, creating a permanent record of the images to enable reexamination without repeating the procedure.

CT scans are helpful in defining the lesions causing spinal cord compression. Metastatic disease and discogenic disease with osteophyte formation and calcification are examples of pathologic processes diagnosed by CT scans. Since the advent of magnetic resonance imaging, CT scans are used less frequently to diagnose infection, abscesses, hematomas, and some disk herniations.

## PURPOSE

● To diagnose spinal lesions and abnormalities

● To monitor the effects of spinal surgery or therapy

## PATIENT PREPARATION

● Explain to the patient that spinal CT allows visualization of his spine.

● If contrast medium isn't ordered, tell the patient that he need not restrict food and fluids. If contrast medium is ordered, instruct him to fast for 4 hours before the test.

● Tell the patient that a series of scans will be taken of his spine. Explain who will perform the procedure and where it will take place.

● Reassure the patient that the procedure is painless, but that he may find having to remain still for a prolonged period uncomfortable.

● Explain to the patient that he'll be positioned on an X-ray table inside a CT body scanning unit and he'll be told to lie still because movement during the procedure may cause distorted images. The computer-controlled scanner will revolve around him, taking multiple scans.

● If a contrast medium is used, tell the patient that he may feel flushed and warm and may experience a transient headache, a salty taste, and nausea or vomiting after injection of the contrast medium. Reassure him that these reactions are normal.

● Instruct the patient to wear a radiologic examining gown and to remove all metal objects and jewelry.

● Check the patient's history for hypersensitivity reactions to iodine, shellfish, or contrast media. If such reactions have occurred, note them in the patient's chart and notify the physician, who may order prophylactic medications or choose not to use contrast enhancement.

● If the patient appears restless or apprehensive about the procedure, a mild sedative may be prescribed.

● Make sure that the patient or a responsible family member has signed an informed consent form, if required.

## PROCEDURE AND POSTTEST CARE

● Place the patient in a supine position on an X-ray table and tell him to lie as still as possible.

● The table slides into the circular opening of the CT scanner and the scanner revolves around the patient, taking radiographs at pre-selected intervals.

● After the first set of scans is taken, the patient is removed from the scanner. Contrast medium may be administered.

**Alert** *Observe the patient for signs and symptoms of a hypersensitivity reaction, including pruritus, rash, and respiratory difficulty, for 30 minutes after the contrast medium has been injected.*

● After contrast medium injection, the patient is moved back into the scanner, and another series of scans is taken. The images obtained from the scan are displayed on a monitor during the procedure and stored on magnetic tape.

● After testing with contrast enhancement, observe the patient for residual effects, such as headache, nausea, and vomiting.

● Inform the patient that he may resume his usual diet, as ordered.

## PRECAUTIONS

● Know that body CT scanning with contrast enhancement is contraindicated in the patient who's hypersensitive to iodine, shellfish, or contrast media used in radiographic studies.

● Be aware that the patient may experience strong feelings of claustrophobia or anxiety when inside the CT body scanner. In such cases, a mild sedative to help reduce anxiety may be ordered.

● For the patient with significant back pain, administer prescribed analgesics before the scan.

## NORMAL FINDINGS

In the CT image, spinal tissue appears white, black, or gray, depending on its density. Vertebrae, the densest tissues, are white; cerebrospinal fluid is black; and soft tissues appear in shades of gray.

## ABNORMAL FINDINGS

By highlighting areas of altered density and depicting structural malformation, CT scanning can reveal all types of spinal lesions and abnormalities. It's particularly useful in detecting and localizing tumors, which appear as masses varying in density. Measuring this density and noting the configuration and location relative to the spinal cord can usually identify the type of tumor. For example, a neurinoma (schwannoma) appears as a spherical mass dorsal to the cord. A darker,

wider mass lying more laterally or ventrally to the cord may be a meningioma.

CT scans also reveal degenerative processes and structural changes in detail. Herniated nucleus pulposus shows as an obvious herniation of disk material with unilateral or bilateral nerve root compression; if the herniation is midline, spinal cord compression will be evident. Cervical spondylosis shows as cervical cord compression due to bony hypertrophy of the cervical spine; lumbar stenosis, as hypertrophy of the lumbar vertebrae, causing cord compression by decreasing space within the spinal column. Facet disorders show as soft-tissue changes, bony overgrowth, and spurring of the vertebrae, which result in nerve root compression. Fluid-filled arachnoidal and other paraspinal cysts show as dark masses displacing the spinal cord. Vascular malformations, evident after contrast enhancement, show as masses or clusters, usually on the dorsal aspect of the spinal cord.

Congenital spinal malformations, such as meningocele, myelocele, and spina bifida, show as abnormally large, dark gaps between the white vertebrae.

## INTERFERING FACTORS

● Excessive patient movement

● Metallic objects in the scan area (possible poor imaging)

# *Concentration and dilution test*

The kidneys normally concentrate or dilute urine according to fluid intake. When such intake is excessive, the kidneys excrete more water in the urine; when intake is limited, they excrete less. The concentration and dilution test evaluates renal capacity to concentrate urine in response to fluid deprivation or to dilute it in response to fluid overload. This test may also be referred to as the *water loading* or *water deprivation test*.

## PURPOSE

● To evaluate renal tubular function

● To detect renal impairment

● To diagnose disorders such as diabetes insipidus

## PATIENT PREPARATION

- Explain to the patient that the concentration and dilution test evaluates kidney function.
- Tell him the test requires multiple urine specimens. Explain how many specimens will be collected and at what intervals.
- Instruct him to discard urine voided for a specific time, as per laboratory protocol such as all urine collected during the night.
- Withhold diuretics as needed.

### Concentration test

- Provide a high-protein meal and only 200 ml of fluid the night before the test.
- Instruct the patient to restrict food and fluids for at least 14 hours before the test. (Some concentration tests require that water be withheld for 24 hours, but permit relatively normal food intake.)
- Limit salt intake at the evening meal to prevent excessive thirst.
- Emphasize to the patient that his cooperation is necessary to obtain accurate results.

### Dilution test

- Generally, the dilution test directly follows the concentration test and necessitates no additional patient preparation.
- If this test is performed alone, simply withhold breakfast.

## PROCEDURE AND POSTTEST CARE

### Concentration test

- Collect urine specimens at 6 a.m., 8 a.m., and 10 a.m.

### Dilution test

- Instruct the patient to void and discard the first urine sample.
- Give the patient 1,500 ml of water to drink within a 30-minute period.
- Collect urine specimens every half hour or every hour for 4 hours thereafter.

### Both tests

- Provide a balanced meal or a snack after collecting the final specimen.
- Make sure the patient voids within 8 hours after the catheter is removed.

## PRECAUTIONS

- Be aware that testing may be contraindicated in the patient with advanced renal disease or cardiac dysfunction because fluid overload can precipitate water intoxication, sodium diuresis, or heart failure.
- Send each specimen to the laboratory immediately after collection.
- Provide the patient with a clean bedpan, urinal, or toilet specimen pan if he's unable to urinate into the specimen containers.
- Rinse the collection device after each use.
- If the patient is catheterized, empty the drainage bag before the test. Obtain the specimens from the catheter and clamp the catheter between collections.

## REFERENCE VALUES

Normal specific gravity ranges from 1.005 to 1.035; osmolality normally ranges from 300 to 900 mOsm/kg.

### Concentration test

Specific gravity ranges from 1.025 to 1.032, and osmolality rises above 800 mOsm/kg of water (SI, >800 mmol/kg) in the patient with normal renal function.

### Dilution test

Normally, specific gravity falls below 1.003 and osmolality below 100 mOsm/kg for at least one specimen; 80% or more of the ingested water is eliminated in 4 hours.

## ABNORMAL FINDINGS

Decreased renal capacity to concentrate urine in response to fluid deprivation, or to dilute urine in response to fluid overload, may indicate tubular epithelial damage, decreased renal blood flow, loss of functional nephrons, or pituitary or cardiac dysfunction.

*Age alert* *In an elderly person, depressed values can be associated with normal renal function.*

## INTERFERING FACTORS

- Use of radiographic contrast agents within 7 days of test (possible increase in osmolality)
- Diuretics and nephrotoxic drugs (possible increase or decrease in specific gravity and osmolality)
- Glycosuria

# Cortisol, plasma and urine

Cortisol — the principal glucocorticoid secreted by the zona fasciculata of the adrenal cortex — helps metabolize nutrients, mediate physiologic stress, and regulate the immune system. Cortisol secretion normally follows a diurnal pattern: Levels rise during the early morning hours and peak around 8 a.m., and then decline to very low levels in the evening and during the early phase of sleep. (See *Diurnal variations in cortisol secretion,* page 118.) Intense heat or cold, infection, trauma, exercise, obesity, and debilitating disease influence cortisol secretion.

Plasma cortisol level measured quantitatively via radioimmunoassay, is usually ordered for patients with signs of adrenal dysfunction. Dynamic tests, suppression tests for hyperfunction, and stimulation tests for hypofunction are generally required to confirm the diagnosis.

Urine free cortisol is used as a screen for adrenocortical hyperfunction. It measures urine levels of the portion of cortisol not bound to the corticosteroid-binding globulin transcortin. It's one of the best diagnostic tools for detecting Cushing's syndrome.

Unlike a single measurement of plasma cortisol, radioimmunoassay determinations of free cortisol levels in a 24-hour urine specimen reflect overall secretion levels instead of diurnal variations. Concurrent measurements of plasma cortisol and corticotropin, with urine 17-hydroxycorticosteroids and the dexamethasone suppression test, may be used to confirm the diagnosis.

## PURPOSE
● To aid in the diagnosis of Cushing's disease, Cushing's syndrome, and Addison's disease
● To evaluate adrenocortical function

## PATIENT PREPARATION
● Explain to the patient that the plasma and urine cortisol tests help evaluate adrenal gland function.

## Plasma cortisol
● Instruct the patient to maintain a normal salt diet (2 to 3 g/day) for 3 days before the test and to fast and limit physical activity for 10 to 12 hours before the test.
● Tell the patient that the test requires a blood sample. Explain who will perform the venipuncture and when.
● Explain to the patient that he may experience slight discomfort from the tourniquet and needle puncture.
● Withhold all medications that may interfere with plasma cortisol levels, such as estrogens, androgens, and phenytoin, for 48 hours before the test, as ordered. If the patient is receiving replacement therapy and is dependent on exogenous steroids for survival, note this on the laboratory request as well as other medications that must be continued.
● Make sure the patient is relaxed and recumbent for at least 30 minutes before the test.

## Urine cortisol
● Inform the patient that he need not restrict food and fluids, but should avoid stressful situations and excessive physical exercise during the collection period.
● Tell the patient that the test requires collection of urine over a 24-hour period.
● Teach the patient the proper collection technique for a 24-hour urine specimen.
● Notify the laboratory and physician of medications the patient is taking that may affect test results; they may need to be restricted.

## PROCEDURE AND POSTTEST CARE
### Plasma cortisol
● Perform a venipuncture between 6 a.m. and 8 a.m.
● Collect the sample in a 7-ml heparinized tube, label it appropriately, and send it to the laboratory immediately.
● For diurnal variation testing, draw another sample between 4 p.m. and 6 p.m.
● Collect the second sample in a 7-ml heparinized tube, label it appropriately, and send it to the laboratory immediately.
● Apply direct pressure to the venipuncture site until bleeding stops.
● If a hematoma develops at the venipuncture site, apply pressure.

### Urine cortisol
● Collect the patient's urine over a 24-hour period, discarding the first specimen and re-

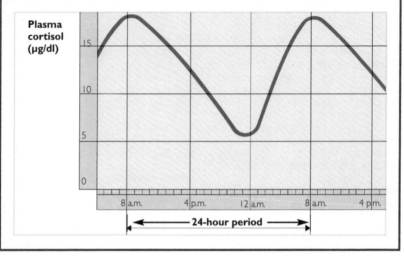

# DIURNAL VARIATIONS IN CORTISOL SECRETION

Cortisol secretion rises in the early morning, peaking after the patient awakens. Levels decline sharply in the evening and during the early phase of sleep. They rise again during the night and peak by the next morning.

**Plasma cortisol (µg/dl)**

15

10

5

0

8 a.m.    4 p.m.    12 a.m.    8 a.m.    4 p.m.

← **24-hour period** →

taining the last specimen. Use a bottle containing a preservative to keep the specimen at a pH of 4.0 to 4.5.
● Instruct the patient that he may resume his usual activities and medications, as ordered.

### Both tests
● Instruct the patient that he may resume his usual diet, activities, and medications discontinued before the test, as ordered.

### PRECAUTIONS
● Handle the blood sample gently to prevent hemolysis.
● Record the collection time of the blood specimen on the laboratory request.
● Refrigerate the urine specimen or place it on ice during the collection period.

### REFERENCE VALUES
Normally, plasma cortisol levels range from 9 to 35 µg/dl (SI, 250 to 690 nmol/L) in the morning and from 3 to 12 µg/dl (SI, 80 to 330 nmol/L) in the afternoon. The afternoon level is usually half the morning level.

Normal free cortisol values are less than 50 µg/24 hours (SI, < 138 mmol/24 hours).

### ABNORMAL FINDINGS
Increased plasma cortisol levels may indicate adrenocortical hyperfunction in Cushing's disease (a rare disease due to basophilic adenoma of the pituitary gland) or Cushing's syndrome (glucocorticoid excess from any cause). In most patients with Cushing's syndrome, the adrenal cortex secretes independently of a natural rhythm. Thus, absence of diurnal variation in cortisol secretion is a significant finding in almost all patients with Cushing's syndrome; in these patients, little difference in values is found between morning and afternoon samples. Diurnal variations may also be absent in otherwise healthy people who are under considerable emotional or physical stress.

Decreased plasma cortisol levels may indicate primary adrenal hypofunction (Addison's disease), usually due to idiopathic glandular atrophy (a presumed autoimmune process). Tuberculosis, fungal invasion, and hemorrhage can cause adrenocortical destruction. Low cortisol levels resulting from secondary adrenal insufficiency may occur in conditions of impaired corticotropin secretion, such as hypophysectomy, postpartum pituitary necrosis, craniopharyngioma, and chromophobe adenoma.

Elevated urine cortisol levels may indicate Cushing's syndrome resulting from adrenal hyperplasia, adrenal or pituitary tumor, or ectopic corticotropin production. Hepatic disease and obesity, which can raise plasma cortisol levels, generally don't appreciably raise urine levels of free cortisol. Low levels have little diagnostic significance and don't necessarily indicate adrenocortical hypofunction.

## INTERFERING FACTORS
### Plasma cortisol
* Pregnancy or use of hormonal contraceptives because of increase in cortisol-binding plasma proteins (false-high)
* Obesity, stress, and severe hepatic or renal disease (possible increase)
* Androgens and phenytoin due to decrease in cortisol-binding plasma proteins (possible decrease)
* Radioactive scan performed within 1 week before the test

### Urine cortisol
* Emotional or physical stress, pregnancy (possible increase)
* Aldactone, amphetamines, danazol, hormonal contraceptives, morphine, phenothiazines, prolonged steroid therapy, reserpine, and spironolactone (possible increase)
* Dexamethasone, ethacrynic acid, ketoconazole, and thiazides (decrease)

## *C-peptide*

Connecting peptide (C-peptide) is a biologically inactive chain formed during the proteolytic conversion of proinsulin to insulin in the pancreatic beta cells. It has no insulin effect either biologically or immunologically. Circulating insulin is measured by immunologic assay. As insulin is released into the bloodstream, the C-peptide chain splits off from the hormone.

## PURPOSE
* To determine the cause of hypoglycemia

* To indirectly measure insulin secretion in the presence of circulating insulin antibodies
* To detect residual tissue after total pancreatectomy for carcinoma
* To determine beta-cell function in the patient with diabetes mellitus

## PATIENT PREPARATION
* Explain to the patient that the C-peptide test helps to evaluate pancreatic function and determine the cause of hypoglycemia.
* Instruct the patient to fast for 8 to 12 hours before the test, restricting all intake except for water.
* Tell the patient that the test requires a blood sample. Explain who will perform the venipuncture and when.
* Explain to the patient that he may experience slight discomfort from the tourniquet and needle puncture.
* If the patient is scheduled for radioisotope testing, it should take place after blood is drawn for C-peptide levels. Blood glucose levels are usually drawn at the same time as C-peptide levels.
* If the C-peptide stimulation test is done, I.V. glucagon is administered, as ordered, after a baseline blood sample is drawn.
* Withhold drugs that may interfere with test results, as ordered. If they must be continued, note this on the laboratory request.

## PROCEDURE AND POSTTEST CARE
* Perform a venipuncture and collect a 1-ml sample in a chilled clot-activator tube. The blood is separated and frozen to be tested later.
* Collect a sample for glucose level in a tube with sodium fluoride and potassium oxalate, if ordered.
* Apply direct pressure to the venipuncture site until bleeding stops.
* If a hematoma develops at the venipuncture site, apply warm soaks.
* Instruct the patient that he may resume his usual activities, diet, and medications discontinued before the test, as ordered.

## PRECAUTIONS
* Pack the sample in ice and send it, along with the glucose sample, to the laboratory immediately.
* Handle the samples gently to prevent hemolysis.

## REFERENCE VALUES

Serum C-peptide levels generally parallel those of insulin. Normal fasting values range between 0.78 and 1.89 ng/ml (SI, 0.26 to 0.63 mmol/L). An insulin C-peptide ratio may be performed to differentiate insulinoma from factitious hypoglycemia. A ratio of 1.0 or less indicates increased, endogenous insulin secretion; a ratio of 1.0 or more indicates exogenous insulin.

## ABNORMAL FINDINGS

Elevated levels may indicate endogenous hyperinsulinism (insulinemia), oral hypoglycemic drug ingestion, pancreas or B-cell transplantation, renal failure, or type 2 diabetes mellitus. Decreased levels may indicate factitious hypoglycemia (surreptitious insulin administration), radical pancreatectomy, or type 1 diabetes.

## INTERFERING FACTORS

● None significant

# C-reactive protein

C-reactive protein (CRP) is an abnormal protein that appears in the blood during an inflammatory process. It's absent from the blood of healthy people. This nonspecific protein is mainly synthesized in the liver and is found in many body fluids (pleural, peritoneal, pericardial, synovial). It appears in the blood 18 to 24 hours after the onset of tissue damage with levels that increase up to 1,000-fold and then decline rapidly when the inflammatory process regresses. CRP has been found to rise before increases in antibody titers and erythrocyte sedimentation rate (ESR) levels occur. It also decreases sooner than ESR levels.

CRP is also a valuable cardiac marker to evaluate a patient with a myocardial infarction (MI). Levels correlate with creatine kinase MB isoenzyme, but typically peak 1 to 3 days after CK-MB. However, if CRP doesn't return to normal, it's highly suggestive of ongoing myocardial tissue damage. A more highly specific test for CRP, the hs-CRP has been developed that's capable of detecting even low levels of CRP. It's extremely helpful in determining the risk for MI in patients with acute coronary syndromes.

## PURPOSE

● To evaluate the inflammatory disease course and severity in conditions, including tissue necrosis (MI, malignancy, rheumatoid arthritis [RA])
● To monitor acute inflammatory phases of RA and rheumatic fever, so early treatment can be initiated
● To monitor the patient's response to treatment or determine if the acute phase is declining
● To help interpret the ESR
● To monitor the wound healing process of internal incisions, burns, and organ transplantation

## PATIENT PREPARATION

● Explain to the patient that the C-reactive protein test is used to identify the presence of infection or to monitor treatment.
● Inform the patient that he needs to restrict all fluids except for water for 8 to 12 hours before the test.
● Tell the patient that the test requires a blood sample. Explain who will perform the venipuncture and when.
● Explain to the patient that he may experience slight discomfort from the tourniquet and needle puncture.
● Notify the laboratory and physician of medications the patient is taking that may affect test results; they may need to be restricted.

## PROCEDURE AND POSTTEST CARE

● Perform a venipuncture and collect the sample in a 5-ml clot-activator tube.
● Apply direct pressure to the venipuncture site until bleeding stops.
● If a hematoma develops at the venipuncture site, apply pressure.
● Instruct the patient that he may resume his usual diet and medications discontinued before the test, as ordered.

## PRECAUTIONS

● Keep the blood sample away from heat.

## REFERENCE VALUES

CRP usually isn't present in the blood. In adults, results may be reported as < 0.8 mg/dl (SI, < 8 mg/L); hs-CRP levels typically range from 0.020 to 0.800 mg/dL (SI, 0.2 to 8 mg/L).

## ABNORMAL FINDINGS

An elevated CRP level may be present in RA, rheumatic fever, MI, cancer (active, widespread), acute bacterial and viral infections, and inflammatory bowel disease, Hodgkin's disease, systemic lupus erythematosus, and postoperatively (declines after the fourth day).

Elevations of hs-CRP indicate an increased risk for cardiac events such as MI.

## INTERFERING FACTORS

● Steroids and salicylates (false normal level)
● Hormonal contraceptives (false increase)
● Intrauterine contraceptive devices (increase) and pregnancy (third trimester)

# Creatine kinase and isoforms

Creatine kinase (CK) is an enzyme that catalyzes the creatine-creatinine metabolic pathway in muscle cells and brain tissue. Because of its intimate role in energy production, CK reflects normal tissue catabolism; increased serum levels indicate trauma to cells.

Fractionation and measurement of three distinct CK isoenzymes — CK-BB (CK1), CK-MB (CK2), and CK-MM (CK3) — have replaced the use of total CK levels to accurately localize the site of increased tissue destruction. CK-BB is most commonly found in brain tissue. CK-MM and CK-MB are found primarily in skeletal and heart muscle. In addition, subunits of CK-MB and CK-MM, called *isoforms* or *isoenzymes,* can be assayed to increase the test's sensitivity.

## PURPOSE

● To detect and diagnose an acute myocardial infarction (MI) and reinfarction (CK-MB primarily used)
● To evaluate possible causes of chest pain and to monitor the severity of myocardial ischemia after cardiac surgery, cardiac catheterization, and cardioversion (CK-MB primarily used)
● To detect early dermatomyositis and musculoskeletal disorders that aren't neurogenic in origin such as Duchenne's muscular dystrophy (total CK primarily used)

## PATIENT PREPARATION

● Explain to the patient that the creatine kinase and isoforms test is used to assess myocardial and musculoskeletal function and that multiple blood samples are required to detect fluctuations in serum levels.
● Tell the patient who will be performing the venipunctures and when.
● Explain to the patient that he may experience slight discomfort from the tourniquet and needle puncture.
● If the patient is being evaluated for musculoskeletal disorders, advise him to avoid exercising for 24 hours before the test.
● Notify the laboratory and physician of medications the patient is taking that may affect test results; they may need to be restricted.

## PROCEDURE AND POSTTEST CARE

● Perform a venipuncture and collect the sample in a 4-ml tube without additives.
● Apply direct pressure to the venipuncture site until bleeding stops.
● If a hematoma develops at the venipuncture site, apply pressure.
● Instruct the patient that he may resume exercise and medications discontinued before the test, as ordered.

## PRECAUTIONS

● Draw the sample before giving I.M. injections or 1 hour after giving them because muscle trauma increases the total CK level.
● Obtain the sample on schedule. Note on the laboratory request the time the sample was drawn and the hours elapsed since the onset of chest pain.
● Handle the sample gently to prevent hemolysis.
● Send the sample to the laboratory immediately because CK activity diminishes significantly after 2 hours at room temperature.

## REFERENCE VALUES

Total CK values determined by ultraviolet or kinetic measurement range from 55 to 170 U/L (SI, 0.94 to 2.89 µkat/L) for men and from 30 to 135 U/L (SI, 0.51 to 2.3 µkat/L) for women. CK levels may be significantly higher in muscular people.

*Age alert Infants up to age 1 have levels two to four times higher than adult levels, possibly reflecting birth trauma and striated muscle development.*

# RELEASE OF CARDIAC ENZYMES AND PROTEINS

Because they're released by damaged tissue, serum proteins and isoenzymes (catalytic proteins that vary in concentration in specific organs) can help identify the compromised organ and assess the extent of damage. After an acute myocardial infarction, cardiac enzymes and proteins rise and fall in a characteristic pattern, as shown in the graph below.

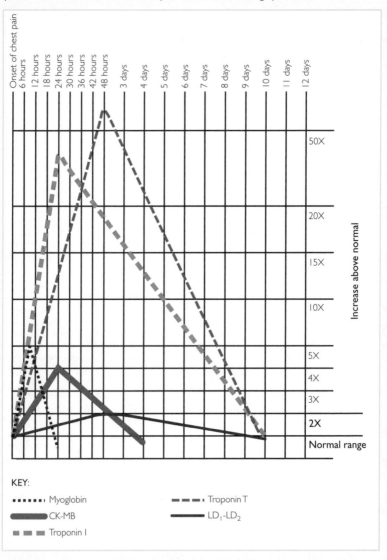

KEY:

∙∙∙∙∙∙∙ Myoglobin

━━━ CK-MB

▬ ▬ ▬ Troponin I

▬ ▬ ▬ Troponin T

━━━ LD$_1$-LD$_2$

Normal ranges for isoenzyme levels are as follows: CK-BB, undetectable; CK-MB, less than 5% (SI, < 0.05); CK-MM, 90% to 100% (SI, 0.9 to 1.0).

## ABNORMAL FINDINGS

CK-MM makes up 99% of total CK normally present in serum. Detectable CK-BB isoenzyme may indicate, but doesn't confirm, a diagnosis of brain tissue injury, widespread malignant tumors, severe shock, or renal failure.

CK-MB levels greater than 5% of the total CK level indicate an MI, especially if the lactate dehydrogenase (LD) isoenzyme ratio is more than 1 (flipped LD). In an acute MI and after cardiac surgery, CK-MB begins to increase within 2 to 4 hours, peaks within 12 to 24 hours, and usually returns to normal within 24 to 48 hours; persistent elevations and increasing levels indicate ongoing myocardial damage. Total CK follows roughly the same pattern, but increases slightly later. CK-MB levels may not increase in heart failure or during angina pectoris not accompanied by myocardial cell necrosis. Serious skeletal muscle injury that occurs in certain muscular dystrophies, polymyositis, and severe myoglobinuria may produce a mild CK-MB increase because a small amount of this isoenzyme is present in some skeletal muscles.

Increasing CK-MM values follow skeletal muscle damage from trauma, such as surgery and I.M. injections, and from diseases, such as dermatomyositis and muscular dystrophy (values may be 50 to 100 times normal). A moderate increase in CK-MM levels develops in a patient with hypothyroidism; sharp increases occur with muscle activity caused by agitation such as during an acute psychotic episode.

Total CK levels may be increased in patients with severe hypokalemia, carbon monoxide poisoning, malignant hyperthermia, and alcoholic cardiomyopathy. They may also be increased after seizures and, occasionally, in patients who have suffered pulmonary or cerebral infarctions. Troponin I and cardiac troponin C are present in the contractile cells of cardiac myocardial tissue, and are released with injury to the myocardial tissue. Troponin levels increase within 1 hour of the infarction and may remain elevated for up to 14 days. (See *Release of cardiac enzymes and proteins.*) Studies have shown that people with unstable angina and high troponin levels, but with normal CK, CK-MB, and myoglobin levels, are at increased risk for MI or other serious heart problems in the months following diagnosis and after blood levels were obtained.

## INTERFERING FACTORS
- Halothane and succinylcholine, gemfibrozil, amphotericin B, chlorthalidone, clofibrate, alcohol, lithium, large doses of aminocaproic acid, I.M. injections, cardioversion, invasive diagnostic procedures, recent vigorous exercise or muscle massage, severe coughing, and trauma (increase in total CK)
- Surgery through skeletal muscle (increase in total CK)

# *Creatinine*

Analysis of serum creatinine levels provides a more sensitive measure of renal damage than do blood urea nitrogen levels. Creatinine is a nonprotein end product of creatine metabolism that appears in serum in amounts proportional to the body's muscle mass.

## PURPOSE
- To assess glomerular filtration
- To screen for renal damage

## PATIENT PREPARATION
- Explain to the patient that the serum creatinine test is used to evaluate kidney function.
- Tell the patient that the test requires a blood sample. Explain who will perform the venipuncture and when.
- Explain to the patient that he may experience slight discomfort from the tourniquet and needle puncture.
- Instruct the patient that he need not restrict food and fluids.
- Notify the laboratory and physician of medications the patient is taking that may affect test results; they may need to be restricted.

## PROCEDURE AND POSTTEST CARE
- Perform a venipuncture and collect the sample in a 3- or 4-ml clot-activator tube.

- Apply direct pressure to the venipuncture site until bleeding stops.
- If a hematoma develops at the venipuncture site, apply pressure.
- Inform the patient that he may resume his usual medications discontinued before the test, as ordered.

## PRECAUTIONS
- Handle the sample gently to prevent hemolysis.
- Send the sample to the laboratory immediately.

## REFERENCE VALUES
Creatinine concentrations normally range from 0.8 to 1.2 mg/dl (SI, 62 to 115 µmol/L) in males and 0.6 to 0.9 mg/dl (SI, 53 to 97 µmol/L) in females.

## ABNORMAL FINDINGS
Elevated serum creatinine levels generally indicate renal disease that has seriously damaged 50% or more of the nephrons. Elevated levels may also be associated with gigantism and acromegaly.

## INTERFERING FACTORS
- Ascorbic acid, barbiturates, and diuretics (possible increase)
- Exceptionally large muscle mass, such as that found in athletes (possible increase despite normal renal function)
- Phenolsulfonphthalein (given within the previous 24 hours can elevate creatinine levels if the test is based on Jaffé's reaction)

# Creatinine clearance

An anhydride of creatine, creatinine is formed and excreted in constant amounts by an irreversible reaction and functions solely as the main end product of creatine. Creatinine production is proportional to tota muscle mass and is relatively unaffected by urine volume or normal physical activity or diet.

An excellent diagnostic indicator of renal function, the creatinine clearance test determines how efficiently the kidneys are clearing creatinine from the blood. The rate of clearance is expressed in terms of the volume of blood (in milliliters) that can be cleared of creatinine in 1 minute. Creatinine levels become abnormal when more than 50% of the nephrons have been damaged.

## PURPOSE
- To assess renal function (primarily glomerular filtration)
- To monitor progression of renal insufficiency

## PATIENT PREPARATION
- Explain to the patient that the creatinine clearance test assesses kidney function.
- Inform the patient that he may need to avoid meat, poultry, fish, tea, or coffee for 6 hours before the test.
- Advise the patient that he should avoid strenuous physical exercise during the collection period.
- Tell the patient that the test requires a timed urine specimen and at least one blood sample.
- Tell the patient how the urine specimen will be collected. Also inform him who will perform the venipuncture and when and that he may feel some discomfort from the needle puncture.
- Explain that more than one venipuncture may be necessary.
- Notify the laboratory and physician of medications the patient is taking that may affect test results; they may need to be restricted.

## PROCEDURE AND POSTTEST CARE
- Collect a timed urine specimen at 2, 6, 12, or 24 hours in a bottle containing a preservative to prevent creatinine degradation.
- Perform a venipuncture anytime during the collection period and collect the sample in a 7-ml tube without additives.
- Apply direct pressure to the venipuncture site until bleeding stops.
- If a hematoma develops at the venipuncture site, apply warm soaks.
- Instruct the patient that he may resume his usual activities, diet, and medications, as ordered.

## PRECAUTIONS
- Refrigerate the urine specimen or keep it on ice during the collection period.
- Send the specimen to the laboratory as soon as the collection is completed.

## REFERENCE VALUES

Normal creatinine clearance varies with age; in males, it ranges from 94 to 140 ml/sec/1.73 m² (SI, 0.91 to 1.35 ml/s/m²); in females, 72 to 110 ml/sec/1.73 m² (SI, 0.69 to 1.06 ml/s/m²).

**Age alert** *With each decade after age 20, creatinine clearance decreases 6.5 ml/min/1.73m² or 0.06 ml/sec/m².*

## ABNORMAL FINDINGS

Low creatinine clearance may result from reduced renal blood flow (associated with shock or renal artery obstruction), acute tubular necrosis, acute or chronic glomerulonephritis, advanced bilateral chronic pyelonephritis, advanced bilateral renal lesions (which may occur in polycystic kidney disease, renal tuberculosis, and cancer), nephrosclerosis, heart failure, or severe dehydration.

High creatinine clearance can suggest poor hydration.

## INTERFERING FACTORS

● Amphotericin B, aminoglycosides, furosemide, and thiazide diuretics (possible decrease)

● High-protein diet or strenuous exercise (increase)

## *Creatinine, urine*

The urine creatinine test measures urine levels of creatinine, the chief metabolite of creatine. Produced in amounts proportional to total body muscle mass, creatinine is removed from the plasma primarily by glomerular filtration and is excreted in the urine. Because the body doesn't recycle it, creatinine has a relatively high, constant clearance rate, making it an efficient indicator of renal function. However, the creatinine clearance test, which measures urine and plasma creatinine clearance, is a more precise index than this test. A standard method for determining urine creatinine levels is based on Jaffé's reaction, in which creatinine treated with an alkaline picrate solution yields a bright orange-red complex.

## PURPOSE

● To help assess glomerular filtration

● To check the accuracy of 24-hour urine collection, based on the relatively constant levels of creatinine excretion

## PATIENT PREPARATION

● Explain to the patient that the urine creatinine test helps evaluate kidney function.

● Inform the patient that he need not restrict fluids, but that he shouldn't eat an excessive amount of meat (protein) before the test.

● Advise the patient that he should avoid strenuous physical exercise during the collection period.

● Tell the patient that the test usually requires urine collection over a 24-hour period, and teach him the proper collection technique.

● Notify the laboratory and physician of medications the patient is taking that may affect test results; they may need to be restricted.

## PROCEDURE AND POSTTEST CARE

● Collect the patient's urine over a 24-hour period, discarding the first specimen and retaining the last. Use a specimen bottle that contains a preservative to prevent creatinine degradation.

● Instruct the patient that he may resume his usual activities, diet, and medications, as ordered.

## PRECAUTIONS

● Refrigerate the specimen or keep it on ice during the collection period.

● Send the specimen to the laboratory immediately after the collection is completed.

## REFERENCE VALUES

Normally, urine creatinine levels range from 14 to 26 mg/kg body weight/24 hours (SI, 124 to 230 µmol/kg body weight/d) in males and from 11 to 20 mg/kg body weight/24 hours (SI, 97 to 177 µmol/kg body weight/d) in females.

## ABNORMAL FINDINGS

Decreased urine creatinine levels may result from impaired renal perfusion (associated with shock, for example) or from renal disease due to urinary tract obstruction. Chronic bilateral pyelonephritis, acute or chronic glomerulonephritis, and polycystic kidney disease may also depress creatinine levels.

Increased levels generally have little diagnostic significance.

## INTERFERING FACTORS

• Amphotericin B, corticosteroids, diuretics, gentamicin, and tetracyclines (possible decrease)

# Cryoglobulins

Cryoglobulins are abnormal serum proteins that precipitate at low laboratory temperatures (39.2° F [4° C]) and redissolve after being warmed. Their presence in the blood (cryoglobulinemia) is usually associated with immunologic disease, but can also occur without known immunopathology. (See *Diseases associated with cryoglobulinemia*.)

If patients with cryoglobulinemia are subjected to cold, they may experience Raynaud-like symptoms (pain, cyanosis, and cold fingers and toes), which generally result from cryoglobulin precipitation in cooler parts of the body. In some patients, for example, cryoglobulins may precipitate at temperatures as high as 86° F (30° C); such temperatures are possible in some peripheral blood vessels.

The cryoglobulin test involves refrigerating a serum sample at 33.8° F (1° C) for 24 hours and observing for formation of a heat-reversible precipitate. Such a precipitate requires further study by immunoelectrophoresis or double diffusion to identify cryoglobulin components.

## DISEASES ASSOCIATED WITH CRYOGLOBULINEMIA

| TYPE OF CRYOGLOBULIN | SERUM LEVEL | ASSOCIATED DISEASES |
|---|---|---|
| **TYPE I** | | |
| Monoclonal cryoglobulin | > 5 mg/ml | ◆ Myeloma<br>◆ Waldenström's macroglobulinemia<br>◆ Chronic lymphocytic leukemia |
| **TYPE II** | | |
| Mixed cryoglobulin | > 1 mg/ml | ◆ Rheumatoid arthritis<br>◆ Sjögren's syndrome<br>◆ Mixed essential cryoglobulinemia<br>◆ Human immunodeficiency virus-1 infection |
| **TYPE III** | | |
| Mixed polyclonal cryoglobulin | < 1 mg/ml<br>(50% below<br>80 mcg/ml) | ◆ Systemic lupus erythematosus<br>◆ Rheumatoid arthritis<br>◆ Sjögren's syndrome<br>◆ Infectious mononucleosis<br>◆ Cytomegalovirus infection<br>◆ Acute viral hepatitis<br>◆ Chronic active hepatitis<br>◆ Primary biliary cirrhosis<br>◆ Poststreptococcal glomerulonephritis<br>◆ Infective endocarditis<br>◆ Leprosy<br>◆ Kala-azar<br>◆ Tropical splenomegaly syndrome |

## PURPOSE

● To detect cryoglobulinemia in the patient with Raynaud-like vascular symptoms

## PATIENT PREPARATION

● Explain to the patient that the cryoglobulins test detects antibodies in blood that may cause sensitivity to low temperatures.
● Instruct the patient to fast for 4 to 6 hours before the test.
● Tell the patient that the test requires a blood sample. Explain who will perform the venipuncture and when.
● Explain to the patient that he may experience slight discomfort from the tourniquet and needle puncture.

## PROCEDURE AND POSTTEST CARE

● Perform a venipuncture and collect the sample in a prewarmed 10-ml tube without additives.
● Instruct the patient that he may resume his usual diet.
● Tell the patient to avoid cold temperatures or contact with cold objects if the test is positive for cryoglobulins, as ordered.
● Apply direct pressure to the venipuncture site until bleeding stops.
● If a hematoma develops at the venipuncture site, apply pressure.
● Observe for signs of intravascular coagulation, such as decreased color and temperature in distal extremities, and increased pain.

## PRECAUTIONS

● Warm the syringe and collection tube to 98.6° F (37° C) before venipuncture and keep the tube at that temperature to prevent cryoglobulin loss.
● Send the sample to the laboratory immediately.

## NORMAL FINDINGS

Normally, serum is negative for cryoglobulins. Positive results are reported as a percentage based on the amount of sample cryoprecipitation.

## ABNORMAL FINDINGS

The presence of cryoglobulins in the blood confirms cryoglobulinemia. This finding doesn't always indicate the presence of clinical disease.

## INTERFERING FACTORS

● Nonadherence to dietary restrictions
● Failure to keep the sample at 98.6° F (37° C) before centrifugation (possible loss of cryoglobulins)
● Reading the sample before the 72-hour precipitation period ends (possible incorrect analysis of results because some cryoglobulins take several days to precipitate)

# *Cystometry*

Cystometry assesses the bladder's neuromuscular function by measuring the efficiency of the detrusor muscle reflex, intravesical pressure and capacity, and the bladder's reaction to thermal stimulation. Because results from cystometry can be ambiguous, they're typically supported by results of other tests, such as cystourethrography, excretory urography, and voiding cystourethrography.

## PURPOSE

● To evaluate detrusor muscle function and tonicity
● To help determine the cause of bladder dysfunction

## PATIENT PREPARATION

● Explain to the patient that cystometry evaluates bladder function.
● Tell the patient that he need not restrict food and fluids.
● Describe the procedure, including who will perform it, where it will take place, and how long it will last.
● Tell the patient that he'll feel a strong urge to void during the test and that he may feel embarrassed or uncomfortable. Provide reassurance.
● Make sure that the patient or a responsible family member has signed an informed consent form.
● Check the patient's medication history for drugs that may affect test results such as antihistamines.
● Tell the patient to urinate just before the procedure.

*(Text continues on page 130.)*

# NORMAL AND ABNORMAL CYSTOMETRY FINDINGS

Because cystometry assesses micturition and vesical function, it can aid diagnosis of neurogenic bladder dysfunction. The five main types of neurogenic bladder, as presented in the following chart, result from lesions of the central or peripheral nervous system. Uninhibited neurogenic bladder results from a lesion to the upper motor neuron and causes frequent, usually uncontrollable micturition in the presence of even a small amount of urine. A complete upper motor neuron lesion characterizes reflex neurogenic bladder and causes total loss of conscious sensation and vesical control.

| FEATURE OR RESPONSE | NORMAL BLADDER FUNCTION | UNINHIBITED NEUROGENIC BLADDER (MILDLY SPASTIC, INCOMPLETE UPPER MOTOR NEURON LESION) | REFLEX NEUROGENIC BLADDER (COMPLETELY SPASTIC, COMPLETE UPPER MOTOR NEURON LESION) |
|---|---|---|---|
| Micturition | | | |
| Start | + | +/0 | 0 |
| Stop | + | 0 | 0 |
| Residual urine | 0 | 0 | + |
| Vesical sensation | + | + | 0 |
| First urge to void | 150 to 200 ml | E (<150 ml) | 0 |
| Bladder capacity | 400 to 500 ml | ↓ | ↓ |
| Bladder contractions | 0 | + | + |
| Intravesical pressure | L | ↑ | ↑ |
| Bulbocavernosus reflex | + | + | ↑ |
| Saddle sensation | + | + | 0 |
| Bethanechol test (exaggerated response) | 0 | + | 0 |
| Ice water test | + | + | + |
| Anal reflex | + | + | + |
| Heat sensation and pain | + | + | 0 |

KEY:
+ = Present/positive
0 = Absent/negative
↑ = Increased
↓ = Decreased
V = Variable
E = Early
D = Delayed
L = Low

# NORMAL AND ABNORMAL CYSTOMETRY
## FINDINGS (continued)

In autonomous neurogenic bladder, a lower motor neuron lesion produces a flaccid bladder that fills without contracting. The patient can't perceive bladder fullness or initiate and maintain urination without applying external pressure. Lower motor neuron lesions can cause sensory or motor paralysis of the bladder. In sensory paralysis, the patient experiences chronic urine retention because he can't perceive bladder fullness. In motor paralysis, the patient has full sensation, but can't initiate or control urination.

| FEATURE OR RESPONSE | AUTONOMOUS NEUROGENIC BLADDER (FLACCID, INCOMPLETE LOWER MOTOR NEURON LESION) | SENSORY PARALYTIC BLADDER (LOWER MOTOR NEURON LESION) | MOTOR PARALYTIC BLADDER (LOWER MOTOR NEURON LESION) |
|---|---|---|---|
| Micturition Start Stop | 0 0 | + + | 0 0 |
| Residual urine | + | + | ++ |
| Vesical sensation | 0 | 0 | + |
| First urge to void | 0 | D | + |
| Bladder capacity | ↑ | ↑/ (< I L) | V |
| Bladder contractions | 0 | 0 | 0 |
| Intravesical pressure | ↓ | ↓ | L |
| Bulbocavernosus reflex | 0 | +/↓/0 | + |
| Saddle sensation | 0 | V | + |
| Bethanechol test (exaggerated response) | + | + | 0 |
| Ice water test | 0 | 0 | 0 |
| Anal reflex | 0 | V | V |
| Heat sensation and pain | 0 | 0 | + |

KEY:
+ = Present/positive    V = Variable
0 = Absent/negative    E = Early
↑ = Increased    D = Delayed
↓ = Decreased    L = Low

## PROCEDURE AND POSTTEST CARE

● Place the patient in a supine position on the examination table.

● A catheter is passed into the bladder to measure the residual urine level. Any difficulty with insertion of the catheter may reflect meatal or urethral obstruction.

● To test the patient's response to thermal sensation, 30 ml of room-temperature physiologic saline solution or sterile water is instilled into the bladder. Then an equal volume of warm (110° F to 115° F [43.3° C to 46.1° C]) fluid is instilled into the bladder. The patient is asked to report his sensations, such as the need to void, nausea, flushing, discomfort, and a feeling of warmth.

● After the fluid is drained from the patient's bladder, the catheter is connected to the cystometer, and normal saline solution, sterile water, or gas (usually carbon dioxide) is slowly introduced into the bladder. The flow of gas is adjusted automatically to the desired reading (100 ml/minute) by a four-channel cystometer.

● The patient is asked to indicate when he first feels an urge to void and then when he feels he must urinate. The related pressure and volume are automatically plotted on the graph.

● When the bladder reaches its full capacity, the patient is asked to urinate so that the maximal intravesical voiding pressure can be recorded. The patient's bladder is then drained and, if no additional tests are required, the catheter is removed; otherwise, the catheter is left in place to measure urethral pressure profile or to provide supplemental findings.

● If abnormal bladder function is caused by muscle incompetence or disrupted innervation, an anticholinergic (atropine) or cholinergic (bethanechol) medication may be injected and the study repeated in 20 to 30 minutes.

● Encourage the patient to drink lots of fluids, unless contraindicated, to relieve burning on urination, a common adverse effect of the procedure.

● Short-term antibiotics are commonly given to prevent infection.

● Administer a sitz bath or warm tub bath if the patient experiences discomfort after the test.

● Measure fluid intake and urine output for 24 hours. Watch for hematuria that persists after the third voiding and for signs of sepsis (such as fever or chills).

## PRECAUTIONS

● Be aware that cystometry is contraindicated in the patient with an acute urinary tract infection because uninhibited contractions may cause erroneous readings and the test may lead to pyelonephritis and septic shock.

● Tell the patient not to strain at voiding; it can cause ambiguous cystometric readings.

● If the patient has a spinal cord injury that has caused motor impairment, transport him on a stretcher so that the test can be performed without transferring him to the examination table.

## FINDINGS

For characteristic findings, see *Normal and abnormal cystometry findings,* pages 128 and 129.

## INTERFERING FACTORS

● Inability to urinate in the supine position

● Concurrent use of drugs such as antihistamines (possible interference with bladder function)

● Cystometry performed within 6 to 8 weeks after surgery for spinal cord injury (inconclusive results)

## *Cystourethroscopy*

Cystourethroscopy, a test that combines two endoscopic techniques, allows visual examination of the bladder and urethra. One of the instruments used in this test is the cystoscope, which has a fiber-optic light source, a magnification system, a right-angled telescopic lens, and an angled beak for smooth passage into the bladder. The other instrument, the urethroscope (or panendoscope), is similar, but has a straight-ahead lens and is used for examination of the bladder neck and urethra. The lenses of the cystoscope and urethroscope use a common sheath inserted into the urethra to obtain the desired view.

Other invasive procedures, such as biopsy, lesion resection, calculi removal, dilatation of a constricted urethra, and catheterization of the ureteral orifices for retrograde

## Using a cystourethroscope

This cross-sectional illustration shows how a urologic examination is performed with a cystourethroscope, a device that allows direct visualization of the tissues of the lower urinary tract. The sheath of the cystourethroscope permits passage of a cystoscope and urethroscope for illuminating the urethra, bladder, and ureters. This instrument also provides a channel for minor surgical procedures, such as biopsy, excision of small lesions, and calculi removal.

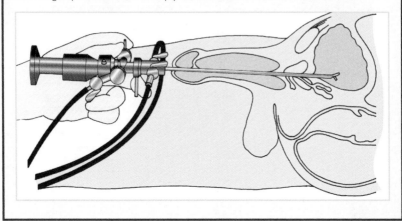

pyelography, may also be performed through this sheath.

Kidney-ureter-bladder radiography and excretory urography usually precede this test.

### PURPOSE
● To diagnose and evaluate urinary tract disorders by direct visualization of urinary structures

### PATIENT PREPARATION
● Explain to the patient that cystourethroscopy permits examination of the bladder and urethra.
● Unless a general anesthetic has been ordered, inform the patient that he need not restrict food and fluids. If a general anesthetic will be administered, instruct the patient to fast for 8 hours before the test.
● Tell the patient who will perform the test, where it will take place, and that it takes about 20 to 30 minutes.
● Inform the patient that he may experience some discomfort after the procedure, including a slight burning when he urinates.
● Make sure that the patient or a responsible family member has signed an informed consent form.

● Before the procedure, administer a sedative, if ordered, and instruct the patient to urinate.

### PROCEDURE AND POSTTEST CARE
● After a general or regional anesthetic (as required) has been administered, the patient is placed in the lithotomy position on a cystoscopic table. The genitalia are cleaned with an antiseptic solution, and the patient is draped. (Local anesthetic is instilled at this point.)
● The instrument is moved toward the bladder to visually examine the urethra. A urethroscope is inserted into the well-lubricated sheath (instead of an obturator), and both are passed gently through the urethra into the bladder. The urethroscope is then removed, and a cystoscope is inserted through the sheath into the bladder.
● After the bladder is filled with irrigating solution, the scope is rotated to inspect the entire surface of the bladder wall and ureteral orifices with the right-angled telescopic lens.
● The cystoscope is then removed, the urethroscope reinserted, and the urethroscope and sheath are slowly withdrawn (see *Using a cystourethroscope*), permitting examination of

the bladder neck and the various portions of the urethra, including the internal and external sphincters.

• During cystourethroscopy, a urine specimen is routinely taken from the bladder for culture and sensitivity testing, and residual urine is measured.

• If a tumor is suspected, a urine specimen is sent to the laboratory for cytologic examination; if a tumor is found, biopsy may be performed. If a urethral stricture is present, urethral dilatation may be necessary before cystourethroscopy.

• If the patient has received only a local anesthetic, he may complain of a burning sensation when the instrument is passed through the urethra. He may also feel an urgent need to urinate as the bladder fills with irrigating solution. Reassure the patient that these sensations are common and generally transient.

• Monitor the patient's vital signs for 15 minutes for the first hour after the test, and then every hour until they stabilize.

• If local anesthesia was used, keep the patient supine for several minutes, and then help him to sit or stand. Watch for orthostatic hypotension.

• Instruct the patient to drink plenty of fluids (or increase I.V. fluids, if ordered) and to take the prescribed analgesic. Reassure him that burning and frequency will soon subside.

• Administer antibiotics, as ordered, to prevent bacterial sepsis due to urethral tissue trauma. Inform the patient about the signs and symptoms of urinary sepsis and to report them immediately.

• Report flank or abdominal pain, chills, fever, an elevated white blood cell count, or low urine output to the physician immediately.

• Record the patient's intake and output for 24 hours, and observe him for distention. If he doesn't void within 8 hours after the test or if bright red blood continues to appear after three voidings, notify the physician.

• Instruct the patient to abstain from alcohol for 48 hours.

• Apply heat to the lower abdomen to relieve pain and muscle spasm (if ordered). A warm sitz bath may be ordered.

## PRECAUTIONS
• Be aware that cystourethroscopy is contraindicated in the patient with acute forms of urethritis, prostatitis, or cystitis because instrumentation can lead to sepsis.

• Know that the test is also contraindicated in the patient with bleeding disorders because instrumentation can lead to increased bleeding.

## NORMAL FINDINGS
The urethra, bladder, and ureteral orifices appear normal in size, shape, and position. The mucosa lining the lower urinary tract should appear smooth and shiny, with no evidence of erythema, cysts, or other abnormalities. The bladder should be free from obstructions, tumors, and calculi.

## ABNORMAL FINDINGS
One of the most common abnormal findings detected in cystourethroscopy is an enlarged prostate gland in older men. In males and females, urethral stricture, calculi, tumors, diverticula, ulcers, and polyps are also common findings. This test may also detect bladder wall trabeculation and various congenital anomalies, such as ureteroceles, duplicate ureteral orifices, or urethral valves in children.

## INTERFERING FACTORS
• None significant

# Cytomegalovirus antibody screen

After primary infection, cytomegalovirus (CMV) remains latent in white blood cells (WBCs). The presence of CMV antibodies indicates past infection with this virus. In an immunocompromised patient, CMV can be reactivated to cause active infection. Administration of blood or tissue from a seropositive donor may cause active CMV infection in a CMV-seronegative organ transplant recipient or neonate, especially one born prematurely.

Antibodies to CMV can be detected by several methods, including passive hemagglutination, latex agglutination, enzyme immunoassay, and indirect immunofluorescence. The complement fixation test is only 60% sensitive compared with other assays and shouldn't be used to screen for CMV antibodies. Screening tests for CMV antibodies are qualitative; they detect the presence of antibody at a single low dilution. In quantitative methods, several dilutions of the serum sample are tested to indicate acute CMV infection.

## PURPOSE
- To detect CMV infection in donors and recipients of organs and blood and in immunocompromised patients
- To screen for CMV infection in infants who require blood transfusions or tissue transplants

## PATIENT PREPARATION
*Age alert* *Explain the purpose of the CMV antibody screen to the patient or the parents of an infant, as appropriate.*
- Tell the patient that the CMV antibody screen requires a blood sample. Explain who will perform the venipuncture and when.
- Explain to the patient that he may experience slight discomfort from the tourniquet and needle puncture.

## PROCEDURE AND POSTTEST CARE
- Perform a venipuncture and collect the sample in a 5-ml tube designated by the laboratory.
- Allow the blood to clot for at least 1 hour at room temperature.
- Apply direct pressure to the venipuncture site until bleeding stops.
- If a hematoma develops at the venipuncture site, apply pressure.

## PRECAUTIONS
- Handle the sample gently to prevent hemolysis.
- Transfer the serum to a sterile tube or vial and send it to the laboratory.
- If transfer must be delayed, store the serum at 39.2° F (4° C) for 1 to 2 days or at –4° F (–20° C) for longer periods to avoid contamination.
- Because the patient may have a compromised immune system, keep the venipuncture site clean and dry.

## REFERENCE VALUES
The patient who has never been infected with CMV has no detectable antibodies to the virus. Immunoglobulin (Ig) G and IgM are normally negative.

## ABNORMAL FINDINGS
A serum sample collected early during the acute phase or late in the convalescent stage may not contain detectable IgG or IgM antibodies to CMV. Therefore, a negative result doesn't preclude recent infection. More than a single sample is needed to ensure accurate results.

A serum sample that tests positive for antibodies at this single dilution indicates that the patient has been infected with CMV and that his WBCs contain latent virus capable of being reactivated in an immunocompromised host. An immunosuppressed patient who lacks antibodies to CMV should receive blood products or organ transplants from a donor who's also seronegative. The patient with CMV antibodies doesn't require seronegative blood products.

## INTERFERING FACTORS
- None significant

# D-dimer

A D-dimer is an asymmetrical carbon compound fragment formed after thrombin converts fibrinogen to fibrin, factor XIIIa stabilizes it into a clot, and plasma acts on the cross-linked, or clotted, fibrin. The D-dimer test is specific for fibrinolysis because it confirms the presence of fibrin split products.

## PURPOSE
● To diagnose disseminated intravascular coagulation (DIC)
● To differentiate subarachnoid hemorrhage from a traumatic lumbar puncture in spinal fluid analysis

## PATIENT PREPARATION
● Obtain the patient's history of hematologic diseases, recent surgery, and the results of other tests performed.
● Explain to the patient that the D-dimer test is used to determine if the blood is clotting normally.
● Tell the patient that the test requires a blood sample. Explain who will perform the venipuncture and when.
● Explain to the patient that he may feel slight discomfort from the tourniquet and needle puncture.

## PROCEDURE AND POSTTEST CARE
● Perform a venipuncture and collect the sample in a 4.5-ml tube with sodium citrate added.
● For a spinal fluid analysis, the sample is collected during a lumbar puncture and placed in a plastic vial. See "Cerebrospinal fluid analysis," pages 92 to 95, for details of the procedure.
● Apply pressure to the venipuncture site for 5 minutes or until bleeding stops.
● If a hematoma develops at the venipuncture site, apply pressure.

## PRECAUTIONS
● Completely fill the collection tube, invert it gently several times, and send it to the laboratory immediately.
● For a patient with coagulation problems, be aware that you may need to apply additional pressure at the venipuncture site to control bleeding.

## REFERENCE VALUES
Normal D-dimer test results are negative or less than 250 µg/L (SI, < 250 µg/L).

## ABNORMAL FINDINGS
Increased D-dimer values may indicate DIC, pulmonary embolism, arterial or venous thrombosis, neoplastic disease, pregnancy (late and postpartum), surgery occurring up to 2 days before testing, subarachnoid hemorrhage (spinal fluid only), or secondary fibrinolysis.

## INTERFERING FACTORS
● High rheumatoid factor titers or increased CA-125 levels (possible false-positive)
● Spinal fluid analysis in an infant under age 6 months (possible false-negative)

# Delayed hypersensitivity skin tests

Skin testing for delayed-type hypersensitivity (DTH) is an important method for evaluating T-cell mediated immune response in a patient. (However, positive reactions don't indicate protection against the antigen.) This response requires previous exposure to the antigen and an intact immune system. After initial exposure to the antigen, the body produces antibodies and sensitized T cells. When reexposed to the antigen (recall antigen), the antibodies react immediately, causing a hypersensitivity reaction; however, the T cells respond over the next few days, causing a delayed hypersensitivity reaction. The immediate response is typically erythema, while the delayed response is induration (hardening). The lack of response to a recall antigen is termed *anergy* and, in the absence of underlying disease or immunosuppressive therapy, may indicate T-cell immunodeficiency disease.

The most commonly used recall antigen is *Mycobacterium tuberculosis* (purified protein derivative [PPD] Mantoux test). Other antigens used in the clinical setting include *Candida, Trichophyton,* and mumps. Some antigens previously used for DTH testing, such as fungi and streptococci, are no longer available or recommended for clinical use.

DTH-like reactions may occur with topical contact to Rhus species plants (poison ivy, oak, and sumac), nickel, dinitrochlorobenzene (DNCB), dinitrofluorobenzene (DNFB), and picryl chloride. Contact sensitivity to Rhus and nickel is determined clinically, and skin testing isn't considered necessary. There's a risk of local tissue necrosis when using chemical antigens, specifically DNCB and DNFB, so their use is discouraged; in vitro assessment of cell-mediated immunity is preferred in those circumstances.

DTH testing can be used to assess the status of an individual's immune system in severe infection, cancer, pretransplantation, and malnutrition. Antigens used for this testing must be antigens the patient has been previously exposed to. For example, *C. albicans,* tetanus, or mumps can be used.

DTH testing is performed by injecting a small amount of antigenic material intradermally or applying it topically and measuring the reaction after 48 to 72 hours. Skin testing has limited value in infants due to their immature immune system and lack of previous sensitization. In addition, patch testing may be used. This test involves applying antigenic material topically to the skin, helping to confirm allergic contact sensitization and isolate the causative agent. (See *Performing a patch test,* page 136.)

## PURPOSE

● To assess for exposure to or activation of certain diseases, most commonly tuberculosis (TB)
● To assess the status of a patient's immune system during illness (cancer, transplantation)
● To evaluate sensitivity to environmental antigens in the patient with persistent symptoms (for example, asthma, seasonal rhinitis, recurrent or persistent urticaria)

## PATIENT PREPARATION

● Explain to the patient that a small amount of antigenic material will be injected superficially or applied to the skin.
● Inform the patient that testing takes only a few minutes for each antigen. Reactions will be evaluated 48 to 72 hours later. Occasionally, the test must be repeated in 2 to 3 weeks when a negative result is initially displayed. The first test "reminds" the body that it was previously exposed to the antigen and a response is noted on retesting. This reminder is commonly done for TB testing and is called the *two-step test.*
● Be sure to ask the patient about sensitivity to the test antigens, whether he has had previous skin testing, and what the outcomes of that testing were. When performing TB testing, ask about previous TB disease or exposure and bacille Calmette-Guérin vaccination.
● Be aware that the U.S. Food and Drug Administration hasn't approved all vaccines for use in skin testing, though nonapproved substances are commonly used. Currently approved antigens include PPD to *M. tuberculosis* and mumps.

# PERFORMING A PATCH TEST

A patch test confirms allergic contact sensitivity and can help identify its cause. In this test, a sample series of common allergens (antigens) is applied to the skin in the hope that one or more will produce a positive reaction. A positive patch test proves that the patient has a contact sensitivity, but doesn't necessarily confirm that the test substance caused the clinical eruption.

If the patient has an acute inflammation, the patch test should be postponed until the inflammation subsides to avoid exacerbating the inflammation.

## KEEP THE FOLLOWING POINTS IN MIND WHEN PERFORMING A PATCH TEST:

♦ Use only potentially irritating substances for a patch test. Testing with primary irritants isn't possible.

♦ To avoid skin irritation, dilute substances that may be irritating to 1% to 2% in petroleum jelly, mineral oil or, as a last choice, water. When there are no clues to a likely allergen in a person with possible contact dermatitis, use a series of common allergens available in standard patch tests.

♦ Apply the allergens to normal, hairless skin on the back or on the ventral surface of the forearm. First, apply them to a small disk of filter paper attached to aluminum and coated with plastic. Tape the paper to the skin, or use a small square of soft cotton and cover it with occlusive tape. Apply liquids and ointments to the disk or cotton. Apply volatile liquids to the skin and allow the areas to dry before covering. Before application, powder solids and moisten powders and fabrics.

♦ Make sure that patches remain in place for 48 hours. However, remove the patch immediately if pain, pruritus, or irritation develops. Positive reactions may take time to develop, so check findings 20 to 30 minutes after removing the patch and again 96 hours (4 days) after the application.

♦ To relieve the effects of a positive reaction, tell the patient to apply topical corticosteroids, as ordered.

## PROCEDURE AND POSTTEST CARE

● Inject each antigen being tested intradermally, using a separate tuberculin syringe, on the patient's forearm. (See *Administering test antigens*.)

● Circle each injection site with a pen, and label each according to the antigen given.

● Instruct the patient to avoid washing off the circles until the test is completed.

● Inject the control allergy diluent on the other forearm.

● Inspect the injection sites for reactivity after 48 to 72 hours. Record induration and erythema in millimeters. A negative test at the first concentration of antigen should be confirmed using a higher concentration.

*Alert* *Watch the patient closely for severe local reactions that may occur at the test site, such as pain, blistering, swelling, induration, itching, and ulceration. Scarring or hyperpigmentation may also result. Also observe for swelling and tenderness in the lymph nodes at the elbow or axillary region. Check for tachycardia and fever, although these rarely occur. Symptoms typically appear in 15 to 30 minutes.*

● Tell the patient experiencing hypersensitivity that steroids will control the reaction, but that skin lesions may persist for 10 to 14 days. Instruct him to avoid scratching or otherwise disturbing the affected area.

## PRECAUTIONS

● If appropriate, store antigens in lyophilized (freeze-dried) form at 39.2° F (4° C) and protected from light. Reconstitute them shortly before use and check their expiration dates. If the patient is suspected of being hypersensitive to the antigens, apply them first in low concentrations.

● If the forearms are not free from disease (for example, if the patient has atopic dermatitis), use other sites such as the back.

*Alert* *Observe the patient carefully for signs of anaphylactic shock — urticaria, respiratory distress, and hypotension. If such signs develop, administer epinephrine, as ordered, and notify the physician immediately.*

## NORMAL FINDINGS

In the recall antigen test, a positive response (5 mm or more of induration at the test site) appears 48 hours after injection.

## ADMINISTERING TEST ANTIGENS

The illustration here shows the arm of a patient undergoing a recall antigen test, which determines whether he has previously been exposed to certain antigens. A sample panel of four test antigens has been injected into his forearm, and the test site has been marked and labeled for each antigen.

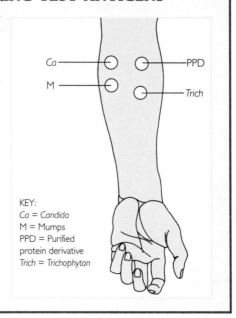

KEY:
Ca = Candida
M = Mumps
PPD = Purified
protein derivative
Trich = Trichophyton

## ABNORMAL FINDINGS

In the recall antigen test, a positive response to less than two of the test antigens, a persistent unresponsiveness to intradermal injection of higher-strength antigens, or a generalized diminished reaction (causing less than 10 mm combined induration) indicates diminished delayed hypersensitivity.

Diminished delayed hypersensitivity can result from Hodgkin's disease (common); sarcoidosis; liver disease; congenital immunodeficiency disease, such as ataxia-telangiectasia, DiGeorge syndrome, and Wiskott-Aldrich syndrome; uremia; acute leukemia; viral diseases, such as influenza, infectious mononucleosis, measles, mumps, and rubella; fungal diseases, such as coccidioidomycosis and cryptococcosis; bacterial diseases, such as leprosy and TB; and terminal cancer. Diminished delayed hypersensitivity can also result from immunosuppressive or steroid therapy or viral vaccination.

## INTERFERING FACTORS

- Use of antigens that have expired or that have been exposed to heat and light or to bacterial contamination
- Poor injection technique (subcutaneous instead of intradermal injection)
- Inaccurate dilution of antigens or an error in reading or timing test results
- A strong immediate reaction to the antigen at the injection site
- Hormonal contraceptives (may cause false-negative results by inhibiting lymphocyte mitosis)

## Dexamethasone suppression

The dexamethasone suppression test requires administration of dexamethasone, an oral steroid. Dexamethasone suppresses levels of circulating adrenal steroid hormones in normal people, but fails to suppress them in patients with Cushing's syndrome and some forms of clinical depression.

## PURPOSE

- To diagnose Cushing's syndrome
- To aid in the diagnosis of clinical depression

## PATIENT PREPARATION

● Explain to the patient the purpose of the dexamethasone suppression test.
● Inform the patient that the test requires two blood samples drawn after administration of dexamethasone. Explain who will perform the venipunctures and when.
● Explain to the patient that he may experience discomfort from the needle punctures and the tourniquet.
● Restrict food and fluids for 10 to 12 hours before the test.

## PROCEDURE AND POSTTEST CARE

● On the first day, give the patient 1 mg of dexamethasone at 11 p.m. On the next day, collect blood samples at 4 p.m. and 11 p.m. More frequent sampling may increase the likelihood of measuring a nonsuppressed cortisol peak.
● If a hematoma develops at the venipuncture site, apply pressure.

## PRECAUTIONS

● Check patient's medication history and have patient withhold medications for 24 to 48 hours if possible.

## NORMAL FINDINGS

A cortisol level of 5 g/dl (140 nmol/L) or greater indicates failure of dexamethasone suppression.

## ABNORMAL FINDINGS

A normal test result doesn't rule out major depression, but an abnormal result strengthens a clinically based diagnosis. Failure of suppression occurs in the patient with Cushing's syndrome, severe stress, and depression that's likely to respond to treatment with antidepressants.

## INTERFERING FACTORS

● Diabetes mellitus, pregnancy, and severe stress, such as trauma, severe weight loss, dehydration, and acute alcohol withdrawal (possible false-positive)
● Certain drugs, particularly barbiturates or phenytoin, within 3 weeks of the test (possible false-positive)
● Caffeine consumed after midnight the night before the test (possible false-positive)
● Use of corticosteroids, hormonal contraceptives, lithium, methadone, aspirin, diuretics, morphine, or monoamine oxidase inhibitors

# *Digital subtraction angiography*

Digital subtraction angiography (DSA) is a sophisticated radiographic technique that uses video equipment and computer-assisted image enhancement to examine the vascular systems. As in conventional angiography, X-ray images are obtained after injecting a contrast medium. However, unlike conventional angiography, in which images of bone and soft tissue commonly obscure vascular detail, DSA provides a high-contrast view of blood vessels without interfering images or shadows.

This unique view is made possible by digital subtraction, in which fluoroscopic images are taken before and after injection of a contrast medium. A computer converts these images into digital information and then "subtracts" the first image from the second, eliminating most information (mainly bone and soft tissue) common to both images. The result is a better image of the contrast-enhanced vasculature.

In addition to superior image quality, DSA has other advantages over conventional angiography. Because the digital subtraction process allows I.V., rather than intra-arterial, injection of the contrast medium, DSA avoids the risk of stroke associated with conventional angiography and reduces the pain and discomfort associated with arterial catheterization.

Although DSA has been used to study peripheral and renal vascular disease, it's probably most useful in diagnosing cerebrovascular disorders, such as carotid stenosis and occlusion, arteriovenous malformation, aneurysms, and vascular tumors. It's also useful in visualizing displacement of vasculature by other intracranial abnormalities or traumatic injuries and in detecting lesions typically missed by computed tomography scans such as thrombosis of the superior sagittal sinus.

## PURPOSE

● To visualize extracranial and intracranial cerebral blood flow

To detect and evaluate cerebrovascular abnormalities

To aid postoperative evaluation of cerebrovascular surgery, such as arterial grafts and endarterectomies

## PATIENT PREPARATION

Explain to the patient that DSA visualizes cerebral blood vessels.

Tell the patient that he'll need to fast for 4 hours before the test, but he need not restrict fluids.

Explain to the patient that he'll receive an injection of a contrast medium, either by needle or through a venous catheter inserted in his arm, and that a series of X-rays will be taken of his head. Tell him who will perform the test, where it will take place, and that it takes 30 to 90 minutes.

Inform the patient that he'll be positioned on an X-ray table with his head immobilized and will be asked to lie still.

*Age alert* *Some patients — especially children — may be given a sedative to prevent movement during the procedure.*

Instruct the patient to remove all jewelry, dentures, and other radiopaque objects from the X-ray field.

Tell the patient that he'll probably feel some transient pain from insertion of the needle or catheter and that he may experience a feeling of warmth, a headache, a metallic taste, and nausea or vomiting after the contrast agent is injected.

Make sure that the patient or a responsible family member has signed an informed consent form, if required.

Check the patient's history for hypersensitivity to iodine; iodine-containing substances such as shellfish; and contrast media. If he's had such reactions, note them on the chart and inform the physician, who may order prophylactic medications or choose not to perform the test.

## PROCEDURE AND POSTTEST CARE

Place the patient in the supine position on an X-ray table and tell him to lie still with his arms at his sides.

After an initial series of fluoroscopic pictures (mask images) of the patient's head is taken, the injection site — most commonly the antecubital basilic or cephalic vein — is shaved and cleaned with an antiseptic solution.

If catheterization is ordered, a local anesthetic is administered, a venipuncture is performed, and a catheter is inserted and advanced to the superior vena cava.

After placement is verified by X-ray, I.V. lines from a bag of normal saline solution and from an automatic contrast medium injector are connected. While the saline is administered, the injector delivers the contrast medium at a rate of about 14 ml/second. If a simple injection of the contrast medium is ordered, a bolus of 40 to 60 ml is administered I.V. by needle.

Monitor the patient's vital signs and neurologic status and observe for signs of a hypersensitivity reaction, such as urticaria, flushing, and respiratory distress.

After allowing time for the contrast medium to clear the pulmonary circulation and enter the cerebral vasculature, a second series of fluoroscopic images (contrast images) is taken. The computer digitizes the information received from both series and compares mask and contrast images, subtracting the information (images of bone and soft tissue) common to both. A detailed image of the contrast medium-filled vessels is displayed on a video monitor; the image may be stored on videotape or a videodisc for future reference.

Because the contrast medium acts as a diuretic, encourage the patient to increase his fluid intake for 24 hours after this test. Advise him that extra fluid intake will also speed excretion of the contrast medium. Monitor his intake and output, as ordered.

Check the venipuncture site for signs of extravasation, such as redness or swelling. If bleeding occurs, apply firm pressure to the puncture site. If a hematoma develops, elevate the arm and apply pressure.

Observe the patient for a delayed hypersensitivity reaction to the contrast medium. A delayed reaction can occur up to 18 hours after the procedure.

Tell the patient that he may resume his usual diet.

## PRECAUTIONS

Know that DSA may be contraindicated in the patient with a hypersensitivity to iodine or contrast media; poor cardiac function; renal, hepatic, or thyroid disease; diabetes; or multiple myeloma.

## NORMAL FINDINGS

The contrast medium should fill and opacify all superficial and deep arteries, arterioles, and veins, allowing visualization of normal cerebral vasculature. The digital subtraction process may intensify areas that should receive only contrast medium. However, conventional angiography provides a more detailed image of the carotid arteries than does DSA.

## ABNORMAL FINDINGS

Vascular filling defects, seen as areas of increased vascular opacity, may indicate arteriovenous occlusion or stenosis, possibly due to vasospasm, vascular malformation or angiomas, arteriosclerosis, or cerebral embolism or thrombosis. Outpouchings in vessel lumina may reflect cerebral aneurysms; such aneurysms frequently rupture, causing subarachnoid hemorrhage. Vessel displacement or vascular masses may indicate an intracranial tumor. DSA can clearly depict the vascular supply of some tumors, reflecting the tumor's position, size, and nature.

## INTERFERING FACTORS

● Patient movement
● Radiopaque objects in the fluoroscopic field

# Doppler ultrasonography

Doppler ultrasonography is a noninvasive test used to evaluate blood flow in the major veins and arteries of the arms and legs and in the extracranial cerebrovascular system. An alternative to arteriography and venography, it's safer, less costly, and faster than invasive tests.

In Doppler ultrasonography, a handheld transducer directs high-frequency sound waves to the artery or vein being tested. The sound waves strike moving red blood cells and are reflected back to the transducer, allowing direct listening and graphic recording of blood flow.

Measurement of systolic pressure during this test is used to detect the presence, location, and extent of peripheral arterial occlusive disease. Changes in sound wave frequency during respiration are observed to

detect venous occlusive disease. Compression maneuvers detect occlusion of the veins and occlusion or stenosis of carotid arteries.

Pulse volume recorder testing may be performed with Doppler ultrasonography to record changes in blood volume or flow in an extremity or organ.

## PURPOSE

● To aid in the diagnosis of venous insufficiency and superficial and deep vein thrombosis (popliteal, femoral, iliac)
● To aid in the diagnosis of peripheral artery disease and arterial occlusion
● To monitor the patient who has had arterial reconstruction and bypass grafts
● To detect abnormalities of carotid artery blood flow associated with conditions such as aortic stenosis
● To evaluate possible arterial trauma

## PATIENT PREPARATION

● Explain to the patient that Doppler ultrasonography is used to evaluate blood flow in the arms and legs or neck.
● Tell the patient who will perform the test.
● Reassure the patient that the test doesn't involve risk or discomfort.
● Tell the patient that he'll be asked to move his arms to different positions and to perform breathing exercises as measurements are taken. A small ultrasonic probe resembling a microphone is placed at various sites along veins or arteries, and blood pressure is checked at several sites.
● Check with the vascular laboratory about special equipment or instructions.

## PROCEDURE AND POSTTEST CARE

● Water-soluble conductive gel is applied to the tip of the transducer.

### Peripheral arterial evaluation

● Peripheral arterial evaluation is always performed bilaterally. The usual test sites in each leg are the common femoral, superficial femoral, popliteal, posterior tibial, and dorsalis pedis arteries; in each arm, the test sites are usually the subclavian, brachial, radial, ulnar and, occasionally, the palmar arch and digital arteries.
● The patient is instructed to remove all clothing above or below the waist, depending on the test site, and he's placed in a

supine position on the examining table or bed, with his arms at his sides.

● Brachial blood pressure is measured, and the transducer is placed at various points along the test arteries.

● The signals are monitored and the waveforms recorded for later analysis.

● Segmental limb blood pressure is obtained to localize arterial occlusive disease.

● During lower extremity tests, a blood pressure cuff is wrapped around the calf, pressure readings are obtained, and waveforms are recorded from the dorsalis pedis and posterior tibial arteries. Then the cuff is wrapped around the thigh, and waveforms are recorded at the popliteal artery.

● In upper extremity tests, examination is performed on one arm, with the patient first placed in a supine position and then sitting; it's then repeated on the other arm. A blood pressure cuff is wrapped around the forearm, pressure readings are taken, and waveforms are recorded over the radial and ulnar arteries. Then the cuff is wrapped around the upper arm, pressure readings are taken, and waveforms are recorded with the transducer over the brachial artery.

● Blood pressure readings and waveform recordings are repeated with the arm in extreme hyperextension and hyperabduction to check for possible compression factors that may interfere with arterial blood flow. The upper extremity examination is performed on one arm, with the patient first placed in a supine position and then sitting; it's then repeated on the other arm.

### Peripheral venous evaluation

● Usual test sites for peripheral venous evaluation include the popliteal, superficial femoral, and common femoral veins in the leg and the posterior tibial vein at the ankle; the brachial, axillary, and subclavian veins in the arm; jugular veins; and, occasionally, the inferior and superior vena cava.

● The patient is instructed to remove all clothing above or below the waist, depending on the test site.

● He's placed in a supine position and instructed to breathe normally.

● The transducer is placed over the appropriate vein, waveforms and compressibility are recorded, and respiratory modulations are noted.

● Proximal limb compression maneuvers are performed and augmentation is noted af-

ter release of compression, to evaluate venous valve competency.

● Changes in respiration are monitored.

● During lower extremity tests, the patient is asked to perform Valsalva's maneuver, and venous blood flow is recorded.

● The procedure is repeated for the other arm or leg.

### Extracranial cerebrovascular evaluation

● Usual test sites for extracranial cerebrovascular evaluation include the supraorbital, common carotid, external carotid, internal carotid, and vertebral arteries.

● The patient is placed in a supine position on the examining table or bed, with a pillow beneath his head for support.

● Brachial blood pressure is then recorded using the Doppler probe.

● The transducer is positioned over the test artery, and blood flow velocity is monitored and recorded.

● The influence of compression maneuvers on blood flow velocity is measured, and the procedure is repeated on the opposite side. (See *How to detect thrombi with a Doppler probe,* page 142.)

### All procedures

● Remove the conductive gel from the patient's skin.

### PRECAUTIONS

● Don't place the Doppler probe over an open or draining lesion.

### NORMAL FINDINGS

Arterial waveforms of the arms and legs are triphasic, with a prominent systolic component and one or more diastolic sounds. The ankle-arm pressure index—the ratio between ankle systolic pressure and brachial systolic pressure—is normally equal to or greater than 1. (The ankle-arm pressure index is also known as the *arterial ischemia index,* the *ankle-brachial index,* or the *pedal-brachial index.*) Proximal thigh pressure is normally 20 to 30 mm Hg higher than arm pressure, but pressure measurements at adjacent sites are similar. In the arms, pressure readings should remain unchanged despite postural changes.

Venous blood flow velocity is normally phasic with respiration and is of a lower pitch than arterial flow. Distal compression or release of proximal limb compression in-

# HOW TO DETECT THROMBI WITH A DOPPLER PROBE

The Doppler probe is typically used to detect venous thrombi by first positioning the transducer and then occluding the blood vessel by compression (as shown in the illustration of the normal leg below). Water-soluble conductive gel is applied to the tip of the transducer to provide coupling between the skin and transducer.

When pressure is released, allowing blood flow to resume, the transducer picks up the sudden augmentation of the flow sound and permits graphic recording of blood flow. If a thrombus is present, a compression maneuver fails to produce the augmented flow sound because the blood flow (as shown below in the femoral vein) is significantly impaired.

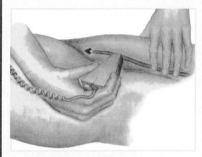

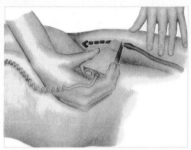

creases blood flow velocity. In the legs, abdominal compression eliminates respiratory variations, but release increases blood flow; Valsalva's maneuver also interrupts venous flow velocity.

In cerebrovascular testing, a strong velocity signal is present. In the common carotid artery, blood flow velocity increases during diastole due to low peripheral vascular resistance of the brain. The direction of periorbital arterial flow is normally anterograde out of the orbit.

## ABNORMAL FINDINGS

Arterial stenosis or occlusion diminishes the blood flow velocity signal, with no diastolic sound and a less prominent systolic component distal to the lesion. At the lesion, the signal is high-pitched and, occasionally, turbulent. If complete occlusion is present and collateral circulation hasn't taken over, the velocity signal may be absent.

A pressure gradient exceeding 20 mm Hg at adjacent sites of measurement in the leg may indicate occlusive disease. Specifically, low proximal thigh pressure signifies common femoral or aortoiliac occlusive disease. An abnormal gradient between the proximal

thigh and the above- or below-knee cuffs indicates superficial femoral or popliteal artery occlusive disease; an abnormal gradient between the below-knee and ankle cuffs indicates tibiofibular disease. Abnormal gradients of arm and forearm pressure readings may indicate brachial artery occlusion.

An abnormal ankle-arm pressure index is directly proportional to the degree of circulatory impairment: mild ischemia, 1.0 to 0.75; claudication, 0.75 to 0.50; pain at rest, 0.50 to 0.25; and pregangrene, 0.25 to 0.

If venous blood flow velocity is unchanged by respirations, doesn't increase in response to compression or Valsalva's maneuver, or is absent, venous thrombosis is indicated. In chronic venous insufficiency and varicose veins, the flow velocity signal may be reversed. Confirmation of results may require venography.

Inability to identify Doppler signals during cerebrovascular examination implies total arterial occlusion. Reversed periorbital arterial flow indicates significant arterial occlusive disease of the extracranial internal carotid artery. In addition, the audible signal may take on the acoustic characteristics of a normal peripheral artery. Internal carotid artery stenosis causes turbulent signals. Collateral circulation can be assessed by compression maneuvers.

Oculoplethysmography, carotid phono-angiography, or carotid imaging can further evaluate cerebrovascular disease. Retrograde blood velocity in the vertebral artery can indicate subclavian steal syndrome. A weak velocity signal on comparison of contralateral vertebral arteries can indicate diffuse vertebral artery disease.

## INTERFERING FACTORS
● Inability of the patient to cooperate

## Ductal lavage of breast tissue

Ductal lavage of breast tissue is a minimally invasive method for assessing a woman's risk for developing breast cancer. This test permits the collection of cells from inside the milk ducts of the breast. Research has demonstrated that the majority of breast cancers begin in the cells that line the breast ducts. These cells may take 8 to 10 years to develop into a tumor that's visible with a mammogram or palpated with a breast examination. This test helps to determine if the woman has atypical cells in her milk ducts that have the potential for becoming malignant. The belief is that the earlier the abnormal cells are found, the more treatment options are available.

This test may be referred to as the "pap smear" for the breasts. It's indicated only in those women who are considered to be at high risk for developing breast cancer based on personal and family factors. It's commonly performed in a physician's office.

## PURPOSE
● To identify a woman's risk for developing breast cancer

## PATIENT PREPARATION
● Describe the procedure to the patient, and explain that ductal lavage of breast tissue helps to identify cells that have the potential to become cancerous.
● Offer her emotional support, and assure her that evidence of atypical cells doesn't necessarily indicate cancer.

● Tell the patient that she need not restrict food, fluids, and medication.
● Tell her who will perform the test and where it will be done.
● Warn the patient that she may feel a sensation of breast fullness similar to lactation, tingling, or pinching. Also inform her that the discomfort is similar to that of a mammogram.
● Check the patient's history for hypersensitivity to local anesthetics.

## PROCEDURE AND POSTTEST CARE
● Apply a topical anesthetic agent, if appropriate, approximately 30 minutes to 1 hour before the test.
● Have the patient apply warmth to the breast and massage if indicated.
● The practitioner places a syringe-like aspirator device on the breast at the nipple area and gently pulls back on the syringe to expel fluid from the ducts. Typically only one or two ducts produce extremely minute amounts (drops) of fluid. (See *Understanding breast ductal lavage,* page 144.)

  *Alert* *Fluid production suggests a higher risk for breast cancer development. If no fluid is aspirated, the lavage is not performed.*
● Once the fluid producing ducts are identified, the practitioner inserts a microcatheter into these ducts and instills an anesthetic followed by saline to rinse the ducts.
● The breasts are massaged gently to move the fluid toward the nipple.
● The practitioner aspirates the fluid into the syringe and then transfers the fluid to specialized vials, which are sent to the laboratory for analysis. The procedure is repeated for other ducts that produced fluid.

## NORMAL FINDINGS
No atypical or malignant cells are noted.

## ABNORMAL FINDINGS
The presence of atypical cells suggests a significant increase in the risk for developing breast cancer. However, evidence of atypical cells doesn't positively indicate that breast cancer will develop. Although rare, malignant cells may be found.

## INTERFERING FACTORS
● Insufficient amount of sample ductal fluid

# UNDERSTANDING BREAST DUCTAL LAVAGE

**1.** A syringe-like aspirator is placed over the breast at the nipple area. Suction is applied to the aspirator to draw out small amounts of fluid from the ducts to the nipple surface. Usually only 1 or 2 ducts produce fluid.

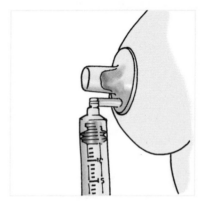

**2.** A microcatheter is then inserted into the ducts from which fluid was obtained.

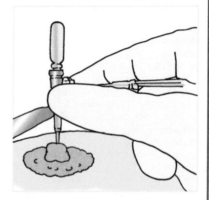

**3.** A small of amount of anesthetic may be instilled followed by a small amount of saline. The breast is massaged and then fluid is withdrawn into the catheter which is attached to a syringe. The sample is then placed in a preservative and sent to the laboratory for analysis.

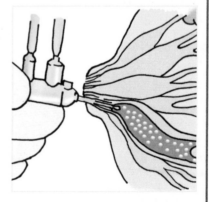

# Echocardiography

Echocardiography is a noninvasive test that shows the size, shape, and motion of cardiac structures. It's useful for evaluating patients with chest pain, enlarged cardiac silhouettes on X-rays, electrocardiographic (ECG) changes unrelated to coronary artery disease (CAD), and abnormal heart sounds on auscultation.

In this test, a transducer directs ultra-high-frequency sound waves toward cardiac structures, which reflect these waves. The echoes are converted to images that are displayed on a monitor and recorded on a strip chart or videotape. Results are correlated with clinical history, physical examination, and findings from additional tests.

The techniques most commonly used in echocardiography are M-mode (motion-mode), for recording the motion and dimensions of intracardiac structures, and two-dimensional (cross-sectional), for recording lateral motion and providing the correct spatial relationship between cardiac structures. (See *M-mode echocardiograms,* page 146.)

## PURPOSE
- To diagnose and evaluate valvular abnormalities
- To measure the size of the heart's chambers
- To evaluate chambers and valves in congenital heart disorders
- To aid in the diagnosis of hypertrophic and related cardiomyopathies
- To detect atrial tumors
- To evaluate cardiac function or wall motion after myocardial infarction
- To detect pericardial effusion
- To detect mucal thrombi

## PATIENT PREPARATION
- Explain to the patient that echocardiography is used to evaluate the size, shape, and motion of various cardiac structures.
- Inform the patient that he need not restrict food and fluids.
- Tell the patient who will perform the test, where it will take place, and that it's safe, painless, and noninvasive.
- Explain that the room may be darkened slightly to aid visualization on the monitor screen and that other procedures (ECG and phonocardiography) may be performed simultaneously to time events in the cardiac cycle.
- Describe the procedure to the patient and instruct him to remain still during the test because movement may distort results.
- Tell the patient that conductive gel will be applied to his chest and a quarter-sized transducer will be placed directly over it. Warn him that he may feel minor discomfort because pressure is exerted to keep the transducer in contact with the skin.
- Explain to the patient that the transducer is angled to observe different areas of the heart and that he may be repositioned on his left side during the procedure.
- Inform the patient that he may be asked to inhale a gas with a slightly sweet odor (amyl nitrite) while changes in heart function are recorded; describe the possible adverse effects (dizziness, flushing, and tachycardia), but assure him that such symptoms quickly subside.

# M-MODE ECHOCARDIOGRAMS

In the normal motion-mode (M-mode) echocardiogram of the mitral valve shown below (top), valve movement appears as a characteristic lopsided, M-shaped tracing. The anterior and posterior mitral valve leaflets separate (D) in early diastole, quickly reach maximum separation (E), and then close during rapid ventricular filling (E-F).

Leaflet separation varies during mid-diastole, and the valve opens widely again (A) following atrial contraction. The valve starts to close with atrial relaxation (A-B) and is completely closed during the start of ventricular systole (C). The steepness of the E-F slope indirectly shows the speed of ventricular filling, which is normally rapid.

## Normal echocardiogram

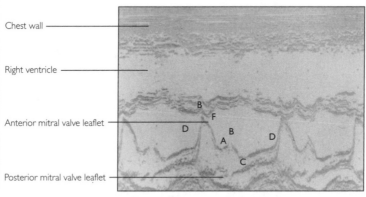

Chest wall

Right ventricle

Anterior mitral valve leaflet

Posterior mitral valve leaflet

## Abnormal echocardiogram

Mitral stenosis is evident in the abnormal echocardiogram shown at right. The E-F slope (line) is very shallow, indicating slowed left ventricular filling.

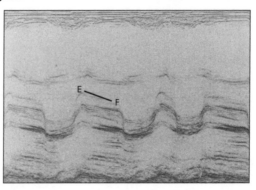

## PROCEDURE AND POSTTEST CARE

● The patient is placed in a supine position.
● Conductive gel is applied to the third or fourth intercostal space to the left of the sternum, and the transducer is placed directly over it.
● The transducer is systematically angled to direct ultrasonic waves at specific parts of the patient's heart.

- During the test, the oscilloscope screen, which displays the returning echoes, is observed.
- Significant findings are recorded on a strip chart recorder (M-mode echocardiography) or on a videotape recorder (two-dimensional echocardiography).
- For a different view of the heart, the transducer is placed beneath the xiphoid process or directly above the sternum.
- For a left lateral view, the patient may be positioned on his left side.
- To record heart function under various conditions, the patient is asked to inhale and exhale slowly, to hold his breath, or to inhale amyl nitrite.
- Doppler echocardiography may be used in this examination to assess speed and direction of blood flow. The sound of blood flow may be heard as the continuous-wave and pulsed-wave Doppler sampling of cardiac valves is performed. This technique is used primarily to assess heart sounds and murmurs as they relate to cardiac hemodynamics.
- When the test is completed, remove the conductive gel from the patient's skin.

## PRECAUTIONS

- Be aware that some laboratories require specific protocols for individualized preparation, including a signed informed consent. Check with your facility's policy.

## NORMAL FINDINGS

An echocardiogram can reveal the motion pattern and structure of the four cardiac valves. Anterior and posterior mitral valve leaflets normally separate in early diastole, with the anterior leaflet moving toward the chest wall and the posterior leaflet moving away from it. The leaflets attain maximum excursion rapidly, and then move toward each other during ventricular diastole; after atrial contraction, they come together and remain so during ventricular systole. On an M-mode echocardiogram, the leaflets appear as two fine lines within the echo-free, blood-filled left ventricular cavity.

The aortic valve cusps lie between the parallel walls of the aortic root, which move anteriorly during systole and posteriorly during diastole. During ventricular systole, these cusps separate and appear as a boxlike configuration on an M-mode echocardiogram. They remain open throughout systole and normally demonstrate a characteristic fine fluttering motion. During diastole, the cusps come together and appear as a single or double line within the aortic root on an M-mode echocardiogram.

The motion of the tricuspid valve resembles that of the mitral valve. The motion of the pulmonic valve — particularly the posterior cusp — is different: During diastole, this cusp gradually moves posteriorly; during atrial systole, it's displaced posteriorly; during ventricular systole, it quickly moves posteriorly; and during right ventricular ejection, the cusp moves anteriorly, attaining its most anterior position during diastole.

The left ventricular cavity normally appears as an echo-free space between the interventricular septum and the posterior left ventricular wall. Echoes produced by the chordae tendineae and the mitral leaflet appear within this cavity. The right ventricular cavity normally appears as an echo-free space between the anterior chest wall and the interventricular septum.

## ABNORMAL FINDINGS

Valvular abnormalities readily appear on the echocardiogram. In mitral stenosis, the valve narrows abnormally due to the leaflets' thickening and disordered motion. Instead of moving in opposite directions during diastole, both mitral valve leaflets move anteriorly. (See *Real-time echocardiograms,* pages 148 and 149.) In mitral valve prolapse, one or both leaflets balloon into the left atrium during systole.

Aortic valve abnormalities — especially aortic insufficiency — can also affect the mitral valve because the anterior mitral leaflet is just below the aortic cusps. When blood regurgitates through the aortic valve during diastole, it strikes this leaflet, causing the flutter seen in M-mode echocardiography. Although the aortic valve may appear normal, this characteristic fluttering confirms aortic insufficiency. In stenosis, due to conditions, such as rheumatic fever or bacterial endocarditis, the aortic valve thickens and thus generates more echoes. However, in rheumatic fever, the valve may thicken slightly and allow normal motion during systole, or it may thicken severely and curtail motion. In bacterial endocarditis, valve motion is disrupted, and shaggy or fuzzy echoes usually appear on or near the valve.

*(Text continues on page 150.)*

# REAL-TIME ECHOCARDIOGRAMS

The real-time (showing motion) echocardiograms shown below are short-axis, cross-sectional views of the mitral valve from a normal patient (top) and a pat ient with mitral stenosis (bottom). In the latter, note the greatly reduced mitral valve orifice caused by stenotic, calcified valve leaflets.

**Normal**

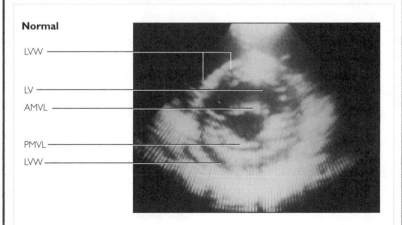

**Mitral stenosis**

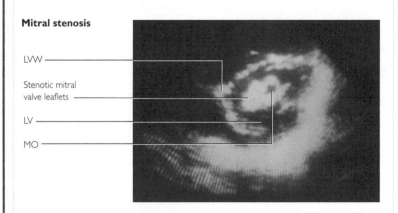

KEY:
AMVL = Anterior mitral valve leaflet
LV = Left ventricle
LVW = Left ventricular wall

MO = Mitral orifice
PMVL = Posterior mitral valve leaflet

## REAL-TIME ECHOCARDIOGRAMS *(continued)*

The echocardiograms shown below are long-axis, cross-sectional views of the mitral valve from a normal patient (top) and a patient with hypertrophic cardiomyopathy, also known as *idiopathic hypertrophic stenosis* (bottom). Note the markedly thickened left ventricular wall in the latter.

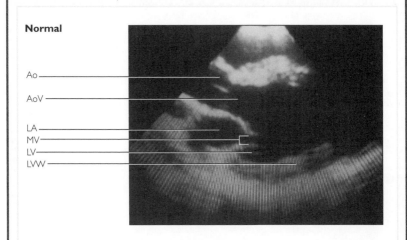

**Normal**

Ao
AoV
LA
MV
LV
LVW

**Hypertrophic cardiomyopathy**

AoV
Ao
LV
LA
LVW

KEY:
Ao = Aorta
AoV = Aortic valve
LA = Left atrium

LV = Left ventricle
LVW = Left ventricular wall
MV = Mitral valve

Other chamber or valve abnormalities may indicate a congenital heart disorder, such as aortic stenosis, which may require further tests. A large chamber size may indicate cardiomyopathy, valvular disorders, or heart failure; a small chamber, restrictive pericarditis.

Hypertrophic obstructive cardiomyopathy can also be identified by the echocardiogram, with systolic anterior motion of the mitral valve and asymmetric septal hypertrophy.

Left atrial tumors are usually on a pedicle and can thus shift in and out of the mitral opening. During diastole, the tumor appears as a mass of echoes against the anterior mitral valve leaflet. During ventricular systole, these echoes shift back into the body of the atrium.

In CAD, ischemia or infarction may cause absent or paradoxical motion in ventricular walls that normally move together and thicken during systole. These affected areas may also fail to thicken or may become thinner, particularly if scar tissue is present.

The echocardiogram is especially sensitive in detecting pericardial effusion. Normally, the epicardium and pericardium are continuous membranes and thus produce a single or near-single echo. When fluid accumulates between these membranes, it causes an abnormal echo-free space to appear. In large effusions, pressure exerted by excess fluid can restrict pericardial motion.

An echocardiogram should be correlated with the patients' history, physical examination findings, and results of additional tests. For a patient with a suboptimal echocardiogram, an agent composed of human albumin microspheres filled with perfluorocarbon gas (Optison) can be used. This agent can enhance the contrast of the ultrasound scans to opacify the left ventricle and improve the delineation of the left ventricular endocardial borders.

## INTERFERING FACTORS

● Incorrect transducer placement and excessive movement
● Thick chest or chest wall abnormalities or chronic obstructive pulmonary disease (possible poor imaging)

# Electrocardiography

A common test for evaluating cardiac status, electrocardiography (ECG) graphically records the electric current (electrical potential) generated by the heart. This current radiates from the heart in all directions and, on reaching the skin, is measured by electrodes connected to an amplifier and strip chart recorder. The standard resting (scalar) ECG uses five electrodes to measure the electrical potential from 12 leads: the standard limb leads (I, II, III), the augmented limb leads ($aV_R$, $aV_L$, and $aV_F$), and the precordial, or chest, leads ($V_1$ through $V_6$).

New computerized ECG machines don't routinely use gel and suction bulbs. The electrodes are small tabs that peel off a sheet and adhere to the patient's skin. The leads coming from the ECG machine are clearly marked and applied to the electrodes with alligator clamps. The entire tracing is displayed on a screen so that abnormalities (loose leads or artifact) can be corrected before the tracing is printed or transmitted to a central computer. The electrode tabs can remain on the patient's chest, arms, and legs to provide continuous lead placement for serial ECG studies.

## PURPOSE

● To help identify primary conduction abnormalities, cardiac arrhythmias, cardiac hypertrophy, pericarditis, electrolyte imbalances, myocardial ischemia, and the site and extent of myocardial infarction (MI)
● To monitor recovery from an MI
● To evaluate the effectiveness of cardiac medication (cardiac glycosides, antiarrhythmics, antihypertensives, and vasodilators)
● To assess pacemaker performance
● To determine the effectiveness of thrombolytic therapy and the resolution of ST-segment depression or elevation and T-wave changes

## PATIENT PREPARATION

● Explain to the patient that an ECG evaluates the heart's electrical activity.
● Tell the patient that he need not restrict food and fluids.

- Describe the test, including who will perform it, where it will take place, and how long it will last.
- Tell the patient that electrodes will be attached to his arms, legs, and chest and that the procedure is painless. Explain that during the test, he'll be asked to relax, lie still, and breathe normally.
- Advise the patient not to talk during the test because the sound of his voice may distort the ECG tracing.
- Check the patient's medication history for use of cardiac drugs and note the use of such drugs on the test request form.

## PROCEDURE AND POSTTEST CARE

- Place the patient in a supine position. If he can't tolerate lying flat, help him to assume semi-Fowler's position.
- Have the patient expose his chest, both ankles, and both wrists for electrode placement. If the patient is a woman, provide a chest drape until the chest leads are applied.
- Turn on the machine and check the paper supply.

## Multichannel ECG

- Place electrodes on the inner aspect of the wrists, the medial aspect of the lower legs, and the chest. If using disposable electrodes, remove the paper backing before positioning.
- Connect the leadwires after all electrodes are in place.
- If frequent ECGs will be necessary, use a marking pen to indicate lead positions on the patient's chest to ensure consistent placement.
- Press the start button and record any required information (for example, the patient's name and room number).
- The machine produces a printout showing all 12 leads simultaneously. Check to make sure all leads are represented in the tracing. If not, determine which one has come loose, reattach it, and restart the tracing.
- Make sure the wave doesn't peak beyond the top edge of the recording grid. If it does, adjust the machine to bring the wave inside the boundaries.
- When the machine finishes the tracing, remove the electrodes and reposition the patient's gown and bed covers.

## Single-channel ECG

- Apply either disposable or standard electrodes to the inner aspect of the wrists and the medial aspect of the lower legs. Connect each leadwire to the corresponding electrode by inserting the wire prong into the terminal post and tightening the screw, if required.
- Set the paper speed, if required (usually 25 mm/second), and calibrate the machine by adjusting the sensitivity to normal. Recalibrate the machine after running each lead to provide a consistent test standard.
- Turn the lead selector to I. Then mark the lead by writing "I" on the paper strip or by depressing the marking button on the machine (some machines do this automatically). Record for 3 to 6 seconds, and then return the machine to the standby mode. Repeat this procedure for leads II, III, $aV_R$, $aV_L$, and $aV_F$.
- Determine proper placement for the chest electrodes. (If frequent ECGs are necessary, mark these spots on the patient's chest to ensure consistent placement.)
- Connect the chest leadwire to the suction bulb, apply gel to each of the six chest positions, and then firmly press the suction bulb to attach the chest lead to the $V_1$ position. Mark the strips as before.
- Turn the lead selector to $V_1$, and record $V_1$ for 3 to 6 seconds. Return the lead selector to standby. Reposition the electrode, and repeat the procedure for $V_2$ through $V_6$.
- After completing $V_6$, obtain a rhythm strip on lead II for at least 6 seconds. Assess the quality of the tracings and repeat any that are unclear.
- Disconnect the equipment, remove the electrodes, and wipe the gel from the patient with a moist cloth towel. Wash the gel from the electrodes and dry them thoroughly.

## Both types

- Label each ECG strip with the patient's name and room number (if applicable), date and time of the procedure, and physician's name. Note whether the ECG was performed during or on resolution of a chest pain episode.
- Disconnect the equipment. The electrode patches are usually left in place if the patient is having recurrent chest pain or if serial ECGs are ordered, as with the use of thrombolytics.

# NORMAL ECG WAVEFORMS

Because each lead takes a different view of heart activity, it generates its own characteristic tracing on an electrocardiogram (ECG). The traces shown here are representative of each of the 12 leads. Leads $aV_R$, $V_1$, $V_2$, $V_3$, and $V_4$ normally show strong negative deflections. Negative deflections indicate that the current is moving away from the positive electrode; positive deflections, that the current is moving toward the positive electrode.

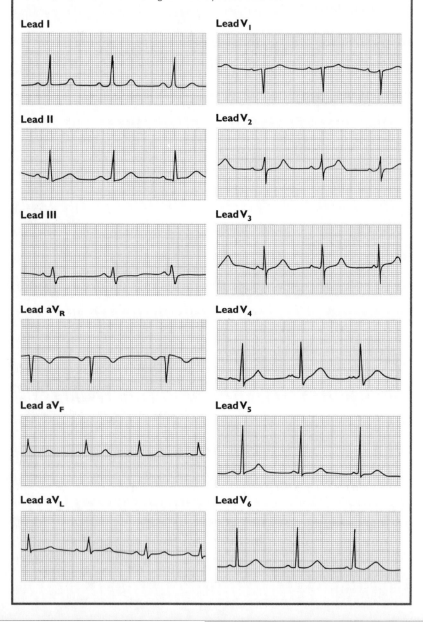

Lead I

Lead $V_1$

Lead II

Lead $V_2$

Lead III

Lead $V_3$

Lead $aV_R$

Lead $V_4$

Lead $aV_F$

Lead $V_5$

Lead $aV_L$

Lead $V_6$

# ABNORMAL ECG WAVEFORMS

Premature ventricular contractions (PVCs) originate in an ectopic focus of the ventricular wall. They can be unifocal (having the same single focus), as shown in this electrocardiogram (ECG) tracing from lead $V_1$, or multifocal (arising from more than one ectopic focus). In PVCs, the P wave is absent and the QRS complex shows considerable distortion, usually deflecting in the opposite direction from the patient's normal QRS complex. The T wave also deflects in the opposite direction from the QRS complex, and the PVC usually precedes a compensatory pause. Some examples of abnormalities causing PVCs include electrolyte imbalances (especially hypokalemia), myocardial infarction (MI), reperfusion of a new MI or injury, hypoxia, and drug toxicity (cardiac glycosides, beta-adrenergics).

**PVC — Lead $V_1$**

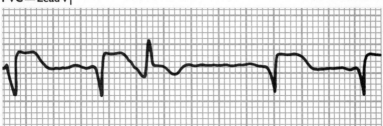

First-degree heart block, the most common conduction disturbance, occurs in healthy hearts as well as diseased hearts and usually is clinically insignificant. It's typically characteristic in elderly patients with chronic degeneration of the cardiac conduction system, and it occasionally occurs in patients receiving cardiac glycosides or antiarrhythmic drugs, such as procainamide and quinidine. In children, first-degree heart block may be the earliest sign of acute rheumatic fever. In this lead $V_1$ tracing, the interval between the P wave and the QRS complex (the PR interval) exceeds 0.20 second.

**First-degree heart block — Lead $V_1$**

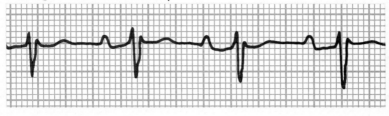

*(continued)*

- Report abnormal ECG findings to the physician.

## PRECAUTIONS
- The recording equipment and other nearby electrical equipment should be properly grounded to prevent electrical interference.
- Double-check color codes and lead markings to be sure connectors match.
- Make sure that the electrodes are firmly attached, and reattach them if loose skin contact is suspected. Don't use cables that are broken, frayed, or bare.

Hypokalemia is a common electrolyte imbalance that's caused by low serum potassium levels and affects the electrical activity of the myocardium. Mild hypokalemia may cause only muscle weakness, fatigue and, possibly, atrial or ventricular irritability; a severe imbalance causes pronounced muscle weakness, paralysis, atrial tachycardia with varying degrees of block, and PVCs that may progress to ventricular tachycardia and fibrillation.

Early signs of hypokalemia, as shown on this lead $V_1$ tracing, include prominent U waves, a prolonged QT interval, and flat or inverted T waves. Usually, T waves don't flatten or invert until potassium depletion becomes severe.

**Hypokalemia — Lead $V_1$**

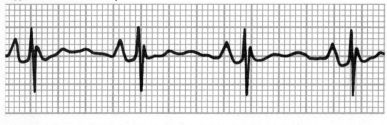

● Make sure that the patient is quiet and motionless during the test because talking and movement distort the recordings.

● If the patient has a pacemaker in place, an ECG may be performed with or without a magnet. Indicate the presence of a pacemaker and whether a magnet is used. (Many pacemakers function only when the heartbeat falls below a preset rate; a magnet makes the pacemaker fire regularly, which permits evaluation of pacemaker performance.)

### NORMAL FINDINGS

The lead II waveform, known as the *rhythm strip,* depicts the heart's rhythm more clearly than does any other waveform. In lead II, the normal P wave doesn't exceed 2.5 mm (0.25 mV) in height or last longer than 0.12 second. The PR interval, which includes the P wave plus the PR segment, persists for 0.12 to 0.2 second for heart rates above 60 beats/minute. The QT interval varies with the heart rate and lasts 0.4 to 0.52 second for heart rates above 60 beats/minute; the voltage of the R wave in the $V_1$ through $V_6$ leads doesn't exceed 27 mm. The total QRS complex lasts 0.06 to 0.1 second. The ST segment is also useful for assessing myocardial ischemia. (See *Normal ECG waveforms,* page 152.)

### ABNORMAL FINDINGS

An abnormal ECG may show an MI, right or left ventricular hypertrophy, arrhythmias, right or left bundle-branch block, ischemia, conduction defects or pericarditis, electrolyte abnormalities (such as hypokalemia), and the effects of cardioactive drugs. Sometimes an ECG may reveal abnormal waveforms only during angina episodes or during exercise. (See *Abnormal ECG waveforms,* pages 153 and 154.)

### INTERFERING FACTORS

● Inaccurate test results because of improper placement of electrodes, patient movement or muscle tremors, strenuous exercise before the test, or medication reactions

● Mechanical difficulties, such as ECG machine malfunction, faulty adherence of electrode patches (for example, due to diaphoresis), and electromagnetic interference (production of artifact)

# Electro-encephalography

In EEG, electrodes attached to areas of the patient's scalp record the brain's electrical activity and transmit this information to an electroencephalograph, which records the resulting brain waves on recording paper. The procedure may be performed in a special laboratory or by a portable unit at the bedside. Ambulatory recording EEGs are available for the patient to wear at home or the workplace to record the patient as he performs his normal daily activities. Continuous-video EEG recording is available on an inpatient basis for identifying epileptic discharges during clinical events or for localization of a seizure focus during surgical evaluation of epilepsy. Intracranial electrodes are surgically implanted to record EEG changes for localization of the seizure focus.

## PURPOSE
- To determine the presence and type of seizure disorder
- To aid in the diagnosis of intracranial lesions, such as abscesses and tumors
- To evaluate the brain's electrical activity in metabolic disease, cerebral ischemia, head injury, meningitis, encephalitis, mental retardation, psychological disorders, and drugs
- To evaluate altered states of consciousness or brain death

## PATIENT PREPARATION
- Explain to the patient that the EEG records the brain's electrical activity.
- Describe the procedure to the patient and his family and answer all their questions.
- Tell the patient that he must forgo caffeine before the test; other than this, there are no food or fluid restrictions. Tell him that skipping the meal before the test can cause relative hypoglycemia and alter the brain wave pattern.
- Inform the patient that smoking is prohibited for at least 8 hours before the test.
- Thoroughly wash and dry the patient's hair to remove hair sprays, creams, and oils.
- Explain to the patient that during the test, he'll relax in a reclining chair or lie on a bed and that electrodes will be attached to his scalp with a special paste. Assure him that the electrodes won't shock him.

**Alert** Check the patient for a history of asthma. The paste has a distinctive odor that may precipitate an asthmatic reaction.

- If needle electrodes are used, explain to the patient that he'll feel a pricking sensation as they're inserted; however, flat electrodes are more commonly used.
- Do your best to allay the patient's fears because nervousness can affect brain wave patterns.
- Check the patient's medication history for drugs that may interfere with test results. Anticonvulsants, tranquilizers, barbiturates, and other sedatives should be withheld for 24 to 48 hours before the test, as ordered by the physician.

**Age alert** Infants and very young children occasionally require sedation to prevent crying and restlessness during the test, but sedation itself may alter test results.

- A patient with a seizure disorder may require a "sleep EEG." In this case, keep the patient awake the night before the test and administer a sedative (such as chloral hydrate) to help him sleep during the test.
- If the test is performed to confirm brain death, provide the patient's family members with emotional support.

## PROCEDURE AND POSTTEST CARE
- Position the patient on the bed or in a reclining chair. Reassure him as the electrodes are attached to his scalp.
- Before the recording procedure begins, instruct the patient to close his eyes, relax, and remain still.
- During the recording, observe the patient carefully; note blinking, swallowing, talking, or other movements and record these findings on the tracing. These activities may cause artifact on the tracing and be misinterpreted as an abnormal tracing.
- The recording may be stopped at intervals to let the patient rest or reposition himself. This is important because restlessness and fatigue can alter brain wave patterns.
- After an initial baseline recording, the patient may be tested under various stress-producing conditions to elicit patterns not observable while he's at rest. For example, he may be asked to breathe deeply and rapidly for 3 minutes (hyperventilation), which may

# COMPARING EEG TRACINGS

The following tracings are examples of regular and irregular brain electrical activity as recorded by an electroencephalogram (EEG).

**Normal (top, right temporal; bottom, parietal-occipital)**

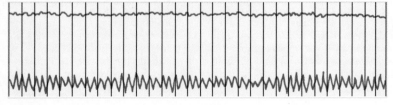

**Absence seizures (spikes and waves, 3/second)**

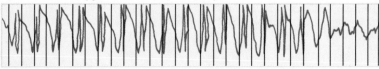

**Generalized tonic-clonic seizures (multiple high-voltage spiked waves)**

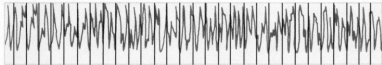

**Right temporal lobe epilepsy (focal spiked waves)**

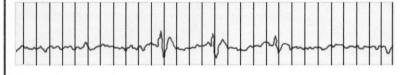

elicit brain wave patterns typical of seizure disorders or other abnormalities. This technique is commonly used to detect absence seizures. Also, photic stimulation tests central cerebral activity in response to bright light, accentuating abnormal activity in absence or myoclonic seizures. In this procedure, a strobe light placed in front of the patient is flashed 1 to 20 times/second; recordings are made with the patient's eyes opened and closed.

● Review carefully the reinstatement of anticonvulsant medication or other drugs withheld before the test.
● Carefully observe the patient for seizure activity and provide a safe environment.
● Help the patient remove electrode paste from his hair.
● If the patient received a sedative before the test, take safety precautions such as raising the bed's side rails.
● If brain death is confirmed, provide the patient's family members with emotional support.

- If clinical events are found to be nonepileptic, a psychological evaluation may be needed.

## PRECAUTIONS

- Observe the patient carefully for seizure activity.
- If seizure activity occurs, record seizure patterns and be prepared to provide assistance. Have suction equipment readily available.

## NORMAL FINDINGS

EEG records a portion of the brain's electrical activity as waves; some are irregular, whereas others demonstrate frequent patterns. Among the basic waveforms are the alpha, beta, theta, and delta rhythms.

Alpha waves occur at a frequency of 8 to 11 cycles/second in a regular rhythm. They're present only in the waking state when the patient's eyes are closed, but he's mentally alert; usually, they disappear with visual activity or mental concentration. Beta waves (13 to 30 cycles/second) — generally associated with anxiety, depression, and use of sedatives — are seen most readily in the frontal and central regions of the brain. Theta waves (4 to 7 cycles/second) are most common in children and young adults and appear in the frontal and temporal regions. Delta waves (0.5 to 3.5 cycles/second) normally occur only in young children and during sleep. (See *Comparing EEG tracings*.)

## ABNORMAL FINDINGS

Usually, about a 100' to 200' (30 to 60 m) strip of recordings is evaluated, with particular attention paid to basic waveforms, symmetry of cerebral activity, transient discharges, and responses to stimulation. A specific diagnosis depends on the patient's clinical status.

In the patient with epilepsy, EEG patterns may identify the specific disorder. In absence seizures, the EEG shows spikes and waves at a frequency of 3 cycles/second. In generalized tonic-clonic seizures, it generally shows multiple, high-voltage, spiked waves in both hemispheres. In temporal lobe epilepsy, the EEG usually shows spiked waves in the affected temporal region. In the patient with focal seizures, it usually shows localized, spiked discharges.

In the patient with an intracranial lesion, such as a tumor or abscess, the EEG may show slow waves (usually delta waves but possibly unilateral beta waves). Vascular lesions, such as cerebral infarcts and intracranial hemorrhages, generally produce focal abnormalities in the injured area.

Generally, any condition that causes a diminishing level of consciousness alters the EEG pattern in proportion to the degree of consciousness lost. For example, in a patient with a metabolic disorder, an inflammatory process (such as meningitis or encephalitis), or increased intracranial pressure, the EEG shows generalized, diffuse, and slow brain waves.

The most pathologic finding of all is an absent EEG pattern — a "flat" tracing (except for artifact), which may indicate brain death.

## INTERFERING FACTORS

- Interference from extraneous electrical activity; head, body, eye, or tongue movement; or muscle contractions (possible production of excessive artifact)
- Anticonvulsants, barbiturates, tranquilizers, and other sedatives (possible masking of seizure activity)
- Acute drug intoxication or severe hypothermia, resulting in loss of consciousness (flat EEG)

# *Electromyography*

Electromyography (EMG) records the electrical activity of selected skeletal muscle groups at rest and during voluntary contraction. It involves percutaneous insertion of a needle electrode into a muscle. The electrical discharge of the muscle is then measured by an oscilloscope. Nerve conduction time is often measured simultaneously. (See *Nerve conduction studies,* page 158.)

## PURPOSE

- To aid in differentiating between primary muscle disorders, such as the muscular dystrophies, and secondary disorders
- To help assess diseases characterized by central neuronal degeneration such as amyotrophic lateral sclerosis (ALS)

# NERVE CONDUCTION STUDIES

Nerve conduction studies aid in the diagnosis of peripheral nerve injuries and diseases affecting the peripheral nervous system such as peripheral neuropathies. To measure nerve conduction time, a nerve is stimulated electrically through the skin and underlying tissues. The patient experiences a mild electric shock with each stimulation. At a known distance from the point of stimulation, a recording electrode detects the response from the stimulated nerve.

The time between stimulation of the nerve and the detected response is measured on an oscilloscope. The speed of conduction along the nerve is then calculated by dividing the distance between the point of stimulation and the recording electrode by the time between stimulus and response. In peripheral nerve injuries and diseases, such as peripheral neuropathies, nerve conduction time is abnormal.

- To aid in the diagnosis of neuromuscular disorders such as myasthenia gravis
- To aid in the diagnosis of radiculopathies

## PATIENT PREPARATION
- Explain to the patient that EMG measures the electrical activity of his muscles.
- Tell the patient that there are usually no restrictions on food and fluids (in some cases, cigarettes, coffee, tea, and cola may be restricted for 2 to 3 hours before the test).
- Describe the test, including who will perform it and where it will take place.
- Tell the patient that he may wear a gown or comfortable clothing that permits access to the muscles to be tested.
- Advise the patient that a needle will be inserted into selected muscles and that he may experience discomfort. Reassure him that adverse effects and complications are rare.
- Make sure that the patient or a responsible family member has signed an informed consent form, if required.
- Check the patient's history for medications that may interfere with the results of

the test—for example, cholinergics, anticholinergics, and skeletal muscle relaxants. If the patient is receiving such medications, note this on the chart and withhold medications, as ordered.

## PROCEDURE AND POSTTEST CARE
- Position the patient on a stretcher or bed or in a chair, depending on the muscles to be tested. Position his arm or leg so that the muscle to be tested is at rest.
- The skin is cleaned with alcohol, the needle electrodes are quickly inserted, and a metal plate is placed under the patient to serve as a reference electrode. Then the muscle's electrical signal (motor unit potential), recorded during rest and contraction, is amplified 1 million times and displayed on an oscilloscope or computer screen.
- The recorder lead wires are attached to an audio amplifier so that the fluctuation of voltage within the muscle can be heard.
- If the patient experiences residual pain, apply warm compresses and administer prescribed analgesics.
- Tell the patient that he may resume his usual medications, as ordered.

## PRECAUTIONS
- Know that EMG is contraindicated in the patient with a bleeding disorder.

## NORMAL FINDINGS
At rest, a normal muscle exhibits minimal electrical activity. During voluntary contraction, electrical activity increases markedly. A sustained contraction or one of increasing strength causes a rapid "train" of motor unit potentials that can be heard as a crescendo of sounds over the audio amplifier.

At the same time, the monitor displays a sequence of waveforms that vary in amplitude (height) and frequency. Waveforms that are close together indicate a high frequency, whereas waveforms that are far apart signify a low frequency.

## ABNORMAL FINDINGS
In primary muscle diseases, such as muscular dystrophy, motor unit potentials are short (low amplitude), with frequent, irregular discharges. In disorders, such as ALS (as well as in peripheral nerve disorders), motor unit potentials are isolated and irregular, but show

increased amplitude and duration. In myasthenia gravis, motor unit potentials initially may be normal, but progressively diminish in amplitude with continuing contractions. The interpreter distinguishes between waveforms that indicate a muscle disorder and those that indicate denervation. Findings must be correlated with the patient's history, clinical features, and the results of other neurodiagnostic tests.

## INTERFERING FACTORS

● The patient's inability to comply with instructions
● Drugs affecting myoneural junctions, such as anticholinergics, cholinergics, and skeletal muscle relaxants

# Electro-nystagmography and videonystagmography

In electronystagmography (ENG) testing and videonystagmography (VNG) testing, eye movements in response to specific stimuli are recorded and used to evaluate the interactions of the vestibular system and the muscles controlling eye movement in what is known as the *vestibulo-ocular reflex.* Nystagmus, the involuntary back-and-forth eye movements caused by this reflex, results from the vestibular system's attempts to maintain visual function during head movement. When the patient turns his head in one direction, the eyes deviate slowly in the opposite direction; on reaching their deviation limit, they quickly return to the center. If the head continues to turn, the pattern of eye movement continues. (See *Understanding eye movement patterns,* page 160.)

The nystagmus cycle has two parts: Slow deviation against the direction of the turn (the slow phase) is controlled by the vestibular system; rapid return to center (the fast phase) is controlled by the central nervous system (CNS). Nystagmus is described as "beating" in the direction of the fast phase. Thus, a head turn to the right yields a right-beating nystagmus, with its slow phase to the left and its fast phase to the right.

Nystagmus accompanying a head turn is normal; prolonged nystagmus after a head turn or nystagmus when the patient isn't turning his head is abnormal. Because of the interaction of the vestibular and ocular systems, abnormal nystagmus can result from lesions of either system; such lesions can be peripheral (end organ or vestibular nerve involvement) or central (cerebellar or brain stem involvement). Abnormal nystagmus is the main sign of vestibular disturbances, such as dizziness and vertigo.

Nystagmography is a technique for monitoring nystagmus and other eye movements. The eye movements can be monitored using electrodes placed near the eyes. Traditional ENG records the corneoretinal potential— the difference of 1 mV between the positive charge of the cornea and the negative charge of the retina—to record nystagmus through electrodes placed near the eyes. As the eyes move horizontally or vertically, the electrodes pick up the corneoretinal potential and chart it. This method permits the recordings of nystagmus in dimly lit surroundings, with the patient's eyes open or closed. (See *ENG eye movements,* page 161.)

In VNG, goggles are placed over the patient's eyes, and eye movements are recorded with an infrared camera. The lenses of the goggles can be closed, excluding outside light and preventing the patient from visually fixating. Additional information about eye movement, such as torsion of the eyes, is also observable. Tracings representing eye movements are obtained.

The ENG/VNG test battery includes oculomotor and caloric tests. The tests seek to determine whether the disorder is peripheral (inner ear or related to cranial nerve VIII involvement) or central (originating from problems of the CNS, brain stem, cerebellum, or cerebrum).

## PURPOSE

● To help identify the cause of dizziness and vertigo
● To confirm the presence and location (central or oculomotor, peripheral, or both) of a lesion
● To assess neurologic disorders

## PATIENT PREPARATION

● Make sure that the patient's ear canals are free from cerumen before referring him for

ENG testing. The caloric testing portion of the ENG can't be conducted safely or accurately if he has cerumen accumulation or a tympanic membrane perforation.

● Inform the patient that tympanometry will be conducted before caloric testing to ensure tympanic membrane integrity.

● Tell the patient that his dizziness problems will be assessed by recording eye movements.

● Inform the patient that the procedure will require approximately 1 1/2 hours to complete.

● Reassure the patient that the test isn't painful and someone will be present to ensure that he doesn't fall, but that some portions may briefly make him dizzy. Because of this, advise him not to eat or drink for 3 to 4 hours before the test.

● Suggest that someone accompany the patient to the evaluation, as occasionally the patient doesn't feel well enough to drive after the appointment. Avoid overemphazing the risk of discomfort because patient anxi-

ety increases the risk of nausea and vomiting during the procedure.

● Encourage the patient to wear comfortable clothing.

● If testing involves traditional ENG with attachment of recording electrodes, inform the patient that his skin will need to be cleaned, so ideally make-up or facial creams shouldn't be used on the day of the test. VNG testing, likewise, is compromised by mascara, so a woman should refrain from wearing make-up on the day of the test.

● Instruct the patient not to smoke or drink caffeinated beverages the day of the test. He should refrain from taking nonessential medication for 48 hours before the test.

● Ask the patient to bring a list of his medications to the evaluation. He must not take these agents 48 hours before the test because they prevent accurate collection and interpretation of the results.

● Alert the health care facility performing the test if the patient has a history of back or

# ENG EYE MOVEMENTS

Traditional electronystagmography (ENG) involves electrodes that are placed above and below (vertical channel), and at the inner and outer canthi (horizontal channel) of one or both of the patient's eyes. Video-nystagmography records the patient's eye movements optically. Both systems create traces of eye movement over time. The horizontal and vertical eye movements over time are shown separately here. The top illustration depicts a right beating nystagmus, and the bottom illustration shows an upbeating nystagmus. The direction of the more rapid portion of the nystagmus determines the labeled direction.

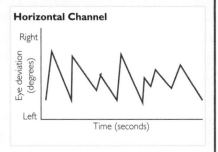

**Horizontal Channel**

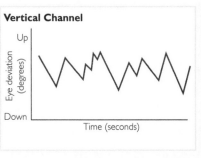

**Vertical Channel**

---

neck problems that would be exacerbated by head or neck movement.
● If the patient wears glasses, tell him to bring them to the test. The patient who wears contact lenses should bring eyeglasses to the examination, if possible.
● Tell the patient that the audiologist will ask for a description of the dizziness and to describe when it began. It's helpful if the patient thinks about what situations creates or makes the dizziness worse. Additionally, find out about the progression of the patient's symptoms by asking him to think about words that might describe the dizziness other than the word "dizzy."

## PROCEDURE AND POSTTEST CARE

● After the device is set up, light bars are connected to the equipment.
● The patient is positioned a calibrated distance from the light source and asked to follow the movement of the lights using eye movement only. The eye movements are recorded and graphed.
● After testing is complete, the patient may resume his usual diet.

## Oculomotor testing
### Saccade testing
● The patient is asked to watch the movement of a dot on the light bar. The dot position will move varying amounts, which correspond to eye deviations in degrees. The accuracy and velocity of the eye tracking of the rapidly moving light is measured. The traces are analyzed to determine if there's symmetrical (right versus left and up versus down) eye movement or dysmetria such as excessive overshoot or undershoot. Glissades, a slowing of the eye movement as it approaches a target, is also ruled out.
### Gaze nystagmus testing
● The patient is asked to look at the light on the light bar and hold the gaze steady. Gaze is directed left, right, up, and down.

The patient is also asked to close his eyes and retain the gaze direction in traditional ENG testing. When VNG recordings are made, the goggles exclude light and the recordings are made with the eyes open. Nystagmus shouldn't occur with the patient's eyes open while he fixates on the target and should be minimal with his eyes closed or when goggles exclude light.

## Smooth pursuit (sinusoidal) tracking testing

- The patient watches the dot on the light bar as it moves smoothly back and forth at varying rates.
- The eye movement is observed to determine if the patient can track the target accurately.
- Tracings are analyzed for left/right symmetry and "smoothness" of the eye's tracking (pursuit) of the target.

## Optokinetics testing

- The patient is instructed to look at the light bar as a series of dots moves across the screen, first in one direction (for example, right to left), and then in the other direction.
- The patient's eyes rapidly move back to center and track another dot. This creates a tracing that looks like nystagmus: the patient follows a dot for a brief period; the eyes rapidly move back to center and track another moving dot. This test assesses the CNS's ability to control rapid eye movement and will be affected by an existing nystagmus.

## Positional and positioning testing

- The patient's eye movements are recorded as he's moved into various body positions and as he remains in these body positions. Recordings note whether nystagmus is present, and if so, the positions that elicit the nystagmus are noted and have diagnostic significance.
- In the Dix-Hallpike test, diagnostic for benign paroxysmal positional vertigo (BPPV), the patient is initially seated. He's then rapidly moved into a supine, head hanging position, with the head deviated to the side and then returned to a sitting position.
- If torsional eye movements are observed, time-locked to the subjective report of dizziness, the findings are positive for BPPV. The test is repeated to establish fatigability, also classic in BPPV. The direction of the rotational eye movement assists in diagnosing which semicircular canal is involved and helps to establish the appropriate BPPV repositioning treatment.

## Caloric testing

- The patient lies supine with his head elevated 30 degrees so that the horizontal semicircular canals are perpendicular to the floor.
- The patient's ear is irrigated with water or air (depending upon the system used) for approximately 60 seconds per irrigation. Four irrigations are completed (both temperatures for each ear).
- Heating and cooling the outer ear causes a change in temperature of the middle ear. The horizontal semicircular canal is located behind the medial wall of the middle ear. The fluid in the semicircular canal moves when the temperature of the fluid is changed, eliciting nystagmus. Thus, for caloric testing, nystagmus is normal.
- The patient is instructed to open his eyes during one portion of each recording. Visual fixation reduces nystagmus if the CNS is normal.
- The symmetry of the nystagmus elicited by irrigation of each ear is assessed. The different temperatures produce different directions of nystagmus. The symmetry of the left beating nystagmus and the right beating nystagmus is analyzed.
- If the patient fails to respond to standard caloric stimulation, ice calorics may be used. A small quantity of ice water or very cold air is introduced into the ear canal to determine if there's residual functioning of that ear's vestibular system.

## PRECAUTIONS

- If the patient has a back or neck condition that could be aggravated by rapid changes in position, check with the physician to determine if any of the positional tests should be omitted.
- Be aware that water caloric testing can't be safely used if the patient has a perforated tympanic membrane. Air caloric test results won't be accurate.
- Know that after testing, the audiologist monitors the patient's status and advises him to remain in a position that reduces dizziness, if present after the procedure.
- Make sure that the patient knows not to drive until all symptoms of imbalance have subsided.

## NORMAL FINDINGS

For normal ENG findings, see *Results of electronystagmography*.

# RESULTS OF ELECTRONYSTAGMOGRAPHY

| TEST AND NORMAL FINDINGS | ABNORMAL FINDINGS | USUAL UNDERLYING CONDITIONS |
|---|---|---|
| **SACCADIC PURSUIT TESTING** | | |
| Square-wave patterns of differing amplitudes mimicking the target, minimal latency and good accuracy of eye movements | *Ocular dysmetria:* significant undershoots, overshoots, glissades, or pulsion; reduced eye velocity, accuracy, prolonged latency | Central nervous system (CNS) pathology: possible involvement of brain stem, cerebellum, or cortex Nonlocalizing: spontaneous or gaze nystagmus may be cause |
| **GAZE TESTING** | | |
| No nystagmus with eyes open, weak or no nystagmus with eyes closed | *Spontaneous nystagmus:* significant amount noted when eyes are closed or when tested in complete darkness under goggles while gazing forward | Nonlocalizing abnormality of the vestibular system: in acute peripheral disorders, horizontal and initially beats away from the affected ear; if present with eyes open, viewing a target, or if the nystagmus changes direction, it's consistent with CNS involvement |
| | *Gaze nystagmus:* presence of nystagmus only when the eyes are deviated from midline | Generally consistent with CNS involvement: the patient with spontaneous nystagmus due to peripheral lesions having stronger nystagmus when looking in the direction of the nystagmus fast phase |
| | *Up-beating nystagmus:* upward deviation of eye movement | Cerebellar or brain stem involvement |
| | *Down-beating nystagmus:* downward deviation of eye movement | Cerebellar or cervico-medullary junction involvement |
| | *Rotary nystagmus:* not classic benign paroxysmal positional vertigo (BPPV) | Brain stem or vestibular nuclei |
| **POSITIONAL TESTING (HEAD IN POSITION)** | | |
| Eyes open, no nystagmus; eyes closed or wearing light-excluding goggles, no more than weak nystagmus in one or more positions | *Nystagmus:* either changes direction across positions or positioning or remains in the same direction, but isn't spontaneous nystagmus | Nonlocalizing: suppression with visual fixation suggests peripheral involvement; enhancement of nystagmus or failure to suppress with visual fixation suggesting central etiology |
| **POSITIONING TESTING (HEAD IN MOVEMENT TOWARD THE POSITION)** | | |
| Eyes open, no nystagmus; eyes closed or wearing light-excluding goggles, no more than weak nystagmus in one or more positions | *Transient, fatigable torsional eye movement:* during Dix-Hallpike procedure, occurring in concert with subjective dizziness | BPPV: responding well to repositioning maneuvers |

*(continued)*

| TEST AND NORMAL FINDINGS | ABNORMAL FINDINGS | USUAL UNDERLYING CONDITIONS |
|---|---|---|
| **SMOOTH PURSUIT TRACKING** | | |
| Volitional smooth tracking of the target, accuracy within age norms | *Sinusoidal tracking:* with superimposed nystagmus | Nonlocalizing: spontaneous or gaze nystagmus may be cause |
| | *Break-up in tracings or saccades:* jerking, rather than smooth movements; reduced velocity, accuracy, prolonged latency that isn't accounted for by advanced age or poor cooperation | CNS involvement if peripheral vision problems ruled out |
| **OPTOKINETIC TESTING** | | |
| Eye movement follows stimulus at speeds to 30 degrees per second; clear triangular wave pattern; similar pattern for stimuli traveling in both directions | *Significant asymmetry:* not explained by spontaneous or gaze nystagmus | CNS involvement |
| | *Reduced eye velocity:* when compared to age-appropriate norms | CNS involvement if peripheral vision problems ruled out |
| **CALORIC TESTING** | | |
| Eyes closed, nystagmus occurring in all conditions; suppressed by visual fixation with cold stimuli, nystagmus beats to opposite ear; with warm stimuli, it beats to same ear (To help recall this phenomenon, use the acronym COWS—cold, opposite, warm, same.) | *Unilateral weakness:* over 20% to 30% difference in maximum slow phase velocities (averaged across temperatures) between ears | Peripheral lesion of weaker side |
| | *Bilateral weakness:* slow-phase velocity of the sum of the four caloric irrigations is reduced, typically below 20 degrees (average of each irrigation ≤ 5 degrees/second) | Bilateral peripheral or CNS involvement |
| | *Directional preponderance:* more than 30% difference in maximum slow-phase velocities for right-versus left-beating nystagmus | Nonlocalizing, usually due to underlying spontaneous nystagmus |
| | *Failure to suppress fixation:* visual fixation fails to reduce nystagmus by at least 40% | CNS involvement |

## ABNORMAL FINDINGS

ENG/VNG results are reported as normal, vestibular (peripheral), CNS, or multifactorial. A peripheral lesion may involve the end organ or the vestibular branch of the eighth cranial nerve and may result from conditions, such as Ménière's disease, multiple sclerosis, ischemic damage to the cochlea, autoimmune disease, and vestibular ototoxity and eighth nerve tumors. A central lesion may involve the brain stem, cerebellum, cerebrum, or any of the connecting structures and may result from demyelinating diseases, tumors, or circulatory disorders.

## INTERFERING FACTORS

● Alcoholic beverages, antihistamines, antivertigo agents, opioids, sleeping pills, and tranquilizers and other medications, which can create dizziness, including certain aminoglycoside antibiotics, antidepressants, diuretics, salicylates, and stimulants
● Poor eyesight or extraocular muscle weakness
● Drowsiness and level of alertness
● Poor patient cooperation

# Electrophysiology studies

Electrophysiology studies (also known as *bundle of His electrography*) permit measurement of discrete conduction intervals by recording electrical conduction during the slow withdrawal of a bipolar or tripolar electrode catheter from the right ventricle through the bundle of His to the sinoatrial node. The catheter is introduced into the femoral vein, passing through the right atrium and across the septal leaflet of the tricuspid valve.

## PURPOSE

● To diagnose arrhythmias and conduction anomalies
● To determine the need for an implanted pacemaker, an internal cardioverter-defibrillator, and cardioactive drugs and to evaluate their effects on the conduction system and ectopic rhythms
● To locate the site of a bundle-branch block, especially in an asymptomatic patient with conduction disturbances
● To determine the presence and location of accessory conducting structures

## PATIENT PREPARATION

● Explain to the patient that electrophysiology studies help to evaluate his heart's conduction system.
● Tell the patient not to eat or drink anything for at least 6 hours before the test.
● Describe the test, including who will perform it and where it will take place.
● Inform the patient that after the groin area is shaved, a catheter will be inserted into the femoral vein and an I.V. line may be started. Assure him that the electrocardiography (ECG) electrodes attached to his chest during the test will cause no discomfort.
● Explain to the patient that he'll experience a stinging sensation when a local anesthetic is injected to numb the incision site for catheter insertion and that he may experience pressure on catheter insertion.
● Inform the patient that he'll be conscious during the test, and urge him to report any discomfort or pain.
● Make sure that the patient or a responsible family member has signed an informed consent form.
● Check the patient's history, and inform the physician of any ongoing drug therapy.
● Just before the procedure, ask the patient to void and to put on a gown.

## PROCEDURE AND POSTTEST CARE

● Help the patient into the supine position on a padded table.
● Limb electrodes and precordial leads are applied for continuous monitoring. If not already in place, an I.V. line is started and dextrose 5% in water or normal saline solution is administered at a keep-vein-open rate.
● After a local anesthetic is injected at the catheterization site, a small incision or percutaneous puncture is made, and a J-tip electrode is introduced I.V. into the femoral vein (or into the antecubital fossa). The catheter is guided to the cardiac chambers using fluoroscopy. It's advanced until it crosses the tricuspid valve and enters the right ventricle. Then the catheter is slowly withdrawn from the tricuspid area, and recordings of conduction intervals are made from each pole of the catheter, either simultaneously or sequentially.
● Monitor the patient's vital signs frequently during the test, noting especially a drop in blood pressure during an arrhythmia.
● The catheter is removed, and a pressure dressing is applied after completion of the procedure.
● Monitor the patient's vital signs every 15 minutes for 1 hour after the procedure and then every hour for 4 hours until he's stable. If he's unstable, check every 15 minutes and notify the physician.
● Observe the patient for shortness of breath, chest pain, pallor, or changes in pulse or blood pressure.
● Enforce bed rest for 4 to 6 hours.

- Check the catheter insertion site for bleeding, as ordered, usually every 30 minutes for 8 hours. If bleeding occurs, notify the physician and apply a pressure bandage until the bleeding stops.
- Advise the patient that he may resume his usual diet.
- Make sure a 12-lead resting ECG is scheduled to assess for changes.

## PRECAUTIONS
- Be aware that electrophysiology studies are contraindicated in the patient with severe coagulopathy, recent thrombophlebitis, or acute pulmonary embolism.

**Alert** *Have emergency medication and resuscitation equipment available in case the patient develops arrhythmias during the electrophysiology study.*

## NORMAL FINDINGS
Normal conduction intervals in an adult are as follows: HV (the conduction time from the bundle of His to the Purkinje fibers) interval, 35 to 55 msec; AH (atrioventricular nodal) interval, 45 to 150 msec; and PA (intra-atrial) interval, 20 to 40 msec.

## ABNORMAL FINDINGS
Abnormalities in electrophysiology studies may reveal a prolonged HV interval that can result from acute or chronic disease. AH interval delays can also occur that stem from atrial pacing, chronic conduction system disease, carotid sinus pressure, recent myocardial infarction, and taking certain drugs. In addition, PA interval delays can result from acquired, surgically induced, or congenital atrial disease and atrial pacing.

## INTERFERING FACTORS
- Malfunctioning recording equipment
- Improper catheter positioning

# Endoscopic retrograde cholangio-pancreatography

Endoscopic retrograde cholangiopancreatography (ERCP) is the radiographic examination of the pancreatic ducts and hepatobiliary tree after injection of a contrast medium into the duodenal papilla. It's indicated in the patient with confirmed or suspected pancreatic disease or obstructive jaundice of unknown etiology. Complications may include cholangitis and pancreatitis.

## PURPOSE
- To evaluate obstructive jaundice
- To diagnose cancer of the duodenal papilla, pancreas, and biliary ducts
- To locate calculi and stenosis in the pancreatic ducts and hepatobiliary tree
- To identify leaks from trauma or surgery
- To evaluate abdominal pain of unknown etiology

## PATIENT PREPARATION
- Explain to the patient that ERCP permits examination of the liver, gallbladder, and pancreas through X-ray films taken after injection of a contrast medium.
- Instruct the patient to fast after midnight before the test.
- Describe the test, including who will perform it and where it will take place.
- Inform the patient that a local anesthetic will be sprayed into his mouth to calm the gag reflex. Warn him that the spray has an unpleasant taste and makes the tongue and throat feel swollen, causing difficulty swallowing.
- Instruct the patient to let saliva drain from the side of his mouth and tell him that suction may be used to remove saliva. Tell him a mouth guard will be inserted to protect his teeth and the endoscope; assure him that it won't obstruct his breathing.
- Tell the patient that he'll receive a sedative before insertion of the endoscope to help him relax, but that he'll remain conscious.
- Tell the patient that he'll also receive an anticholinergic or I.V. glucagon after endoscope insertion. Describe the possible adverse effects of anticholinergics (dry mouth, thirst, tachycardia, urine retention, and blurred vision) or of glucagon (nausea, vomiting, urticaria, and flushing).
- Warn the patient that he may experience transient flushing on injection of the contrast medium. Advise him that he may have a sore throat for 3 or 4 days after the examination.
- Make sure that the patient or a responsible family member has signed an informed consent form.

- Check the patient's history for hypersensitivity to iodine, seafood, or contrast media used for other diagnostic procedures and inform the physician of sensitivities.
- Just before the procedure, obtain the patient's baseline vital signs. Instruct him to remove all metallic or other radiopaque objects and constricting undergarments. Then tell him to void to minimize the discomfort of urine retention that may follow the procedure.

## PROCEDURE AND POSTTEST CARE

- An I.V. infusion is started with 150 ml of normal saline solution. The local anesthetic is then administered and usually takes effect in about 10 minutes.
- If an anesthetic spray is used, ask the patient to hold his breath while his mouth and throat are sprayed.
- Place the patient in a left lateral position and give him an emesis basin; provide tissues. Because the anesthetic causes the patient to lose some control of his secretions and thus increases the risk of aspiration, encourage him to allow saliva to drain from the side of his mouth.
- Insert a mouth guard.
- While the patient remains in the left lateral position, 5 to 20 mg of I.V. diazepam or midazolam is administered as well as an opioid analgesic, if needed.
- When ptosis or dysarthria develops, the patient's head is bent forward and he's asked to open his mouth.
- The examiner inserts his left index finger in the patient's mouth and guides the tip of the endoscope along his finger to the back of the patient's throat. The scope is then deflected downward with the left index finger and advanced. As the endoscope passes through the posterior pharynx and cricopharyngeal sphincter, the patient's head is slowly extended to assist the advance of the endoscope. The patient's chin must be kept midline. When the endoscope has passed the cricopharyngeal sphincter, the scope is advanced under direct vision. When it's well into the esophagus, the patient's chin is moved toward the table so saliva can drain from the mouth. The endoscope is advanced through the remainder of the esophagus and into the stomach under direct vision.
- When the pylorus is located, a small amount of air is insufflated, and the tip of the endoscope is angled upward and passed into the duodenal bulb.
- After the endoscope is rotated clockwise to enter the descending duodenum, the patient is assisted to a prone position.
- An anticholinergic or I.V. glucagon is administered to induce duodenal atony and to relax the ampullary sphincter.
- A small amount of air is insufflated, and the endoscope is manipulated until the optic lies opposite the duodenal papilla. Then the cannula filled with contrast medium is passed through the biopsy channel of the endoscope, the duodenal papilla, and into the ampulla of Vater.
- The pancreatic duct is visualized first under fluoroscopic guidance with injection of contrast medium.
- The cannula is repositioned at a more cephalad angle, and the hepatobiliary tree is visualized with injection of contrast medium.
- After each injection, rapid-sequence X-ray films are taken.
- Instruct the patient to remain prone while the films are developed and reviewed. If necessary, additional films may be taken.
- When the required radiographs have been obtained, the cannula is removed. Before the endoscope is withdrawn, a tissue specimen may be obtained or fluid aspirated for histologic and cytologic examination, respectively.
- Observe the patient closely for signs of cholangitis and pancreatitis. Hyperbilirubinemia, fever, and chills are the immediate signs of cholangitis; hypotension associated with gram-negative septicemia may develop later. Left-upper-quadrant pain and tenderness, elevated serum amylase levels, and transient hyperbilirubinemia are the usual signs of pancreatitis. Draw blood samples for amylase and bilirubin determinations, if necessary, but remember that these levels usually rise after ERCP.
- Observe the patient for signs of perforation, such as abdominal pain, bleeding, and fever.
- Tell the patient that he may experience a feeling of fullness, some cramping, and passage of flatus several hours after the test.
- Continue to watch the patient for signs of respiratory depression, apnea, hypotension, excessive diaphoresis, bradycardia, and laryngospasm. Check his vital signs every 15 minutes for 1 hour, every 30 minutes for the

# ABNORMAL ERCP

This endoscopic retrograde cholangiopancreatographic (ERCP) view shows a dilated pancreatic duct secondary to stenosis. Stenosis was caused by carcinoma at the head of the pancreas.

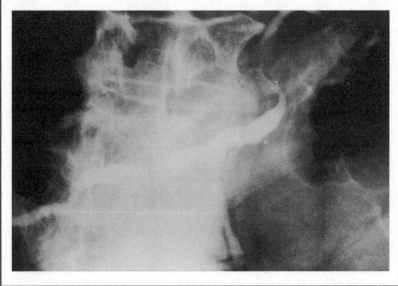

next 2 hours, every hour for the next 4 hours, and then every 4 hours for 48 hours.

⚜ *Alert* *Withhold food and fluids until the patient's gag reflex returns. Test the gag reflex by touching the back of his throat with a tongue blade.*

● When the gag reflex returns, allow fluids and a light meal.

● Discontinue or maintain the I.V. infusion, as ordered.

● Check for signs of urine retention. Notify the physician if the patient hasn't voided within 8 hours.

● If the patient has a sore throat, provide soothing lozenges and warm saline gargles to ease discomfort.

● If a tissue biopsy or polypectomy occurred, a small amount of blood in the patient's first stool is normal.

⚜ *Alert* *Immediately report excessive bleeding to the primary care provider.*

● If this test is performed on an outpatient basis, be sure that transportation is available. The patient who has undergone anesthesia or sedation shouldn't operate an automobile

for at least 12 hours postprocedure. Alcohol should be avoided for 24 hours.

## PRECAUTIONS

● Be aware that ERCP is contraindicated in the pregnant patient, due to risk of fetal harm secondary to radiation exposure.

● Know that ERCP is also contraindicated in the patient with infectious disease, pancreatic pseudocysts, stricture or obstruction of the esophagus or duodenum, or acute pancreatitis, cholangitis, or cardiorespiratory disease.

● Be aware that the patient receiving anticoagulants has an increased risk of bleeding.

● Monitor the patient's vital signs and airway patency throughout the procedure. Watch him for signs of respiratory depression, apnea, hypotension, excessive diaphoresis, bradycardia, and laryngospasm. Be sure to have available emergency resuscitation equipment and an opioid antagonist such as naloxone.

● If the patient has known cardiac disease, continuous electrocardiographic monitoring should be instituted. Continuing periodic pulse oximetry is advisable, particularly in the patient with pulmonary compromise.

## NORMAL FINDINGS

The duodenal papilla appears as a small, red (or sometimes pale) erosion protruding into the lumen. Its orifice is commonly bordered by a fringe of white mucosa, and a longitudinal fold running perpendicular to the deep circular folds of the duodenum helps mark its location. Although the pancreatic and hepatobiliary ducts usually unite in the ampulla of Vater and empty through the duodenal papilla, separate orifices are sometimes present.

The contrast medium uniformly fills the pancreatic duct, hepatobiliary tree, and gallbladder.

## ABNORMAL FINDINGS

Obstructive jaundice may result from various abnormalities of the hepatobiliary tree and pancreatic duct. Examination of the hepatobiliary tree may reveal stones, strictures, or irregular deviations that suggest biliary cirrhosis, primary sclerosing cholangitis, or carcinoma of the bile ducts. (See *Abnormal ERCP*.)

Examination of the pancreatic ducts may also show stones, strictures, and irregular deviations that may indicate pancreatic cysts and pseudocysts, a pancreatic tumor, carcinoma of the head of the pancreas, chronic pancreatitis, pancreatic fibrosis, carcinoma of the duodenal papilla, and papillary stenosis.

Depending on test findings, a definitive diagnosis may require further studies. In addition, certain interventions, such as stent placement to allow drainage or a papillotomy to decrease scar tissue and allow light drainage, may be indicated.

## INTERFERING FACTORS

● Barium in the GI tract from previous studies (possible poor imaging)

# Epstein-Barr virus antibodies

Epstein-Barr virus (EBV), a member of the herpesvirus group, is the causative agent of heterophil-positive infectious mononucleosis, Burkitt's lymphoma, and nasopharyngeal carcinoma. Although the virus doesn't replicate in standard cell cultures, most EBV infections can be recognized by testing the patient's serum for heterophil antibodies (monospot test), which usually appear within the first 3 weeks of illness and then decline rapidly within a few weeks.

In about 10% of adults and a larger percentage of children, the monospot test is negative despite primary infection with EBV. Further, EBV has been associated with lymphoproliferative processes in immunosuppressed patients. These disorders occur with reactivated, rather than primary, EBV infections and, therefore, are also monospot-negative.

Alternatively, EBV-specific antibodies, which develop to several antigens of the virus during active infection, can be measured with a high level of sensitivity and specificity by indirect immunofluorescence.

## PURPOSE

● To provide a laboratory diagnosis of heterophil- (or monospot-) negative cases of infectious mononucleosis
● To determine the antibody status to EBV of immunosuppressed patients with lymphoproliferative processes

## PATIENT PREPARATION

● Explain the purpose of the EBV antibodies test to the patient.
● Tell the patient that the test requires a blood sample. Explain who will perform the venipuncture and when.
● Explain to the patient that he may experience slight discomfort from the tourniquet and needle puncture.

## PROCEDURE AND POSTTEST CARE

● Perform a venipuncture and collect 5 ml of sterile blood in a clot-activator tube.
● Allow the blood to clot for at least 1 hour at room temperature.
● Apply direct pressure to the venipuncture site until bleeding stops.
● If a hematoma develops at the venipuncture site, apply pressure.

## PRECAUTIONS

● Handle the sample gently to prevent hemolysis.
● Transfer the serum to a sterile tube or vial and send it to the laboratory immediately.

- If transfer must be delayed, store the serum at 39.2° F (4° C) for 1 to 2 days or at –4° F (–20° C) for longer periods to prevent contamination.

## NORMAL FINDINGS

Sera from patients who have never been infected with EBV have no detectable antibodies to the virus as measured by either the monospot test or the indirect immunofluorescence test. The monospot test is positive only during the acute phase of infection with EBV; the indirect immunofluorescence test detects and discriminates between acute and past infection with the virus.

## ABNORMAL FINDINGS

EBV infection can be ruled out if no antibodies to EBV antigens are detected in the indirect immunofluorescence test. A positive monospot test or an indirect immunofluorescence test that's either immunoglobulin (Ig) M-positive or Epstein-Barr nuclear antigen (EBNA)-negative indicates acute EBV infection.

A monospot-negative result doesn't necessarily rule out acute or past infection with EBV. Conversely, IgG class antibody to viral capsid antigen and EBNA antigens (IgM-negative) indicates remote (more than 2 months) infection with EBV. Recognize that most cases of monospot-negative infectious mononucleosis are caused by cytomegalovirus infections.

## INTERFERING FACTORS
- None significant

## *Erythrocyte sedimentation rate*

The erythrocyte sedimentation rate (ESR) measures the degree of erythrocyte settling in a blood sample during a specified period. The ESR is a sensitive but nonspecific test that's commonly the earliest indicator of disease when other chemical or physical signs are normal. The ESR usually increases significantly in widespread inflammatory disorders; elevations may be prolonged in localized inflammation and malignant disease.

## PURPOSE
- To monitor inflammatory or malignant disease
- To aid detection and diagnosis of occult disease, such as tuberculosis, tissue necrosis, or connective tissue disease

## PATIENT PREPARATION
- Explain to the patient that the ESR test is used to evaluate the condition of red blood cells.
- Tell the patient that a blood sample will be taken. Explain who will perform the venipuncture and when.
- Explain to the patient that he may feel slight discomfort from the tourniquet and needle puncture.
- Inform the patient that he need not restrict food and fluids.

## PROCEDURE AND POSTTEST CARE
- Perform a venipuncture and collect the sample in a 4.5-ml tube with EDTA added or a tube with sodium citrate added. (Check with the laboratory to determine its preference.)
- Ensure subdermal bleeding has stopped before removing pressure.
- If a hematoma develops at the venipuncture site, apply pressure. If the hematoma is large, monitor pulses distal to the phlebotomy site.

## PRECAUTIONS
- Completely fill the collection tube and invert it gently several times to thoroughly mix the sample and the anticoagulant.
- Because prolonged standing decreases the ESR, examine the sample for clots or clumps and send it to the laboratory immediately. It must be tested within 2 to 4 hours.
- Handle the sample gently to prevent hemolysis.

## REFERENCE VALUES

The ESR normally ranges from 0 to 10 mm/hour (SI, 0 to 10 mm/hour) in males, and 0 to 20 mm/hour (SI, 0 to 20 mm/hour) in females. Rates gradually increase with age.

## ABNORMAL FINDINGS

The ESR rises in pregnancy, anemia, acute or chronic inflammation, tuberculosis, paraproteinemias (especially multiple myeloma and Waldenström's macroglobulinemia), rheumatic fever, rheumatoid arthritis, and some cancers.

Polycythemia, sickle cell anemia, hyperviscosity, and low plasma fibrinogen or globulin levels tend to depress the ESR.

## INTERFERING FACTORS

● Failure to use the proper anticoagulant, to adequately mix the sample and the anticoagulant, or to send the sample to the laboratory immediately

● Hemoconcentration due to prolonged tourniquet constriction

## Erythropoietin

The erythropoietin (EPO) test of renal hormone production measures EPO by immunoassay. It's used to evaluate anemia, polycythemia, and kidney tumors. It's also used to evaluate abuse of commercially prepared EPO by athletes who believe that the drug enhances performance.

A glycoprotein hormone, EPO is secreted by the liver of fetuses, but by the kidneys in adults. The hormone acts on stem cells in the bone marrow to stimulate production of red blood cells (RBCs). It's regulated by a feedback loop involving red cell volume and oxygen saturation of the blood, especially in the brain.

## PURPOSE

● To aid diagnosis of anemia and polycythemia

● To aid diagnosis of kidney tumors

● To detect EPO abuse by athletes

## PATIENT PREPARATION

● Explain to the patient that the EPO test determines if hormonal secretion is causing changes in his RBCs.

● Instruct the patient to fast for 8 to 10 hours before the test.

● Tell the patient that the test requires a blood sample. Explain who will perform the venipuncture and when.

● Explain to the patient that he may experience slight discomfort from the tourniquet and needle puncture.

● Keep the patient relaxed and recumbent for 30 minutes before the test.

## PROCEDURE AND POSTTEST CARE

● Perform a venipuncture and collect the sample in a 5-ml clot-activator tube.

● If requested, a hematocrit (HCT) may be drawn at the same time by collecting an additional sample in a 2-ml tube.

● Apply direct pressure to the venipuncture site until bleeding stops.

● If a hematoma develops at the venipuncture site, apply warm soaks.

## PRECAUTIONS

● Handle the sample gently to prevent hemolysis.

## REFERENCE VALUES

The reference range for EPO is 5 to 36 mU/ml (SI, 5 to 36 IU/L).

## ABNORMAL FINDINGS

Low levels of EPO appear in the patient with anemia who has inadequate or absent hormone production. Congenital absence of EPO can occur. Severe renal disease may decrease EPO production.

Elevated EPO levels occur in anemias as a compensatory mechanism in the reestablishment of homeostasis. Inappropriate elevations (when HCT is normal to high) are seen in polycythemia and EPO-secreting tumors.

Some athletes use EPO to enhance performance. The increased RBC volume conveys additional oxygen-carrying capacity to the blood. Adverse reactions include clotting abnormalities, headache, seizures, hypertension, nausea, vomiting, diarrhea, and rash.

## INTERFERING FACTORS

● Failure to collect a sample in the fasting state

## Esophageal acidity

The esophageal acidity test evaluates the competence of the lower esophageal sphincter—the major barrier to reflux—by measuring intraesophageal pH with an electrode attached to a manometric catheter.

Recently, a newer method for measuring esophageal pH, called the *Bravo pH monitoring system,* was developed. This method uses a small capsule to monitor a patient's pH levels. (See *Monitoring pH with the Bravo system*.)

## PURPOSE
- To evaluate the competence of the lower esophageal sphincter

## PATIENT PREPARATION
- Explain to the patient that the esophageal acidity test evaluates the function of the sphincter between the esophagus and the stomach. Tell him to fast and avoid smoking after midnight before the test.
- Describe the test, including who will perform it and where it will take place.
- Tell the patient that a tube will be passed through his mouth into his stomach and that he may experience slight discomfort, a desire to cough, or a gagging sensation.
- Just before the test, check the patient's pulse rate and blood pressure and instruct him to void.
- Withhold antacids, anticholinergics, cholinergics, beta-adrenergic blockers, alcohol, corticosteroids, cimetidine, and reserpine for 24 hours before the test. If they must be continued, note this on the laboratory request.
- Make sure that the patient or a responsible family member has signed an informed consent form.

## PROCEDURE AND POSTTEST CARE
- After the patient is placed in high Fowler's position, the catheter with the electrode is introduced into his mouth.
- The patient is instructed to swallow when the electrode reaches the back of his throat.

- Using a manometer, the examiner locates the lower esophageal sphincter. The catheter is raised ³/₄" (1.9 cm). The patient is told to perform Valsalva's maneuver or lift his legs to stimulate reflux. After he does so, intraesophageal pH is measured.
- If the pH is normal, the catheter is passed into the patient's stomach. A prescribed acid solution (300 ml of 0.1 sodium hydrochloride) is instilled over 3 minutes (100 ml/minute). Then the catheter is raised ³/₄" above the sphincter. Again, the patient is asked to perform Valsalva's maneuver or lift his legs, and intraesophageal pH is measured.
- Tell the patient that he may resume his usual diet and medications, as ordered.
- Provide lozenges if the patient complains of a sore throat.

## PRECAUTIONS
- During insertion, be aware that the catheter may enter the trachea instead of the esophagus. If the patient develops cyanosis or paroxysmal coughing, move the catheter immediately.
- Observe the patient closely during insertion because arrhythmias may develop.
- Clamp the catheter before removing it to prevent fluid aspiration into the lungs.

## REFERENCE VALUES
pH of the esophagus normally exceeds 5.0.

## ABNORMAL FINDINGS
An intraesophageal pH of 1.5 to 2.0 indicates gastric acid reflux resulting from incompetence of the lower esophageal sphincter. Persistent reflux leads to chronic reflux esophagitis. Additional studies, such as barium swallow and esophagogastroduodenoscopy,

are necessary to diagnose and determine the extent of esophagitis.

## INTERFERING FACTORS

- Antacids, anticholinergics, histamine-2 blockers, and proton pump inhibitors (possible lowering of intraesophageal pH because of decrease in gastric secretions or acidity)
- Adrenergic blockers, alcohol, cholinergics, corticosteroids, and reserpine (possible elevation of intraesophageal pH because of reflux from a relaxed lower esophageal sphincter or an increase in gastric secretions)

# Esophagogastro-duodenoscopy

Esophagogastroduodenoscopy (EGD) permits visual examination of the lining of the esophagus, stomach, and upper duodenum using a flexible fiber-optic or video endoscope. It's indicated for patients with GI bleeding, hematemesis, melena, substernal or epigastric pain, gastroesophageal reflux disease, dysphagia, anemia, strictures, or peptic ulcer disease; those requiring foreign body retrieval; and postoperative patients with recurrent or new symptoms.

EGD eliminates the need for extensive exploratory surgery and can be used to detect small or surface lesions missed by radiography. Because the scope provides a channel for biopsy forceps or a cytology brush, it permits laboratory evaluation of abnormalities detected by radiography. Similarly, it allows for the removal of foreign bodies by suction (for small, soft objects) or by electrocautery snare or forceps (for large, hard objects).

## PURPOSE

- To diagnose inflammatory disease, malignant and benign tumors, ulcers, Mallory-Weiss syndrome, and structural abnormalities
- To evaluate the stomach and duodenum postoperatively
- To obtain emergency diagnosis of duodenal ulcer or esophageal injury such as that caused by chemical ingestion

## PATIENT PREPARATION

- Explain to the patient that EGD permits visual examination of the lining of the esophagus, stomach, and upper duodenum.
- Check the patient's medical history for allergies, medications, and information pertinent to the current complaint. Check for hypersensitivity to the medications and anesthetics ordered for the test.
- Instruct the patient to fast for 6 to 12 hours before the test.
- Tell the patient that a flexible instrument with a camera on the end will be passed through his mouth; explain who will perform this procedure, where it will take place, and that it takes about 30 minutes.
- If emergency EGD is to be performed, tell the patient that stomach contents may be aspirated through a nasogastric tube.
- Inform the patient that a bitter-tasting local anesthetic will be sprayed into his mouth and throat to calm the gag reflex and that his tongue and throat may feel swollen, making swallowing seem difficult. Advise him to let the saliva drain from the side of his mouth; a suction machine may be used to remove saliva if necessary.
- Explain that a mouth guard will be inserted to protect his teeth and the endoscope; assure him that the guard won't obstruct his breathing.
- Inform the patient that an I.V. line will be started and a sedative will be administered before the endoscope is inserted to help him relax. If the procedure is being done on an outpatient basis, advise the patient to arrange for someone to drive him home because he may feel drowsy from the sedative. Drugs that retard peristalsis of the upper GI tract may be administered in some circumstances.
- Tell the patient that he may experience pressure in the stomach as the endoscope is moved about and a feeling of fullness when air or carbon dioxide is insufflated. If he's apprehensive, administer meperidine or another analgesic I.M. about 30 minutes before the test as ordered; also administer atropine sulfate subcutaneously at this time, as ordered, to decrease gastric secretions, which would interfere with test results.
- Make sure that the patient or a responsible family member has signed an informed consent form.
- Just before the procedure, instruct the patient to remove dentures, eyeglasses, and constricting undergarments.

## PROCEDURE AND POSTTEST CARE

- Obtain the patient's baseline vital signs and leave the blood pressure cuff in place for monitoring throughout the procedure.
- If the patient has known cardiac disease, continuous electrocardiographic monitoring should be instituted. Continuous or periodic pulse oximetry is advisable, particularly in the patient with pulmonary compromise.
- Ask the patient to hold his breath while his mouth and throat are sprayed with a local anesthetic, if requested by the physician.
- Remind the patient to let saliva drain from the side of his mouth. Provide an emesis basin to spit out saliva and tissues to wipe saliva from his mouth or use oropharyngeal suction as needed.
- Place the patient in a left lateral position, bend his head forward, and ask him to open his mouth.
- The examiner guides the tip of the endoscope to the back of the patient's throat and downward. As the endoscope passes through the posterior pharynx and the cricopharyngeal sphincter, the patient's neck is slowly extended. His chin must be kept at midline. The endoscope is then passed along the esophagus under direct vision.
- When the endoscope is well into the esophagus (about 12″ [30 cm]), the patient's head is positioned with his chin toward the table so that saliva can drain out of his mouth.
- After examination of the esophagus and the cardiac sphincter, the endoscope is rotated clockwise and advanced to allow examination of the stomach and duodenum. During the examination, air or water may be introduced through the endoscope to aid visualization, and suction may be applied to remove insufflated air and secretions.
- A camera may be attached to the endoscope to photograph areas for later study, or a measuring tube may be passed through the endoscope to determine the size of a lesion.
- Biopsy forceps or a cytology brush may be passed through the scope to obtain specimens for histologic or cytologic study.
- The endoscope is slowly withdrawn, and suspicious-looking areas of the gastric and esophageal lining are reexamined.
- Specimens should be collected in accordance with laboratory and pathology guidelines. Place tissue specimens immediately in a specimen bottle containing 10% formalin solution; cell specimens are smeared on glass slides and placed in a Coplin jar containing 95% ethyl alcohol.

⚜ *Alert* Observe the patient for possible perforation. Perforation in the cervical area of the esophagus produces pain on swallowing and with neck movement, thoracic perforation causes substernal or epigastric pain that increases with breathing or movement of the trunk, diaphragmatic perforation produces shoulder pain and dyspnea, and gastric perforation causes abdominal or back pain, cyanosis, fever, and pleural effusion.

- Observe the patient for evidence of aspiration of gastric contents, which could precipitate aspiration pneumonia.
- Monitor the patient's vital signs and document them according to facility policy.
- Test the patient's gag reflex by touching the back of the throat with a tongue blade. Withhold food and fluids until the gag reflex returns (usually in 1 hour), and then allow fluids and a light meal.
- Tell the patient that he may burp some insufflated air and have a sore throat for 3 to 4 days. Throat lozenges and warm saline gargles may ease his discomfort.
- If the patient experiences soreness at the I.V. site, apply warm soaks.
- Because of sedation, an outpatient should avoid alcohol for 24 hours and shouldn't drive for 12 hours. Make sure the patient has transportation home.
- Instruct the patient to notify the physician immediately if he experiences persistent difficulty with swallowing, pain, fever, black stools, or bloody vomitus.

## PRECAUTIONS

- If tissue or cell specimens are obtained during the procedure, label and send them to the appropriate laboratory immediately.
- Be aware that this procedure is generally safe, but it can cause perforation of the esophagus, stomach, or duodenum, especially if the patient is restless or uncooperative.
- Know that EGD is usually contraindicated in the patient with Zenker's diverticulum, a large aortic aneurysm, recent ulcer perforation (known as *suspected viscus perforation*), or an unstable cardiac or pulmonary condition.
- Know that EGD shouldn't be performed within 2 days after an upper GI series.
- Be aware that the patient requiring dental prophylaxis may also require antibiotics before this procedure.

**Alert** *Observe closely for adverse effects of the sedative: respiratory depression, apnea, hypotension, excessive diaphoresis, bradycardia, and laryngospasm. Have emergency resuscitation equipment and an opioid antagonist, such as naloxone, available. Be prepared to intervene as necessary.*

## NORMAL FINDINGS

The smooth mucosa of the esophagus is normally yellow-pink and marked by a fine vascular network. A pulsation on the anterior wall of the esophagus between 8″ and 10″ (20 and 25.5 cm) from the incisor teeth represents the aortic arch. The orange-red mucosa of the stomach begins the "Z" line, an irregular transition line slightly above the esophagogastric junction.

Unlike the esophagus, the stomach has rugal folds, and its blood vessels aren't visible beneath the gastric mucosa. The reddish mucosa of the duodenal bulb is marked by a few shallow longitudinal folds. The mucosa of the distal duodenum has prominent circular folds, is lined with villi, and appears velvety.

## ABNORMAL FINDINGS

EGD, coupled with the results of histologic and cytologic tests, may indicate acute or chronic ulcers, benign or malignant tumors, and inflammatory disease, including esophagitis, gastritis, and duodenitis. This test may demonstrate diverticula, varices, Mallory-Weiss syndrome, esophageal rings, esophageal and pyloric stenoses, and esophageal hiatal hernia. Although EGD can evaluate gross abnormalities of esophageal motility, as occur in achalasia, manometric studies are more accurate.

## INTERFERING FACTORS

● Anticoagulants (increased risk for bleeding)
● Patient's inability to cooperate, preventing optimal visualization

## Estrogens

Estrogens (and progesterone) are secreted by the ovaries under the influence of the pituitary gonadotropins, follicle-stimulating hormone (FSH), and luteinizing hormone (LH).

Estrogens — in particular, estradiol, the most potent estrogen — interact with the hypothalamic-pituitary axis through negative and positive feedback mechanisms. Slowly rising or sustained high levels inhibit secretion of FSH and LH (negative feedback), but a rapid rise in estrogen just before ovulation seems to stimulate LH secretion (positive feedback).

Estrogens are responsible for the development of secondary female sexual characteristics and for normal menstruation; levels are usually undetectable in children. These hormones are secreted by ovarian follicular cells during the first half of the menstrual cycle and by the corpus luteum during the luteal phase and during pregnancy. In menopause, estrogen secretion drops to a constantly low level.

This radioimmunoassay measures serum levels of estradiol, estrone, and estriol (the only estrogens that appear in serum in measurable amounts) and has diagnostic significance in evaluating female gonadal dysfunction. Tests of hypothalamic-pituitary function may be required to confirm the diagnosis.

## PURPOSE

● To determine sexual maturation and fertility
● To aid diagnosis of gonadal dysfunction, such as precocious or delayed puberty, menstrual disorders (especially amenorrhea), and infertility
● To determine fetal well-being
● To aid diagnosis of tumors known to secrete estrogen

## PATIENT PREPARATION

● Explain to the patient that the estrogens radioimmunoassay helps determine if secretion of female hormones is normal and that the test may be repeated during the various phases of the menstrual cycle.
● Tell the patient that she need not restrict food and fluids.
● Tell the patient that the test requires a blood sample. Explain who will perform the venipuncture and when.
● Explain to the patient that she may experience slight discomfort from the tourniquet and needle puncture.
● Withhold all steroid and pituitary-based hormones, as ordered. If they must be continued, note this on the laboratory request.

## PROCEDURE AND POSTTEST CARE

Care may vary slightly, depending on whether plasma or serum is being measured.

● Perform a venipuncture and collect the sample in a 10-ml clot-activator tube.

● If the patient is premenopausal, indicate the phase of her menstrual cycle on the laboratory request.

● Apply direct pressure to the venipuncture site until bleeding stops.

● If a hematoma develops at the venipuncture site, apply pressure.

● Instruct the patient that she may resume medications discontinued before the test, as ordered.

## PRECAUTIONS

● Handle the sample gently to prevent hemolysis.

● Send the sample to the laboratory immediately.

## REFERENCE VALUES

Normal serum estrogen levels for premenopausal women vary widely during the menstrual cycle, ranging from 26 to 149 pg/ml (SI, 90 to 550 pmol/L). The range for postmenopausal women is 0 to 34 pg/ml (SI, 0 to 125 pmol/L).

Serum estrogen levels in men range from 12 to 34 pg/ml (SI, 40 to 125 pmol/ L).

★ *Age alert  In children younger than age 6, the normal level of serum estrogen is 3 to 10 pg/ml (SI, 10 to 36 pmol/L). Estriol is secreted in large amounts by the placenta during pregnancy. Levels range from 2 ng/ml (SI, 7 nmol/L) by 30 weeks' gestation to 30 ng/ml (SI, 105 nmol/L) by week 40.*

## ABNORMAL FINDINGS

Decreased estrogen levels may indicate primary hypogonadism, or ovarian failure, as in Turner's syndrome or ovarian agenesis; secondary hypogonadism, such as in hypopituitarism; or menopause.

Abnormally high estrogen levels may occur with estrogen-producing tumors, in precocious puberty, and in severe hepatic disease, such as cirrhosis, that prevents clearance of plasma estrogens. High estrogen levels may also result from congenital adrenal hyperplasia, which is the increased conversion of androgens to estrogen.

## INTERFERING FACTORS

● Pregnancy and pretest use of estrogens such as hormonal contraceptives (possible increase)

● Clomiphene, an estrogen antagonist (possible decrease)

● Steroids and pituitary-based hormones such as dexamethasone

# *Evoked potential studies*

Evoked potential studies evaluate the integrity of visual, somatosensory, and auditory nerve pathways by measuring evoked potentials — the brain's electrical response to stimulation of the sensory organs or peripheral nerves. Evoked potentials are recorded as electronic impulses by surface electrodes attached to the scalp and skin over various peripheral sensory nerves. A computer extracts these low-amplitude impulses from background brain wave activity and averages the signals from repeated stimuli. (See *Visual evoked potentials.*)

Three types of responses are measured:

● Visual evoked potentials, produced by exposing the eye to a rapidly reversing checkerboard pattern, help evaluate demyelinating diseases, traumatic injury, and puzzling visual complaints.

● Somatosensory evoked potentials, produced by electrically stimulating a peripheral sensory nerve, help diagnose peripheral nerve disease and locate brain and spinal cord lesions.

● Auditory brain stem-evoked potentials, produced by delivering clicks to the ear, help locate auditory lesions and evaluate brain stem integrity. (See *Auditory evoked potentials,* page 40.)

Evoked potential studies are also useful for monitoring comatose or anesthetized patients, monitoring spinal cord function during spinal cord surgery, and evaluating neurologic function in an infant whose sensory system normally can't be adequately assessed.

## PURPOSE

● To aid in the diagnosis of nervous system lesions and abnormalities

# VISUAL EVOKED POTENTIALS

## VISUAL (PATTERN-SHIFT) EVOKED POTENTIALS

In the visual (pattern-shift) evoked potentials test, visual neural impulses are recorded as they travel along the pathway from the eye to the occipital cortex. Wave P100 is the most significant component of the resultant waveform. Normal P100 latency is about 100 msec after the application of a visual stimulus, as shown in the top diagram. Increased P100 latency, shown in the bottom diagram, is an abnormal finding, indicating a lesion along the visual pathway.

**Normal tracing**

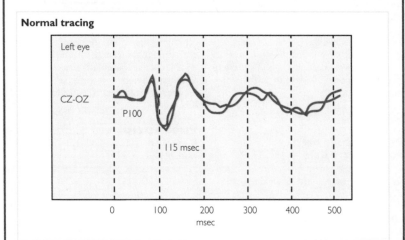

**Tracing in multiple sclerosis**

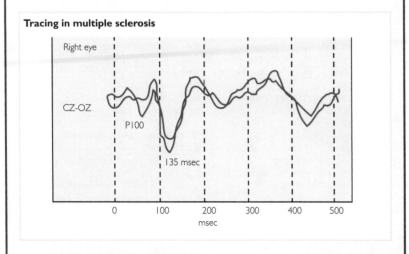

KEY: CZ = vertex; OZ = midocciput

● To assess the patient's neurologic function

## PATIENT PREPARATION
● Tell the patient that evoked potential studies measure the electrical activity of his nervous system. Explain who will perform the test and where it will take place.
● Tell the patient that he'll sit in a reclining chair or lie on a bed. If visual evoked potentials will be measured, electrodes will be attached to his scalp; if somatosensory evoked potentials will be measured, electrodes will be placed on his scalp, neck, lower back, wrist, knee, and ankle.
● Assure the patient that the electrodes won't hurt him. Encourage him to relax; tension can affect neurologic function and interfere with test results.
● Have the patient remove all jewelry and other metal objects.

## PROCEDURE AND POSTTEST CARE
● Position the patient in a reclining chair or on a bed and tell him to relax and remain still.

### For visual evoked potentials
● Electrodes are attached to the patient's scalp at occipital, parietal, and vertex sites; a reference electrode is placed on the midfrontal area or ear.
● The patient is positioned 3′ (1 m) from the pattern-shift stimulator.
● One eye is occluded, and the patient is instructed to fix his gaze on a dot in the center of the screen.
● A checkerboard pattern is projected and then rapidly reversed or shifted 100 times, once or twice per second.
● A computer amplifies and averages the brain's response to each stimulus, and the results are plotted as a waveform.
● The procedure is repeated for the other eye.

### For somatosensory evoked potentials
● Electrodes are attached to the patient's skin over somatosensory pathways — typically the wrist, knee, and ankle — to stimulate peripheral nerves. Recording electrodes are placed on the scalp over the sensory cortex of the hemisphere opposite the limb to be stimulated. Additional electrodes may be placed at Erb's point (above the clavicle overlying the brachial plexus), at the second cervical vertebra, and over the lower lumbar vertebrae. Midfrontal or noncephalic electrodes are placed for reference.
● Painless electrical stimulation is delivered to the peripheral nerve through the electrode. The intensity is adjusted to produce a minor muscle response such as a thumb twitch on median nerve stimulation at the wrist.
● Electrical stimuli are delivered 500 or more times at a rate of 5 per second.
● A computer measures and averages the time it takes for the electric current to reach the cortex; the results, expressed in milliseconds (msec), are recorded as waveforms.
● The test is repeated once to verify results, and then the electrodes are repositioned and the entire procedure is repeated for the other side.

## PRECAUTIONS
● Know that the patient's hair should be washed and rinsed before testing. No other hair products should be applied once the hair is clean.

## NORMAL FINDINGS
### Visual evoked potentials
On the waveform, the most significant wave is P100, a positive wave appearing about 100 msec after the pattern-shift stimulus is applied. The most clinically significant measurements are absolute P100 latency (the time between stimulus application and peaking of the P100 wave) and the difference between the P100 latencies of each eye. Because many physical and technical factors affect P100 latency, normal results vary greatly among laboratories and patients.

### Somatosensory evoked potentials
Waveforms obtained vary, depending on locations of the stimulating and recording electrodes. The positive and negative peaks are labeled in sequence, based on normal time of appearance. For example, N19 is a negative peak normally recorded 19 msec after application of the stimulus. Each wave peak arises from a discrete location: N19 is generated mainly from the thalamus, P22 from the parietal sensory cortex, and so on. Interwave latencies (time between waves), rather than absolute latencies, are used as a basis for

clinical interpretation. Latency differences between sides are significant.

## ABNORMAL FINDINGS

Information from evoked potential studies is useful, but insufficient to confirm a specific diagnosis. Test data must be interpreted in light of clinical information.

### Visual evoked potentials

Generally, abnormal (extended) P100 latencies confined to one eye indicate a visual pathway lesion anterior to the optic chiasm. A lesion posterior to the optic chiasm usually doesn't produce abnormal P100 latencies. Because each eye projects to both occipital lobes, the unaffected pathway transmits sufficient impulses to produce a normal latency response. Bilateral abnormal P100 latencies have been found in patients with multiple sclerosis, optic neuritis, retinopathies, amblyopia (although abnormal latencies don't correlate well with impaired visual acuity), spinocerebellar degeneration, adrenoleukodystrophy, sarcoidosis, Parkinson's disease, and Huntington's disease.

### Somatosensory evoked potentials

Because somatosensory evoked potential components are assumed to be linked in series, an abnormal interwave latency indicates a conduction defect between the generators of the two peaks involved. This defect commonly identifies a precise location of a neurologic lesion. Abnormal upper-limb interwave latencies may indicate cervical spondylosis, intracerebral lesions, or sensorimotor neuropathies. Abnormalities in the lower limb demonstrate peripheral nerve and root lesions, such as those in Guillain-Barré syndrome, compressive myelopathies, multiple sclerosis, transverse myelitis, and traumatic spinal cord injury.

## INTERFERING FACTORS

- Incorrect electrode placement or equipment failure
- Patient tension, inability to relax, or failure to cooperate
- Poor patient vision

## Examination of urogenital secretions

Microscopic examination of urine or vaginal, urethral, or prostatic secretions can detect urogenital infection by *Trichomonas vaginalis,* a parasitic, flagellate protozoan that's usually transmitted sexually. This test is more commonly performed on women than on men because women are more likely to exhibit symptoms of trichomoniasis; men may exhibit symptoms of urethritis or prostatitis.

## PURPOSE

- To confirm trichomoniasis

## PATIENT PREPARATION

- Explain to the patient that the microscopic examination of urogenital secretion test can identify the cause of urogenital infection.
- If the patient is a woman, tell her that the test requires a specimen of vaginal secretions or urethral discharge and ask her not to douche before the test.
- If the patient is a man, tell him the test requires a specimen of urethral or prostatic secretions.
- Inform the patient who will perform the procedure and when.

## PROCEDURE AND POSTTEST CARE
### Vaginal secretions

- With the patient in the lithotomy position, an unlubricated vaginal speculum is inserted, and discharge is collected with a cotton swab. The swab is then placed in a tube containing normal saline solution and the speculum is removed.
- Another method is to smear the specimen on a glass slide, allow it to air-dry, and then transport it to the laboratory.

### Prostatic material

- After prostatic massage, collect secretions with a cotton swab, and place the swab in normal saline solution.

### Urethral discharge

- Collect the discharge with a cotton swab, and place the swab in normal saline solution.

### Urine
- Include the first portion of a voided random specimen (not midstream).

### All procedures
- Label the specimen container appropriately, including the date and time of collection.
- Provide perineal care.

## PRECAUTIONS
- Remember to use gloves when performing procedures and handling specimens.
- If possible, obtain the urogenital specimen before treatment with a trichomonacide begins.
- Send the specimen to the laboratory immediately after collection because trichomonads can be identified only while they're still motile.

## NORMAL FINDINGS
Trichomonads are normally absent from the urogenital tract.

## ABNORMAL FINDINGS
Trichomonads confirm trichomoniasis. In approximately 25% of women and in most infected men, trichomonads may be present without associated pathology.

## INTERFERING FACTORS
- Improper collection technique
- Failure to send the specimen to the laboratory immediately after collection, causing trichomonads to lose motility
- Collection of the specimen after trichomonacide therapy begins (fewer trichomonads in the specimen)

## *Excretory urography*

The cornerstone of a urologic workup, excretory urography (also called *I.V. pyelography*) requires I.V. administration of a contrast medium and allows visualization of the renal parenchyma, calyces, and pelvis as well as the ureters, bladder and, in some cases, the urethra.

In some facilities, a nonenhanced computed tomography scan of the urinary tract is commonly performed instead of this test if urinary tract stones are suspected.

## PURPOSE
- To evaluate the structure and excretory function of the kidneys, ureters, and bladder
- To support a suspected differential diagnosis of renovascular hypertension

## PATIENT PREPARATION
- Explain to the patient that excretory urography helps to evaluate the structure and function of the urinary tract.
- Make sure that the patient is well hydrated; then instruct him to fast for 8 hours before the test. Tell him who will perform the test and where it will take place. Obtain blood urea nitrogen (BUN) and creatinine levels, as ordered.
- Inform the patient that he may experience a transient burning sensation and metallic taste when the contrast medium is injected. Tell him to report other sensations he may experience.
- Warn the patient that the X-ray machine may make loud, clacking sounds during the test.
- Make sure that the patient or a responsible family member has signed an informed consent form.
- Check the patient's history for hypersensitivity to iodine, iodine-containing foods, or contrast media containing iodine. Mark sensitivities on the chart and notify the physician.
- Administer a laxative, if necessary, the night before the test, to minimize poor resolution of X-ray films due to stool and gas in the GI tract.

## PROCEDURE AND POSTTEST CARE
- The patient is placed in a supine position on the X-ray table.
- A kidney-ureter-bladder X-ray is exposed, developed, and studied for gross abnormalities of the urinary system. Contrast medium is injected (dosage varies according to age), and the patient is observed for signs of hypersensitivity (flushing, nausea, vomiting, hives, or dyspnea).
- The first X-ray, visualizing the renal parenchyma, is obtained about 1 minute after the injection, possibly supplemented by tomography if small space-occupying masses, such as cysts or tumors, are suspected.
- X-rays are then exposed at regular intervals — usually 5, 10, and 15 or 20 minutes after the injection.

# Abnormal excretory urogram

In a patient with suspected renal hypertension, an excretory urogram taken 8 minutes after injection of a contrast medium shows normal filling of the right kidney but delayed filling of the left kidney and ureter (at right). This impaired excretion of the contrast material commonly results from narrowing of the renal artery feeding the subject kidney. Constriction hinders blood flow to the glomerulus and leads to increased renal absorption of water and decreased urine output. Demonstration of delayed filling can distinguish unilateral renal hypertension from essential hypertension.

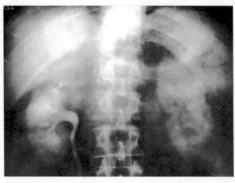

● Ureteral compression is performed after the 5-minute film is exposed. This compression can be accomplished through inflation of two small rubber bladders placed on the abdomen on both sides of the midline, secured by a fastener wrapped around the patient's torso. The inflated bladders occlude the ureters without causing the patient discomfort and facilitate retention of the contrast medium by the upper urinary tract. (Ureteral compression is contraindicated by ureteral calculi, aortic aneurysm, pregnancy, or recent abdominal trauma or surgical procedure.)

● After the 10-minute film is exposed, ureteral compression is released. As the contrast flows into the lower urinary tract, another film is taken of the lower halves of both ureters and then, finally, one is taken of the bladder.

● At the end of the procedure, the patient voids, and another film is made immediately to visualize residual bladder content or mucosal abnormalities of the bladder or urethra.

● If a hematoma develops at the injection site, apply warm soaks.

● Observe the patient for delayed reactions to the contrast medium.

● Continue I.V. fluids or provide oral fluid to increase hydration.

● Administer medications, as ordered.

## PRECAUTIONS

● Be aware that premedication with corticosteroids may be indicated for the patient with severe asthma or a history of sensitivity to the contrast medium.

● Know that this test may be contraindicated in the patient with abnormal renal function (as evidenced by increased creatinine and BUN levels) and in a child or an elderly patient with actual or potential dehydration.

## NORMAL FINDINGS

The kidneys, ureters, and bladder show no gross evidence of soft- or hard-tissue lesions. Prompt visualization of the contrast medium in the kidneys demonstrates bilateral renal parenchyma and pelvicalyceal systems of normal conformity. The ureters and bladder should be outlined, and the postvoiding radiograph should show no mucosal abnormalities and minimal residual urine.

## ABNORMAL FINDINGS

Excretory urography can demonstrate many abnormalities of the urinary system, including renal or ureteral calculi; abnormal size, shape, or structure of kidneys, ureters, or bladder; a supernumerary or an absent kidney; polycystic kidney disease associated with renal hypertrophy; a redundant pelvis or ureter; a space-occupying lesion; pyelonephrosis; renal tuberculosis; hydronephrosis; and renovascular hypertension. (See *Abnormal excretory urogram*.)

## INTERFERING FACTORS

● End-stage renal disease or stool or gas in the colon (possible poor imaging)
● Insufficient injection of contrast medium, a recent barium enema, or GI or gallbladder series (possible poor imaging)

# Exercise electrocardiography

Also referred to as a *stress test,* an exercise electrocardiogram (ECG) evaluates the heart's response to physical stress, providing important diagnostic information that can't be obtained from a resting ECG alone.

An ECG and blood pressure readings are taken while the patient walks on a treadmill or pedals a stationary bicycle, and his response to a constant or an increasing workload is observed. Unless complications develop, the test continues until the patient reaches the target heart rate (determined by an established protocol) or experiences chest pain, fatigue, or sustained ventricular arrhythmias. The patient who has recently had a myocardial infarction (MI) or coronary artery surgery may walk the treadmill at a slow pace to determine his activity tolerance before discharge.

## PURPOSE

● To help diagnose the cause of chest pain or other possible cardiac pain
● To determine the functional capacity of the heart after surgery or an MI
● To screen for asymptomatic coronary artery disease (CAD), particularly in men over age 35
● To help set limitations for an exercise program
● To identify arrhythmias that develop during physical exercise
● To evaluate the effectiveness of antiarrhythmic or antianginal therapy
● To evaluate myocardial perfusion

## PATIENT PREPARATION

● Explain to the patient that the exercise ECG records the heart's electrical activity and performance under stress.
● Instruct the patient not to eat, smoke, or drink alcoholic or caffeinated beverages for 3 hours before the test, but to continue his prescribed drug regimen unless directed otherwise.
● Describe to the patient who will perform the test, where it will take place, and how long it will last.
● Tell the patient that the test will cause fatigue and that he'll be slightly breathless and sweaty, but assure him that the test poses few risks. He may, in fact, stop the test if he experiences fatigue or chest pain.
● Advise the patient to wear comfortable socks and shoes and loose, lightweight shorts or slacks. Men usually don't wear a shirt during the test, and women generally wear a bra and a lightweight short-sleeved blouse or a patient gown with a front closure.
● Explain to the patient that electrodes will be attached to several areas on his chest and, possibly, his back after the skin areas are cleaned and abraded. Reassure him that he won't feel current from the electrodes; however, they may itch slightly.
● Tell the patient that his blood pressure will be checked periodically throughout the procedure and assure him that his heart rate and ECG will be monitored continuously.
● If the patient is scheduled for a multistage treadmill test, explain that the speed and incline of the treadmill will increase at predetermined intervals and that he'll be informed of each adjustment.
● If the patient is scheduled for a bicycle ergometer test, explain that the resistance he experiences in pedaling increases gradually as he tries to maintain a specific speed.
● Encourage the patient to report his feelings during the test. Tell him that his blood pressure and ECG will be monitored for 5 to 10 minutes after the test.
● Check the patient's history for a recent physical examination (within 1 week) and for baseline 12-lead ECG results.
● Make sure that the patient or a responsible family member has signed an informed consent form.

## PROCEDURE AND POSTTEST CARE

● The electrode sites are cleaned with an alcohol swab, and superficial epidermal cell layers and excess skin oils are removed with a gauze pad or fine sandpaper. After thorough cleaning and abrading, adequately prepared sites will appear slightly red.

Chest electrodes are placed according to the lead system selected and are secured with adhesive tape, if necessary. The leadwire cable is placed over the patient's shoulder, and the leadwire box is placed on his chest. The cable is secured by pinning it to the patient's clothing or taping it to his shoulder or back. Then the leadwires are connected to the chest electrodes.

The monitor is started, and a stable baseline tracing is obtained and checked for arrhythmias. A blood pressure reading is taken, and the patient is auscultated for the presence of third heart sound ($S_3$) or fourth heart sound ($S_4$) gallops or crackles.

In a treadmill test, the treadmill is turned on to a slow speed, and the patient is shown how to step onto it and how to use the support railings to maintain balance, but not support weight. Then the treadmill is turned off. The patient is instructed to step onto the treadmill, and it's turned on to slow speed until he gets used to walking on it. Exercise intensity is then increased every 3 minutes by slightly increasing the speed of the machine and at the same time increasing the incline by 3%.

For a bicycle ergometer test, the patient is instructed to sit on the bicycle while the seat and handlebars are adjusted to comfortable positions. He's instructed not to grip the handlebars tightly, but to use them only for maintaining balance and to pedal until he reaches the desired speed, as shown on the speedometer.

In both tests, a monitor is observed continuously for changes in the heart's electrical activity. The rhythm strip is checked at preset intervals for arrhythmias, premature ventricular contractions (PVCs), and ST-segment and T-wave changes. The test level and the time elapsed in the test level are marked on each strip. Blood pressure is monitored at predetermined intervals, usually at the end of each test level, and changes in systolic readings are noted. Some common responses to maximal exercise are dizziness, light-headedness, leg fatigue, dyspnea, diaphoresis, and a slightly ataxic gait. If symptoms become severe, the test is stopped.

Usually, testing stops when the patient reaches the target heart rate. As the treadmill speed slows, he may be instructed to continue walking for several minutes to cool down. Then the treadmill is turned off, the patient is helped to a chair, and his blood pressure and

ECG are monitored for 5 to 10 minutes or until the ECG returns to baseline.

Auscultate for the presence of an $S_3$ or $S_4$ gallop. An $S_4$ gallop commonly develops after exercise because of increased blood flow volume and turbulence. An $S_3$ gallop is more significant than an $S_4$ gallop, indicating transient left ventricular dysfunction.

Tell the patient that he may resume any activities and medications discontinued before the test, as ordered.

Remove the electrodes and clean the electrode sites before the patient leaves.

## PRECAUTIONS

Because an exercise ECG places considerable stress on the heart, know that it may be contraindicated in the patient with ventricular aneurysm, dissecting aortic aneurysm, uncontrolled arrhythmias, pericarditis, myocarditis, severe anemia, uncontrolled hypertension, unstable angina, or heart failure.

*Alert* Stop the test immediately if the ECG shows frequent PVCs or a significant increase in ectopy, if the systolic blood pressure falls below resting level, if the heart rate falls to 10 beats/minute below resting level, or if the patient becomes exhausted. Depending on the patient's condition, the test may be stopped if the ECG shows bundle branch block, ST-segment depression that exceeds 1.5 mm, persistent ST-segment elevation, or frequent or complicated PVCs; if blood pressure fails to rise above the resting level; if systolic pressure exceeds 220 mm Hg; or if the patient experiences angina.

## NORMAL FINDINGS

In a normal exercise ECG, the P and T waves, the QRS complex, and the ST segment change minimally; a slight ST-segment depression occurs in some patients, especially women. The heart rate rises in direct proportion to the workload and metabolic oxygen demand; blood pressure also rises as workload increases. The patient attains the endurance levels predicted by his age and the appropriate exercise protocol. (See *Exercise ECG tracings,* page 184.)

## ABNORMAL FINDINGS

Although criteria for judging test results vary, two findings strongly suggest an abnormality: a flat or downsloping ST-segment depression of 1 mm or more for at least 0.08 second after the junction of the QRS and ST segments (J point) and a markedly depressed

# Exercise ECG tracings

These tracings are from an abnormal exercise electrocardiogram (ECG) obtained during a treadmill test performed on a patient who had just undergone a triple coronary artery bypass graft. The first tracing shows the heart at rest, with a blood pressure reading of 124/80 mm Hg. In the second tracing, the patient worked up to a 10% grade at 1.7 miles per hour before experiencing angina at 2 minutes, 25 seconds. The tracing shows a depressed ST segment; heart rate was 85 beats/minute, and blood pressure was 140/70 mm Hg. The third tracing shows the heart at rest 6 minutes after the test; blood pressure was 140/90 mm Hg.

**Resting**

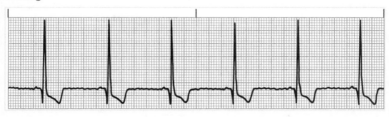

**Angina**

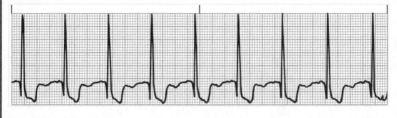

**Recovery**

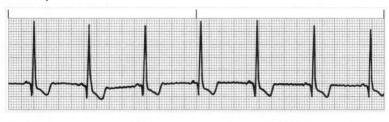

J point, with an upsloping but depressed ST segment of 1.5 mm below the baseline 0.08 second after the J point. T-wave inversion also signifies ischemia. Initial ST-segment depression on the resting ECG must be further depressed by 1 mm during exercise to be considered abnormal.

Hypotension resulting from exercise, ST-segment depression of 3 mm or more, downsloping ST segments, and ischemic ST segments appearing within the first

3 minutes of exercise and lasting 8 minutes into the posttest recovery period may indicate multivessel or left CAD. ST-segment elevation may indicate dyskinetic left ventricular wall motion or severe transmural ischemia.

The predictive value of this test for CAD varies with the patient's history and sex; false-negative and false-positive test results are common. This discrepancy is usually related to the effects of drugs, such as digoxin, or caffeine ingestion before testing. To detect CAD accurately, nuclear imaging and stress testing, exercise multiple-gated acquisition scanning, or coronary angiography may be necessary.

## INTERFERING FACTORS

● The patient's inability to exercise to the target heart rate due to fatigue or failure to cooperate

● Wolff-Parkinson-White syndrome (anomalous atrioventricular excitation), electrolyte imbalance, or use of a cardiac glycoside (possible false-positive)

● Conditions that affect left ventricular hypertrophy, such as congenital abnormalities and hypertension (possible interference with testing for ischemia)

● Beta-adrenergic blockers (may make test results difficult to interpret)

# *External sphincter electromyography*

External sphincter electromyography (EMG) measures electrical activity of the external urinary sphincter using needle electrodes inserted in perineal or periurethral tissues, electrodes in an anal plug, or skin electrodes. Skin electrodes are the most common method used.

Incontinence is the primary indication for external sphincter EMG. Usually, the test is done with cystometry and voiding urethrography as part of a full urodynamic study.

## PURPOSE

● To assess neuromuscular function of the external urinary sphincter

● To assess the functional balance between bladder and sphincter muscle activity

## PATIENT PREPARATION

● Explain to the patient that external sphincter EMG will determine how well his bladder and sphincter muscles work together.

● Describe the test, including who will perform it, where it will take place, and how long it will last.

● If skin electrodes are used, describe their placement and explain the preparatory procedure, which may include shaving a small area.

● If needle electrodes are used, describe their placement to the patient and explain that the discomfort is equivalent to an I.M. injection. Assure him that he'll feel discomfort only during insertion. Explain that wires connect the needles to the recorder, but pose no danger of electric shock. If the patient is a woman, tell her that she may notice slight bleeding at the first voiding.

● If an anal plug is used, tell the patient that only the tip of the plug will be inserted into the rectum and that he may feel fullness, but no discomfort.

● Check the patient's history for use of cholinergic or anticholinergic drugs and note such use.

● Make sure that the patient or a responsible family member has signed an informed consent form.

## PROCEDURE AND POSTTEST CARE

● Place the patient in the lithotomy position for electrode placement. After placement, he may lie in the supine position. Record the patient's position, the type of electrode and measuring equipment used, and other tests done at the same time.

● Electrode paste is applied to the ground plate, which is taped to the thigh and grounded. The electrodes are positioned and connected to electrode adapters.

● When using skin electrodes, clean the skin with antiseptic solution and then dry the area. If necessary, shave a small area to optimize electrode contact. Apply electrode paste and tape the electrodes in place. For a woman, electrodes are placed in the periurethral area; for a man, in the perineal area beneath the scrotum.

● To position needle electrodes on a male patient, a gloved finger is inserted in the rectum. The needles and wires are inserted through the perineal skin toward the apex of the prostate. Needle positions are 3 o'clock and 9 o'clock. The needles are withdrawn, and the wires are held in place and then taped to the thigh.

● To position needle electrodes on a female patient, the labia are spread and the needles and wires are inserted periurethrally at the 2 o'clock and 10 o'clock positions. The needles are withdrawn, and the wires are taped to the thigh.

● When using anal plug electrodes, the plug is lubricated, and the patient is asked to breathe slowly and deeply and to relax the anal sphincter to accommodate the plug by bearing down.

● After electrode placement, the adapters are inserted in the preamplifier, and recording starts. The patient is asked to alternately relax and tighten the sphincter.

● When sufficient data have been recorded, the patient is asked to bear down and exhale while the anal plug and needle electrodes are removed. Remove skin electrodes gently to avoid pulling hair and tender skin.

● Clean and dry the area before the patient dresses.

● In some urodynamic laboratories, cystometrography is done with EMG for a thorough evaluation of detrusor and sphincter coordination.

● For women, watch for and report hematuria after the first voiding if needle electrodes were used.

● Watch for and report symptoms of mild urethral irritation, such as dysuria, hematuria, and urinary frequency.

● Advise the patient to take a warm sitz bath and encourage him to drink 2 to 3 qt (2 to 3 L) of fluids daily, unless contraindicated.

## PRECAUTIONS

● Insert the needles quickly to minimize discomfort.

● Make sure that the ground plate is properly applied and anchored; wires should be taped securely to prevent artifacts.

## NORMAL FINDINGS

The EMG shows increased muscle activity when the patient tightens the external urinary sphincter and decreased muscle activity when he relaxes it. If EMG and cystometrography are performed simultaneously, a comparison of results shows that muscle activity of the normal sphincter increases as the bladder fills. During voiding and bladder contrac-

tion, muscle activity decreases as the sphincter relaxes. This comparison is important in assessing external sphincter efficiency and functional balance between bladder and sphincter muscle activity.

## ABNORMAL FINDINGS

Failure of the sphincter to relax or increased muscle activity during voiding demonstrates detrusor–external sphincter dyssynergia. Confirmation of such muscle activity by EMG may indicate neurogenic bladder, spinal cord injury, multiple sclerosis, Parkinson's disease, or stress incontinence.

## INTERFERING FACTORS

● Patient movement (possible distortion)

● Effect of anticholinergic or cholinergic drugs on detrusor and sphincter activity

● Improperly placed and anchored electrodes

## *Extractable nuclear antigen antibodies*

Extractable nuclear antigen (ENA) is a complex of at least four antigens. One of them—ribonucleoprotein (RNP)—is susceptible to degradation by ribonuclease. The second—Smith (Sm) antigen—is an acidic nuclear protein that resists ribonuclease degradation. The third and fourth antigens that are sometimes included in this group—Sjögren's syndrome A (SS-A) antigen and Sjögren's syndrome B (SS-B) antigen—form a precipitate when an antibody is present.

Antibodies to these antigens are associated with certain autoimmune disorders. Tests to detect ENA antibodies help differentiate autoimmune disorders with similar signs and symptoms.

The RNP antibody test detects RNP autoantibodies, which are associated with systemic lupus erythematosus (SLE), progressive systemic sclerosis, and other rheumatic disorders. This test aids in the differential diagnosis of systemic rheumatic disease and is a useful follow-up test for collagen vascular autoimmune disease.

The anti-Sm antibody test detects Sm autoantibodies, which are a specific marker for SLE; thus, positive results strongly suggest a diagnosis of SLE. This test, too, helps monitor collagen vascular autoimmune disease. The Sjögren's antibody test detects the SS-B autoantibodies produced by Sjögren's syndrome, an immunologic abnormality sometimes associated with rheumatic arthritis and SLE. However, this test doesn't confirm a diagnosis of Sjögren's syndrome.

## PURPOSE

● To aid in the differential diagnosis of autoimmune disease
● To distinguish between anti-RNP and anti-Sm antibodies
● To screen for anti-RNP antibodies (common in mixed connective tissue disease)
● To screen for anti-Sm antibodies (common in SLE)
● To support the diagnosis of collagen vascular autoimmune diseases
● To monitor the patient's response to therapy

## PATIENT PREPARATION

● Explain to the patient that the ENA antibody test detects certain antibodies and that test results help determine diagnosis and treatment.
● Explain that the test assesses the effectiveness of treatment, when appropriate.
● Inform the patient that he need not restrict food and fluids.
● Tell the patient that the test requires a blood sample. Explain who will perform the venipuncture and when.
● Explain to the patient that he may experience slight discomfort from the tourniquet and needle puncture.

## PROCEDURE AND POSTTEST CARE

● Perform a venipuncture and collect the sample in a 7-ml tube without additives.
● Because a patient with an autoimmune disease has a compromised immune system, check the venipuncture site for infection, and report changes promptly.
● Keep a clean, dry bandage over the site for at least 24 hours.
● Apply direct pressure to the venipuncture site until bleeding stops.
● If a hematoma develops at the venipuncture site, apply pressure.

## PRECAUTIONS

● Send the sample to the laboratory immediately.

## REFERENCE VALUES

Serum should be negative for anti-RNP, anti-Sm, and SS-B antibodies.

## ABNORMAL FINDINGS

Anti-RNP antibodies are elevated in SLE (35% to 40% of cases) and in mixed connective tissue disease. Anti-Sm antibodies are specific for SLE. Anti-SS-A and anti-SS-B antibodies are elevated in Sjögren's syndrome (40% to 45% of cases). Anti-SS-B antibodies are also elevated in SLE.

## INTERFERING FACTORS

● None significant

# Fasting plasma glucose

The fasting plasma glucose (or fasting blood sugar) test is used to measure plasma glucose levels after a 12 to 14 hour fast. This test is commonly used to screen for diabetes mellitus, in which absence or deficiency of insulin allows persistently high glucose levels.

## PURPOSE
● To screen for diabetes mellitus
● To monitor drug or diet therapy in the patient with diabetes mellitus

## PATIENT PREPARATION
● Explain to the patient that the fasting plasma glucose test is used to detect disorders of glucose metabolism and aids in the diagnosis of diabetes.
● Tell the patient that the test requires a blood sample. Explain who will perform the venipuncture and when.
● Explain to the patient that he may experience slight discomfort from the tourniquet and needle puncture.
● Instruct the patient to fast for 12 to 14 hours before the test.
● Notify the laboratory and physician of medications the patient is taking that may affect test results; they may need to be restricted.
● Alert the patient to the symptoms of hypoglycemia (weakness, restlessness, nervousness, hunger, and sweating) and tell him to report such symptoms immediately.

## PROCEDURE AND POSTTEST CARE
● Perform a venipuncture and collect the sample in a 5ml clot-activator tube.
● Apply direct pressure to the venipuncture site until bleeding stops.
● If a hematoma develops at the venipuncture site, apply pressure.
● Provide a balanced meal or a snack.
● Instruct the patient that he may resume his usual medications discontinued before the test, as ordered.

## PRECAUTIONS
● Send the sample to the laboratory immediately. If transport is delayed, refrigerate the sample.
● Note on the laboratory request when the patient last ate, the sample collection time, and when the last pretest dose of insulin or oral antidiabetic drug (if applicable) was given.

## REFERENCE VALUES
The normal range for fasting plasma glucose varies according to the laboratory procedure. Generally, normal values after at least an 8-hour fast are 70 to 110 mg (SI, 3.9 to 6.1 mmol/L) of true glucose per deciliter of blood.

## ABNORMAL FINDINGS
Confirmation of diabetes mellitus requires fasting plasma glucose levels of 126 mg/dl (SI, 7 mmol/L) or more obtained on two or more occasions. Levels ranging from 110 to 125 mg/dL are considered impaired fasting glucose or impaired glucose tolerance. In the patient with borderline or transient elevated

levels, a 2 hour postprandial plasma glucose test or oral glucose tolerance test may be performed to confirm the diagnosis.

Increased fasting plasma glucose levels can also result from pancreatitis, recent acute illness (such as myocardial infarction), Cushing's syndrome, acromegaly, and pheochromocytoma. Hyperglycemia may also stem from hyperlipoproteinemia (especially type III, IV, or V), chronic hepatic disease, nephrotic syndrome, brain tumor, sepsis, or gastrectomy with dumping syndrome and is typical in eclampsia, anoxia, and seizure disorders.

Low plasma glucose levels can result from Addison's disease, hyperinsulinism, insulinoma, von Gierke's disease, functional and reactive hypoglycemia, myxedema, adrenal insufficiency, congenital adrenal hyperplasia, hypopituitarism, malabsorption syndrome, and some cases of hepatic insufficiency.

## INTERFERING FACTORS

- Recent illness, infection, or pregnancy (possible increase)
- Glycolysis due to failure to refrigerate the sample or to send it to the laboratory immediately (possible false-negative)
- Acetaminophen, if using the glucose oxidase or hexokinase method (possible false-positive)
- Arginine, benzodiazepines, chlorthalidone, corticosteroids, dextrothyroxine, diazoxide, epinephrine, furosemide, hormonal contraceptives, phenothiazines, lithium, phenolphthalein, phenytoin, recent I.V. glucose infusions, large doses of nicotinic acid, thiazide diuretics, and triamterene (Dyrenium) (increase)
- Ethacrynic acid (may cause hyperglycemia); large doses in patients with uremia (can cause hypoglycemia)
- Alcohol, beta-adrenergic blockers, insulin, monoamine oxidase inhibitors, and oral antidiabetic agents (possible decrease)
- Strenuous exercise (decrease)

## Febrile agglutination tests

Sometimes bacterial infections (such as tularemia, brucellosis, and the disorders caused by Salmonella) and rickettsial infections (such as Rocky Mountain spotted fever and typhus) cause puzzling fevers, called fevers of undetermined origin (FUO). In these infections and others in which microorganisms are difficult to isolate from blood or excreta, febrile agglutination tests can provide important diagnostic information.

The Weil-Felix test for rickettsial disease, Widal's test for Salmonella, and tests for brucellosis and tularemia are essentially the same. In these tests, a serum sample is mixed with a few drops of prepared antigens in normal saline solution on a slide and the reaction is observed.

The Weil-Felix test establishes rickettsial antibody titers. It uses three forms of *Proteus* antigens (OX-19, OX-2, and OX-K) that cross-react with the various strains of rickettsiae. Antibodies to certain rickettsial strains react with more than one *Proteus* antigen, whereas antibodies to other strains fail to react with any *Proteus* antigens.

Widal's test establishes the titers for flagellar (H) and somatic (O) antigens, which may indicate Salmonella gastroenteritis and extraintestinal focal infections, caused by *S. enteritidis,* or enteric (typhoid) fever, caused by *S. typhosa*. A third antigen, the Vi or envelope antigen, may indicate typhoid carrier status, which commonly tests negative for H and O antigens. Widal's test isn't recommended for diagnosing Salmonella gastroenteritis.

Slide agglutination and tube dilution tests, using killed suspensions of the disease organisms as antigens, establish titers for the gram-negative coccobacilli *Brucella* and *Francisella tularensis,* which cause brucellosis and tularemia, respectively.

## PURPOSE

- To support clinical findings in diagnosis of disorders caused by Salmonella, Rickettsia, *F. tularensis,* and *Brucella* organisms
- To identify the cause of FUO

## PATIENT PREPARATION

- Explain to the patient that the febrile agglutination test detects and quantifies microorganisms that may cause fever and other symptoms.
- Inform the patient that he need not restrict food, fluids, or medications.
- Tell the patient that the test requires a blood sample. Explain who will perform the venipuncture and when.

- Explain to the patient that he may experience slight discomfort from the tourniquet and needle puncture.
- Explain to the patient that this test requires a series of blood samples to detect a pattern of titers characteristic of the suspected disorder, if appropriate. Reassure him that a positive titer only suggests a disorder.
- Note on the laboratory request when antimicrobial therapy began, if appropriate.

## PROCEDURE AND POSTTEST CARE
- Perform a venipuncture and collect the sample in a 7-ml clot-activator tube.
- Apply direct pressure to the venipuncture site until bleeding stops.
- If a hematoma develops at the venipuncture site, apply pressure.
- In FUO and suspected infection, contact the facility's infection control department. Infection control measures may be necessary.

## PRECAUTIONS
- Use standard precautions when collecting and handling samples.
- Send samples to the laboratory immediately.

## REFERENCE VALUES
Results are reported as negative or positive, and positive results are titered. Normal dilutions are:
- Salmonella antibody: < 1:80
- Brucellosis antibody: < 1:80
- Tularemia antibody: < 1:40
- Rickettsial antibody: < 1:40.

## ABNORMAL FINDINGS
Observed rise and fall of titers is crucial for detecting active infection. If this isn't possible, certain titer levels can suggest the disorder. For all febrile agglutinins, a fourfold increase in titers is strong evidence of infection.

The Weil-Felix test is positive for rickettsiae with antibodies to *Proteus* 6 to 12 days after infection; titers peak in 1 month and usually drop to negative in 5 to 6 months. This test can't be used to diagnose rickettsialpox or Q fever because the antibodies of these diseases don't cross-react with *Proteus* antigens; the test shows positive titers in Proteus infections and, in such cases, is nonspecific for rickettsiae.

In Salmonella infection, H and O agglutinins usually appear in serum after 1 week, and titers rise for 3 to 6 weeks. O agglutinins usually fall to insignificant levels in 6 to 12 months. Agglutinin titers may remain elevated for years.

In brucellosis, titers usually rise after 2 to 3 weeks and reach their highest levels between 4 and 8 weeks. The absence of *Brucella* agglutinins doesn't rule out brucellosis. In tularemia, titers usually become positive during the second week of infection, exceed 1:320 by the third week, peak within 4 to 7 weeks, and usually decline gradually 1 year after recovery.

## INTERFERING FACTORS
- Vaccination or continuous exposure to bacterial or rickettsial infection, resulting in immunity (high titers)
- Antibody cross-reaction with bacteria causing other infectious diseases such as tularemia antibodies cross-reacting with *Brucella* antigens
- Immunodeficiency (negative titers even during symptom-producing infection due to inability to form antibodies)
- Antibiotics (low titers early in the course of infection)
- Elevated immunoglobulin levels due to hepatic disease or excessive drug use (high Salmonella titers)
- Skin tests with *Brucella* antigen (possible high *Brucella* titers)
- *Proteus* infections (possible positive Weil-Felix titers for rickettsial disease)

# Fecal lipids

Lipids excreted in stools include monoglycerides, diglycerides, triglycerides, phospholipids, glycolipids, soaps (fatty acids and fatty acid salts), sterols, and cholesterol esters. When biliary and pancreatic secretions are adequate, emulsified dietary lipids are almost completely absorbed in the small intestine.

Excessive excretion of fecal lipids (steatorrhea) occurs in several malabsorption syndromes. Qualitative and quantitative tests are used to detect excessive excretion of lipids in patients exhibiting signs of malabsorption, such as weight loss, abdominal distention, and scaly skin.

The qualitative test involves staining a stool specimen with Sudan III dye and then examining it microscopically for evidence of malabsorption, such as undigested muscle fibers and various fats. The quantitative test involves drying and weighing a 72-hour specimen and then using a solvent to extract the lipids, which are subsequently evaporated and weighed. Only the quantitative test confirms steatorrhea.

## PURPOSE
- To confirm steatorrhea

## PATIENT PREPARATION
- Explain to the patient that the fecal lipid test evaluates fat digestion.
- Instruct the patient to abstain from alcohol and to maintain a high-fat diet (100 g/day) for 3 days before the test and during the collection period.
- Tell the patient that the test requires a 72-hour stool collection.
- Notify the laboratory and physician of medications the patient is taking that may affect test results; they may need to be restricted.
- Teach the patient how to collect a timed stool specimen, and provide him with the necessary equipment.
- Inform the patient that the laboratory requires 1 or 2 days to complete the analysis.

## PROCEDURE AND POSTTEST CARE
- Collect a 72-hour stool specimen.
- Instruct the patient that he may resume his usual diet and medications, as ordered.

## PRECAUTIONS
- Don't use a waxed collection container because the wax may become incorporated in the stool and interfere with accurate testing.
- Tell the patient to avoid contaminating the stool specimen with toilet tissue or urine.
- Refrigerate the collection container and keep it tightly covered.

## NORMAL FINDINGS
Fecal lipids normally comprise less than 20% of excreted solids, with excretion more than 7 g/24 hours.

## ABNORMAL FINDINGS
Digestive and absorptive disorders cause steatorrhea. Digestive disorders may affect the production and release of pancreatic lipase or bile; absorptive disorders may affect the intestine's integrity.

In pancreatic insufficiency, impaired lipid digestion may result from insufficient lipase production. Pancreatic resection, cystic fibrosis, chronic pancreatitis, or ductal obstruction by stone or tumor may prevent the normal release or action of lipase.

In impaired hepatic function, faulty lipid digestion may result from inadequate bile salt production. Biliary obstruction, which may accompany gallbladder disease, may prevent the normal release of bile salts into the duodenum. Extensive small-bowel resection or bypass may also interrupt normal enterohepatic bile salt circulation.

Diseases of the intestinal mucosa affect the normal absorption of lipids. Regional ileitis and atrophy due to malnutrition cause gross structural changes in the intestinal wall; celiac disease and tropical sprue produce mucosal abnormalities.

Scleroderma, radiation enteritis, fistulas, intestinal tuberculosis, small intestine diverticula, and altered intestinal flora may also cause steatorrhea. Whipple's disease and lymphomas cause lymphatic obstruction that may inhibit fat absorption.

## INTERFERING FACTORS
- A contaminated or incomplete stool specimen (total weight < 300 g)
- Alcohol, aluminum hydroxide, azathioprine (Imuran), bisacodyl, calcium carbonate (Caltrate), cholestyramine (Questran), colchicine, kanamycin (Kantrex), mineral oil, neomycin (Mycifradin), and potassium chloride (possible increase or decrease due to inhibited absorption or altered chemical digestion)

# Fecal occult blood test

Fecal occult blood is detected by microscopic analysis or by chemical tests for hemoglobin, such as the guaiac test. Normally, stools contain small amounts of blood (2 to 2.5 ml/day); therefore, tests for occult blood detect quantities larger than this. Testing is indicated when clinical symptoms and preliminary blood studies suggest GI bleeding. Additional tests are required to pinpoint the origin of

# COMMON SITES AND CAUSES OF GI BLOOD LOSS

Illustrated here are potential areas that can cause blood loss, resulting in positive fecal occult blood testing. Further clinical assessment and testing is necessary to determine the specific area involved.

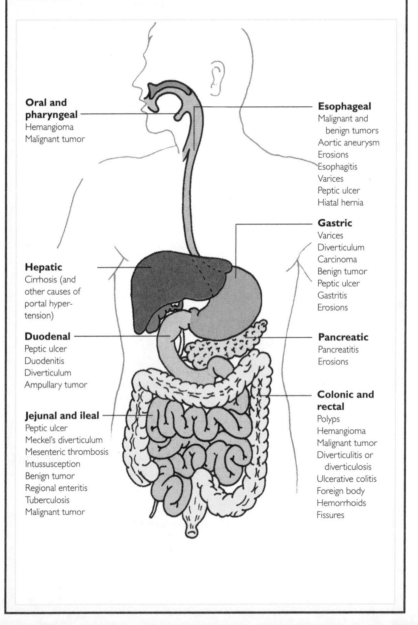

**Oral and pharyngeal**
Hemangioma
Malignant tumor

**Esophageal**
Malignant and
   benign tumors
Aortic aneurysm
Erosions
Esophagitis
Varices
Peptic ulcer
Hiatal hernia

**Gastric**
Varices
Diverticulum
Carcinoma
Benign tumor
Peptic ulcer
Gastritis
Erosions

**Hepatic**
Cirrhosis (and
other causes of
portal hyper-
tension)

**Duodenal**
Peptic ulcer
Duodenitis
Diverticulum
Ampullary tumor

**Pancreatic**
Pancreatitis
Erosions

**Colonic and rectal**
Polyps
Hemangioma
Malignant tumor
Diverticulitis or
   diverticulosis
Ulcerative colitis
Foreign body
Hemorrhoids
Fissures

**Jejunal and ileal**
Peptic ulcer
Meckel's diverticulum
Mesenteric thrombosis
Intussusception
Benign tumor
Regional enteritis
Tuberculosis
Malignant tumor

the bleeding. (See *Common sites and causes of GI blood loss*.)

## PURPOSE
- To detect GI bleeding
- To aid in the early diagnosis of colorectal cancer

## PATIENT PREPARATION
- Explain to the patient that the fecal occult blood test helps detect abnormal GI bleeding.
- Instruct the patient to maintain a high fiber diet and to refrain from eating red meats, turnips, and horseradish for 48 to 72 hours before the test as well as throughout the collection period.
- Tell the patient that the test requires the collection of three stool specimens. Occasionally, only a random specimen is collected.
- Notify the laboratory and physician of medications the patient is taking that may affect test results; they may need to be restricted. If these drugs must be continued, note this on the laboratory request.

## PROCEDURE AND POSTTEST CARE
- Collect three stool specimens or a random stool specimen, as ordered. Obtain specimens from two different areas of each stool. Testing may take place in the laboratory or in a utility room on the nursing unit, depending on the facility's policy. Two of the most commonly used screening tests are Hematest and Hemoccult. Hematest uses orthotoluidine to detect hemoglobin and Hemoccult uses guaiac.
- After any of the tests described here are performed, tell the patient that he may resume his usual diet and medications, as ordered.

## Hematest reagent tablet test
- Use a wooden applicator to smear a bit of the stool specimen on the filter paper supplied with the kit. Alternatively, after performing a digital rectal examination, wipe the finger you used for the examination on a square of the filter paper. Place the filter paper with the stool smear on a glass plate.
- Remove a reagent tablet from the bottle, and immediately replace the cap tightly. Place the tablet in the center of the stool smear on the filter paper. Add one drop of

water to the tablet, and allow it to soak in for 5 to 10 seconds. Add a second drop, letting it run from the tablet onto the specimen and filter paper. If necessary, tap the plate gently to dislodge any water from the top of the tablet.
- After 2 minutes, the filter paper will turn blue if the test is positive. Don't read the color that appears on the tablet itself or develops on the filter paper after the 2-minute period. Note the results and discard the filter paper. Remove and discard your gloves and wash your hands thoroughly.

## Hemoccult slide test
- Open the flap on the slide pack and use a wooden applicator to apply a thin smear of the stool specimen to the guaiac-impregnated filter paper exposed in box A. Alternatively, after performing a digital rectal examination, wipe the finger you used for the examination on a square of filter paper. Apply a second smear from another part of the specimen to the filter paper exposed in box B because some parts of the specimen may not contain blood.
- Allow the specimen to dry for 3 to 5 minutes. Open the flap at the rear of the slide package and place 2 drops of Hemoccult developing solution on the paper over each smear. A blue reaction will appear in 30 to 60 seconds if the test is positive. Record the results and discard the slide package. Remove and discard your gloves and wash your hands thoroughly.

## Instant-view fecal occult blood test
- Add a stool specimen to the collection tube. Shake it to mix the specimen with the extraction buffer, and then dispense 4 drops into the sample well of the cassette. Results will appear on the test region and the control region of the cassette in 5 to 10 minutes, indicating whether the level of hemoglobin is greater than 0.05 µg/ml of stool. Results will also indicate if the device is performing properly.

## PRECAUTIONS
- Instruct the patient to avoid contaminating the stool specimen with toilet tissue or urine.
- Send the specimen to the laboratory or perform the test immediately.

## NORMAL FINDINGS

Less than 2.5 ml of blood should be present in stools, resulting in a green reaction.

## ABNORMAL FINDINGS

A positive test indicates GI bleeding, which may result from many disorders, such as varices, a peptic ulcer, carcinoma, ulcerative colitis, dysentery, or hemorrhagic disease. This test is particularly important for the early diagnosis of colorectal cancer. Further tests, such as barium swallow, analyses of gastric contents, and endoscopic procedures, are necessary to define the site and extent of bleeding.

## INTERFERING FACTORS

● Bromides, colchicine, indomethacin (Indocin), iron preparations, phenylbutazone, rauwolfia derivatives, and steroids (possible increase due to association with GI blood loss)
● Ascorbic acid (false-normal, even with significant bleeding)
● Ingestion of 2 to 5 ml of blood such as from bleeding gums
● Active bleeding from hemorrhoids (possible false-positive results)

## *Fecal urobilinogen*

Urobilinogen, the end product of bilirubin metabolism, is a brown pigment formed by bacterial enzymes in the small intestine. It's excreted in stools or reabsorbed into portal blood, where it's returned to the liver and excreted in bile. A small amount is excreted in urine. Proper bilirubin metabolism depends on normal hepatobiliary system functioning and a normal erythrocyte life span.

Although measuring fecal urobilinogen is a useful indicator of hepatobiliary and hemolytic disorders, the test is rarely performed because it's easier to measure serum bilirubin and urine urobilinogen.

## PURPOSE

● To aid in the diagnosis of hepatobiliary and hemolytic disorders

## PATIENT PREPARATION

● Explain to the patient that the fecal urobilinogen test evaluates liver and bile duct function or detects red blood cell disorders.
● Inform the patient that he need not restrict food and fluids.
● Tell the patient that the test requires collection of a random stool specimen.
● Notify the laboratory and physician of medications the patient is taking that may affect test results; they may need to be restricted.

## PROCEDURE AND POSTTEST CARE

● Collect a random stool specimen.
● Tell the patient that he may resume his usual medications, as ordered.

## PRECAUTIONS

● Tell the patient not to contaminate the stool specimen with toilet tissue or urine.
● Use a light-resistant collection container because urobilinogen breaks down to urobilin when exposed to light.
● Send the specimen to the laboratory immediately after collection.
● Refrigerate the specimen if transport or testing is delayed more than 30 minutes; freeze the specimen if the test is to be performed by an outside laboratory.

## REFERENCE VALUES

Normally, fecal urobilinogen values range from 50 to 300 mg/24 hours (SI, 100 to 400 EU/100 g).

## ABNORMAL FINDINGS

Absent or low levels of urobilinogen in stools indicate obstructed bile flow, the result of intrahepatic disorders (such as hepatocellular jaundice due to cirrhosis or hepatitis) or extrahepatic disorders (such as choledocholithiasis or tumor of the head of the pancreas, ampulla of Vater, or bile duct). Low fecal urobilinogen levels are also characteristic of depressed erythropoiesis such as in aplastic anemia.

## INTERFERING FACTORS

● Broad-spectrum antibiotics (possible decrease due to inhibition of bacterial growth in the colon)
● Sulfonamides, which react with the reagent used by the laboratory in this test,

and large doses of salicylates (possible increase)

# Ferritin, serum

Ferritin, a major iron-storage protein, normally appears in small quantities in serum. In healthy adults, serum ferritin levels are directly related to the amount of available iron stored in the body and can be measured accurately by radioimmunoassay.

## PURPOSE
- To screen for iron deficiency and iron overload
- To measure iron storage
- To distinguish between iron deficiency (a condition of low iron storage) and chronic inflammation (a condition of normal storage)

## PATIENT PREPARATION
- Explain to the patient that the serum ferritin test is used to assess the available iron stored in the body.
- Tell the patient that a blood sample will be taken. Explain who will perform the venipuncture and when.
- Explain to the patient that he may feel slight discomfort from the tourniquet and needle puncture.
- Review the patient's history for blood transfusion within the past 4 months.
- Inform the patient that he need not restrict food, fluids, or medications.

## PROCEDURE AND POSTTEST CARE
- Perform a venipuncture, collecting the sample in a 10-ml tube without additives.
- If a hematoma develops at the venipuncture site, apply pressure.

## PRECAUTIONS
- Handle the sample gently to prevent hemolysis.
- Send the sample to the laboratory immediately.

## REFERENCE VALUES
Normal serum ferritin values in adults vary with age and sex, as follows:
- adult males — 20 to 300 ng/ml (SI, 20 to 300 µg/L)
- adult females — 20 to 120 ng/ml (SI, 20 to 120 µg/L).

*Age alert* *Normal values in infants and children also vary with age:*
- *neonates — 25 to 200 ng/ml (SI, 25 to 200 µg/L)*
- *age 1 month — 200 to 600 ng/ml (SI, 200 to 600 µg/L)*
- *age 2 to 5 months — 50 to 200 ng/ml (SI, 50 to 200 µg/L)*
- *age 6 months to 15 years — 7 to 140 ng/ml (SI, 7 to 140 µg/L).*

## ABNORMAL FINDINGS
High serum ferritin levels may indicate acute or chronic hepatic disease, iron overload, leukemia, acute or chronic infection or inflammation, Hodgkin's disease, or chronic hemolytic anemias. In these disorders, iron stores in the bone marrow may be normal or significantly increased.

Serum ferritin levels are characteristically normal or slightly elevated in patients with chronic renal disease. Low serum ferritin levels indicate chronic iron deficiency.

## INTERFERING FACTORS
- Recent blood transfusion (possible false-high)

# Fibrinogen, plasma

Fibrinogen (factor I) originates in the liver and is converted to fibrin by thrombin during clotting. Because fibrin is necessary for clot formation, fibrinogen deficiency can produce mild to severe bleeding disorders.

## PURPOSE
- To aid the diagnosis of suspected clotting or bleeding disorders caused by fibrinogen abnormalities

## PATIENT PREPARATION
- Explain to the patient that the plasma fibrinogen test is used to determine if blood clots normally.
- Tell the patient that a blood sample will be taken. Explain who will perform the venipuncture and when.
- Explain to the patient that he may feel slight discomfort from the tourniquet and needle puncture.

- Notify the laboratory and physician of medications the patient is taking that may affect test results; they may need to be restricted.
- Inform the patient that he need not restrict food and fluids.

## PROCEDURE AND POSTTEST CARE
- Perform a venipuncture and collect the sample in a 3- or 4.5-ml tube with sodium citrate added.
- If a hematoma develops at the site, apply pressure.
- Instruct the patient that he may resume any medications discontinued before the test, as ordered.

## PRECAUTIONS
- Be aware that the plasma fibrinogen test is contraindicated in the patient with active bleeding or acute infection or illness and in a patient who has had a blood transfusion within the past 4 weeks.
- Avoid excessive probing during venipuncture and handle the sample gently.
- Completely fill the collection tube, invert it gently several times, and send it to the laboratory immediately or place it on ice.

## REFERENCE VALUES
Fibrinogen levels normally range from 200 to 400 mg/dl (SI, 2 to 4 g/L).

## ABNORMAL FINDINGS
Depressed fibrinogen levels may indicate congenital afibrinogenemia; hypofibrinogenemia or dysfibrinogenemia; disseminated intravascular coagulation; fibrinolysis; severe hepatic disease; cancer of the prostate, pancreas, or lung; or bone marrow lesions. Obstetric complications or trauma may cause low levels. Markedly decreased fibrinogen levels impede the accurate interpretation of coagulation tests that have a fibrin clot as an end point.

Elevated levels may indicate cancer of the stomach, breast, or kidney or inflammatory disorders, such as pneumonia or membranoproliferative glomerulonephritis.

Prolonged partial thromboplastin time, prothrombin time, and thrombin time may also indicate a fibrinogen deficiency.

## INTERFERING FACTORS
- Diets rich in omega-3 fatty acids and omega-6 fatty acids (decreased levels)
- Estrogens and hormonal contraceptives (increased levels)
- Anabolic steroids, asparaginase (Elspar), androgens, phenobarbital, streptokinase, urokinase, and valproic acid (Depakene) (decreased levels)

# 5-hydroxyindoleacetic acid, urine

The quantitative analysis of urine levels of 5-hydroxyindoleacetic acid (5-HIAA) is used mainly to screen for carcinoid tumors (argentaffinomas). Such tumors, found generally in the intestine or appendix, secrete an excessive amount of serotonin, which is reflected by high 5-HIAA levels. This test measures 5-HIAA levels by the colorimetric technique and is most accurate when performed with a 24-hour urine specimen, which can detect small or intermittently secreting carcinoid tumors.

## PURPOSE
- To aid in the diagnosis of carcinoid tumors (argentaffinomas)

## PATIENT PREPARATION
- Explain to the patient what serotonin is and why the urine 5-HIAA test is important.
- Instruct the patient not to eat foods containing serotonin, such as bananas, plums, pineapples, avocados, eggplants, tomatoes, and walnuts, for 4 days before the test.
- Tell the patient that the test requires collection of urine over a 24-hour period, and teach him the proper collection technique.
- Notify the laboratory and physician of medications the patient is taking that may affect test results; they may need to be restricted.

## PROCEDURE AND POSTTEST CARE
- Collect the patient's urine over a 24-hour period, discarding the first specimen and retaining the last. Use a bottle containing a preservative to keep the specimen at a pH of 2 to 4.

- Instruct the patient that he may resume his usual diet and medications, as ordered.

## PRECAUTIONS
- Refrigerate the specimen or keep it on ice during the collection period.
- Send the specimen to the laboratory as soon as collection is complete.

## REFERENCE VALUES
Normally, urine 5-HIAA values are qualitatively reported as negative; quantitative results are 2 to 7 mg/24 hours (SI, 10.4 to 36.6 μmol/d).

## ABNORMAL FINDINGS
Marked elevation of urine 5-HIAA levels, possibly as high as 200 to 600 mg/24 hours (SI, 1,040 to 3,120 μmol/d), indicates a carcinoid tumor. However, because these tumors vary in their capacity to store and secrete serotonin, some patients with carcinoid syndrome (metastatic carcinoid tumors) may not show elevated levels. Repeated testing is usually necessary.

## INTERFERING FACTORS
- Severe GI disturbance or diarrhea
- Fluorouracil, melphalan, methamphetamine, and reserpine (increase)
- Alcohol, isoniazid, methyldopa, monoamine oxidase inhibitors, and tricyclic antidepressants (decrease in most cases)
- Acetaminophen, guaifenesin, methenamine compounds, methocarbamol, phenothiazines, and salicylates (possible increase or decrease)

# Fluorescein angiography

In fluorescein angiography, a special camera takes rapid-sequence photographs of the fundus following I.V. injection of sodium fluorescein (a contrast medium), thereby recording the appearance of blood vessels within the eye. This technique provides enhanced visibility of the microvascular structures of the retina and choroid, which permits the evaluation of the entire retinal vascular bed, including retinal circulation.

## PURPOSE
- To document retinal circulation when evaluating intraocular abnormalities, such as retinopathy, tumors, and circulatory or inflammatory disorders

## PATIENT PREPARATION
- Explain that fluorescein angiography takes about 30 minutes and evaluates the small blood vessels in the eyes.
- Make sure the patient or a responsible family member has signed an informed consent form.
- Check the patient's history for glaucoma and hypersensitivity reactions or allergies, especially to contrast media and dilating eyedrops. If necessary, tell a patient with glaucoma not to use miotic eyedrops on the day of the test.
- Explain that eyedrops will be instilled to dilate his pupils and that a dye will be injected into his arm. Tell him that his eyes will be photographed with a special camera before and after the injection. Stress that these are photographs, not X-rays.
- Warn the patient that his skin may be discolored and his urine may appear orange for 24 to 48 hours after the procedure.

## PROCEDURE AND POSTTEST CARE
- Administer mydriatic eyedrops. Usually, two instillations are necessary to achieve maximum mydriasis within 15 to 40 minutes.
- Following mydriasis, seat the patient comfortably in the examining chair facing the camera.
- Have the patient loosen or remove any restrictive clothing around his neck.
- Tell the patient to place his chin in the chin rest and his forehead against the bar. Tell him to open his eyes wide and stare straight ahead, while keeping his teeth together and maintaining normal breathing and blinking.
- The antecubital vein is prepared and punctured; however, dye isn't injected yet. At this time, a few photographs may be taken. Make sure the patient keeps his arm extended; if necessary, use an arm board.
- Warn the patient that the dye will be injected rapidly. Remind him to maintain his position and to continue to stare straight ahead, and then inject the dye.

- The patient may experience nausea and a feeling of warmth. Provide reassurance and observe him for hypersensitivity reactions, such as vomiting, dry mouth, metallic taste, suddenly increased salivation, sneezing, light-headedness, fainting, or hives. In rare instances, anaphylactic shock may occur.
- As the dye is injected, 25 to 30 photographs are taken in rapid sequence. Each photograph is taken 1 second after the other.
- The needle and syringe are removed carefully; pressure and a dressing are applied to the injection site.
- If late-phase photographs are needed, tell the patient to sit and relax for 20 minutes, and then reposition him for 5 to 10 photographs. If necessary, photographs may be taken up to 1 hour after the injection.
- Remind the patient that his skin and urine will be slightly discolored for 24 to 48 hours after the test. Encourage the patient to drink increased amounts of fluids to help excrete the dye.
- Explain to the patient that his near vision will be blurred for up to 12 hours and that he should avoid direct sunlight and refrain from driving during this time.

## PRECAUTIONS

- Don't leave the patient unattended because he may experience mild adverse reactions, such as nausea, vomiting, sneezing, paresthesia of the tongue, and dizziness.

*Age alert* Have emergency resuscitation equipment at hand. Serious adverse effects (laryngeal edema, bronchospasm, and respiratory arrest) are possible. If a reaction occurs, note it on the patient's allergy history.
- Keep in mind that the needle must be placed in the vein correctly; extravasation of dye around the injection site is painful.

## NORMAL FINDINGS

After rapid injection into the antecubital vein, sodium fluorescein reaches the retina in 12 to 15 seconds (filling phase). As the choroidal vessels and choriocapillaries fill, the background of the retina fluoresces, taking on an evenly mottled appearance known as the choroidal flush. Then the dye fills the arteries (arterial phase). The arteriovenous (AV) phase lasts from the complete filling of the arteries and capillaries to the earliest evidence of dye in the veins. The time the arteries begin to empty to the time the veins fill

and empty is known as the venous phase. Finally, the recirculation phase occurs 30 to 60 minutes after the injection, when the fluorescein — if at all present — is barely detectable in the retinal vessels. Normally, there's no leakage from the retinal vessels.

## ABNORMAL FINDINGS

The varying and complex findings after fluorescein angiography require interpretation by a highly skilled ophthalmologist with extensive experience in diagnosing retinal disorders.

Abnormalities detected in the early filling phase may include microaneurysms, AV shunts, and neovascularization. The test may identify arterial occlusion by showing delayed or absent flow of the dye through the arteries, stenosis, and prolonged venous drainage. Venous occlusion may be associated with vessel dilation and fluorescein leakage. Chronic obstruction may produce recanalization and collateral circulation.

In hypertensive retinopathy, abnormalities may include areas of increased vascular tortuosity, microaneurysms around zones of capillary nonperfusion, and generalized suffusion of the dye in the retina. Aneurysms and capillary hemangiomas may leak fluorescein and are typically surrounded by hard yellow exudate. Tumors exhibit variable fluorescein patterns, depending on the histologic type. Retinal edema or inflammation and fibrous tissue may show variable degrees of fluorescence. Papilledema produces vascular leakage in the disk area.

## INTERFERING FACTORS

- Inadequate view of the fundus due to insufficient pupillary dilation (possible poor imaging)
- Cataract, media opacity, or inability to keep eyes open and to maintain fixation (possible poor imaging)

## *Fluorescent treponemal antibody absorption*

The fluorescent treponemal antibody absorption (FTA-ABS or simply FTA) test uses indirect immunofluorescence to detect antibodies to the spirochete *Treponema pallidum* in serum. This spirochete causes syphilis.

In this test, prepared *T. pallidum* is fixed on a slide, and the patient's serum is added after the addition of an absorbed preparation of Reiter treponema. This addition to the test serum prevents interference by antibodies from nonsyphilitic treponemas; Reiter treponema combines with most nonsyphilitic antibodies, making the FTA-ABS test specific for *T. pallidum*.

If syphilitic antibodies are present in the test serum, they'll coat the treponemal organisms. The slide is then stained with fluorescein-labeled antiglobulin. This antiglobulin attaches to the coated spirochetes, which fluoresce when viewed under an ultraviolet microscope.

Although the FTA-ABS test is generally performed on a serum sample to detect primary or secondary syphilis, a cerebrospinal fluid (CSF) specimen is required to detect tertiary syphilis. Because antibody levels remain constant for long periods, the FTA-ABS test isn't recommended for monitoring the patient's response to therapy. (See *Two tests for* Treponema pallidum.)

## PURPOSE
- To confirm primary and secondary syphilis
- To screen for suspected false-positive results of Venereal Disease Research Laboratories tests

## PATIENT PREPARATION
- Explain to the patient that the FTA-ABS test can confirm or rule out syphilis.
- Inform the patient that he need not restrict food, fluids, or medications.
- Tell the patient that the test requires a blood sample. Explain who will perform the venipuncture and when.
- Explain to the patient that he may experience slight discomfort from the tourniquet and needle puncture.

## PROCEDURE AND POSTTEST CARE
- Perform a venipuncture and collect the sample in a 7-ml clot-activator tube.
- Apply direct pressure to the venipuncture site until bleeding stops.

---

## TWO TESTS FOR *TREPONEMA PALLIDUM*

The microhemagglutination assay for the *Treponema pallidum* antibody increases the specificity of syphilis testing by eliminating methodologic interference. In this assay, tanned sheep red blood cells are coated with *T. pallidum* antigen and combined with absorbed test serum. Hemagglutination occurs in the presence of specific anti-*T. pallidum* antibodies in the serum.

In the enzyme-linked immunosorbent assay, tubes coated with *T. pallidum* are washed and then treated with enzyme-labeled antihuman globulin. After the substrate for the enzymes is added to the tubes, the enzymatic activity is measured by quantitating the reaction product formed.

---

- If a hematoma develops at the venipuncture site, apply pressure.
- If the test is reactive, explain the nature of syphilis and stress the importance of proper treatment and the need to find and treat the patient's sexual contacts.
- Provide the patient with additional information about syphilis and how it's spread; emphasize the need for antibiotic therapy, if appropriate. Report positive results to state public health authorities and prepare the patient for mandatory inquiries.
- If the test is nonreactive or findings are borderline, but syphilis hasn't been ruled out, instruct the patient to return for follow-up testing; explain that inconclusive results don't necessarily indicate that he's free from the disease.

## PRECAUTIONS
- Handle the sample gently to prevent hemolysis.

## NORMAL FINDINGS
Normally, results of the FTA-ABS test are nonreactive.

## ABNORMAL FINDINGS
The presence of treponemal antibodies in the serum—a reactive test result—doesn't indi-

cate the stage or severity of infection. (The presence of these antibodies in CSF is strong evidence of tertiary neurosyphilis.) Elevated antibody levels appear in most patients with primary syphilis and in almost all patients with secondary syphilis. Higher antibody levels persist for several years, with or without treatment.

The absence of treponemal antibodies—a nonreactive test result—doesn't necessarily rule out syphilis. *T. pallidum* causes no detectable immunologic changes in the blood for 14 to 21 days after initial infection. Organisms may be detected earlier by examining suspicious lesions with a dark-field microscope. Low antibody levels and other nonspecific factors produce borderline findings. In such cases, repeated testing and a thorough review of the patient's history may be productive.

Although the FTA-ABS test is specific, some patients with nonsyphilitic conditions, such as systemic lupus erythematosus, genital herpes, and increased or abnormal globulins, or those who are pregnant may show minimally reactive levels. In addition, the FTA-ABS test doesn't always distinguish between *T. pallidum* and certain other treponemas, such as those that cause pinta, yaws, and bejel.

## INTERFERING FACTORS
- None significant

## Folic acid

The folic acid test is a quantitative analysis of serum folic acid levels (also called *pteroylglutamic acid, folacin,* or *folate*) by radioisotope assay of competitive binding. It's commonly performed concomitantly with measurement of serum vitamin $B_{12}$ levels. Like vitamin $B_{12}$, folic acid is a water soluble vitamin that influences hematopoiesis, deoxyribonucleic acid synthesis, and overall body growth.

Normally, diet supplies folic acid in organ meats, such as liver or kidneys, yeast, fruits, leafy vegetables, fortified breads and cereals, eggs, and milk. Inadequate dietary intake may cause a deficiency, especially during pregnancy. Because of folic acid's vital role in

hematopoiesis, the usual indication for this test is a suspected hematologic abnormality.

## PURPOSE
- To aid in the differential diagnosis of megaloblastic anemia, which may result from folic acid or vitamin $B_{12}$ deficiency
- To assess folate stores in pregnancy

## PATIENT PREPARATION
- Explain to the patient that the folic acid test determines the folic acid level in the blood.
- Instruct the patient to fast overnight before the test.
- Tell the patient that the test requires a blood sample. Explain who will perform the venipuncture and when.
- Explain to the patient that he may experience slight discomfort from the tourniquet and needle puncture.
- Notify the laboratory and physician of medications the patient is taking that may affect test results; they may need to be restricted.

## PROCEDURE AND POSTTEST CARE
- Perform a venipuncture and collect the sample in a 4.5ml tube without additives.
- Apply direct pressure to the venipuncture site until bleeding stops.
- If a hematoma develops at the venipuncture site, apply pressure.
- Instruct the patient that he may resume his usual diet and medications, as ordered.

## PRECAUTIONS
- Handle the sample gently to prevent hemolysis.
- Protect the sample from light.
- Send the sample to the laboratory immediately.

## REFERENCE VALUES
Normally, serum folic acid values are 1.8 to 9 ng/ml (SI, 4 to 20 nmol/L).

## ABNORMAL FINDINGS
Low serum levels may indicate hematologic abnormalities, such as anemia (especially megaloblastic anemia), leukopenia, and thrombocytopenia. The Schilling test is usually performed to rule out vitamin $B_{12}$ deficiency, which also causes megaloblastic ane-

...mia. Decreased folic acid levels can also result from hypermetabolic states (such as hyperthyroidism), inadequate dietary intake, small bowel malabsorption syndrome, hepatic or renal diseases, chronic alcoholism, or pregnancy.

Serum levels greater than normal may indicate excessive dietary intake of folic acid or folic acid supplements. Even when taken in large doses, this vitamin is nontoxic.

## INTERFERING FACTORS
● Alcohol, anticonvulsants such as primidone (Mysoline), antimalarials; antineoplastics, hormonal contraceptives, and phenytoin (Dilantin) (possible decrease)

## Follicle-stimulating hormone, serum

The follicle stimulating hormone (FSH) test of gonadal function, performed more commonly on females than on males, measures FSH levels and is vital in infertility studies. Its overall diagnostic significance typically depends on the results of related hormone tests (for luteinizing hormone, estrogen, or progesterone, for example).

A glycoprotein secreted by the anterior pituitary gland, FSH stimulates gonadal activity in both sexes. In females, it spurs development of primary ovarian follicles into graafian follicles for ovulation. Secretion varies diurnally and fluctuates during the menstrual cycle, peaking at ovulation. In males, continuous secretion of FSH (and testosterone) stimulates and maintains spermatogenesis. Plasma levels fluctuate widely in females; to obtain a true baseline level, daily testing may be necessary (for 3 to 5 days), or multiple samples may be drawn on the same day.

## PURPOSE
● To aid in the diagnosis and treatment of infertility and disorders of menstruation such as amenorrhea
● To aid in the diagnosis of precocious puberty in girls (before age 9) and in boys (before age 10)
● To aid in the differential diagnosis of hypogonadism

## PATIENT PREPARATION
● Explain to the patient, or her parents if she's a minor, that the serum FSH test helps determine if her hormonal secretion is normal.
● Tell the patient that the test requires a blood sample. Explain who will perform the venipuncture and when.
● Explain to the patient that she may experience slight discomfort from the tourniquet and needle puncture.
● Inform the patient that she need not restrict food and fluids.
● Withhold medications that may interfere with accurate determination of test results for 48 hours before the test, as ordered. If they must be continued (for example, for infertility treatment), note this on the laboratory request.
● Make sure the patient is relaxed and recumbent for 30 minutes before the test.

## PROCEDURE AND POSTTEST CARE
● Perform a venipuncture, preferably between 6 a.m. and 8 a.m., and collect the sample in a 7 ml clot-activator tube. Send the sample to the laboratory immediately.
● Apply direct pressure to the venipuncture site until bleeding stops.
● If a hematoma develops at the venipuncture site, apply pressure.
● Instruct the patient that she may resume medications discontinued before the test, as ordered.

## PRECAUTIONS
● Handle the sample gently to prevent hemolysis.
*Age alert* If the patient is female, indicate the phase of her menstrual cycle on the laboratory request. If she's menopausal, note this on the laboratory request.

## REFERENCE VALUES
Reference values vary greatly, depending on the patient's age, stage of sexual development, and — for a female — phase of her menstrual cycle. For the menstruating female, approximate FSH values are as follows:
● follicular phase — 5 to 20 mIU/ml (SI, 5 to 20 IU/L)
● ovulatory phase — 15 to 30 mIU/ml (SI, 15 to 30 IU/L)

- luteal phase — 5 to 15 mIU/ml (SI, 5 to 15 IU/L).

Approximate FSH values for men range from 5 to 20 mIU/ml (SI, 5 to 20 IU/L); for menopausal women, 50 to 100 mIU/ml (SI, 50 to 100 IU/L).

## ABNORMAL FINDINGS

Decreased FSH levels may cause male or female infertility: aspermatogenesis in men and anovulation in women. Low FSH levels may indicate secondary hypogonadotropic states, which can result from anorexia nervosa, panhypopituitarism, or hypothalamic lesions.

High FSH levels in women may indicate ovarian failure associated with Turner's syndrome (primary hypogonadism) or Stein Leventhal syndrome (polycystic ovary syndrome). Elevated levels may occur in patients with precocious puberty (idiopathic or with central nervous system lesions) and in postmenopausal women. In men, abnormally high FSH levels may indicate destruction of the testes (from mumps orchitis or X-ray exposure), testicular failure, seminoma, or male climacteric. Congenital absence of the gonads and early stage acromegaly may cause FSH levels to rise in both sexes.

## INTERFERING FACTORS

- Ovarian steroid hormones, such as estrogen and progesterone, related compounds, and phenothiazines such as chlorpromazine (Thorazine) (possible decrease through negative feedback by inhibiting FSH flow from the hypothalamus and pituitary gland)
- Radioactive scan performed within 1 week before the test

# Free thyroxine and free triiodothyronine

The free thyroxine ($FT_4$) and free triiodothyronine ($FT_3$) tests, commonly done simultaneously, measure serum levels of $FT_4$ and $FT_3$, the minute portions of thyroxine ($T_4$) and triiodothyronine ($T_3$) not bound to thyroxine binding globulin (TBG) and other serum proteins. These unbound hormones are responsible for the thyroid's effects on cellular metabolism. Measurement of free

hormone levels is the best indicator of thyroid function.

Because of disagreement as to whether $FT_4$ or $FT_3$ is the better indicator, laboratories commonly measure both. The disadvantages of these tests include a cumbersome and difficult laboratory method, inaccessibility, and cost. This test may be useful in the 5% of patients in whom the standard $T_3$ or $T_4$ tests fail to produce diagnostic results.

## PURPOSE

- To measure the metabolically active form of the thyroid hormones
- To aid diagnosis of hyperthyroidism and hypothyroidism when TBG levels are abnormal

## PATIENT PREPARATION

- Explain to the patient that the $FT_4$ and $FT_3$ tests help to evaluate thyroid function.
- Tell the patient that the test requires a blood sample. Explain who will perform the venipuncture and when.
- Instruct the patient that he need not restrict food and fluids.
- Check the patient's medical history for use of any thyroid therapy. Notify the physician; therapy may need to be restricted.
- Explain to the patient that he may experience slight discomfort from the tourniquet and needle puncture.

## PROCEDURE AND POSTTEST CARE

- Perform a venipuncture and collect the sample in a 7ml clot-activator tube.
- Apply direct pressure to the venipuncture site until bleeding stops.
- If a hematoma develops at the venipuncture site, apply pressure.

## PRECAUTIONS

- Handle the sample gently to prevent hemolysis.

## REFERENCE VALUES

Normal range for $FT_4$ is 0.9 to 2.3 ng/dl (SI, 10 to 30 nmol/L); for $FT_3$, 0.2 to 0.6 ng/dl (SI, 0.003 to 0.009 nmol/L). Values vary, depending on the laboratory.

## ABNORMAL FINDINGS

Elevated $FT_4$ and $FT_3$ levels indicate hyperthyroidism, unless peripheral resistance to thyroid hormone is present. $T_3$ toxicosis, a distinct form of hyperthyroidism, yields high $FT_3$ levels with normal or low $FT_4$ values. Low $FT_4$ levels usually indicate hypothyroidism, except in patients receiving replacement therapy with $T_3$. Patients receiving thyroid therapy may have varying levels of $FT_4$ and $FT_3$, depending on the preparation used and the time of sample collection.

## INTERFERING FACTORS
● Thyroid therapy, depending on dosage (possible increase)

# Fungal serology

Most fungal organisms enter the body as spores inhaled into the lungs or infiltrated through wounds in the skin or mucosa. If the body's defenses can't destroy the organisms initially, the fungi multiply to form lesions; blood and lymph vessels may then spread the mycoses throughout the body. Most healthy people easily overcome initial mycotic infection, but elderly people and others with a deficient immune system are more susceptible to acute or chronic mycotic infection and to disorders secondary to such infection. Mycosis may be deep-seated or superficial. Deep-seated mycosis occurs primarily in the lungs; superficial mycosis, in the skin or mucosal linings.

Although cultures are usually performed to diagnose mycoses by identifying the causative organism, serologic tests occasionally provide the sole evidence for mycosis. Such serologic tests use immunodiffusion, complement fixation, precipitin, latex agglutination, or agglutination methods to demonstrate the presence of specific mycotic antibodies. (See *Serum test methods for fungal infections,* pages 204 and 205.)

## PURPOSE
● To rapidly detect the presence of antifungal antibodies, aiding in the diagnosis of mycoses
● To monitor the effectiveness of therapy for mycoses

## PATIENT PREPARATION
● Explain to the patient that the fungal serology test aids in the diagnosis of certain fungal infections. If appropriate, tell him that this test monitors his response to antimycotic therapy and that it may be necessary to repeat the test.
● Instruct him to restrict food and fluids for 12 to 24 hours before the test.
● Tell the patient that the test requires a blood sample. Explain who will perform the venipuncture and when.
● Explain to the patient that he may experience slight discomfort from the tourniquet and needle puncture.

## PROCEDURE AND POSTTEST CARE
● Perform a venipuncture and collect the sample in a 10-ml sterile clot-activator tube.
● Apply direct pressure to the venipuncture site until bleeding stops.
● If a hematoma develops at the venipuncture site, apply pressure.
● Instruct the patient to resume his usual diet, as ordered.

## PRECAUTIONS
● Send the sample to the laboratory immediately.
● If transport to the laboratory is delayed, store the sample at 39.2° F (4° C).

## NORMAL FINDINGS
Depending on the test method, a negative finding, or normal titer, usually indicates the absence of mycosis.

## ABNORMAL FINDINGS
The chart on pages 205 and 206 explains the significance of findings for specific organisms.

## INTERFERING FACTORS
● Cross-reaction of antibodies with other antigens, such as blastomycosis and histoplasmosis antigens (possible false-positive or high titers)
● Recent skin testing with fungal antigens (possible high titers)
● Mycosis-caused immunosuppression (low titers or false-negative)

# SERUM TEST METHODS FOR FUNGAL INFECTIONS

| DISEASE AND NORMAL VALUES | CLINICAL SIGNIFICANCE OF ABNORMAL RESULTS |
|---|---|
| **BLASTOMYCOSIS** | |
| Complement fixation: titers < 1:8 | Titers ranging from 1:8 to 1:16 suggest infection; titers > 1:32 denote active disease. A rising titer in serial samples taken every 3 to 4 weeks indicates disease progression; a falling titer indicates regression. This test has limited diagnostic value because of a high percentage of false-negatives. |
| Immunodiffusion: negative | A more sensitive test for blastomycosis; detects 80% of infected people. |
| **COCCIDIOIDOMYCOSIS** | |
| Complement fixation: titers < 1:2 | Most sensitive test for this fungus. Titers ranging from 1:2 to 1:4 suggest active infection; titers > 1:16 usually denote active disease. Test may remain active in mild infections. |
| Immunodiffusion: negative | Most useful for screening, followed by complement fixation test for confirmation. |
| Precipitin: titers < 1:16 | Good screening test; titers > 1:16 usually indicate infection. About 80% of infected people show positive titers by 2 weeks; most revert to negative by 6 months. Early primary disease is shown by positive precipitin and negative complement fixation test. A positive complement fixation and negative precipitin test indicate chronic disease. |
| **HISTOPLASMOSIS** | |
| Complement fixation (histoplasmin): titers < 1:8 | Titers ranging from 1:8 to 1:16 suggest infection; titers > 1:32 indicate active disease. Antibodies generally appear 10 to 21 days after initial infection. Test is positive in 10% to 15% of cases. |
| Complement fixation: titers < 1:18 | Titers ranging from 1:8 to 1:16 suggest infection; titers > 1:32 indicate active disease. More sensitive than histoplasmin complement fixation test; gives positive results in 75% to 80% of cases. (Histoplasmin and yeast antigens are positive in 10% of cases.) A rising titer in serial samples taken every 2 to 3 weeks indicates progressive infection; a decreasing titer indicates regression. |
| Immunodiffusion (histoplasmin): negative | Appearance of H and M bands indicates active infection. If the M band appears first and lasts longer than the H band, the infection may be regressing. The M band alone may indicate early infection, chronic disease, or a recent skin test. |
| **ASPERGILLOSIS** | |
| Complement fixation: titers < 1:8 | Titers > 1:8 suggest infection; 70% to 90% of patients with known pulmonary aspergillosis or aspergillus allergy present antibodies. This test can't detect invasive aspergillosis because patients with this disease don't have antibodies; biopsy is required. |

# Gallium scanning

Gallium scan is a total body scan used to assess certain neoplasms and inflammatory lesions that attract gallium. It's usually performed 24 to 48 hours after the I.V. injection of radioactive gallium (67Ga) citrate; occasionally, it's performed 72 hours after the injection or, in acute inflammatory disease, 4 to 6 hours after the injection.

Because gallium has an affinity for benign and malignant neoplasms and inflammatory lesions, exact diagnosis requires additional confirming tests, such as ultrasonography and computed tomography scanning. Also, be aware that many neoplasms and a few inflammatory lesions may fail to demonstrate abnormal gallium activity.

## PURPOSE

 To detect primary or metastatic neoplasms and inflammatory lesions when the site of the disease hasn't been clearly defined
 To evaluate malignant lymphoma and identify recurrent tumors following chemotherapy or radiation therapy
 To clarify focal defects in the liver when liver-spleen scanning and ultrasonography prove inconclusive
 To evaluate bronchogenic carcinoma

## PATIENT PREPARATION

 Explain to the patient that gallium scanning helps detect abnormal or inflammatory tissue.
 Tell the patient that he need not restrict food and fluids.

● Explain to the patient that the test requires a total body scan (usually performed 24 to 48 hours after the I.V. injection of 67Ga citrate).
● Tell the patient who will perform the test and where it will take place.
● Warn the patient that he may experience transient discomfort from the needle puncture during injection of the 67Ga citrate. Reassure him, however, that the dosage is only slightly radioactive and isn't harmful.
● If a gamma scintillation camera is to be used, assure the patient that although the uptake probe and detector head may touch his skin, he'll experience no discomfort.
● If a rectilinear scanner is to be used, mention to the patient that it makes a soft, irregular clicking noise as it registers the radiation emissions.
● Make sure that the patient or a responsible family member has signed an informed consent form.
● Administer a laxative, an enema, or both, as ordered.

## PROCEDURE AND POSTTEST CARE

● The patient may be positioned erect or recumbent or in an appropriate combination of these positions, depending on his physical condition.
● Scans or scintigrams of the patient are taken 24 to 48 hours after 67Ga citrate injection, from anterior and posterior views and, occasionally, lateral views.
● If the initial gallium scan suggests bowel disease and additional scans are necessary, give the patient a cleaning enema before continuing the test.

## SERUM TEST METHODS FOR FUNGAL INFECTI
### (continued)

| DISEASE AND NORMAL VALUES | CLINICAL SIGNIFICANCE OF ABNORMAL RESULTS |
|---|---|

**ASPERGILLOSIS (continued)**

| Immunodiffusion: negative | One or more precipitin bands suggests infection. The numbe related to complement fixation titers; the more precipitin ba er the titer. |
|---|---|

**SPOROTRICHOSIS**

| Agglutination: titers < 1:40 | Titers > 1:80 usually indicate active infection. The test usually in cutaneous infections and positive in extracutaneous infectio |
|---|---|

**CRYPTOCOCCOSIS**

| Latex agglutination for cryptococcal antigen: negative | About 90% of patients with cryptococcal meningitis exhibit p agglutination in cerebrospinal fluid. Culturing is definitive becau positives do occur. (Presence of rheumatoid factor may cause reaction.) Serum antigen tests are positive in 33% of patients pulmonary cryptococcosis; biopsy is usually required. |
|---|---|

## PRECAUTIONS

● Be aware that the gallium scanning test should precede barium studies because barium retention may hinder visualization of gallium activity in the bowel.

● Know that gallium scanning is usually contraindicated in a child and during pregnancy or lactation; however, it may be performed if the potential diagnostic benefit outweighs the risks of exposure to radiation.

## NORMAL FINDINGS

Gallium activity is normally demonstrated in the liver, spleen, bones, and large bowel. Activity in the bowel results from mucosal uptake of gallium and fecal excretion of gallium.

## ABNORMAL FINDINGS

Gallium scanning may reveal inflammatory lesions — discrete abscesses or diffuse infiltration. In pancreatic or perinephric abscess, gallium activity is relatively localized; in bacterial peritonitis, gallium activity is spread diffusely within the abdomen.

Abnormally high gallium accumulation is characteristic in inflammatory bowel diseases, such as ulcerative colitis and regional ileitis (Crohn's disease), and in carcinoma of the colon. However, because gallium normally accumulates in the colon, the detection of inflammatory and neoplastic diseases is sometimes difficult.

Abnormal gallium activity may be present in various sarcomas, Wilms' tumor, and neuroblastomas; carcinoma of the kidney, uterus, vagina, and stomach; and testicular tumors, such as seminoma, embryonal carcinoma, choriocarcinoma, and teratocarcinoma, which commonly metastasize via the lymphatic system. In Hodgkin's disease and malignant lymphoma, gallium scanning can demonstrate abnormal activity in one or more lymph nodes or in extranodal locations. However, gallium scanning supported by results of lymphangiography can gauge the extent of metastasis more accurately than either test alone because neither test consistently identifies all neoplastic nodes.

After chemotherapy or radiation therapy, gallium scanning may be used to detect new or recurrent tumors. However, these forms of therapy tend to diminish tumor affinity for gallium without necessarily eliminating the tumor.

In the differential diagnosis of focal hepatic defects, abnormal gallium activity may help narrow the diagnostic possibilities. Gallium localizes in hepatomas, but not in pseudotumors; in abscesses, but not in pleural effusions; and in tumors, but not in cysts or hematomas.

In examining patients with suspected bronchogenic carcinoma, abnormal activity confirms the presence of a tumor. However, because gallium also localizes in inflammatory pulmonary diseases, such as pneumonia and sarcoidosis, a chest X-ray should be performed to distinguish a tumor from an inflammatory lesion.

## INTERFERING FACTORS

● Hepatic and splenic intake (possible false-negative scans due to possible obscuring of abnormal para-aortic nodes in Hodgkin's disease)

● Fecal accumulation in the bowel (poor imaging of retroperitoneal space)

● Residual barium from other tests done 1 week before the scan (possible poor imaging)

# *Gamma glutamyl transferase*

Also called gamma glutamyl transpeptidase, gamma glutamyl transferase (GGT) participates in the transfer of amino acids across cellular membranes and, possibly, in glutathione metabolism. The highest concentrations of GGT exist in the renal tubules, but the enzyme also appears in the liver, biliary tract, epithelium, pancreas, lymphocytes, brain, and testes. The GGT test is used to measure serum GGT levels.

Because GGT isn't elevated in bone growth or pregnancy, this test is a somewhat more sensitive indicator of hepatic necrosis than the aspartate aminotransferase assay and is as sensitive as or more sensitive than the alkaline phosphatase (ALP) assay. However, the test is nonspecific, providing little data about the type of hepatic disease because increased levels also occur in renal, cardiac, and prostatic disease and with the use of certain medications. GGT is particularly sensitive to the effects of alcohol on the liver, and levels may be elevated after moderate alcohol intake and in chronic alcoholism, even without clinical evidence of hepatic injury.

## PURPOSE

● To provide information about hepatobiliary diseases, to assess liver function, and to detect alcohol ingestion
● To distinguish between skeletal and hepatic disease when the serum ALP level is elevated (A normal GGT level suggests that such elevation stems from skeletal disease.)

## PATIENT PREPARATION

● Explain to the patient that the GGT test is used to evaluate liver function.
● Tell the patient that the test requires a blood sample. Explain who will perform the venipuncture and when.
● Explain to the patient that he may experience slight discomfort from the tourniquet and needle puncture.
● Inform the patient that he need not restrict food, fluids, or medications.

## PROCEDURE AND POSTTEST CARE

● Perform a venipuncture and collect the sample in a 4-ml tube without additives.
● Apply direct pressure to the venipuncture site until bleeding stops.
● If a hematoma develops at the venipuncture site, apply pressure.

## PRECAUTIONS

● Handle the sample gently to prevent hemolysis.
● GGT activity is stable in serum at room temperature for 2 days.

## REFERENCE VALUES

Normal serum GGT levels range as follows:
● males — age 16 and older, 6 to 38 U/L (SI, 0.10 to 0.63 μkat/L)
● females — ages 16 to 45, 4 to 27 U/L (SI, 0.08 to 0.46 μKat/L).

   *Age alert*   *Normal serum GGT levels range as follows:*
● *females — age 45 and older, 6 to 37 U/L (SI, 0.10 to 0.63 μkat/L)*
● *children — younger than age 16, 3 to 30 U/L (SI, 0.05 to 0.51 μkat/L).*

## ABNORMAL FINDINGS

Serum GGT levels rise in acute hepatic disease because enzyme production increases in response to hepatocellular injury. Moderate increases occur in acute pancreatitis, renal disease, and prostatic metastasis; postoperatively; and in some patients with epilepsy or brain tumors. Levels also increase after alcohol ingestion because of enzyme induction. The sharpest elevations occur in patients with obstructive jaundice and hepatic metastatic infiltrations.

GGT levels may also increase 5 to 10 days after acute myocardial infarction, either as a result of tissue granulation and healing or as an indication of the effects of cardiac insufficiency on the liver.

## INTERFERING FACTORS

● Hormonal contraceptives (decrease)
● Aminoglycosides, barbiturates, glutethimide, and phenytoin (Dilantin) (increase)
● Moderate alcohol intake (increase for at least 60 hours)

# Gastric acid stimulation test

The gastric acid stimulation test measures the secretion of gastric acid for 1 hour after subcutaneous injection of pentagastrin or a similar drug that stimulates gastric acid output. This test is indicated when the basal secretion test suggests abnormal gastric secretion and is commonly performed immediately afterward. Although this test detects abnormal gastric secretion, radiographic studies and endoscopy are necessary to determine the cause.

## PURPOSE

● To aid in the diagnosis of a duodenal ulcer, Zollinger-Ellison syndrome, pernicious anemia, and gastric carcinoma

## PATIENT PREPARATION

● Explain to the patient that the gastric acid stimulation test determines if the stomach is secreting acid properly.
● Instruct the patient to refrain from eating, drinking, and smoking after midnight before the test.
● Tell the patient who will perform the test, where it will take place, and that it takes 1 hour.

- Explain that the test requires passing a tube through the nose and into the stomach and a subcutaneous injection of pentagastrin.
- Describe the possible adverse effects of the test, such as abdominal pain, nausea, vomiting, flushing, and transitory dizziness, faintness, and numbness in the extremities. Instruct the patient to report such symptoms immediately.
- Check the patient's history for hypersensitivity to pentagastrin.
- Notify the laboratory and the physician of medications the patient is taking that may affect test results; they may need to be restricted. If these drugs must be continued, however, note this on the laboratory request.
- Record the patient's baseline vital signs before beginning the procedure.

## PROCEDURE AND POSTTEST CARE
- After basal gastric secretions have been collected, the nasogastric (NG) tube remains in place.
- Pentagastrin is injected S.C.; after 15 minutes, collect a specimen every 15 minutes for 1 hour.
- Record the color and odor of each specimen, and note the presence of food, mucus, bile, or blood.
- Label the specimens stimulated contents, and number them 1 through 4.
- If the NG tube is kept in place, it should be clamped or attached to low intermittent suction, as ordered.
- Watch the patient for nausea, vomiting, and abdominal distention and pain after the NG tube is removed.
- If the patient complains of a sore throat, provide soothing lozenges.
- Instruct the patient that he may resume his usual diet and medications, as ordered.

## PRECAUTIONS
- Know that the gastric acid stimulation test is contraindicated in the patient with hypersensitivity to pentagastrin or with conditions that prohibit NG intubation.
- Observe the patient for adverse effects of pentagastrin.
- To prevent contamination of the specimens with saliva, instruct the patient to expectorate excess saliva.
- Send the specimens to the laboratory immediately after the collection is completed.

## REFERENCE VALUES
Following stimulation, gastric acid secretion ranges from 18 to 28 mEq/hour for males and from 11 to 21 mEq/hour for females.

## ABNORMAL FINDINGS
Elevated gastric secretion may indicate a duodenal ulcer; markedly elevated secretion suggests Zollinger-Ellison syndrome. Depressed secretion may indicate gastric carcinoma; achlorhydria may indicate pernicious anemia.

## INTERFERING FACTORS
- Adrenergic blockers and cholinergics (increase)
- Antacids, anticholinergics, histamine-2 blockers, and proton pump inhibitors (decrease)

# Gastrin

Gastrin is a polypeptide hormone produced and stored primarily in the antrum of the stomach and to a lesser degree in the islets of Langerhans. Its main function is to facilitate food digestion by triggering gastric acid secretion. It also stimulates the release of pancreatic enzymes and the gastric enzyme pepsin, increases gastric and intestinal motility, and stimulates bile flow from the liver. Abnormal secretion of gastrin can result from tumors (gastrinomas) and pathologic disorders that affect the stomach, pancreas and, less commonly, the esophagus and small bowel.

This radioimmunoassay, a quantitative analysis of gastrin levels, is especially useful in patients suspected of having gastrinomas (Zollinger-Ellison syndrome). In doubtful situations, provocative testing may be necessary.

## PURPOSE
- To confirm a diagnosis of gastrinoma, the gastrin-secreting tumor in Zollinger-Ellison syndrome
- To aid differential diagnosis of gastric and duodenal ulcers and pernicious anemia (Gastrin estimation has limited value in the patient with a duodenal ulcer.)

## PATIENT PREPARATION

- Explain to the patient that the gastrin test helps determine the cause of GI symptoms.
- Instruct the patient to abstain from alcohol for at least 24 hours before the test and to fast and avoid caffeinated drinks for 12 hours before the test, although he may drink water.
- Tell the patient that the test requires a blood sample. Explain who will perform the venipuncture and when.
- Explain to the patient that he may experience slight discomfort from the tourniquet and needle puncture.
- Withhold all drugs that may interfere with test results, especially insulin and anticholinergics, such as atropine and belladonna, as ordered. If they must be continued, note this on the laboratory request.
- Tell the patient to lie down and relax for at least 30 minutes before the test.

## PROCEDURE AND POSTTEST CARE

- Perform a venipuncture and collect the sample in a 10 to 15ml clot-activator tube.
- Apply direct pressure to the venipuncture site until bleeding stops.
- If a hematoma develops at the venipuncture site, apply pressure.
- Instruct the patient that he may resume his usual diet and medications discontinued before the test, as ordered.

## PRECAUTIONS

- Handle the sample gently to prevent hemolysis.
- To prevent destruction of serum gastrin by proteolytic enzymes, immediately send the sample to the laboratory to have the serum separated and frozen.

## REFERENCE VALUES

Normal serum gastrin levels are 50 to 150 pg/ml (SI, 50 to 150 ng/L).

## ABNORMAL FINDINGS

Strikingly high serum gastrin levels (> 1,000 pg/ml [SI, > 1,000 ng/L]) confirm Zollinger-Ellison syndrome. (Levels as high as 450,000 pg/ml [SI, 450,000 ng/L] have been reported.)

Increased serum levels of gastrin may occur in a few patients with duodenal ulceration (< 1%) and in patients with achlorhydria (with or without pernicious anemia) or extensive stomach carcinoma (because of hyposecretion of gastric juices and hydrochloric acid).

## INTERFERING FACTORS

- Acetylcholine, alcohol, amino acids (especially glycine), calcium carbonate, and calcium chloride (increase)
- Anticholinergics, such as atropine, as well as hydrochloric acid and secretin, a strongly basic polypeptide (decrease)
- Insulin-induced hypoglycemia (increase)

# Gastroesophageal reflux scanning

When the results of a barium swallow X-ray are inconclusive, gastroesophageal reflux scanning may be done to test esophageal function and identify evidence of reflux. This test delivers less radiation than a barium swallow and is a much more sensitive indicator of reflux. It also allows reflux to be measured without insertion of an esophageal tube.

## PURPOSE

- To identify reflux
- To evaluate for esophageal disorders such as regurgitation
- To aid in identifying the cause of persistent nausea and vomiting

*Age alert* *To aid in differentiating reflux from vomiting in infants*

## PATIENT PREPARATION

- Explain the purpose of the gastroesophageal reflux scanning test in evaluating the patient's complaints of reflux and identifying possible causes of his complaints.
- Tell the patient that the test will be performed in the nuclear medicine department and that the test is painless and safe.
- Inform the patient that a binder with a balloonlike compression device will be applied to his abdomen. The binder will fit snugly and the balloon may be inflated to apply pressure.
- Tell the patient that he'll be required to drink a solution such as orange juice or eat a small portion of scrambled eggs that contains a radioisotope. Check for any patient allergies to eggs.

**Age alert** *Inform the parents of an infant that the radioisotope will be given with milk.*

- Tell the patient that after ingesting the solution or eggs, a machine will be passed over his chest to monitor the radioisotope's passage.
- Tell the patient to fast beginning at midnight on the day before the test.
- Explain that images will usually be obtained in approximately 2 hours.
- Inform the patient that he can resume his usual diet after the procedure, as ordered.

## PROCEDURE AND POSTTEST CARE

- The patient is placed in a supine or upright position and a binder is applied to the abdomen. The patient is then asked to swallow the solution containing a radiopharmaceutical such as technetium 99m ($^{99m}$Tc) sulfur colloid. The radiopharmaceutical may be mixed with orange juice or with scrambled eggs.

**Age alert** *For an infant, the radiopharmaceutical is mixed with milk. A portion of the milk solution is given and then the infant is burped. Then the remainder of the milk is given, followed by some radiopharmaceutical-free milk to clear the esophagus.*

- The radiopharmaceutical also may be administered via a nasogastric (NG) tube.

**Alert** *Be sure to remove the NG tube before images are taken to prevent false-positive results.*

- The binder may be inflated to exert abdominal pressure at specific intervals while a gamma counter is passed over the patient's chest to record the passage of the radiopharmaceutical through the esophagus and into the stomach to determine transit time and evaluate esophageal function.
- The patient may be repositioned as his stomach distends with continuous recordings to visualize events.
- A computer analysis is done to calculate the percentage of reflux (using a mathematical formula).

## PRECAUTIONS

- Endoscopic tube insertion is used with patients who have esophageal motor dysfunction, hiatal hernia, or difficulty swallowing.

- The patient needs to be able to tolerate abdominal compression. The binder must be applied below the ribs to avoid fractures.
- Gastroesophageal reflux scanning is contraindicated during pregnancy and lactation.

## NORMAL FINDINGS

Normally, $^{99m}$Tc sulfur colloid descends through the esophagus in about 6 seconds. Radioactivity is then detected only in the stomach and small bowel.

Typically, less than 4% gastric reflux is considered normal.

## ABNORMAL FINDINGS

Diffuse spasm of the esophagus, achalasia, or other esophageal motility disorder may prolong transit time. With gastroesophageal reflux, the radioactivity may be detected in the esophagus.

## INTERFERING FACTORS

- Previous X-rays of the upper GI tract
- Presence of an NG tube (false-positive result)

# Given Diagnostic Imaging System (camera pill)

The Given Diagnostic Imaging System (also called the *camera pill*) is a tiny video camera with a light source and transmitter inside a capsule, allowing recording of images along its path. The "capsule endoscope" measures 11 × 30 mm and is propelled along the digestive tract by peristalsis. The clear end records images of the stomach walls and, particularly, the small intestine, where many other diagnostic techniques may not reach or otherwise visualize. (See *Detecting disorders in the stomach and small intestine,* page 212.) The images are transmitted to a data recorder on a belt placed around the patient's waist. After swallowing the pill, the patient doesn't need to stay at the hospital and can return to work or other activities of daily living.

## PURPOSE

- To detect polyps or cancer
- To detect causes of bleeding and anemia

# Detecting disorders in the stomach and small intestine

In the Given Diagnostic Imaging System, the patient swallows the capsule, which then travels through the body by the natural movement of the digestive tract. A receiver worn outside the body records the images. The strength of the signal indicates the capsule's location.

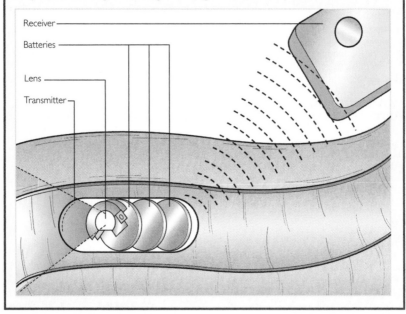

## PATIENT PREPARATION

- Explain to the patient that this test helps visualize the stomach and small intestine, helping to detect disorders.
- Tell the patient who will perform the test and where it will take place.
- Inform the patient that he may need to fast for 12 hours before the test but may have fluids for up to 2 hours before the test, unless ordered otherwise. (Usually no preparation is involved, but some patients may benefit from it.)
- Explain to the patient that he'll need to swallow the camera pill and that it will send information to a receiver he'll wear on his belt.
- Tell the patient that the procedure is painless and after swallowing the pill he can go home or go to work.
- Explain to the patient that walking helps facilitate movement of the pill.
- Tell the patient that he'll need to return to the facility in 24 hours (or as directed) so the recorder can be removed from his belt.
- Tell the patient that the pill will be excreted in his stool in 8 to 72 hours.

## PROCEDURE AND POSTTEST CARE

- The patient ingests the camera pill, as ordered, and a receiver is attached to his belt.
- The pill records images for up to 6 hours along its path of the stomach, small intestine, and mouth of the large intestine, transmitting the information to the receiver.
- The patient returns to the facility, as ordered, so the images can be transmitted into the computer, where they're displayed on the screen.
- Tell the patient that he may resume his usual diet after the images are obtained, as ordered.
- The pill is excreted normally in stool.

## PRECAUTIONS

**Alert** The procedure is contraindicated in the patient with a suspected obstruction, fistula, or stricture and in the patient who can't swallow (an infant, a young child, or someone with a swallowing impairment).

● Know that the battery is short-lived, so images of the large intestine are unobtainable.

● Be aware that the pill can't be used to stop bleeding, take tissue samples, remove growths, or repair any problems detected. Other invasive studies may be needed.

## NORMAL FINDINGS

The camera illustrates normal anatomy of the stomach and small intestine.

## ABNORMAL FINDINGS

The camera may detect bleeding sites or abnormalities of the stomach and small bowel, such as erosions, Crohn's disease, celiac disease, benign and malignant tumors of the small intestine, vascular disorders, medication-related small-bowel injuries, and pediatric small-bowel disorders.

## INTERFERING FACTORS

● Narrowing or obstruction of the intestine, causing the pill to become lodged

## Glucagon, plasma

Glucagon, a polypeptide hormone secreted by the alpha cells of the islets of Langerhans in the pancreas, acts primarily on the liver to promote glucose production and control glucose storage. Glucagon is secreted in response to hypoglycemia; secretion is inhibited by the other pancreatic hormones, insulin and somatostatin. Normally, the coordinating release of glucagon, insulin, and somatostatin ensures an adequate and constant fuel supply while maintaining blood glucose levels within relatively stable limits.

This test, a quantitative analysis of plasma glucagon by radioimmunoassay, evaluates patients suspected of having glucagonoma (alpha cell tumor) or hypoglycemia due to idiopathic glucagon deficiency or pancreatic dysfunction. Glucagon is usually measured concomitantly with serum glucose and insulin because glucose and insulin levels influence glucagon secretion.

## PURPOSE

● To aid diagnosis of glucagonoma and hypoglycemia due to chronic pancreatitis or idiopathic glucagon deficiency

## PATIENT PREPARATION

● Explain to the patient that the plasma glucagon test helps to evaluate pancreatic function.

● Instruct the patient to fast for 10 to 12 hours before the test.

● Tell the patient that the test requires a blood sample. Explain who will perform the venipuncture and when.

● Explain to the patient that he may experience slight discomfort from the tourniquet and needle puncture.

● Withhold insulin, catecholamines, and other drugs that could influence the test results, as ordered. If they must be continued, note this on the laboratory request.

● Have the patient lie down and relax for 30 minutes before the test.

## PROCEDURE AND POSTTEST CARE

● Perform a venipuncture and collect the sample in a chilled 10-ml EDTA tube.

● Apply direct pressure to the venipuncture site until bleeding stops.

● If a hematoma develops at the venipuncture site, apply pressure.

● Instruct the patient that he may resume his usual diet and medications discontinued before the test, as ordered.

## PRECAUTIONS

● Handle the sample gently to prevent hemolysis.

● Place the sample on ice and send it to the laboratory immediately.

## REFERENCE VALUES

Fasting glucagon levels are normally less than 60 pg/ml (SI, < 60 ng/L).

## ABNORMAL FINDINGS

Elevated fasting glucagon levels (900 to 7,800 pg/ml [SI, 900 to 7,800 ng/L]) can occur in glucagonoma, diabetes mellitus, acute pancreatitis, and pheochromocytoma.

Abnormally low glucagon levels are associated with idiopathic glucagon deficiency and hypoglycemia due to chronic pancreatitis.

## INTERFERING FACTORS
- Exercise, stress, prolonged fasting, insulin, or catecholamines (increase)
- Radioactive scans and tests performed within 48 hours of the test

# Gonorrhea culture

Gonorrhea almost always results from sexual transmission of *Neisseria gonorrhoeae*. A stained smear of genital exudate can confirm gonorrhea in 90% of males with characteristic symptoms, but a culture is usually necessary, especially in asymptomatic females. Possible culture sites include the urethra (usual site in males), endocervix (usual site in females), anal canal, and oropharynx.

## PURPOSE
- To confirm gonorrhea

## PATIENT PREPARATION
- Describe the procedure to the patient. Explain that this test is used to confirm gonorrhea.
- Inform the patient who will perform the test and when.
- Instruct the female patient not to douche for 24 hours before the test.
- Tell the male patient not to void during the hour preceding the test. Warn him that males sometimes experience nausea, sweating, weakness, and fainting due to stress or discomfort when the cotton swab or wire loop is introduced into the urethra.

## PROCEDURE AND POSTTEST CARE
### Endocervical culture
- Place the patient in the lithotomy position, drape her appropriately, and instruct her to take deep breaths.
- Using gloved hands, insert a vaginal speculum that has been lubricated only with warm water. Clean mucus from the cervix, using cotton balls in ring forceps.
- Insert a dry, sterile cotton swab into the endocervical canal and rotate it from side to side. Leave the swab in place for several seconds for optimum absorption of organisms.

- In cases of deep pelvic inflammatory disease, cultures of the endometrium or aspirations by laparoscopy or culdoscopy may be necessary. Endometrial specimens are obtained by inserting stents through a narrow-bore catheter introduced into the cervical canal.

### Urethral culture
- Place the patient in a supine position, and drape him appropriately.
- Clean the urethral meatus with sterile gauze or a cotton swab, and then insert a thin urogenital alginate swab or a wire bacteriologic loop $3/8''$ to $3/4''$ (1 to 2 cm) into the urethra, and rotate the swab or loop from side to side. Leave it in place for several seconds for optimum absorption of organisms. If permitted, the patient may milk the urethra, bringing urethral secretions to the meatus for collection on a cotton swab.

### Rectal culture
- After obtaining an endocervical or a urethral specimen (while the patient is still on the examination table), insert a sterile cotton swab into the anal canal about 1" (2.5 cm), move the swab from side to side, and leave it in place for several seconds for optimum absorption.
- If the swab is contaminated with stools, discard it and repeat the procedure with a clean swab.

### Throat culture
- Position the patient with his head tilted back.
- Check his throat for inflamed areas using a tongue blade. Rub a sterile swab from side to side over the tonsillar areas, including inflamed or purulent sites. Be careful not to touch the teeth, cheeks, or tongue with the swab.

### After specimen collection
- Roll the swab in a Z pattern in a plate containing MTM medium. Then cross streak the medium with a sterile wire loop or the tip of the swab and cover the plate. (See *Culturing for* Neisseria gonorrhoeae.)
- Label the specimen with the patient's name and room number (if applicable), the physician's name, and the date and time of collection.
- Direct smears of obtained material should be made immediately to prepare the

# CULTURING FOR *NEISSERIA GONORRHOEAE*

Culturing for *Neisseria gonorrhoeae* requires use of a modified Thayer-Martin (MTM) medium. If a laboratory isn't readily available, you may use Transgrow medium.

## MODIFIED THAYER-MARTIN MEDIUM

MTM medium is a combination of hemoglobin, gonococcal growth-enhancing chemicals, and antimicrobial agents for culturing endocervical, urethral, and rectal specimens. To inoculate a culture plate treated with MTM medium and to spread organisms out of their associated mucus, take these steps:

◆ Roll the swab in a Z pattern (as shown),
◆ Using the swab or a sterile wire loop, immediately crossstreak the plate (as shown).

Incubate within 15 minutes of streaking.

## TRANSGROW MEDIUM

A modification of MTM medium, Transgrow is available in a screw-cap bottle containing air and carbon dioxide. Transgrow bottles are used to transport suspect cultures when laboratory facilities aren't available at the site of specimen collection. Use this procedure:

◆ To prevent loss of carbon dioxide, inoculate the specimen bottle while it's upright.
◆ After uncapping the bottle, immediately insert the swab and soak up all excess moisture.
◆ Starting at the bottom of the bottle, roll the swab from side to side across the medium (as shown).
◆ Recap the bottle, and send it to the laboratory immediately. Subculturing should begin within 24 to 48 hours.

**Two-step method of streaking Thayer-Martin medium**

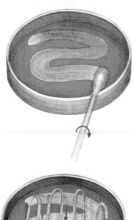

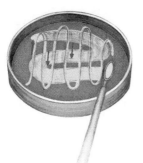

**One-step method of streaking Transgrow medium**

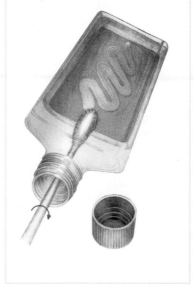

Gram stain. Remaining material must be quickly inoculated into selective culture media or into a transport system. A culturette transport tube or a swab transport medium containing charcoal can be used. Charcoal helps neutralize toxic materials in the specimen.

● If laboratory facilities aren't readily available, do the following: Uncap the Transgrow medium specimen bottle just before inserting the swab of test material into the bottle. Keep the bottle upright to minimize loss of carbon dioxide. With the swab, absorb the excess moisture within the bottle, and then roll the swab across the Transgrow medium. Discard the swab. Place the lid on the bottle, and label it appropriately.

● Advise the patient to avoid all sexual contact until test results are available.

● Explain that treatment usually begins after confirming a positive culture, except in a person who has symptoms of gonorrhea or who has had intercourse with someone known to have gonorrhea.

● Advise the patient that a repeat culture is required 1 week after completion of treatment to evaluate the effectiveness of therapy.

● Inform the patient that positive culture findings must be reported to the local health department.

## PRECAUTIONS

● Wear gloves when performing the procedures and handling the specimens.

  **Alert** *Place the male patient in the supine position to prevent him from falling if vasovagal syncope occurs when the cotton swab or wire loop is introduced into the urethra. Observe for profound hypotension, bradycardia, pallor, and sweating.*

● Collect a urethral specimen at least 1 hour after the patient has voided to prevent loss of urethral secretions.

● After collecting the specimens, carefully dispose of gloves, swabs, and speculum to prevent staff exposure.

● Send the specimens to the laboratory immediately, or arrange for transport of the Transgrow bottle because the specimen must be subcultured within 24 to 48 hours.

## NORMAL FINDINGS

Normally, no *N. gonorrhoeae* appears in the culture.

## ABNORMAL FINDINGS

A positive culture confirms gonorrhea.

## INTERFERING FACTORS

● Pretest antimicrobial therapy
● Contamination due to fecal material in a rectal culture
● Failure to use the proper collection technique (may provide a nonrepresentative or contaminated specimen)
● In males, voiding within 1 hour of specimen collection; in females, douching within 24 hours of specimen collection (fewer organisms available for culture)

# *Growth hormone suppression test*

Also called *glucose loading,* the growth hormone suppression test evaluates excessive baseline levels of human growth hormone (hGH) from the anterior pituitary gland. Normally, hGH raises plasma glucose and fatty acid concentrations; in response, insulin secretion increases to counteract these effects. Consequently, a glucose load should suppress hGH secretions. In a patient with excessive hGH levels, failure of suppression indicates anterior pituitary dysfunction and confirms a diagnosis of acromegaly or gigantism.

## PURPOSE

● To assess elevated baseline levels of hGH
● To confirm diagnosis of gigantism in children and acromegaly in adults and adolescents

## PATIENT PREPARATION

● Explain to the patient, or his parents if the patient is a child, that this test helps determine the cause of his abnormal growth.

● Instruct the patient to fast and limit physical activity for 10 to 12 hours before the test.

● Tell him that two blood samples will be drawn. Warn him that he may experience nausea after drinking the glucose solution and some discomfort from the tourniquet and needle punctures.

● Withhold all steroids and other pituitary-based hormones. If they or other medications must be continued, note this on the laboratory request.

● Tell the patient to lie down and relax for 30 minutes before the test.

## PROCEDURE AND POSTTEST CARE

● Perform a venipuncture and collect 6 ml of blood (basal sample) in a 7-ml clot-activator tube between 6 a.m. and 8 a.m.

● Administer 100 g of glucose solution by mouth. To prevent nausea, advise the patient to drink the glucose slowly.

● About 1 hour later, draw venous blood into a 7-ml clot-activator tube. Label the tubes appropriately, and send them to the laboratory immediately.

● Apply direct pressure to the venipuncture site until bleeding stops.

● If a hematoma develops at the venipuncture site, apply pressure.

● Instruct the patient that he may resume his usual diet, activities, and medications discontinued before the test, as ordered.

## PRECAUTIONS

● Handle the samples gently to prevent hemolysis.

● Send each sample to the laboratory immediately because hGH has a half life of only 20 to 25 minutes.

## REFERENCE VALUES

Normally, glucose suppresses hGH to levels ranging from undetectable to 3 ng/ml (SI, 3 µg/L) in 30 minutes to 2 hours.

**Age alert**  *In children, rebound stimulation may occur after 2 to 5 hours.*

## ABNORMAL FINDINGS

In a patient with active acromegaly, elevated baseline hGH levels (5 ng/ml [SI, 5 µg/L]) aren't suppressed to be less than 5 ng/ml during the test. Unchanged or rising hGH levels in response to glucose loading indicate hGH hypersecretion and may confirm suspected acromegaly and gigantism. This response may be verified by repeating the test after a 1-day rest.

## INTERFERING FACTORS

● Corticosteroids and phenothiazines such as chlorpromazine (Thorazine) (possible decrease in hGH secretion)

● Amphetamines, arginine, estrogens, glucagon, levodopa, and niacin (possible increase in hGH secretion)

● Radioactive scan performed within 1 week before the test

# Haptoglobin

The haptoglobin test is used to measure serum levels of haptoglobin, a glycoprotein produced in the liver. In acute intravascular hemolysis, the haptoglobin concentration decreases rapidly and may remain low for 5 to 7 days, until the liver synthesizes more glycoprotein.

## PURPOSE
● To serve as an index of hemolysis
● To distinguish between hemoglobin and myoglobin in plasma because haptoglobin doesn't bind with myoglobin
● To investigate hemolytic transfusion reactions
● To establish proof of paternity using genetic (phenotypic) variations in haptoglobin structure

## PATIENT PREPARATION
● Explain to the patient that the haptoglobin test is used to determine the condition of red blood cells.
● Tell the patient that the test requires a blood sample. Explain who will perform the venipuncture and when.
● Explain to the patient that he may experience slight discomfort from the tourniquet and needle puncture.
● Inform the patient that he need not restrict food and fluids.
● Notify the laboratory and physician of medications the patient is taking that may affect test results; they may need to be restricted.

## PROCEDURE AND POSTTEST CARE
● Perform a venipuncture and collect the sample in a 7ml clot-activator tube.
● Apply direct pressure to the venipuncture site until bleeding stops.
● If a hematoma develops at the venipuncture site, apply pressure.
● Inform the patient that he may resume his usual medications discontinued before the test, as ordered.

## PRECAUTIONS
● Handle the sample gently to prevent hemolysis.

## REFERENCE VALUES
Normally, serum haptoglobin concentrations, measured in terms of the protein's hemoglobin binding capacity, range from 40 to 180 mg/dl (SI, 0.4 to 1.8 g/L). Nephelometric procedures yield lower results.

**Age alert** *Haptoglobin is absent in 90% of neonates, but in most cases, levels gradually increase to normal by age 4 months.*

## ABNORMAL FINDINGS
Markedly decreased serum haptoglobin levels are characteristic in acute and chronic hemolysis, severe hepatocellular disease, infectious mononucleosis, and transfusion reactions. Hepatocellular disease inhibits haptoglobin synthesis. In hemolytic transfusion reactions, haptoglobin levels begin decreasing after 6 to 8 hours and drop to 40% of pretransfusion levels after 24 hours.

If serum haptoglobin values are very low, watch for symptoms of hemolysis: chills, fever, back pain, flushing, distended jugular veins, tachycardia, tachypnea, and hypotension.

In about 1% of the population, including 4% of blacks, haptoglobin is permanently absent; this disorder is known as congenital ahaptoglobinemia.

Strikingly elevated serum haptoglobin levels occur in diseases marked by chronic inflammatory reactions or tissue destruction, such as rheumatoid arthritis and malignant neoplasms.

### INTERFERING FACTORS
● Androgens and corticosteroids (possible increase; may mask hemolysis in patients with inflammatory disease)

# Helicobacter pylori antibodies

*Helicobacter pylori* is a spiral, gram-negative bacterium associated with chronic gastritis and idiopathic chronic duodenal ulceration. Although a gastric specimen can be obtained by endoscopy and cultured for *H. pylori,* the *H. pylori* antibody blood test is a more useful noninvasive screening procedure and may be performed using the enzyme-linked immunosorbent assay. (See *Additional tests for* Helicobacter pylori.)

### PURPOSE
● To help diagnose *H. pylori* infection in the patient with GI symptoms

### PATIENT PREPARATION
● Inform the patient that the *H. pylori* antibodies test is used to diagnose the infection that may cause ulcers.
● Inform the patient that he need not restrict food and fluids.
● Tell the patient that the test requires a blood sample. Explain who will perform the venipuncture and when.
● Explain to the patient that he may experience slight discomfort from the tourniquet and needle puncture.

### PROCEDURE AND POSTTEST CARE
● Perform a venipuncture and collect the sample in a 7-ml clot-activator tube.
● Send the sample to the laboratory immediately.
● Apply direct pressure to the venipuncture site until bleeding stops.
● If a hematoma develops at the venipuncture site, apply pressure.

---

## ADDITIONAL TESTS FOR *HELICOBACTER PYLORI*

*Helicobacter pylori* is diagnosed through blood, breath, stool, and tissue tests. Blood tests are the most common. They detect antibodies to *H. pylori* bacteria.

Urea breath tests are an effective diagnostic tool for *H. pylori*. They're also used after treatment to see whether it has been effective. In the physician's office, the patient swallows a capsule or drinks a urea solution that contains a special carbon atom. If *H. pylori* is present, it breaks down the urea, releasing the carbon. The blood carries the carbon to the lungs, where the patient exhales it. The breath test is 96% to 98% accurate.

A stool antigen test detects substances that trigger the immune system to fight an *H. pylori* infection. Stool antigen testing is less expensive and results can be obtained in about 3 hours.

Tissue tests are usually done using the biopsy specimen taken with the endoscope. There are three types:
◆ The rapid urease detects the enzyme disease produced by *H. pylori*.
◆ A histology test allows the physician to find and examine the actual bacteria.
◆ A culture test involves allowing *H. pylori* to grow in the tissue specimen.

In diagnosing *H. pylori,* blood, breath, and stool tests are commonly done before tissue tests because they're less invasive. However, blood tests aren't used to detect *H. pylori* following treatment because a patient's blood can show positive results even after *H. pylori* has been eliminated.

## PRECAUTIONS

- This test should be performed only on a patient with GI symptoms because of the many healthy people who have *H. pylori* antibodies.

## NORMAL FINDINGS

Normally, no antibodies to *H. pylori* are revealed. Test results are reported as negative or positive.

## ABNORMAL FINDINGS

A positive *H. pylori* test result indicates that the patient has antibodies to the bacterium. The serologic results should be interpreted in light of the clinical findings.

## INTERFERING FACTORS

- None significant

---

# Hematocrit

A hematocrit (HCT) test may be done separately or as part of a complete blood count. It measures percentage by volume of packed red blood cells (RBCs) in a whole blood sample; for example, an HCT of 40% indicates that a 100-ml sample of blood contains 40 ml of packed RBCs. Packing is achieved by centrifuging anticoagulated whole blood in a capillary tube so that red cells are tightly packed without hemolysis. Test results may be used to calculate two erythrocyte indices; mean corpuscular volume and mean corpuscular hemoglobin concentration.

## PURPOSE

- To aid diagnosis of polycythemia, anemia, or abnormal states of hydration
- To aid calculation of erythrocyte indices

## PATIENT PREPARATION

- Explain to the patient that HCT is tested to detect anemia and other abnormal blood conditions.
- Tell the patient that the test requires a blood sample. Explain who will perform the venipuncture and when.
- Explain to the patient that he may feel slight discomfort from the tourniquet and needle puncture.
- Inform the patient that he need not restrict food and fluids.

*Age alert* If the patient is a child, explain to him (if he's old enough) and his parents that a small amount of blood will be taken from his finger or earlobe.

## PROCEDURE AND POSTTEST CARE

- Perform a fingerstick using a heparinized capillary tube with a red band on the anticoagulant end.
- Fill the capillary tube from the red-banded end to about two-thirds capacity; seal this end with clay.
- Alternatively, perform a venipuncture and fill a 3- or 4.5-ml EDTA tube.
- Ensure subdermal bleeding has stopped before removing pressure.
- If a hematoma develops at the venipuncture site, apply pressure.

## PRECAUTIONS

- If you perform the test, place the tube in the centrifuge with the red end pointing outward.
- Fill the collection tube completely.
- Invert the tube gently several times to mix the sample.
- Send the sample to the laboratory immediately.

## REFERENCE VALUES

HCT is usually measured electronically. The results are 3% lower than manual measurements, which trap plasma in the column of packed RBCs.

Reference values for adults vary, depending on the type of sample, the laboratory performing the test, and the patient's age and sex, as follows:
- adult males — 42% to 52% (SI, 0.42 to 0.52)
- adult females — 36% to 48% (SI, 0.36 to 0.48).

*Age alert* Reference values for children also vary depending on age:
- neonates — 55% to 68% (SI, 0.55 to 0.68)
- neonates age 1 week — 47% to 65% (SI, 0.47 to 0.65)
- infants age 1 month — 37% to 49% (SI, 0.37 to 0.49)
- infants age 3 months — 30% to 36% (SI, 0.3 to 0.36)
- age 1 year — 29% to 41% (SI, 0.29 to 0.41)
- age 10 years — 36% to 40% (SI, 0.36 to 0.4).

## ABNORMAL FINDINGS

Low HCT suggests anemia, hemodilution, or massive blood loss. High HCT indicates polycythemia or hemoconcentration due to blood loss and dehydration.

## INTERFERING FACTORS

● Hemoconcentration due to tourniquet constriction for longer than 1 minute (increase, typically 2.5% to 5%)
● Hemodilution due to drawing the blood from the arm above an I.V. infusion

# Hemoglobin electrophoresis

Hemoglobin (Hb) electrophoresis is probably the most useful laboratory method for separating and measuring normal and abnormal Hb. Through electrophoresis, different types of Hb are separated to form a series of distinctly pigmented bands in a medium. Results are then compared with those of a normal sample.

Hb A, A$_2$, S, and C are routinely checked, but the laboratory may change the medium or its pH to expand the range of this test.

## PURPOSE

● To measure the amount of Hb A and to detect abnormal Hb
● To aid diagnosis of thalassemia

## PATIENT PREPARATION

● Explain to the patient that the Hb electrophoresis test is used to evaluate Hb.
● Tell the patient that a blood sample will be taken. Explain who will perform the venipuncture and when.
● Explain to the patient that he may feel slight discomfort from the tourniquet and needle puncture.

*Age alert* *If the patient is an infant or child, explain to the parents that a small amount of blood will be taken from his finger.*
● Inform the patient that he need not restrict food and fluids.

## VARIATIONS OF HEMOGLOBIN TYPE AND DISTRIBUTION

| HEMOGLOBIN | PERCENTAGE OF TOTAL HEMOGLOBIN | CLINICAL IMPLICATIONS |
| --- | --- | --- |
| Hb A | 95% to 100% (SI, 0.95 to 1.0) | Normal |
| Hb A$_2$ | 4% to 5.8% (SI, 0.04 to 0.058)<br>1.5% to 3% (SI, 0.015 to 0.03)<br>Under 1.5% (SI, < 0.015) | ß-thalassemia minor<br>Normal<br>Hb H disease |
| Hb F | Under 1% (SI, < 0.01)<br>2% to 5% (SI, 0.02 to 0.05)<br>10% to 90% (SI, 0.1 to 0.9)<br>5% to 15% (SI, 0.05 to 0.15)<br>5% to 35% (SI, 0.05 to 0.35)<br><br>100% (SI, 1.0)<br>15% (SI, 0.15) | Normal<br>ß-thalassemia minor<br>ß-thalassemia major<br>ß-thalassemia minor<br>Heterozygous hereditary persistence of fetal Hb (HPFH)<br>Homozygous HPFH<br>Homozygous Hb S |
| Homozygous Hb S | 70% to 98% (SI, 0.7 to 0.98) | Sickle cell disease |
| Homozygous Hb C | 90% to 98% (SI, 0.9 to 0.98) | Hb C disease |
| Heterozygous Hb C | 24% to 44% (SI, 0.24 to 0.44) | Hb C trait |

## PROCEDURE AND POSTTEST CARE

● Ask the patient if he has received a blood transfusion within the past 4 months.

● Perform a venipuncture and collect the sample in a 3- or 4.5-ml EDTA tube.

★ *Age alert  For young children, collect capillary blood in a microcollection device.*

● If a hematoma develops at the venipuncture site, apply pressure.

## PRECAUTIONS

● Completely fill the collection tube and invert it gently several times to mix the sample and the anticoagulant.

● Don't shake the tube vigorously.

## REFERENCE VALUES

In adults, Hb A accounts for 95% (SI, 0.95) of all Hb; Hb A$_2$, 1.5% to 3% (SI, 0.15 to 0.030); and Hb F, < 2% (SI, < 0.02).

★ *Age alert  In neonates, Hb F normally accounts for one-half of the total. Hb S and Hb C are normally absent.*

## ABNORMAL FINDINGS

Hb electrophoresis allows identification of various types of Hb. Certain types may indicate a hemolytic disease. (See *Variations of hemoglobin type and distribution,* page 221.)

## INTERFERING FACTORS

● Blood transfusion within the past 4 months

---

# Hemoglobin, urine

---

An abnormal finding, free hemoglobin (Hb) in the urine may occur in hemolytic anemias, infection, strenuous exercise, or severe intravascular hemolysis from a transfusion reaction. Contained in red blood cells (RBCs), Hb consists of an iron-protoporphyrin complex (heme) and a polypeptide (globin). Usually, RBC destruction occurs within the reticuloendothelial system. However, when RBC destruction occurs within the circulation, free Hb enters the plasma and binds with haptoglobin. If the plasma level of Hb exceeds that of haptoglobin, the excess of unbound Hb is excreted in the urine (hemoglobinuria).

Heme proteins act like enzymes that catalyze oxidation of organic substances. This reaction produces a blue coloration; the intensity of color varies with the amount of Hb present. Microscopic examination is required to identify intact RBCs in urine (hematuria), which can occur in the presence of unbound Hb.

## PURPOSE

● To aid in the diagnosis of hemolytic anemias, infection, or severe intravascular hemolysis from a transfusion reaction

## PATIENT PREPARATION

● Explain to the patient that the urine Hb test detects excessive RBC destruction.

● Inform the patient that he need not restrict food and fluids.

● Tell the patient that the test requires a random urine specimen, and teach him the proper collection technique.

● If the female patient is menstruating, reschedule the test, as results may be altered.

● Notify the laboratory and physician of medications the patient is taking that may affect test results; they may need to be restricted.

## PROCEDURE AND POSTTEST CARE

● Collect a random urine specimen. (See *Bedside testing for urine blood pigments.*)

● Instruct the patient that he may resume his usual medications, as ordered.

## PRECAUTIONS

● Have a female patient who's menstruating reschedule her test because contamination of the specimen with menstrual blood alters results.

● Send the specimen to the laboratory immediately after collection.

## NORMAL FINDINGS

Normally, Hb isn't present in the urine.

## ABNORMAL FINDINGS

Hemoglobinuria may result from severe intravascular hemolysis due to a blood transfusion reaction, burns, or a crush injury. It may result from acquired hemolytic anemias caused by chemical or drug intoxication or malaria; congenital hemolytic anemias, such as hemoglobinopathies or enzyme defects; or paroxysmal nocturnal hemoglobinuria (another type of hemolytic anemia). Less commonly, it may signal cystitis, ureteral calculi, or urethritis.

Hemoglobinuria and hematuria occur in renal epithelial damage (which may result from acute glomerulonephritis or pyelonephritis), renal tumor, and tuberculosis.

## INTERFERING FACTORS
● Nephrotoxic drugs and anticoagulants (positive results)
● Large doses of vitamin C or drugs that contain vitamin C as a preservative (false-negative)
● Lysis of RBCs in stale or alkaline urine and contamination of the specimen by menstrual blood
● Bacterial peroxidases in highly infected specimens (false-positive)

## Hemosiderin, urine

The test for hemosiderin measures the urine level of hemosiderin — a colloidal iron oxide and one of the two forms of iron that are stored and deposited in body tissue.

When iron storage mechanisms fail to manage iron overload, excess iron may escape to cells unaccustomed to high iron concentrations and may produce toxic effects. Toxicity may affect the liver, myocardium, bone marrow, pancreas, kidneys, and skin. Subsequent tissue damage is referred to as hemochromatosis. Hemochromatosis may occur in a rare hereditary form (primary hemochromatosis) and in exogenous forms.

## PURPOSE
● To aid in the diagnosis of hemochromatosis, hemolytic anemia associated with intravascular hemolysis

## PATIENT PREPARATION
● Explain to the patient that the urine hemosiderin test helps determine if the body is accumulating excessive amounts of iron.
● Inform the patient that no restrictions are necessary and that the test requires a urine specimen.

## PROCEDURE AND POSTTEST CARE
● Collect a random urine specimen of approximately 30 ml, preferably the first void of the morning.

## PRECAUTIONS

- Seal the container securely, and send the specimen to the laboratory immediately after collection.

## NORMAL FINDINGS

Normally, hemosiderin isn't found in urine.

## ABNORMAL FINDINGS

The presence of hemosiderin, appearing as yellow-brown granules in urinary sediment, indicates hemochromatosis; liver or bone marrow biopsy is necessary to confirm primary hemochromatosis. Hemosiderin may also suggest pernicious anemia, chronic hemolytic anemia, multiple blood transfusions, and paroxysmal nocturnal hemoglobinuria, the result of excessive iron injections or dietary iron intake.

## INTERFERING FACTORS

- None significant

# Hepatitis B surface antigen

Hepatitis B surface antigen (HBsAg), also called hepatitis-associated antigen or Australia antigen, appears in the serum of the patient with hepatitis B virus. It can be detected by radioimmunoassay or, less commonly, reverse passive hemagglutination during the extended incubation period and usually during the first 3 weeks of acute infection or if the patient is a carrier.

Because hepatitis transmission is one of the gravest complications associated with blood transfusion, all donors must be screened for hepatitis B before their blood is stored. This screening, required by the U.S. Food and Drug Administration's Bureau of Biologics, has helped reduce the incidence of hepatitis. This test doesn't screen for hepatitis A virus (infectious hepatitis).

For information on related tests, see *Viral hepatitis test panel*.

## PURPOSE

- To screen blood donors for hepatitis B
- To screen people at high risk for contracting hepatitis B such as hemodialysis health care workers

- To aid in the differential diagnosis of viral hepatitis

## PATIENT PREPARATION

- Explain to the patient that the HBsAg test helps identify a type of viral hepatitis.
- Inform the patient that he need not restrict food and fluids.
- Tell the patient that the test requires a blood sample. Explain who will perform the venipuncture and when.
- Explain to the patient that he may experience slight discomfort from the tourniquet and needle puncture.
- Check the patient's history for administration of hepatitis B vaccine.
- If the patient is giving blood, explain the donation procedure to him.

## PROCEDURE AND POSTTEST CARE

- Perform a venipuncture and collect the sample in a 10-ml clot-activator tube.
- Apply direct pressure to the venipuncture site until bleeding stops.
- If a hematoma develops at the venipuncture site, apply pressure.

**Alert** *Report confirmed viral hepatitis to public health authorities. This is a reportable disease in most states.*

## PRECAUTIONS

- Wash your hands carefully after the procedure.
- Remember to wear gloves when drawing blood and dispose of the needle properly.

## NORMAL FINDINGS

Normal serum is negative for HBsAg.

## ABNORMAL FINDINGS

The presence of HBsAg in patients with hepatitis confirms hepatitis B. In chronic carriers and in people with chronic active hepatitis, HBsAg may be present in the serum several months after the onset of acute infection. It may also occur in more than 5% of patients with certain diseases other than hepatitis, such as hemophilia, Hodgkin's disease, and leukemia. If HBsAg is found in donor blood, that blood must be discarded because it carries a risk of transmitting hepatitis. Blood samples that test positive should be retested because inaccurate results do occur. (See *Serodiagnosis of acute viral hepatitis*.)

# VIRAL HEPATITIS TEST PANEL

The six types of viral hepatitis produce similar symptoms but differ in transmission mode, course of treatment, prognosis, and carrier status. When the clinical history is insufficient for differentiation, serologic tests can aid in diagnosis. Testing helps to identify antibodies specific to the causative virus and establish the type of hepatitis:

◆ Type A—Detection of an antibody to hepatitis A, confirming the diagnosis
◆ Type B—The presence of hepatitis B surface antigens and hepatitis B antibodies, confirming the diagnosis
◆ Type C—Diagnosis depends on serologic testing for the specific antibody 1 or more months after the onset of acute illness: until then, diagnosis principally established by obtaining negative test results for hepatitis A, B, and D
◆ Type D—Detection of intrahepatic delta antigens or immunoglobulin (Ig) M antidelta antigens in acute disease (or IgM and IgG in chronic disease), confirming the diagnosis

◆ Type E—Detection of hepatitis E antigens confirming the diagnosis; however, possibly ruling out hepatitis C
◆ Type G—Detection of hepatitis G ribonucleic acid confirming the diagnosis (serologic assays are being developed).

Additional findings from liver function studies supporting the diagnosis include:
◆ Serum aspartate aminotransferase and serum alanine aminotransferase levels increased in the prodromal stage of acute viral hepatitis
◆ Serum alkaline phosphatase levels slightly increased
◆ Serum bilirubin levels elevated; levels possibly remaining elevated late in the disease, especially with severe disease
◆ Prothrombin time (PT) prolonged (PT of more than 3 seconds longer than normal, indicating severe liver damage)
◆ White blood cell counts commonly revealing transient neutropenia and lymphopenia followed by lymphocytosis.

# SERODIAGNOSIS OF ACUTE VIRAL HEPATITIS

The chart below helps evaluate positive test results in acute viral hepatitis.

| TEST RESULTS | | | INTERPRETATION |
|---|---|---|---|
| HBsAg | Anti-HBC IgM | Anti-HAV IgM | |
| – | – | + | Recent acute hepatitis A infection |
| + | + | – | Acute hepatitis B infection |
| + | – | – | Early acute hepatitis B infection or chronic hepatitis B |
| – | + | – | Confirms acute or recent infection with hepatitis B virus |
| – | – | – | Possible hepatitis C infection, other viral infection, or liver toxin |
| + | + | + | Recent probable hepatitis A infection and superimposed acute hepatitis B infection; uncommon profile |

**KEY:**   + = positive   – = negative

Reprinted with permission of Abbott Laboratories, Abbott Park, Ill.

• Hepatitis B vaccine (possible positive)

# Herpes simplex antibodies

Herpes simplex virus (HSV), a member of the herpesvirus group, causes various clinically severe manifestations, including genital lesions, keratitis or conjunctivitis, generalized dermal lesions, and pneumonia. Severe involvement is associated with intrauterine or neonatal infections and encephalitis; such infections are most severe in immunosuppressed patients. Of the two closely related antigenic types, type 1 usually causes infections above the waistline; type 2 infections predominantly involve the external genitalia. Primary contact with this virus occurs in early childhood as acute stomatitis or, more commonly, as an inapparent infection. More than 50% of adults have antibodies to HSV.

Sensitive assays, such as indirect immunofluorescence and enzyme immunoassay, are used to demonstrate immunoglobulin (Ig) M class antibodies to HSV or to detect a fourfold or greater increase in IgG class antibodies between acute- and convalescent-phase sera.

## PURPOSE
• To confirm infections caused by HSV
• To detect recent or past HSV infection

## PATIENT PREPARATION
• Explain the purpose of the herpes simplex antibodies test to the patient.
• Tell the patient that the test requires a blood sample. Explain who will perform the venipuncture and when.
• Explain to the patient that he may experience slight discomfort from the tourniquet and needle puncture.

## PROCEDURE AND POSTTEST CARE
• Perform a venipuncture and collect 5 ml of sterile blood in a tube designated by the laboratory.
• Allow the blood to clot for at least 1 hour at room temperature.
• Apply direct pressure to the venipuncture site until bleeding stops.

• If a hematoma develops at the venipuncture site, apply pressure.
• If the patient's immune system is compromised, check the venipuncture site for changes and report them promptly.

## PRECAUTIONS
• Handle the sample gently to prevent hemolysis.
• Transfer the serum to a sterile tube or vial and send it to the laboratory promptly.
• If transfer must be delayed, store the serum at 39.2° F (4° C) for 1 to 2 days or at –4° F (–20° C) for longer periods to avoid contamination.
• Because the patient may have a compromised immune system, keep the venipuncture site clean and dry.

## REFERENCE VALUES
Sera from patients who have never been infected with HSV have no detectable antibodies (less than 1:5).

## ABNORMAL FINDINGS
HSV infection can be ruled out in patients whose serum shows no detectable antibodies to the virus. The presence of IgM or a fourfold or greater increase in IgG antibodies indicates active HSV infection.

## INTERFERING FACTORS
• None significant

# Herpes simplex virus culture

Herpes simplex virus (HSV) produces a wide spectrum of clinical manifestations, including keratitis, gingivostomatitis, and encephalitis. In the immunocompromised individual, it may lead to disseminated illness. The herpesvirus group includes Epstein Barr virus, cytomegalovirus (CMV), varicella zoster virus (VZV), human herpesvirus 6, herpesvirus-7, herpesvirus-8, and the two closely related serotypes of HSV — type 1 and type 2. Only CMV, VZV, and HSV replicate in the standard cell cultures used in diagnostic laboratories.

About 50% of HSV strains can be detected by characteristic cytopathic effects (CPE) within 24 hours after the laboratory receives the specimen; 5 to 7 days are required to detect the remaining HSV strains. Alternatively, early HSV antigens can be detected by monoclonal antibodies in shell vial cell cultures within 16 hours after receipt of the specimen with the same sensitivity and specificity as standard tube cell cultures.

## PURPOSE

● To confirm diagnosis of HSV infection by culturing the virus from specimens

## PATIENT PREPARATION

● Explain to the patient that the HSV culture test is performed to detect HSV infection.
● Explain to the patient that specimens will be collected from suspected lesions during the prodromal and acute stages of clinical infection.

## PROCEDURE AND POSTTEST CARE

● Collect a specimen for culture in the appropriate collection device. Vesicle fluid can be obtained with a 27G needle or a tuberculin syringe. If the fluid is scant, the base of the ulcer can be scraped with a swab to remove cells.
● For the throat, skin, eye, or genital area, use a microbiologic transport swab.
● For body fluids or other respiratory specimens (washings, lavage), use a sterile screw-capped jar.
● Transport the specimen to the laboratory as soon as possible after collection. If the anticipated time between collection and inoculation of cell cultures is more than 3 hours, the specimen should be stored and transported at 39.2° F (4° C).

## PRECAUTIONS

● Wear gloves when obtaining and handling all specimens.
● Don't allow the specimen to dry up.

## NORMAL FINDINGS

HSV is seldom recovered from an immunocompetent patient who shows no overt signs of disease.

## ABNORMAL FINDINGS

HSV detected in specimens taken from dermal lesions, the eye, or cerebrospinal fluid is highly significant. Specimens from the upper respiratory tract may be associated with intermittent shedding of the virus, particularly in an immunocompromised patient.

Like other herpesviruses, HSV can be shed from the immunocompromised patient intermittently in the absence of apparent disease. For epidemiologic purposes, HSV detected by CPE in standard tube cell cultures is confirmed and identified as type 1 or 2.

## INTERFERING FACTORS

● Administration of antiviral drugs before specimen collection

# *Hexosaminidase A and B, serum*

This fluorometric test measures the hexosaminidase A and B content of serum samples drawn by venipuncture or collected from a neonate's umbilical cord or of amniotic fluid obtained by amniocentesis.

Hexosaminidase deficiency can also be identified by testing cultured skin fibroblasts; however, this procedure is costly and technically complex. A reference center for congenital disease should be consulted for the preferred screening method and specimen.

Hexosaminidase is a group of enzymes that are necessary for metabolism of gangliosides, water soluble glycolipids found primarily in brain tissue. The hexosaminidase A and B test is used to measure the hexosaminidase A and B content of serum and amniotic fluid.

Deficiency of hexosaminidase A indicates Tay-Sachs disease, which is about 100 times more common in people of eastern European Jewish ancestry than in the general population. Both parents must carry the defective gene to transmit Tay-Sachs disease to their children. Sandhoff's disease, which results from deficiency of hexosaminidase A and B, is uncommon and not prevalent in any ethnic group.

## PURPOSE

● To confirm or rule out Tay-Sachs disease in the neonate
● To screen for a Tay-Sachs carrier
● To establish prenatal diagnosis of hexosaminidase A deficiency

## PATIENT PREPARATION

• Explain to the patient that the serum hexosaminidase A and B test is used to identify carriers of Tay-Sachs disease.

• Tell the patient that the test requires a blood sample. Explain who will perform the venipuncture and when.

• Explain to the patient that he may experience slight discomfort from the tourniquet and needle puncture.

• Inform the patient that he need not restrict food and fluids.

🐾 *Age alert* *When testing a neonate, explain to the parents that the serum hexosaminidase A and B test is used to detect Tay-Sachs disease. Tell them that blood will be drawn from the neonate's arm, neck, or umbilical cord; that the procedure is safe and quickly performed; and that the neonate will have a small bandage on the venipuncture site. Inform them that no pretest restrictions of food or fluid are needed.*

• If the test is being performed prenatally, advise the patient of preparations for amniocentesis.

## PROCEDURE AND POSTTEST CARE

• Perform a venipuncture, collect cord blood, or assist with amniocentesis, as appropriate. Collect the sample in a 7-ml clot-activator tube.

• Apply direct pressure to the venipuncture site until bleeding stops.

• If a hematoma develops at the venipuncture site, apply pressure.

• When testing a neonate, follow laboratory procedure for collecting serum samples.

## PRECAUTIONS

• Handle the sample gently to prevent hemolysis.

• This test can't be done on a pregnant woman's serum (but her leukocytes or amniotic fluid may be tested, if necessary); if the father's blood test result is negative, Tay-Sachs disease won't be transmitted to the child.

• If the test can't be performed immediately, freeze the sample.

## REFERENCE VALUES

Total hexosaminidase levels range from 9.83 to 15.95 U/L (SI, 164 to 266 nkat/L). The percentage of normal total hexosaminidase A ranges from 7.2 to 9.88 U/L (SI, 120 to 165

nkat/L); hexosaminidase A accounts for 56% to 80% of the total.

## ABNORMAL FINDINGS

Absence of hexosaminidase A indicates Tay-Sachs disease (total hexosaminidase levels can be normal). Absence of hexosaminidase A and B indicates Sandhoff's disease, an uncommon, virulent variant of Tay-Sachs disease in which deterioration occurs more rapidly.

## INTERFERING FACTORS

• Hormonal contraceptives (false-high)
• Rifampin (Rifadin) and isoniazid (Nydrazid) (increase)

---

# *Holter monitoring*

Holter monitoring, also called *dynamic monitoring and ambulatory electrocardiography* (ECG), involves the continuous recording of heart activity over a 24 hour period as the patient follows his normal routine. During this period, the patient wears a small reel-to-reel or cassette tape recorder connected to electrodes placed on his chest and keeps a diary of his activities and any associated symptoms. After the recording period, the tape is analyzed by a computer and a physician to correlate cardiac irregularities, such as arrhythmias and ST-segment changes, with the activities noted in the patient's diary.

## PURPOSE

• To detect cardiac arrhythmias
• To evaluate chest pain
• To evaluate cardiac status after an acute myocardial infarction (MI) or a pacemaker implantation
• To evaluate the effectiveness of antiarrhythmic drug therapy
• To assess and correlate dyspnea, central nervous system (CNS) symptoms (such as syncope and light-headedness), and palpitations with actual cardiac events and the patient's activities

## PATIENT PREPARATION

• Explain to the patient that Holter monitoring helps determine how the heart responds to normal activity or, if appropriate, to cardioactive medication. Tell him that electrodes will be attached to his chest, that his chest may be shaved, and that he may experience some discomfort during preparation of the electrode sites.

● Explain to the patient that he'll wear a small tape recorder for 24 hours (for 5 to 7 days, if a patient-activated monitor is being used).

● Mention that a shoulder strap or a special belt will be provided to carry the recorder, which weighs about 2 lb (1 kg). Show him how to position the recorder when he lies down.

● Encourage the patient to continue his routine activities during the monitoring period. Stress the importance of logging his usual activities (such as walking, climbing stairs, urinating, sleeping, and having sex), emotional upsets, physical symptoms (dizziness, palpitations, fatigue, chest pain, and syncope), and ingestion of medication; show the patient a sample diary.

● Tell the patient to wear loose fitting clothing with front-buttoning tops during monitoring.

● Demonstrate the proper use of specific equipment, including how to mark the tape (if applicable) at the onset of symptoms.

● If a patient-activated monitor is being used, show the patient how to press the event button to activate the monitor if he experiences an unusual sensation. Instruct him not to tamper with the monitor or disconnect the leadwires or electrodes.

● Bathing instructions depend on the type of recorder being worn (certain equipment must not get wet).

● Advise the patient to avoid magnets, metal detectors, high-voltage areas, and electric blankets. Show him how to check the recorder to make sure it's working properly. Instruct him how to troubleshoot problems if the monitor alarm sounds. Explain that if the monitor light flashes, one of the electrodes may be loose and he should depress the center of each one. Tell him to notify you if one comes off.

● If the patient won't be returning to the health care facility immediately after the monitoring period, show him how to remove and store the equipment. Remind him to bring the diary when he returns.

## PROCEDURE AND POSTTEST CARE

● Clean and gently abrade the electrode sites. Peel the backings from the electrodes, and apply them to the correct sites, being sure to press the sides and center of each electrode firmly to ensure proper adhesion.

● Attach the electrode cable securely to the monitor.

● Position the monitor and case as the patient will wear it, and then attach the leadwires to the electrodes. There shouldn't be too much slack or pull on the wires.

● Make sure the recorder has a new or fully charged battery, insert the tape, and turn on the recorder.

● Test the electrode attachment circuit by connecting the recorder to a standard ECG machine. Watch for artifacts while the patient moves normally (stands, sits).

● Remove all chest electrodes and clean the electrode sites after the test.

## PRECAUTIONS

● To eliminate muscle artifact, make sure the lead cable is plugged in firmly. Check to ensure that electrodes aren't placed over large muscle masses such as the pectorals.

## NORMAL FINDINGS

When correlated with the patient's diary, the ECG pattern shows normal sinus rhythm with no significant arrhythmias or ST-segment changes. Changes in heart rate normally occur during various activities.

## ABNORMAL FINDINGS

Cardiac abnormalities detected by ambulatory ECG include premature ventricular contractions (PVCs), conduction defects, tachyarrhythmias, bradyarrhythmias, bradytachy syndrome, and atrial arrhythmias, such as atrial fibrillation and atrial flutter. Arrhythmias may be associated with dyspnea and CNS symptoms, such as dizziness and syncope. During recovery from an MI, this test can monitor for PVCs to determine the prognosis and effectiveness of drug therapy.

ST-T wave changes associated with ischemia may coincide with chest pain or increased patient activity. ST-segment changes associated with an acute MI require careful study because smoking, eating, postural changes, certain drugs, Wolff-Parkinson-White syndrome, bundle-branch block, myocarditis, myocardial hypertrophy, anemia, hypoxemia, and abnormal hemoglobin binding can produce a similar tracing on the ECG. Monitoring the patient with an MI for 1 to 3 days before discharge and again 4 to 6 weeks after discharge may detect ST-T wave changes associated with ischemia or arrhythmias; such information aids patient therapy and rehabilitation and refines the prognosis. Monitoring a patient with an artificial pacemaker may detect an arrhythmia, such as bradycardia, that the pacemaker fails to override.

Although ambulatory ECG correlates patient symptoms and ECG changes, it doesn't always identify the symptoms' causes. If initial monitoring proves inconclusive, the test may be repeated.

## INTERFERING FACTORS
● Electrode placement over a large muscle mass, poor electrode contact with skin, or other failure to correctly apply the electrodes (possible muscle or movement artifact)
● Failure of patient to carefully record daily activities and symptoms, to maintain his normal routine, or to turn on the monitor during symptoms (if using a patient-activated monitor)
● Physiologic variation in arrhythmia frequency and severity (possible failure to detect arrhythmias during 24-hour Holter monitoring)

# Homocysteine

Homocysteine (tHcy), a sulfur-containing amino acid, is a transmethylation product of methionine. It's an intermediate in the synthesis of cysteine, which is produced by the enzymatic or acid hydrolysis of proteins. The test is useful for the biochemical diagnosis of inborn errors of methionine, folate, and vitamins $B_6$ and $B_{12}$ metabolism. Elevated homocysteine levels have also been implicated as a risk factor for cardiac disease, cerebrovascular disease, peripheral artery disease, and venous thrombosis. Research has demonstrated that homocysteine plays a role in promoting atherosclerotic changes in the blood vessels. These changes can occur in people without any hyperlipoproteinemia.

## PURPOSE
● To establish a biochemical diagnosis of inborn errors of methionine, folate, and vitamins $B_6$ and $B_{12}$ metabolism
● To establish an indicator of acquired folate or cobalamin deficiency
● To evaluate risk factors for atherosclerotic vascular disease
● To assess contributing factors in the pathogenesis of neural tube defects
● To evaluate the cause of recurrent spontaneous abortions
● To assess delayed child development or failure to thrive in infants

## PATIENT PREPARATION
● Inform the patient that this test detects homocysteine levels in plasma.
● Advise him to fast for 12 to 14 hours before the test.
● Tell him that this test requires a blood sample, who will perform the venipuncture and when, and that he may experience transient discomfort from the pressure of the tourniquet and needle puncture.

## PROCEDURE AND POSTTEST CARE
● Perform a venipuncture, and collect the sample in a 5-ml tube with EDTA added.
● If a hematoma develops at the venipuncture site, apply pressure.

## PRECAUTIONS
● Handle the sample gently to prevent hemolysis.
● Immediately put the sample on ice and send it to the laboratory.

## REFERENCE VALUES
Normal total homocysteine levels are 4 to 17 µmol/L (SI, 0.54 to 2.3 mg/L).

## ABNORMAL FINDINGS
Low homocysteine levels are associated with inborn or acquired folate or cobalamine deficiency and inborn $B_6$ or $B_{12}$ deficiency.

Elevated homocysteine levels are associated with a higher incidence of atherosclerotic vascular disease. Typically, levels ranging from 12 to 15 µmol/L are considered borderline. Levels about 15 µmol/L are associated with an increased risk of atherosclerotic disease. In patients with type 2 diabetes mellitus, studies have shown that homocysteine levels increase with even a modest deterioration in renal function.

**Alert** *A greater muscle mass and higher creatinine levels are usually responsible for higher homocysteine levels in males.*

## INTERFERING FACTORS
- Penicillamine (Cuprimine) (reduced plasma levels)
- Carbamazepine (Tegretol), methotrexate deficiency, nitrous oxide, phenytoin (Dilantin), renal impairment, and smoking (increased plasma levels)
- Hormonal contraceptives (possible alteration in metabolism of homocysteine)
- Low intake of B vitamins

# Homovanillic acid, urine

The urine homovanillic acid (HVA) test is a quantitative analysis of urine HVA levels. HVA is a metabolite of dopamine, one of the three major catecholamines. Synthesized primarily in the brain, dopamine is a precursor to epinephrine and norepinephrine, the other principal catecholamines. The liver breaks down most dopamine into HVA for eventual excretion; a minimal amount of dopamine appears in the urine.

Using two-dimensional chromatography, urine HVA levels are usually measured simultaneously with the major catecholamines and other catecholamine metabolites — metanephrine, normetanephrine, and vanillylmandelic acid (VMA).

## PURPOSE
- To aid in the diagnosis of neuroblastoma and ganglioneuroma
- To rule out pheochromocytoma

## PATIENT PREPARATION
- Explain to the patient that the urine HVA test assesses hormone secretion.
- Inform the patient that he need not restrict food and fluids but should avoid stressful situations and excessive physical exercise during the collection period.

- Tell the patient that the test requires collection of urine over a 24-hour period, and teach him the proper collection technique.
- Notify the laboratory and physician of medications the patient is taking that may affect test results; they may need to be restricted.

## PROCEDURE AND POSTTEST CARE
- Collect the patient's urine over a 24-hour period, discarding the first specimen and retaining the last. Use a bottle containing a preservative to keep the specimen at a pH of 2.0 to 4.0.
- Instruct the patient that he may resume his usual activities and medications, as ordered.

## PRECAUTIONS
- Refrigerate the specimen or keep it on ice during the collection period.
- Send the specimen to the laboratory immediately after the collection is completed.

## REFERENCE VALUES
The normal urine HVA value for adults is less than 10 mg/24 hours (SI, < 55 μmol/d).

## ABNORMAL FINDINGS
Elevated urine HVA levels suggest neuroblastoma, a malignant soft-tissue tumor that develops in infants and young children, or ganglioneuroma, a tumor of the sympathetic nervous system that develops in older children and adolescents and rarely metastasizes. HVA levels don't usually rise in patients with pheochromocytoma because this tumor secretes mainly epinephrine, which metabolizes primarily into VMA. Thus, an abnormally high urine HVA level generally rules out pheochromocytoma.

## INTERFERING FACTORS
- Excessive physical exercise or emotional stress during the collection period (possible increase)
- Monoamine oxidase inhibitors (decrease due to inhibition of dopamine metabolism)
- Aspirin, levodopa, and methocarbamol (Robaxin) (possible increase or decrease)

# Human chorionic gonadotropin

Human chorionic gonadotropin (hCG) is a glycoprotein hormone produced in the placenta. If conception occurs, a specific assay for hCG—commonly called the *beta-subunit assay*—may detect this hormone in the blood 9 days after ovulation. This interval coincides with the implantation of the fertilized ovum into the uterine wall. Although the precise function of hCG is unclear, it appears that hCG, with progesterone, maintains the corpus luteum during early pregnancy.

Production of hCG increases steadily during the first trimester, peaking around 10 weeks' gestation. Levels then fall to less than 10% of first-trimester peak levels during the remainder of the pregnancy. About 2 weeks after delivery, the hormone may no longer be detectable. (See *Production of hCG during pregnancy*.) This serum immunoassay, a quantitative analysis of hCG beta subunit level, is more sensitive (and costlier) than the routine pregnancy test using a urine sample.

## PURPOSE
- To detect early pregnancy
- To determine adequacy of hormonal production in high risk pregnancies (for example, habitual abortion)
- To aid diagnosis of trophoblastic tumors, such as hydatidiform mole and choriocarcinoma, and tumors that ectopically secrete hCG
- To monitor treatment for induction of ovulation and conception

## PATIENT PREPARATION
- Explain to the patient that the hCG test determines if she's pregnant. If detection of pregnancy isn't the diagnostic objective, offer the appropriate explanation.
- Inform the patient that she need not restrict food and fluids.
- Tell the patient that the test requires a blood sample. Explain who will perform the venipuncture and when.

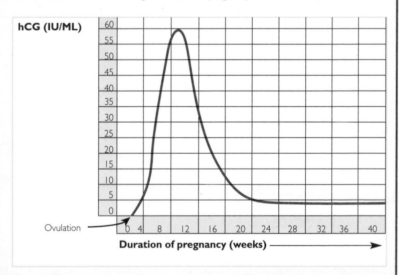

## PRODUCTION OF hCG DURING PREGNANCY

Production of human chorionic gonadotropin (hCG) increases steadily during the first trimester, peaking around 10 weeks' gestation, as shown below. Levels then fall to less than 10% of first-trimester levels during the rest of the pregnancy.

hCG (IU/ML)

Ovulation

Duration of pregnancy (weeks)

- Explain to the patient that she may experience slight discomfort from the tourniquet and needle puncture.

## PROCEDURE AND POSTTEST CARE
- Perform a venipuncture and collect the sample in a 7-ml clot-activator tube.
- Apply direct pressure to the venipuncture site until bleeding stops.
- If a hematoma develops at the venipuncture site, apply pressure.

## PRECAUTIONS
- Handle the sample gently to prevent hemolysis.
- Send the sample to the laboratory immediately.

## REFERENCE VALUES
Normally, hCG levels are less than 4 IU/L (SI, less than 4 mIU/ml). During pregnancy, hCG levels vary widely, depending partly on the number of days after the last normal menstrual period. Typically, levels double every 48 hours during the first 6 weeks of gestation.

## ABNORMAL FINDINGS
Elevated hCG beta subunit levels indicate pregnancy; significantly higher concentrations are present in a multiple pregnancy. Increased levels may also suggest hydatidiform mole, trophoblastic neoplasms of the placenta, and nontrophoblastic carcinomas that secrete hCG (including gastric, pancreatic, and ovarian adenocarcinomas). Low hCG beta-subunit levels can occur in ectopic pregnancy or pregnancy of less than 9 days. Beta-subunit levels can't differentiate between pregnancy and tumor recurrence because they're high in both conditions.

## INTERFERING FACTORS
- Heparin anticoagulants and EDTA (decrease; ask laboratory whether test will be performed on plasma or serum)
- Lipemia and administration of radioisotopes within 1 week of test (possible affect on results)
- Abortion within 1 week (positive results)

# Human chorionic gonadotropin, urine

Qualitative analysis of urine levels of human chorionic gonadotropin (hCG) allows for the detection of pregnancy as early as 14 days after ovulation. Production of hCG, a glycoprotein, which prevents degeneration of the corpus luteum at the end of the normal menstrual cycle, begins after conception. During the first trimester, hCG levels rise steadily and rapidly, peaking around 10 weeks' gestation, subsequently tapering off to less than 10% of peak levels.

The most common method of evaluating hCG in urine is hemagglutination inhibition. This laboratory procedure can provide qualitative and quantitative information. The qualitative urine test is easier and less expensive than the serum hCG test (beta-subunit assay); therefore, it's used more commonly to detect pregnancy.

## PURPOSE
- To detect and confirm pregnancy
- To aid in the diagnosis of hydatidiform mole or hCG-secreting tumors, threatened abortion, or dead fetus

## PATIENT PREPARATION
- If appropriate, explain to the patient that the urine hCG test determines whether she's pregnant or the status of her pregnancy. Alternatively, explain how the test functions as a screen for some types of cancer.
- Tell the patient that she need not restrict food but should restrict fluids for 8 hours before the test.
- Inform the patient that the test requires a first-voided morning specimen or urine collection over a 24-hour period, depending on whether the test is qualitative or quantitative.
- Notify the laboratory and physician of medications the patient is taking that may affect test results; they may need to be restricted.

## PROCEDURE AND POSTTEST CARE
- For verification of pregnancy (qualitative analysis), collect a first-voided morning specimen. If this isn't possible, collect a random specimen.

- For quantitative analysis of hCG, collect the patient's urine over a 24-hour period in the appropriate container, discarding the first specimen and retaining the last.
- Specify the date of the patient's last menstrual period on the laboratory request.
- Instruct the patient that she may resume her usual diet and medications, as ordered.

## PRECAUTIONS
- Refrigerate the 24-hour specimen or keep it on ice during the collection period.
- Make sure the test is performed at least 5 days after a missed period to avoid a false-negative result.

## NORMAL FINDINGS
In a qualitative immunoassay analysis, results are reported as negative (nonpregnant) or positive (pregnant) for hCG. In quantitative analysis, urine hCG levels in the first trimester of a normal pregnancy may be as high as 500,000 IU/24 hours; in the second trimester, they range from 10,000 to 25,000 IU/24 hours; and in the third trimester, from 5,000 to 15,000 IU/24 hours.

Measurable hCG levels don't normally appear in the urine of men or nonpregnant women.

## ABNORMAL FINDINGS
During pregnancy, elevated urine hCG levels may indicate multiple pregnancy or erythroblastosis fetalis; depressed urine hCG levels may indicate threatened abortion or ectopic pregnancy.

Measurable levels of hCG in males and nonpregnant females may indicate choriocarcinoma, ovarian or testicular tumors, melanoma, multiple myeloma, or gastric, hepatic, pancreatic, or breast cancer.

## INTERFERING FACTORS
- Gross proteinuria (> 1 g/24 hours), hematuria, or an elevated erythrocyte sedimentation rate (possible false-positive, depending on the laboratory method)
- Early pregnancy, ectopic pregnancy, or threatened abortion (possible false-negative)
- Chlorpromazine (Thorazine), methadone, and phenothiazines (possible false-positive)

# Human growth hormone, serum

Human growth hormone (hGH), also called *somatotropin,* is a protein secreted by acidophils of the anterior pituitary gland. It's the primary regulator of human growth. Unlike other pituitary hormones, hGH has no easily defined feedback mechanism or single target gland — it affects many body tissues. Like insulin, hGH promotes protein synthesis and stimulates amino acid uptake by cells. It also raises plasma glucose levels by inhibiting glucose uptake and utilization by cells, and increases free fatty acid concentrations by enhancing lipolysis.

Secretion of hGH appears to be regulated by the hypothalamus by means of a growth hormone-releasing factor and a growth hormone release-inhibiting factor (somatostatin). Secretion of hGH is diurnal and varies with such factors as exercise, sleep, stress, and nutritional status.

Hyposecretion or hypersecretion of this hormone may induce pathologic states (such as dwarfism or gigantism). Altered hGH levels are common in the patient with pituitary dysfunction.

This test, a quantitative analysis of plasma hGH levels, is usually performed as part of an anterior pituitary stimulation or suppression test. Such testing is crucial because clinical manifestations of an hGH deficiency can rarely be reversed by therapy.

## PURPOSE
- To aid differential diagnosis of dwarfism because growth retardation can result from pituitary or thyroid hypofunction
- To confirm diagnosis of acromegaly and gigantism in the adult
- To aid diagnosis of pituitary and hypothalamic tumors
- To help evaluate hGH therapy

## PATIENT PREPARATION
- Explain to the patient, or his parents if the patient is a child, that the serum hGH test measures hormone levels and helps determine the cause of abnormal growth.
- Instruct the patient to fast and limit activity for 10 to 12 hours before the test.

- Tell the patient that the test requires a blood sample. Explain who will perform the venipuncture and when. Inform him that another sample may have to be drawn the next day for comparison.
- Explain to the patient that he may experience slight discomfort from the tourniquet and needle puncture.
- Withhold all medications that affect hGH levels such as pituitary-based steroids. If they must be continued, note this on the laboratory request.
- Make sure the patient is relaxed and recumbent for 30 minutes before the test; stress and activity elevate hGH levels.

## PROCEDURE AND POSTTEST CARE

- Between 6 a.m. and 8 a.m. on 2 consecutive days, or as ordered, perform a venipuncture and collect at least 7 ml of blood in a clot-activator tube.
- Apply direct pressure to the venipuncture site until bleeding stops.
- If a hematoma develops at the venipuncture site, apply pressure.
- Instruct the patient that he may resume his usual diet, activities, and medications discontinued before the test, as ordered.

## PRECAUTIONS

- Handle the sample gently to prevent hemolysis.
- Send the sample to the laboratory immediately because hGH has a half-life of only 20 to 25 minutes.

## REFERENCE VALUES

Normal hGH levels for males range from undetectable to 5 ng/ml (SI, 5 µg/L); for females, from undetectable to 10 ng/ml (SI, 10 µg/L).

*Age alert* *Children's values may range from undetectable to 16 ng/ml (SI, 16 µg/L), and are usually higher.*

## ABNORMAL FINDINGS

Increased hGH levels may indicate a pituitary or hypothalamic tumor, usually an adenoma, which causes gigantism in children and acromegaly in adults and adolescents. Some patients with diabetes mellitus have elevated hGH levels without acromegaly. Suppression testing is necessary to confirm diagnosis.

Pituitary infarction, metastatic disease, and tumors may decrease hGH levels. Dwarfism may be due to low hGH levels, although only 15% of all cases of growth failure relate to endocrine dysfunction. Confirming the diagnosis requires stimulation testing with arginine or insulin.

## INTERFERING FACTORS

- Arginine, beta-adrenergic blockers such as propranolol (Inderal), and estrogens (increase)
- Amphetamines, bromocriptine (Parlodel), dopamine (Intropin), histamine, levodopa, methyldopa (Aldoril), and pituitary-based steroids (increase)
- Insulin (induced hypoglycemia), glucagon, and nicotinic acid (increase)
- Phenothiazines (such as chlorpromazine [Thorazine]) and corticosteroids (decrease)
- Radioactive scan performed within 1 week before the test

# Human immunodeficiency virus antibodies

The human immunodeficiency virus (HIV) antibodies test detects antibodies to HIV in serum. HIV is the virus that causes acquired immunodeficiency syndrome (AIDS). Transmission occurs by direct exposure of a person's blood to body fluids containing the virus. The virus may be transmitted from one person to another through exchange of contaminated blood and blood products, during sexual intercourse with an infected partner, when I.V. drugs are shared, and from an infected mother to her child during pregnancy or breast-feeding.

Initial identification of HIV is usually achieved through enzyme-linked immunosorbent assay. Positive findings are confirmed by Western blot test and immunofluorescence. Other tests may also be performed to detect antibodies. (See *Testing for HIV,* page 236.)

## PURPOSE

- To screen for HIV in the high-risk patient
- To screen donated blood for HIV

# Testing for HIV

Newer tests are available to help identify human immunodeficiency virus (HIV)-infected antibodies quicker and more conveniently, including a test to identify genetic changes that may alter the patient's course of treatment.

## OraQuick rapid HIV-1 antibody test

For the many people per year who don't check back for test results, rapid HIV testing may be done in any outpatient setting. The OraQuick rapid HIV-1 antibody test, approved by the U.S. Food and Drug Administration (FDA), allows results to be obtained in less than 20 minutes using 1 drop of blood. A color indicator similar to a home pregnancy test is used. If it's positive, another test must be done to confirm the results.

## Nucleic acid test

The FDA has also approved a nucleic acid test to screen plasma donation for HIV and hepatitis C. This test has been shown to dramatically reduce the waiting time involved until blood and blood products may be used.

## Gene-based test

Spikes of HIV virus in the bloodstream commonly mean that the individual being treated for HIV is growing resistant to the drug treatment being used. The U.S. government has approved the first gene-based test to help determine if an HIV-infected person's virus is mutating, making therapy fail. This test can help the physician to select more appropriate treatment.

## Patient preparation

- Explain to the patient that the HIV antibodies test detects HIV infection.
- Provide adequate counseling about the reasons for performing the test, which is usually requested by the patient's physician.
- If the patient has questions about his condition, be sure to provide full and accurate information.
- Tell the patient that the test requires a blood sample. Explain who will perform the venipuncture and when.
- Explain to the patient that he may experience slight discomfort from the tourniquet and needle puncture.

## Procedure and posttest care

- Perform a venipuncture, and collect the sample in a 10-ml barrier tube. Barrier tubes help prevent contamination when pouring the serum in the laboratory.
- Apply direct pressure to the venipuncture site until bleeding stops.
- If a hematoma develops at the venipuncture site, apply pressure.
- Keep test results confidential.
- When the patient receives the results, give him another opportunity to ask questions.
- Encourage the patient with positive screening tests to seek medical follow-up care, even if he's asymptomatic.

- Tell the patient to report early signs of AIDS, such as fever, weight loss, axillary or inguinal lymphadenopathy, rash, and persistent cough or diarrhea. Women should also report gynecologic symptoms.
- Tell the patient to assume that he can transmit HIV to others until conclusively proved otherwise. To prevent possible virus transmission, advise him about safer sex practices.
- Instruct the patient not to share razors, toothbrushes, or utensils (which may be contaminated with blood) and to clean such items with household bleach diluted 1:10 in water.
- Advise the patient against donating blood, tissues, or an organ.
- Warn the patient to inform his physician and dentist about his condition so that they can take proper precautions.

## Precautions

- Observe standard precautions when drawing a blood sample.
- Use gloves, properly dispose of needles, and use blood-fluid precaution labels on tubes, as necessary.
- Because the patient may have a compromised immune system, keep the venipuncture site clean and dry.

## Normal findings

Test results are normally negative.

## ABNORMAL FINDINGS

The test detects previous exposure to HIV. However, it doesn't identify a patient who has been exposed to the virus but hasn't yet made antibodies. In most cases, the patient with AIDS has antibodies to HIV. A positive test for the HIV antibody can't determine whether a patient harbors actively replicating virus or when the patient will manifest signs and symptoms of AIDS.

Many apparently healthy people have been exposed to HIV and have circulating antibodies. The test results for such people aren't false-positives. Furthermore, patients in the later stages of AIDS may exhibit no detectable antibody in their sera because they can no longer mount an antibody response.

## INTERFERING FACTORS

● None significant

# Human placental lactogen

A polypeptide hormone, human placental lactogen (hPL) — also known as *human chorionic somatomammotropin* — displays lactogenic and somatotropic (growth hormone) properties in a pregnant female. In combination with prolactin, hPL prepares the breasts for lactation. It also indirectly provides energy for maternal metabolism and fetal nutrition. It facilitates protein synthesis and mobilization essential to fetal growth. Secretion is autonomous, beginning at about 5 weeks' gestation and declining rapidly after delivery. According to some evidence, this hormone may not be essential for a successful pregnancy.

This radioimmunoassay measures plasma hPL levels, which are roughly proportional to placental mass. Such assays may be required in high-risk pregnancies (patients with diabetes mellitus or hypertension) and suspected placental tissue dysfunction. Because values vary widely during the latter half of pregnancy, serial determinations over several days provide the most reliable test results. This test, when combined with the measurement of estriol levels, is a reliable indicator of placental function and well-being. It may also be useful as a tumor marker in certain malignant states such as ectopic tumors that secrete hPL.

## PURPOSE

● To assess placental function and fetal well-being (combined with measurement of estriol levels)
● To aid diagnosis of hydatidiform mole and choriocarcinoma (human chorionic gonadotropin levels may be more useful in diagnosing these conditions)
● To aid diagnosis and monitor treatment of nontrophoblastic tumors that ectopically secrete hPL

## PATIENT PREPARATION

● Explain to the patient that the hPL test helps assess placental function and fetal well-being. If assessing fetal well-being isn't the diagnostic objective, offer an appropriate explanation.
● Tell the patient that the test requires a blood sample. Explain who will perform the venipuncture and when.
● Explain to the patient that she may experience slight discomfort from the tourniquet and needle puncture.
● Inform the pregnant patient that this test may be repeated during her pregnancy.

## PROCEDURE AND POSTTEST CARE

● Perform a venipuncture, and collect the sample in a 7ml clot-activator tube.
● Apply direct pressure to the venipuncture site until bleeding stops.
● If a hematoma develops at the venipuncture site, apply pressure.

## PRECAUTIONS

● Handle the sample gently to prevent hemolysis.
● Send the sample to the laboratory immediately.

## REFERENCE VALUES

For pregnant women, normal hPL levels vary with the gestational phase and slowly increase throughout pregnancy, reaching 8.6 µg/ml at term.
● 5 to 27 weeks: < 4.6 µg/ml
● 28 to 31 weeks: 2.4 to 6.1 µg/ml
● 32 to 35 weeks: 3.7 to 7.7 µg/ml
● 36 weeks to term: 5.0 to 8.6 µg/ml

At term, patients with diabetes may have mean levels of 9 to 11 µg/ml. Normal levels for males and nonpregnant females are less than 0.5 µg/ml.

## ABNORMAL FINDINGS

For reliable interpretation, hPL levels must be correlated with gestational age; for example, after 30 weeks' gestation, levels below 4 µg/ml may indicate placental dysfunction. Low hPL concentrations are also characteristically associated with postmaturity syndrome, intrauterine growth retardation, preeclampsia, and eclampsia. Declining concentrations may help differentiate incomplete abortion from threatened abortion.

Be aware that low hPL concentrations don't confirm fetal distress. Conversely, concentrations over 4 µg/ml after 30 weeks' gestation don't guarantee fetal well-being because elevated levels have been reported after fetal death.

An hPL value above 6 µg/ml after 30 weeks' gestation may suggest an unusually large placenta, commonly occurring in a patient with diabetes mellitus, multiple pregnancy, or Rh isoimmunization. The test's usefulness in predicting fetal death in a patient with diabetes mellitus and in managing Rh isoimmunization during pregnancy is limited.

Below-normal concentrations of hPL may be associated with trophoblastic neoplastic disease, such as hydatidiform mole and choriocarcinoma. Abnormal concentrations of hPL have been found in the sera of patients with other neoplastic disorders, including bronchogenic carcinoma, hepatoma, lymphoma, and pheochromocytoma. In these patients, hPL levels are used as tumor markers for evaluating chemotherapy, monitoring tumor growth and recurrence, and detecting residual tissue after excision.

## INTERFERING FACTORS

- Administration of radiopharmaceuticals within 24 hours of testing

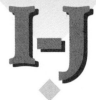

# I-J

## *Immune complex assays*

When immune complexes are produced faster than they can be cleared by the lymphoreticular system, immune complex disease, such as postinfectious syndromes, serum sickness, drug sensitivity, rheumatoid arthritis, and systemic lupus erythematosus (SLE), may occur. Immune complexes can develop when a certain ratio of antigen reacts with antibody of isotopes immunoglobulin (Ig) G 1, 2, 3, or IgM in tissues. These complexes can fix the first component of complement (C1) and activate the complement cascade. Subsequent complement-mediated activity leads to inflammation and local tissue necrosis. In the blood, soluble circulating immune complexes may also activate complement and eventually cause damage, usually in the renal glomeruli, the aorta, and other large blood vessels.

Histologic examination of tissue obtained by biopsy and the use of fluorescence or peroxidase staining with antibodies specific for immunologic types generally detect immune complexes. However, tissue biopsies can't provide information about titers of complexes still in circulation; therefore, serum assays, which detect circulating immune complexes indirectly, may be required. Because of the inherent variability of these complexes, several serum test methods may be appropriate using C1, rheumatoid factor (RF), or cellular substrates, such as Raji cells, as reagents.

Most immune complex assays haven't been standardized, so more than one test may be required to achieve accurate results.

### PURPOSE
- To demonstrate circulating immune complexes in serum
- To monitor the patient's response to therapy
- To estimate disease severity

### PATIENT PREPARATION
- Explain to the patient that the immune complex assay tests help evaluate his immune system.
- Inform the patient that the test will be repeated to monitor his response to therapy, if appropriate.
- Inform the patient that he need not restrict food and fluids.
- Tell the patient that the test requires a blood sample. Explain who will perform the venipuncture and when.
- Explain to the patient that he may experience slight discomfort from the tourniquet and needle puncture.
- If the patient is scheduled for C1q assay (a component of C1), check his history for recent heparin therapy and report such therapy to the laboratory.

### PROCEDURE AND POSTTEST CARE
- Perform a venipuncture and collect the sample in a 7-ml clot-activator tube.
- Because many patients with immune complexes have a compromised immune system, keep the venipuncture site clean and dry.

- Apply direct pressure to the venipuncture site until bleeding stops.
- If a hematoma develops at the venipuncture site, apply pressure.

## PRECAUTIONS
- Send the sample to the laboratory immediately to prevent deterioration of immune complexes.

## NORMAL FINDINGS
Normally, immune complexes aren't detectable in serum.

## ABNORMAL FINDINGS
The presence of detectable immune complexes in serum has etiologic importance in many autoimmune diseases, such as SLE and rheumatoid arthritis. For definitive diagnosis, the presence of these complexes must be considered with the results of other studies. For example, in SLE, immune complexes are associated with high titers of antinuclear antibodies and circulating antinative deoxyribonucleic acid antibodies.

Because of their filtering function, renal glomeruli seem vulnerable to immune complex deposition, although blood vessel walls and choroid plexuses (vascular folds in the ventricles of the brain) can be affected. Renal biopsy to detect immune complexes can provide conclusive evidence for immune complex (type III) glomerulonephritis, differentiating it from other types of glomerulonephritis.

Immune complexes may also occur with infectious diseases, such as bacterial endocarditis or hepatitis C, and neoplastic diseases, such as Hodgkin's disease.

## INTERFERING FACTORS
- Presence of cryoglobulins in the serum
- Inability to standardize RF inhibition tests and platelet aggregation assays

## *Insulin*

The insulin test, a radioimmunoassay, is a quantitative analysis of serum insulin levels. Insulin is usually measured concomitantly with glucose levels because glucose is the primary stimulus for insulin release from pancreatic islet cells. (See *How the pancreas produces insulin.*)

Insulin regulates the metabolism and transport or mobilization of carbohydrates, amino acids, proteins, and lipids. Stimulated by increased plasma levels of glucose, insulin secretion reaches peak levels after meals, when metabolism and food storage are greatest.

## PURPOSE
- To aid diagnosis of hyperinsulinemia as well as hypoglycemia resulting from a tumor or hyperplasia of pancreatic islet cells, glucocorticoid deficiency, or severe hepatic disease
- To aid diagnosis of diabetes mellitus and insulinresistant states

## PATIENT PREPARATION
- Explain to the patient that the insulin test helps determine if the pancreas is functioning normally.
- Instruct the patient to fast for 10 to 12 hours before the test.
- Tell the patient that the test requires a blood sample. Explain who will perform the venipuncture and when.
- Explain to the patient that he may experience slight discomfort from the tourniquet and needle puncture.
- Explain that questionable results may require a repeat test or a simultaneous glucose tolerance test, which requires that the patient drink a glucose solution.
- Withhold corticotropin, corticosteroids (including hormonal contraceptives), thyroid supplements, epinephrine, and other medications that may interfere with test results, as ordered. If they must be continued, note this on the laboratory request.
- Make sure the patient is relaxed and recumbent for 30 minutes before the test.

## PROCEDURE AND POSTTEST CARE
- Perform a venipuncture and collect one sample for insulin level in a 7-ml EDTA tube.
- Collect a sample for glucose level in a tube with sodium fluoride and potassium oxalate.
- Apply direct pressure to the venipuncture site until bleeding stops.
- If a hematoma develops at the venipuncture site, apply pressure.

# HOW THE PANCREAS PRODUCES INSULIN

The pancreas is composed of an exocrine portion—acinar cells, which secrete digestive enzymes—and an endocrine portion—the islets of Langerhans, which secrete insulin and glucagon into the bloodstream in response to changes in blood glucose levels. The islets of Langerhans contain two principal types of cells—beta cells, which produce insulin when blood glucose increases, and alpha cells, which produce glucagon when blood glucose de-creases. Splenic arteries transport oxygenated blood to the pancreas; mesenteric veins transport insulin and glucagon, contained in deoxygenated blood, from the pancreas.

Insulin lowers blood glucose levels by facilitating transport of glucose into cells and by increasing the conversion of glucose into liver and muscle glycogen; it also prevents break-down of liver glycogen to yield glucose. Glucagon exerts the opposite effect.

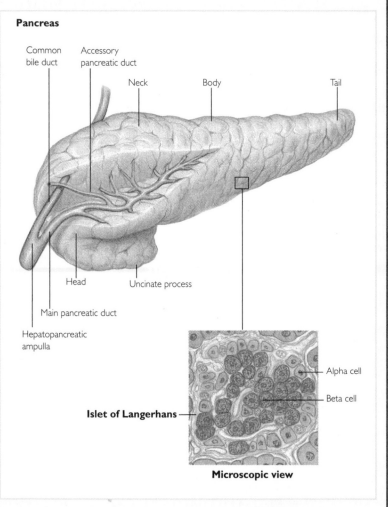

**Pancreas**

Common bile duct

Accessory pancreatic duct

Neck

Body

Tail

Head

Uncinate process

Main pancreatic duct

Hepatopancreatic ampulla

Alpha cell

Beta cell

**Islet of Langerhans**

**Microscopic view**

- Instruct the patient that he may resume his usual activities, diet, and medications discontinued before the test, as ordered.

## PRECAUTIONS
- Pack the insulin sample in ice, and send it, along with the glucose sample, to the laboratory immediately.
- In the patient with an insulinoma, fasting for this test may precipitate dangerously severe hypoglycemia. Keep an ampule of dextrose 50% available to counteract possible hypoglycemia.
- Handle the samples gently to prevent hemolysis.

## REFERENCE VALUES
Serum insulin levels normally range from 0 to 35 μU/ml (SI, 144 to 243 pmol/L).

## ABNORMAL FINDINGS
Insulin levels are interpreted in light of the prevailing glucose concentration. A normal insulin level may be inappropriate for the glucose results. High insulin and low glucose levels after a significant fast suggest the presence of an insulinoma. Prolonged fasting or stimulation testing may be required to confirm the diagnosis. In insulin-resistant diabetes mellitus, insulin levels are elevated; in non–insulin-resistant diabetes, they're low.

## INTERFERING FACTORS
- Agitation and stress
- Corticotropin, corticosteroids (including hormonal contraceptives), thyroid hormones, and epinephrine (possible increase)
- Use of insulin by the patient with type 2 diabetes mellitus (possible increase)
- High levels of insulin antibodies in the patient with type 1 diabetes mellitus

# Insulin tolerance test

The insulin tolerance test measures serum levels of human growth hormone (hGH) and corticotropin after administration of a loading dose of insulin. It's more reliable than direct measurement of hGH and corticotropin because many healthy people have undetectable fasting levels of these hormones. Insulin induced hypoglycemia stimulates hGH and corticotropin secretion in persons with an intact hypothalamic-pituitary-adrenal axis. Failure of stimulation indicates anterior pituitary or adrenal hypofunction and helps confirm an hGH or a corticotropin deficiency.

Because the insulin tolerance test stimulates an adrenergic response, it isn't recommended for patients with cardiovascular or cerebrovascular disorders, epilepsy, or low basal plasma cortisol levels.

## PURPOSE
- To aid diagnosis of hGH and corticotropin deficiency
- To identify pituitary dysfunction
- To aid differential diagnosis of primary and secondary adrenal hypofunction

## PATIENT PREPARATION
- Explain to the patient, or his parents if the patient is a child, that the insulin tolerance test evaluates hormonal secretion.
- Instruct the patient to fast and restrict physical activity for 10 to 12 hours before the test.
- Explain that the test involves I.V. infusion of insulin and the collection of multiple blood samples.
- Warn the patient that he may experience an increased heart rate, diaphoresis, hunger, and anxiety after administration of insulin. Reassure him that these symptoms are transient, and that if they become severe, the test will be discontinued.
- Tell the patient to lie down and relax for 90 minutes before the test.

## PROCEDURE AND POSTTEST CARE
- Between 6 a.m. and 8 a.m., perform a venipuncture and collect three 5-ml samples of blood for basal levels: one in a gray-top tube (for blood glucose) and two in green-top tubes (for hGH and corticotropin).
- Administer an I.V. bolus of U 100 regular insulin (0.15 U/kg, or as ordered) over 1 to 2 minutes.
- Use an indwelling venous catheter to avoid repeated venipunctures. Collect additional blood samples 15, 30, 45, 60, 90, and 120 minutes after insulin administration. At each interval, collect three samples: one in a tube with sodium fluoride and potassium oxidate and two in heparinized tubes. Label the tubes appropriately, and send them to the laboratory immediately.

- Apply direct pressure to the venipuncture site until bleeding stops.
- If a hematoma develops at the I.V. or venipuncture site, apply pressure.
- Instruct the patient that he may resume his usual diet, activities, and medications discontinued before the test, as ordered.

## PRECAUTIONS
- Make sure to have concentrated glucose solution readily available in the event that the patient has a severe hypoglycemic reaction to insulin.
- Handle the samples gently to prevent hemolysis.
- Label the tubes appropriately, including the collection times on the laboratory request, and send all samples to the laboratory immediately.

## REFERENCE VALUES
Normally, blood glucose falls to 50% of the fasting level 20 to 30 minutes after insulin administration. This stimulates a 10- to 20-ng/dl (SI, 10 to 20 μg/L) increase in baseline values for hGH and corticotropin, with peak levels occurring 60 to 90 minutes after insulin administration.

## ABNORMAL FINDINGS
Failure of stimulation or a blunted response suggests dysfunction of the hypothalamic-pituitary-adrenal axis. An hGH increase of less than 10 ng/dl (SI, < 10 μg/L) above baseline suggests hGH deficiency. A definitive diagnosis of hGH deficiency requires a supplementary stimulation test such as the arginine test. Additional testing is necessary to determine the site of the abnormality.

An increase in corticotropin levels of less than 10 ng/dl above baseline suggests adrenal insufficiency. The metyrapone or corticotropin stimulation test then confirms the diagnosis and determines whether the insufficiency is primary or secondary.

## INTERFERING FACTORS
- Corticosteroids and pituitary-based drugs (increase in hGH)
- Beta-adrenergic blockers and glucocorticoids (decrease in hGH)
- Alcohol, amphetamines, calcium gluconate, estrogens, glucocorticoids, methamphetamines, and spironolactone (Aldactone) (decrease in corticotropin)

# International Normalized Ratio

The International Normalized Ratio (INR) system is viewed as the best means of standardizing measurement of prothrombin time to monitor oral anticoagulant therapy. It isn't used as a screening test for coagulopathies.

## PURPOSE
- To evaluate the effectiveness of oral anticoagulant therapy

## PATIENT PREPARATION
- Explain to the patient that the INR test is used to determine the effectiveness of his oral anticoagulant therapy.
- Tell the patient that a blood sample will be taken. Explain who will perform the venipuncture and when.
- Explain to the patient that he may feel slight discomfort from the tourniquet and needle puncture.

## PROCEDURE AND POSTTEST CARE
- Perform a venipuncture, and collect the sample in a 4.5-ml tube with sodium citrate added.
- If a hematoma develops at the venipuncture site, apply pressure.

## PRECAUTIONS
- Completely fill the collection tube; otherwise, an excess of citrate appears in the sample.
- Gently invert the tube several times to thoroughly mix the sample and the anticoagulant.
- To prevent hemolysis, avoid excessive probing during venipuncture and handle the sample gently.
- Put the sample on ice, and send it to the laboratory promptly.

## REFERENCE VALUES
A normal INR for those receiving warfarin therapy is 2.0 to 3.0 (SI, 2.0 to 3.0). For those with mechanical prosthetic heart valves, an INR of 2.5 to 3.5 (SI, 2.5 to 3.5) is suggested.

## ABNORMAL FINDINGS

Increased INR values may indicate disseminated intravascular coagulation, cirrhosis, hepatitis, vitamin K deficiency, salicylate intoxication, uncontrolled oral anticoagulation, or massive blood transfusion.

## INTERFERING FACTORS

● None significant

# Intracranial computed tomography

Intracranial computed tomography (CT) provides a series of tomograms, translated by a computer and displayed on a monitor, representing cross-sectional images of various layers of the brain. This technique can reconstruct cross-sectional, horizontal, sagittal, and coronal plane images. Hundreds of thousands of readings of radiation levels absorbed by brain tissues may be combined to depict anatomic slices of varying thickness. Specificity and accuracy are enhanced by the degree of resolution, which depends on the number of radiation density calculations made by the computer. Although magnetic resonance imaging (MRI) has surpassed CT scanning in diagnosing neurologic conditions, the CT scan is more widely available and cost-effective and can be performed more easily in acute situations.

The increasing availability of CT scanners allows faster and safer diagnosis than in the past. In many cases, intracranial CT scanning eliminates the need for painful and hazardous invasive procedures, such as pneumoencephalography and cerebral angiography. CT scans, which usually use contrast enhancement, are especially valuable in assessing a patient with focal neurologic abnormalities and other clinical features that suggest an intracranial mass. In a patient with a suspected head injury, intracranial CT scans may allow the diagnosis of a subdural hematoma before characteristic symptoms appear.

## PURPOSE

● To diagnose intracranial lesions and abnormalities

● To monitor the effects of surgery, radiation therapy, or chemotherapy on intracranial tumors

● To serve as a guide for cranial surgery

## PATIENT PREPARATION

● Explain to the patient that intracranial CT permits assessment of the brain.

● Unless contrast enhancement is scheduled, inform the patient that there are no food or fluid restrictions. If contrast enhancement is scheduled, instruct him to fast for 4 hours before the test.

● Tell the patient that a series of X-ray films will be taken of his brain. Describe who will perform the test and where it will take place. Explain that the test will cause minimal discomfort.

● Tell the patient that he'll be positioned on a moving CT bed with his head immobilized and his face uncovered. The head of the table will then be moved into the scanner, which rotates around his head and makes loud clacking sounds.

● If a contrast medium is used, tell the patient that he may feel flushed and warm and may experience a transient headache, a salty or metallic taste, or nausea and vomiting after the contrast medium is injected.

● Instruct the patient to wear a gown (outpatients may wear comfortable clothing) and to remove all metal objects from the CT scan field.

● If the patient is restless or apprehensive, a sedative may be prescribed.

● Check the patient's history for hypersensitivity to shellfish, iodine, or contrast media, and mark your findings in his chart. Inform the physician of any sensitivities because he may order prophylactic medications or may choose not to use contrast enhancement.

## PROCEDURE AND POSTTEST CARE

● Place the patient in a supine position on an X-ray table with his head immobilized by straps, if required, and ask him to lie still.

● The head of the table is moved into the scanner, which rotates around the patient's head, taking radiographs at 1-degree intervals in a 180-degree arc.

● When this series of radiographs is completed, contrast enhancement is performed. Usually 50 to 100 ml of contrast medium is administered by I.V. injection or I.V. drip over 1 to 2 minutes.

# Comparing normal and abnormal CT scans

Shown here are two intracranial computed tomography (CT) scans. The scan on the left is normal. The scan on the right shows a large meningioma in the frontal region, represented by the white area.

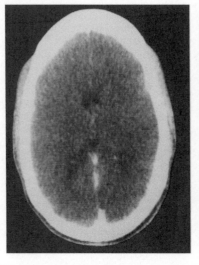 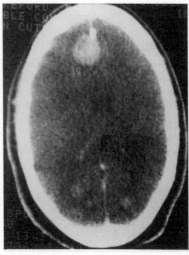

**Alert** *During intracranial CT, monitor the patient for hypersensitivity reactions, such as urticaria, respiratory difficulty, or rash. Reactions usually develop within 30 minutes.*

● After injection of the contrast medium, another series of scans is taken. Information from the scans is stored on magnetic tapes, fed into a computer, and converted into images on an oscilloscope. Photographs of selected views are taken for further study.

● If a contrast medium was used, watch the patient for residual adverse reactions (headache, nausea, and vomiting) and inform him that he may resume his usual diet.

## PRECAUTIONS

● Be aware that intracranial CT scanning with contrast enhancement is contraindicated in the patient who's hypersensitive to iodine or contrast medium.

● Know that iodine or contrast medium may be harmful or fatal to a fetus, especially during the first trimester.

## NORMAL FINDINGS

The tissue density determines the amount of radiation that passes through it. Tissue densities appear as white, black, or shades of gray on the computed image obtained by intracranial CT scanning. Bone, the densest tissue, appears white; ventricular and subarachnoid cerebrospinal fluid, the least dense, appears black. Brain matter appears in shades of gray. Structures are evaluated according to their density, size, shape, and position.

## ABNORMAL FINDINGS

Areas of altered density (they may be lighter or darker) or displaced vasculature or other structures may indicate an intracranial tumor, a hematoma, cerebral atrophy, an infarction, edema, or congenital anomalies such as hydrocephalus. (See *Comparing normal and abnormal CT scans*.)

Intracranial tumors vary significantly in appearance and characteristics. Metastatic tumors generally cause extensive edema in early stages and can usually be defined by contrast enhancement. Primary tumors vary in

# Understanding PET and SPECT

Like computed tomography (CT) scanning and magnetic resonance imaging, positron emission tomography (PET) and single-photon emission computed tomography (SPECT) provide brain images through sophisticated computer reconstruction algorithms. However, PET and SPECT images detail brain function as well as structure and thus differ significantly from the images provided by these other advanced techniques. PET and SPECT combine elements of CT scanning and conventional radionuclide imaging. For example, they measure the emissions of injected radioisotopes and convert them to a tomographic image of the brain. SPECT scanning uses gamma radiation with radionucleotides within the brain, and PET uses radioisotopes of biologically important elements — oxygen, nitrogen, carbon, and fluorine — that emit particles called positrons.

## HOW IT WORKS

During PET and SPECT, pairs of gamma rays are emitted; the scanner detects them and relays the information to a computer for reconstruction as an image. SPECT scanners use radionucleotides labeled with iodine and hexamethylpropyline amineoxime to detect blood flow. PET scanners omit positrons that can be chemically "tagged" to biologically active molecules, such as carbon monoxide, neurotransmitters, hormones, and metabolites (especially glucose), enabling study of their uptake and distribution in brain tissue. For example, blood tagged with $^{11}$C-carbon monoxide allows study of hemodynamic patterns in brain tissue; tagged neurotransmitters, hormones, and drugs allow mapping of receptor distribution.

Isotope-tagged glucose (which penetrates the blood-brain barrier rapidly) allows dynamic study of brain function because PET scans can pinpoint the sites of glucose metabolism in the brain under various conditions. Researchers expect SPECT and PET scanning to prove useful in the diagnosis of psychiatric disorders, transient ischemic attacks, amyotrophic lateral sclerosis, Parkinson's disease, Wilson's disease, multiple sclerosis, seizure disorders, cerebrovascular disease, and Alzheimer's disease. The reason is that all of these disorders may alter the location and patterns of cerebral glucose metabolism.

## COST FACTORS

PET scanning is a costly test because the radioisotopes used have very short half-lives and must be produced at an on-site cyclotron and attached quickly to the desired tracer molecules.

---

density and in their capacity to cause edema, displace ventricles, and absorb the contrast medium in contrast enhancement. Astrocytomas, for example, usually have low densities; meningiomas have higher densities and can generally be defined with contrast enhancement; glioblastomas, usually ill defined, are also enhanced after injection of a contrast medium.

Because the high density of blood contrasts markedly with low-density brain tissue, it's usually easy to detect subdural and epidural hematomas and other acute hemorrhages. Contrast enhancement helps locate subdural hematomas.

Cerebral atrophy customarily appears as enlarged ventricles with large sulci. Cerebral infarction may appear as low-density areas at the obstruction site or may not be apparent, especially within the first 24 hours or if the infarction is small or doesn't cause edema. With contrast enhancement, the infarcted area may not show in the acute phase, but will show clearly after resolution of the lesion. Cerebral edema usually appears as an area of marked generalized decreased density. In children, enlargement of the fourth ventricle generally indicates hydrocephalus.

The cerebral vessels usually don't appear on CT images. However, in the patient with arteriovenous malformation, cerebral vessels may appear with slightly increased density. Contrast enhancement allows a better view of the abnormal area, but MRI is now the preferred procedure for imaging cerebral vessels.

Another technology for obtaining brain images is positron emission tomography. (See *Understanding PET and SPECT.*)

## INTERFERING FACTORS

● Patient's head movement (possible poor imaging)

- Failure to remove metal objects from the scanning field (possible poor imaging)
- Hemorrhage (possible false-negative imaging due to change in hematoma)

# Iron and total iron-binding capacity

Iron is essential to the formation and function of hemoglobin as well as many other heme and nonheme compounds. After iron is absorbed by the intestine, it's distributed to various body compartments for synthesis, storage, and transport. (See *Normal iron metabolism*.)

Serum iron concentration is normally highest in the morning and declines progressively during the day; therefore, the sample should be drawn in the morning.

An iron assay is used to measure the amount of iron bound to transferrin in blood plasma. Total iron-binding capacity (TIBC) measures the amount of iron that would appear in plasma if all the transferrin were saturated with iron.

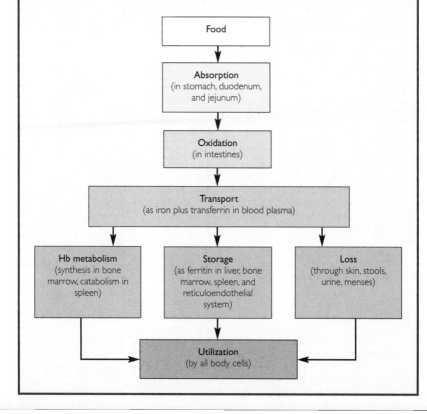

## NORMAL IRON METABOLISM

Ingested iron, absorbed and oxidated in the bowel, bonds with the protein transferrin for circulation to bone marrow, where hemoglobin (Hb) synthesis occurs, and to all iron-hungry body cells. In the spleen, Hb breakdown recycles iron back to the bone marrow or into storage. The body conserves iron, losing small amounts through skin, stools, urine, and menses. Storage areas in the liver, spleen, bone marrow, and reticuloendothelial system hold iron as ferritin until the body needs it; the liver alone stores about 60%.

Food

↓

Absorption
(in stomach, duodenum, and jejunum)

↓

Oxidation
(in intestines)

↓

Transport
(as iron plus transferrin in blood plasma)

↓

Hb metabolism
(synthesis in bone marrow, catabolism in spleen)

Storage
(as ferritin in liver, bone marrow, spleen, and reticuloendothelial system)

Loss
(through skin, stools, urine, menses)

↓

Utilization
(by all body cells)

# SIDEROCYTE STAIN

Siderocytes are red blood cells (RBCs) containing particles of nonhemoglobin iron known as siderocytic granules. In neonates, siderocytic granules are normally present in normoblasts and reticulocytes during hemoglobin synthesis. However, the spleen removes most of these granules from normal RBCs, and they disappear rapidly with age.

In adults, an elevated siderocyte level usually indicates abnormal erythropoiesis, which may occur in congenital spherocytic anemia, chronic hemolytic anemias (such as the thalassemias), pernicious anemia, hemochromatosis, toxicities (such as lead poisoning), infection, or severe burns. Elevated levels may also follow splenectomy because the spleen normally removes siderocytic granules.

## PERFORMING THE TEST
The siderocyte stain test measures the number of circulating siderocytes. Venous blood is drawn into a 3- or 4.5-ml EDTA tube or, for infants and children, collected in a Microtainer

or pipette and smeared directly on a 3″ × 5″ glass slide. When the blood smear is stained, siderocytic granules appear as purple-blue specks clustered around the periphery of mature erythrocytes. Cells containing these granules are counted as a percentage of total RBCs. The results aid differential diagnosis of the anemias and hemochromatosis and help detect toxicities.

## INTERPRETING RESULTS
Normally, neonates have a slightly elevated siderocyte level that reaches the normal adult value of 0.5% (SI, 0.05) of total RBCs in 7 to 10 days. In patients with pernicious anemia, the siderocyte level is 8% to 14% (SI, 0.08 to 0.14); in chronic hemolytic anemia, 20% to 100% (SI, 0.2 to 1.0); in lead poisoning, 10% to 30% (SI, 0.1 to 0.3); and in hemochromatosis, 3% to 7% (SI, 0.03 to 0.07). A high siderocyte level calls for additional testing (including bone marrow examination) to determine the cause of abnormal erythropoiesis.

---

Serum iron and TIBC are of greater diagnostic usefulness when performed with the serum ferritin assay, but together these tests may not accurately reflect the state of other iron compartments, such as myoglobin iron and the labile iron pool. Bone marrow or liver biopsy and iron absorption or excretion studies may yield more information.

## PURPOSE
- To estimate total iron storage
- To aid diagnosis of hemochromatosis
- To help distinguish iron deficiency anemia from anemia of chronic disease (For information on another test used to differentiate anemias, see *Siderocyte stain.*)
- To help evaluate nutritional status

## PATIENT PREPARATION
- Explain to the patient that the iron and total iron-binding capacity test evaluates the body's capacity to store iron.
- Tell the patient that a blood sample will be taken. Explain who will perform the venipuncture and when.

- Explain to the patient that he may feel slight discomfort from the tourniquet and needle puncture.
- Notify the laboratory and physician of medications the patient is taking that may affect test results; they may need to be restricted.
- Inform the patient that he need not restrict food and fluids.

## PROCEDURE AND POSTTEST CARE
- Perform a venipuncture, and collect the sample in a 4.5-ml clot-activator tube.
- If a hematoma develops at the venipuncture site, apply pressure.
- Instruct the patient that he may resume medications discontinued before the test, as ordered.

## PRECAUTIONS
- Handle the sample gently to prevent hemolysis.
- Send the sample to the laboratory immediately.

## REFERENCE VALUES

Normal serum iron and TIBC values are as follows:

- Serum iron
  - males—60 to 170 mcg/dl (SI, 10.7 to 30.4 µmol/L)
  - females—50 to 130 mcg/dl (SI, 9 to 23.3 µmol/L)
- TIBC
  - males and females—300 to 360 mcg/dl (SI, 54 to 64 mcmol/L)
- Saturation
  - males and females—20% to 50% (SI, 0.2 to 0.5).

## ABNORMAL FINDINGS

In iron deficiency, serum iron levels decrease and TIBC increases, decreasing saturation. In cases of chronic inflammation (such as in rheumatoid arthritis), serum iron may be low in the presence of adequate body stores, but TIBC may remain unchanged or may decrease to preserve normal saturation. Iron overload may not alter serum levels until relatively late but, in general, serum iron increases and TIBC remains the same, which increases the saturation.

## INTERFERING FACTORS

- Chloramphenicol and hormonal contraceptives (possible false-positive)
- Corticotropin (ACTH) (possible false-negative)
- Iron supplements (possible false-positive serum iron values but false-negative TIBC)

# Ketone test

In the ketone test, a routine, semiquantitative screening test, a commercially prepared product is used to measure the urine level of ketone bodies. Ketone bodies are the by-products of fat metabolism; they include acetoacetic acid, acetone, and beta-hydroxybutyric acid. Excessive amounts may appear in the patient with carbohydrate dehydration, which may occur in starvation or diabetic ketoacidosis (DKA).

Commercially available tests include the Acetest tablet, Chemstrip K, Ketostix, or Keto-Diastix. Each product measures a specific ketone body. For example, Acetest measures acetone, and Ketostix measures acetoacetic acid.

## PURPOSE
● To screen for ketonuria
● To identify DKA and carbohydrate deprivation
● To distinguish between a diabetic and a nondiabetic coma
● To monitor control of diabetes mellitus, ketogenic weight reduction, and treatment of DKA

## PATIENT PREPARATION
● Explain to the patient that the ketone test evaluates fat metabolism.
● If the patient is newly diagnosed with diabetes, tell him how to perform the test.
  **Alert** *If the patient is taking levodopa or phenazopyridine, use Acetest tablets because reagent strips may produce inaccurate results.*

## PROCEDURE AND POSTTEST CARE
● Instruct the patient to void; then give him a drink of water.
● Collect a second-voided midstream specimen about 30 minutes later.

### Acetest
● Lay the tablet on a piece of white paper, and place one drop of urine on the tablet.
● Compare the tablet color (white, lavender, or purple) with the color chart after 30 seconds.

### Ketostix
● Dip the reagent stick into the specimen, and remove it immediately.
● Compare the stick color (buff or purple) with the color chart after 15 seconds.
● Record the results as negative, small, moderate, or large amounts of ketones.

### Keto-Diastix
● Dip the reagent strip into the specimen, and remove it immediately.
● Tap the edge of the strip against the container or a clean, dry surface to remove excess urine.
● Hold the strip horizontally to prevent mixing the chemicals from the two areas.
● Interpret each area of the strip separately. Compare the color of the ketone section (buff or purple) with the appropriate color chart after exactly 15 seconds; compare the color of the glucose section after 30 seconds.
● Ignore color changes that occur after the specified waiting periods.
● Record the results as negative or positive for small, moderate, or large amounts of ketones.

## PRECAUTIONS

● Test the specimen within 60 minutes after it's obtained, or you must refrigerate it.
● Allow refrigerated specimens to return to room temperature before testing.
● Don't use tablets or strips that have become discolored or darkened.

## NORMAL FINDINGS

Normally, no ketones are present in urine.

## ABNORMAL FINDINGS

Ketonuria may occur in uncontrolled diabetes mellitus or starvation. It also occurs as a metabolic complication of total parenteral nutrition.

## INTERFERING FACTORS

● Failure to keep the reagent container tightly closed to prevent absorption of light or moisture or bacterial contamination of the specimen (false-negative)
● Levodopa and phenazopyridine (Pyridium) (false-positive results when Ketostix or Keto-Diastix is used instead of Acetest)

# Kidney-ureter-bladder radiography

Usually the first step in diagnostic testing of the urinary system, kidney-ureter-bladder (KUB) radiography surveys the abdomen to determine the position of the kidneys, ureters, and bladder and to detect gross abnormalities.

This test doesn't require intact renal function and may aid differential diagnosis of urologic and GI diseases, which commonly produce similar signs and symptoms. However, KUB radiography has many limitations and usually must be followed by more elaborate tests, such as excretory urography or renal computed tomography. KUB radiography shouldn't follow recent instillation of barium.

## PURPOSE

● To evaluate the size, structure, and position of the kidneys
● To screen for abnormalities, such as calcifications, in the region of the kidneys, ureters, and bladder

## PATIENT PREPARATION

● Explain to the patient that KUB radiography helps detect urinary system abnormalities.
● Inform the patient that he need not restrict food and fluids. Tell him who will perform the test, where it will take place, and that it takes only a few minutes.

## PROCEDURE AND POSTTEST CARE

● The patient is placed in a supine position in correct body alignment on an X-ray table. His arms are extended overhead, and the iliac crests are checked for symmetrical positioning.
● If the patient can't extend his arms or stand, he may lie on his left side with his right arm up.
● A single X-ray is taken.

## PRECAUTIONS

● A male patient should have gonadal shielding to prevent irradiation of the testes. A female patient's ovaries can't be shielded because they're too close to the kidneys, ureters, and bladder.

## NORMAL FINDINGS

The shadows of the kidneys appear bilaterally, the right slightly lower than the left. They should be approximately the same size, with the superior poles tilted slightly toward the vertebral column, paralleling the shadows (or stripes) produced by the psoas muscles. The ureters are only visible when an abnormality, such as calcification, is present. Visualization of the bladder depends on the density of its muscular wall and on the amount of urine in it. Generally, the bladder's shadow can be seen, but not as clearly as the kidneys' shadows.

## ABNORMAL FINDINGS

Bilateral renal enlargement may result from polycystic disease, multiple myeloma, lymphoma, amyloidosis, diabetes, hydronephrosis, or compensatory hypertrophy. A tumor, a cyst, or hydronephrosis may cause unilateral enlargement. Abnormally small kidneys may suggest end-stage glomerulonephritis or bilateral atrophic pyelonephritis. An apparent decrease in the size of one kidney suggests possible congenital hypoplasia, atrophic pyelonephritis, or ischemia. Renal displacement may be due to a retroperitoneal tumor such as an adrenal tumor. Obliteration or bulging of a portion of the psoas muscle stripe may result from a tumor, an abscess, or a hematoma.

Congenital anomalies, such as abnormal location or absence of a kidney, may be detected. Horseshoe kidney may be suggested by renal axes that parallel the vertebral column, especially if the inferior poles of the kidneys can't be clearly distinguished. A lobulated edge or border may suggest polycystic kidney disease or patchy atrophic pyelonephritis.

Opaque bodies may reflect calculi or vascular calcification due to aneurysm or atheroma; opacification may also suggest cystic tumors, fecaliths, foreign bodies, or abnormal fluid collection. Calcifications may appear anywhere in the urinary system, but positive identification requires further testing. The lone exception is staghorn calculus, which forms a perfect cast of the renal pelvis and calyces.

## INTERFERING FACTORS

- Contrast medium, foreign bodies, gas, or stools in the intestine (possible poor imaging)
- Calcified uterine fibromas or ovarian lesions
- Ascites or obesity (possible poor imaging)

# Lactate dehydrogenase

Lactate dehydrogenase (LD) catalyzes the reversible conversion of muscle lactic acid into pyruvic acid, an essential step in the metabolic process that ultimately produces cellular energy. Because LD is present in almost all body tissues, cellular damage increases total serum LD, limiting its diagnostic usefulness.

However, five tissue-specific isoenzymes can be identified and measured, using immunochemical separation and quantitation or electrophoresis. Two of these isoenzymes, $LD_1$ and $LD_2$, appear primarily in the heart, red blood cells (RBCs), and kidneys; $LD_3$, primarily in the lungs; and $LD_4$ and $LD_5$, in the liver and the skeletal muscles. Also, the midzone fractions ($LD_2$, $LD_3$, $LD_4$) can be elevated in granulocytic leukemia, lymphomas, and platelet disorders.

The specificity of LD isoenzymes and their distribution pattern is useful in diagnosing hepatic, pulmonary, and erythrocyte damage. However, their widest clinical application is in aiding diagnosis of acute myocardial infarction (MI). An LD isoenzyme assay is useful when creatine kinase (CK) hasn't been measured within 24 hours of an acute MI. The myocardial LD level rises later than CK (12 to 48 hours after infarction begins), peaks in 2 to 5 days, and drops to normal in 7 to 10 days if tissue necrosis doesn't persist. (See *LD isoenzyme variations in disease,* page 254.)

## PURPOSE

- To aid differential diagnosis of an MI, pulmonary infarction, anemias, and hepatic disease
- To support CK isoenzyme test results in diagnosing an MI or to provide diagnosis when CK-MB samples are drawn too late to display increase
- To monitor the patient's response to some forms of chemotherapy

## PATIENT PREPARATION

- Explain to the patient that the LD test is used primarily to detect tissue alterations.
- Tell the patient that the test requires a blood sample. Explain who will perform the venipuncture and when.
- Explain to the patient that he may experience slight discomfort from the tourniquet and needle puncture.
- Inform the patient that he need not restrict food and fluids.
- If an MI is suspected, tell the patient that the test will be repeated on the next two mornings to monitor progressive changes.

## PROCEDURE AND POSTTEST CARE

- Perform a venipuncture, and collect the sample in a 4-ml clot-activator tube.
- Apply direct pressure to the venipuncture site until bleeding stops.
- If a hematoma develops at the venipuncture site, apply pressure.

## PRECAUTIONS

- Draw the samples on schedule to avoid missing peak levels, and mark the collection time on the laboratory request.

# LD ISOENZYME VARIATIONS IN DISEASE

| DISEASE | LD$_1$ | LD$_2$ | LD$_3$ | LD$_4$ | LD$_5$ |
|---|---|---|---|---|---|
| **CARDIOVASCULAR** | | | | | |
| Myocardial infarction (MI) | Diagnostic | Diagnostic | | | Diagnostic |
| MI with hepatic congestion | Diagnostic | Diagnostic | | | |
| Rheumatic carditis | Diagnostic | | | | |
| Myocarditis | Diagnostic | | | | |
| Heart failure (decompensated) | | | | | Diagnostic |
| Shock | Diagnostic | Diagnostic | Diagnostic | Diagnostic | Diagnostic |
| Angina pectoris | Normal | | | | |
| **PULMONARY** | | | | | |
| Pulmonary embolism | Normal | | | | |
| Pulmonary infarction | | | Diagnostic | | |
| **HEMATOLOGIC** | | | | | |
| Pernicious anemia | Diagnostic | Diagnostic | Diagnostic | | |
| Hemolytic anemia | Diagnostic | Diagnostic | Diagnostic | | |
| Sickle cell anemia | Diagnostic | Diagnostic | Diagnostic | | |
| **HEPATOBILIARY** | | | | | |
| Hepatitis | | | | | Diagnostic |
| Active cirrhosis | | | | | Diagnostic |
| Hepatic congestion | | | | | Diagnostic |

**KEY**

| | | |
|---|---|---|
| Normal | Diagnostic | Not diagnostic |

- Handle the sample gently to prevent artifact blood sample hemolysis because RBCs contain LD$_1$.
- Send the sample to the laboratory immediately or, if transport is delayed, keep the sample at room temperature. Changes in temperature reportedly inactivate LD$_5$, thus altering isoenzyme patterns.

## REFERENCE VALUES

Total LD levels normally range from 71 to 207 U/L (SI, 1.2 to 3.52 μkat/L). Normal distribution is as follows:

- $LD_1$ — 14% to 26% (SI, 0.14 to 0.26) of total
- $LD_2$ — 29% to 39% (SI, 0.29 to 0.39) of total
- $LD_3$ — 20% to 26% (SI, 0.20 to 0.26) of total
- $LD_4$ — 8% to 16% (SI, 0.08 to 0.16) of total
- $LD_5$ — 6% to 16% (SI, 0.06 to 0.16) of total.

*Age alert* *LD levels in older adults may be increased slightly due to declining muscle mass and liver function.*

## ABNORMAL FINDINGS

Because many common diseases increase total LD levels, isoenzyme electrophoresis is usually necessary for diagnosis. In some disorders, total LD may be within normal limits, but abnormal proportions of each enzyme indicate specific organ tissue damage. For instance, in an acute MI, the concentration of $LD_1$ is greater than $LD_2$ within 12 to 48 hours after the onset of symptoms; therefore, the $LD_1/LD_2$ ratio is greater than 1. This reversal of the normal isoenzyme pattern is typical of myocardial damage and is known as flipped LD.

Midzone fractions ($LD_2$, $LD_3$, $LD_4$) can be increased in granulocytic leukemia, lymphomas, and platelet disorders.

## INTERFERING FACTORS

- Recent surgery or pregnancy (possible increase)
- Prosthetic heart valve (possible increase due to chronic hemolysis)
- Alcohol, anabolic steroids, anesthetics, opioids, and procainamide (Procanbid) (increase)

# Laparoscopy

Laparoscopy permits visualization of the peritoneal cavity by the insertion of a small fiber-optic telescope (laparoscope) through the anterior abdominal wall. This surgical technique may be used diagnostically to detect abnormalities, such as cysts, adhesions, fibroids, and infection. It can also be used therapeutically to perform procedures, such as adhesion lysis; ovarian biopsy; tubal sterilization; removal of ectopic pregnancies, fibroids, hydrosalpinx, and foreign bodies; and fulguration of endometriotic implants.

Although laparoscopy has largely replaced laparotomy, the latter is usually preferred when extensive surgery is indicated. Potential risks of laparoscopy include a punctured visceral organ, causing bleeding or spilling of intestinal contents into the peritoneum.

## PURPOSE

- To identify the cause of pelvic pain
- To help detect endometriosis, ectopic pregnancy, and pelvic inflammatory disease (PID)
- To evaluate pelvic masses or the fallopian tubes of the infertile patient
- To stage carcinoma in selected cases

## PATIENT PREPARATION

- Explain the procedure to the patient, and tell her that laparoscopy is used to detect abnormalities of the uterus, fallopian tubes, and ovaries.
- Instruct the patient to fast for at least 8 hours before surgery.
- Tell the patient who will perform the procedure and where it will take place.
- Tell the patient whether she'll receive a general anesthetic and whether the procedure will require an outpatient visit or overnight hospitalization.
- Warn the patient that she may experience pain at the puncture site and in the shoulder.
- Make sure that the patient or a responsible family member has signed an informed consent form.
- Check the patient's history for hypersensitivity to the anesthetic.
- Make sure laboratory work is completed and results are reported before the test.
- Instruct the patient to empty her bladder just before the test.

## PROCEDURE AND POSTTEST CARE

- The patient is anesthetized and placed in the lithotomy position.
- The examiner catheterizes the bladder and then performs a bimanual examination of the pelvic area to detect abnormalities that

may contraindicate the test and to ensure that the bladder is empty.

- The tenaculum is placed on the cervix and a uterine manipulator is inserted; an incision is made at the inferior rim of the umbilicus.
- The Veress needle is inserted into the peritoneal cavity, and 2 to 3 L of carbon dioxide or nitrous oxide is insufflated to distend the abdominal wall and provide an organ-free space for trocar insertion; the needle is removed and a trocar and sheath are inserted into the peritoneal cavity; multiple trocars may be inserted at the pubic hairline to allow access for other instruments.
- After removal of the trocar, the laparoscope is inserted through the sheath to examine the pelvis and abdomen.
- To evaluate tubal patency, the examiner infuses a dye through the cervix and observes the tubes for spillage.
- After the examination, minor surgical procedures, such as ovarian biopsy, may be performed.
- Monitor the patient's vital signs and urine output. Report sudden changes immediately; they may indicate complications.
- Monitor the patient for adverse or allergic reactions. After administration of a general anesthetic, monitor her electrolyte balance, hemoglobin level, and hematocrit. Help her ambulate after recovery.
- Tell the patient that she may resume her usual diet, as ordered.
- Instruct the patient to restrict activity for 2 to 7 days, as necessary.
- Reassure the patient that some abdominal and shoulder pain is normal and should disappear within 24 to 36 hours. If pain continues or worsens, notify the physician immediately as this may be a sign of bowel perforation. Provide analgesics, as ordered, and monitor her for adverse effects.

## PRECAUTIONS

- Be aware that laparoscopy is contraindicated in the patient with advanced abdominal wall cancer, advanced pulmonary or cardiovascular disease, intestinal obstruction, palpable abdominal mass, large abdominal hernia, chronic tuberculosis, or a history of peritonitis.
- During the procedure, check for proper catheter drainage.

## NORMAL FINDINGS

The uterus and fallopian tubes are of normal size and shape, free from adhesions, and mobile. The ovaries are of normal size and shape; cysts and endometriosis are absent. Dye injected through the cervix flows freely from the fimbria.

## ABNORMAL FINDINGS

An ovarian cyst appears as a bubble on the surface of the ovary. The cyst may be clear if filled with follicular fluid or serous or mucous material, or it may be red, blue, or brown if filled with blood. Adhesions may appear as thick and fibrous tissue or as almost transparent strands of tissue.

Endometriosis may resemble small, blue powder burns on the peritoneum or the serosa of any pelvic or abdominal structure; however, clear, red lesions are also possible. Fibroids appear as lumps on the uterus, hydrosalpinx as an enlarged fallopian tube, and ectopic pregnancy as an enlarged or ruptured fallopian tube. In PID, infection or abscess is evident.

## INTERFERING FACTORS

- Adhesions or marked obesity (possible obstruction to visualization)
- Tissue or fluid becoming attached to the lens (possible obstruction to visualization)

## *Laryngoscopy, direct*

Direct laryngoscopy allows visualization of the larynx by the use of a fiber-optic endoscope or laryngoscope passed through the mouth or nose and pharynx to the larynx. It's indicated for any condition requiring direct visualization or specimen samples for diagnosis, such as in patients with strong gag reflexes due to anatomic abnormalities, and those who have had no response to short-term therapy for symptoms of pharyngeal or laryngeal disease, such as stridor and hemoptysis. Secretions or tissue may be removed during this procedure for further study. The test is usually contraindicated in patients with epiglottiditis but may be performed on them in an operating room with resuscitative equipment available.

## PURPOSE

- To detect lesions, strictures, or foreign bodies
- To remove benign lesions or foreign bodies from the larynx
- To aid in the diagnosis of laryngeal or upper airway abnormalities
- To examine the larynx when indirect laryngoscopy is inadequate

## PATIENT PREPARATION

- Explain to the patient that direct laryngoscopy is used to detect laryngeal abnormalities.
- Instruct the patient to fast for 6 to 8 hours before the test.
- Tell the patient who will perform the procedure and where it will be done.
- Inform the patient that he'll receive a sedative to help him relax, medication to reduce secretions and, during the procedure, a general or local anesthetic. Reassure him that this procedure won't obstruct his airway.
- Make sure that the patient or a responsible family member has signed an informed consent form.
- Check the patient's history for hypersensitivity to the anesthetic.
- Obtain the patient's baseline vital signs.
- Administer the sedative and other medication (usually 30 minutes to 1 hour before the test), as ordered.
- Instruct the patient to remove dentures, contact lenses, and jewelry and to void before giving him a sedative.

## PROCEDURE AND POSTTEST CARE

- Place the patient in the supine position.
- Encourage the patient to breathe through his nose and to relax with his arms at his sides.
- Assist as appropriate when a general anesthetic is administered or when the patient's mouth and throat are sprayed with a local anesthetic.
- A laryngoscope is introduced through the patient's mouth or nostril, the larynx is examined for abnormalities, and a specimen or secretions may be removed for further study; minor surgery, such as removal of polyps or nodules, may be performed at this time.
- Place the specimens in their respective containers. Specimen collection should be done in accordance with laboratory and pathology guidelines.

- Place the conscious patient in semi-Fowler's position; place the unconscious patient on his side with his head slightly elevated to prevent aspiration.
- Check the patient's vital signs according to facility protocol, or every 15 minutes until the patient is stable and then every 30 minutes for 2 hours, every hour for the next 4 hours, and then every 4 hours for 24 hours. Immediately report to the physician any adverse reaction to the anesthetic or sedative (tachycardia, palpitations, hypertension, euphoria, excitation, and rapid, deep respirations).
- Apply an ice collar to minimize laryngeal edema.
- Provide an emesis basin, and instruct the patient to spit out saliva rather than swallow it. Observe sputum for blood and report excessive bleeding immediately.
- Instruct the patient to refrain from clearing his throat and coughing to prevent hemorrhaging at the biopsy site.
- Advise the patient to avoid smoking until his vital signs are stable and there's no evidence of complications.
- Immediately report subcutaneous crepitus around the patient's face and neck, which may indicate tracheal perforation.
- Listen to the patient's neck with a stethoscope for signs of stridor and airway obstruction.

> **Alert** *Observe the patient with epiglottiditis for signs of airway obstruction and immediately report signs of respiratory difficulty. Keep emergency resuscitation equipment available; keep a tracheotomy tray nearby for 24 hours.*

- Restrict food and fluids to avoid aspiration until the gag reflex returns (usually within 2 hours). Then the patient may resume his usual diet, beginning with sips of water.
- Reassure the patient that voice loss, hoarseness, and sore throat are temporary. Provide throat lozenges or a soothing liquid gargle when his gag reflex returns.

## PRECAUTIONS

- Send the specimens to the laboratory immediately.

## NORMAL FINDINGS

A normal larynx shows no evidence of inflammation, lesions, strictures, or foreign bodies.

## ABNORMAL FINDINGS

The combined results of direct laryngoscopy, biopsy, and radiography may indicate laryngeal carcinoma. Direct laryngoscopy may also show benign lesions, strictures, or foreign bodies and, with a biopsy, may distinguish laryngeal edema from a radiation reaction or tumor. It can also determine vocal cord dysfunction.

## INTERFERING FACTORS

- Inability to pass scope

---

# Leucine aminopeptidase

The leucine aminopeptidase (LAP) test is used to measure serum levels of LAP, an isoenzyme of alkaline phosphatase (ALP) that's widely distributed in body tissues. The greatest concentrations appear in the hepatobiliary tissues, pancreas, and small intestine. Serum LAP levels parallel serum ALP levels in hepatic disease.

## PURPOSE

- To provide information about suspected liver, pancreatic, and biliary diseases
- To differentiate skeletal disease from hepatobiliary or pancreatic disease
- To evaluate neonatal jaundice

## PATIENT PREPARATION

- Explain to the patient that the leucine aminopeptidase test is used to evaluate liver and pancreatic function.
- Tell the patient that the test requires a blood sample. Explain who will perform the venipuncture and when.
- Explain to the patient that he may experience slight discomfort from the tourniquet and needle puncture.
- Tell the patient to fast for at least 8 hours before the test.
- Notify the laboratory and physician of medications the patient is taking that may affect test results; they may need to be restricted.

## PROCEDURE AND POSTTEST CARE

- Perform a venipuncture, and collect the sample in a 4-ml clot-activator tube.

- Apply direct pressure to the venipuncture site until bleeding stops.
- Instruct the patient that he may resume his usual diet and medications discontinued before the test, as ordered.

## PRECAUTIONS

- Handle the sample gently to avoid hemolysis.
- Transport the sample to the laboratory immediately.

## REFERENCE VALUES

Normal values are 80 to 200 U/ml (SI, 80 to 200 kU/L) in males and 75 to 185 U/ml (SI, 75 to 185 kU/L) in females.

## ABNORMAL FINDINGS

Elevated levels can occur in biliary obstruction, tumors, strictures, and atresia; advanced pregnancy; and therapy with drugs containing estrogen or progesterone.

## INTERFERING FACTORS

- Advanced pregnancy (false-high)
- Estrogen or progesterone (false-high)

---

# Lipase, serum

Lipase is produced in the pancreas and secreted into the duodenum, where it converts triglycerides and other fats into fatty acids and glycerol. The destruction of pancreatic cells, which occurs in acute pancreatitis, causes large amounts of lipase to be released into the blood. (See *Blocked enzyme pathway*.) The lipase test is used to measure serum lipase levels; it's most useful when performed with a serum or urine amylase test.

## PURPOSE

- To aid diagnosis of acute pancreatitis

## PATIENT PREPARATION

- Explain to the patient that the serum lipase test is used to evaluate pancreatic function.
- Tell the patient that the test requires a blood sample. Explain who will perform the venipuncture and when.
- Inform the patient that he may experience slight discomfort from the tourniquet and needle puncture.

## BLOCKED ENZYME PATHWAY

The pancreas secretes lipase, amylase, and other enzymes that pass through the pancreatic duct into the duodenum. In pancreatitis and obstruction of the pancreatic duct by a tumor or calculus (shown below), these enzymes can't reach their intended destination. Instead, they're diverted into the bloodstream by a mechanism that isn't fully understood.

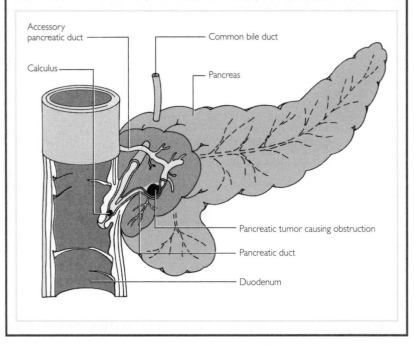

Accessory pancreatic duct

Common bile duct

Calculus

Pancreas

Pancreatic tumor causing obstruction

Pancreatic duct

Duodenum

---

● Instruct the patient to fast overnight before the test.

● Notify the laboratory of medications the patient is taking that may affect test results; they may need to be restricted.

### PROCEDURE AND POSTTEST CARE

● Perform a venipuncture and collect the sample in a 4-ml clot-activator tube.

● Apply direct pressure to the venipuncture site until bleeding stops.

● If a hematoma develops at the venipuncture site, apply pressure.

● Instruct the patient that he may resume his usual diet and medications discontinued before the test, as ordered.

### PRECAUTIONS

● Handle the sample gently to prevent hemolysis.

### REFERENCE VALUES

Serum lipase levels are normally less than 160 U/L (SI, < 2.72 μkat/L).

### ABNORMAL FINDINGS

High lipase levels suggest acute pancreatitis or pancreatic duct obstruction. After an acute attack, levels remain elevated for up to 14 days. Lipase levels may also increase in other pancreatic injuries, such as perforated peptic ulcer with chemical pancreatitis due to gastric juices, and in a patient with high intestinal obstruction, pancreatic cancer, or renal disease with impaired excretion.

## INTERFERING FACTORS

● Cholinergics, codeine, meperidine (Demerol), and morphine (false-high due to spasm of the sphincter of Oddi)

# Lipoprotein electrophoresis

Lipoprotein electrophoresis involves fractionation and phenotyping tests. Fractionation tests are used to isolate and measure the types of cholesterol in serum: low-density lipoproteins (LDLs) and high-density lipoproteins (HDLs). The HDL level is inversely related to the risk of coronary artery disease (CAD); the higher the HDL level, the lower the incidence of CAD. Conversely, the higher the LDL level, the higher the incidence of CAD.

Lipoprotein phenotyping is used to determine levels of the four major lipoproteins: chylomicrons, very-low-density (prebeta) lipoproteins, low-density (beta) lipoproteins, and high-density (alpha) lipoproteins. (See *Familial hyperlipoproteinemias*.) Detecting altered lipoprotein patterns is essential in identifying hyperlipoproteinemia and hypolipoproteinemia.

## PURPOSE

● To assess the risk of CAD
● To assess the efficacy of lipid-lowering drug therapy
● To determine the classification of hyperlipoproteinemia and hypolipoproteinemia (phenotyping)

## PATIENT PREPARATION

● Tell the patient that the fractionation test is used to determine his risk of CAD and that lipoprotein typing is used to determine how the body metabolizes fats.
● Tell the patient that the test requires a blood sample. Explain who will perform the venipuncture and when.
● Explain to the patient that he may experience slight discomfort from the tourniquet and needle puncture.
● Instruct the patient to maintain his normal diet for 2 weeks before the test, to abstain from alcohol for 24 hours before the test, and to fast and avoid exercise for 12 to 14 hours before the test. For the phenotyping

test, provide a low-fat meal the night before the test.
● Notify the laboratory and physician of medications the patient is taking that may affect test results; they may need to be restricted.

### Phenotyping test

● Check the patient's drug history for heparin use. As ordered, withhold antilipemics, such as cholestyramine, about 2 weeks before the test.
● Notify the laboratory if the patient is receiving treatment for another condition that might significantly alter lipoprotein metabolism, such as diabetes mellitus, nephrosis, or hypothyroidism.

## PROCEDURE AND POSTTEST CARE

● Perform a venipuncture and collect the sample. Use a 7-ml EDTA tube for fractionation test and a 4-ml EDTA tube for phenotyping test.
● Apply direct pressure to the venipuncture site until bleeding stops.
● If a hematoma develops at the venipuncture site, apply pressure.
● Instruct the patient that he may resume his usual diet and medications discontinued before the test, as ordered.

## PRECAUTIONS

● When drawing multiple samples, collect the sample for lipoprotein phenotyping first because venous obstruction for 2 minutes can affect test results.
● Fill the collection tube completely and invert it gently several times to mix the sample and the anticoagulant thoroughly.
● Handle the sample gently to prevent hemolysis.
● Send the sample to the laboratory immediately to avoid spontaneous redistribution among the lipoproteins.
● If the sample can't be transported immediately, refrigerate it but don't freeze it.

## REFERENCE VALUES

Normal lipoprotein values vary by age, sex, geographic area, and ethnic group; check the laboratory for reference values. HDL levels range from 37 to 70 mg/dl (SI, 0.96 to 1.8 mmol/L) for males and from 40 to 85 mg/dl (SI, 1.03 to 2.2 mmol/L) for females. LDL levels are less than 130 mg/dl

# FAMILIAL HYPERLIPOPROTEINEMIAS

| TYPE | CAUSES AND INCIDENCE | CLINICAL SIGNS | LABORATORY FINDINGS |
|---|---|---|---|
| I | ◆ Deficient lipoprotein lipase, resulting in increased chylomicrons<br>◆ May be induced by alcoholism<br>◆ Incidence: rare | ◆ Eruptive xanthomas<br>◆ Lipemia retinalis<br>◆ Abdominal pain | ◆ Increased chylomicron, total cholesterol, and triglyceride levels<br>◆ Normal or slightly increased VLDLs<br>◆ Normal or decreased LDLs and high-density lipoproteins<br>◆ Cholesterol-triglyceride ratio < 0.2 |
| IIa | ◆ Deficient cell receptor, resulting in increased low-density lipoproteins (LDL) and excessive cholesterol synthesis<br>◆ May be induced by hypothyroidism<br>◆ Incidence: common | ◆ Premature coronary artery disease (CAD)<br>◆ Arcus cornea<br>◆ Xanthelasma<br>◆ Tendinous and tuberous xanthomas | ◆ Increased LDL<br>◆ Normal VLDL<br>◆ Cholesterol-triglyceride ratio > 2.0 |
| IIb | ◆ Deficient cell receptor, resulting in increased LDL and excessive cholesterol synthesis<br>◆ May be induced by dysgammaglobulinemia, hypothyroidism, uncontrolled diabetes mellitus, and nephrotic syndrome<br>◆ Incidence: common | ◆ Premature CAD<br>◆ Obesity<br>◆ Possible xanthelasma | ◆ Increased LDL, VLDL, total cholesterol, and triglycerides |
| III | ◆ Unknown cause, resulting in deficient very-low-density lipoproteins (VLDL)-to-LDL conversion<br>◆ May be induced by hypothyroidism, uncontrolled diabetes mellitus, and paraproteinemia<br>◆ Incidence: rare | ◆ Premature CAD<br>◆ Arcus cornea<br>◆ Eruptive tuberous xanthomas | ◆ Increased total cholesterol, VLDL, and triglycerides<br>◆ Normal or decreased LDL<br>◆ Cholesteroltriglyceride ratio of > 0.4<br>◆ Broad beta band observed on electrophoresis |
| IV | ◆ Unknown cause, resulting in decreased levels of lipase<br>◆ May be induced by uncontrolled diabetes mellitus, alcoholism, pregnancy, steroid or estrogen therapy, dysgammaglobulinemia, and hyperthyroidism<br>◆ Incidence: common | ◆ Possible premature CAD<br>◆ Obesity<br>◆ Hypertension<br>◆ Peripheral neuropathy | ◆ Increased VLDL and triglycerides<br>◆ Normal LDL<br>◆ Cholesterol-triglyceride ratio of < 0.25 |
| V | ◆ Unknown cause, resulting in defective triglyceride clearance<br>◆ May be induced by alcoholism, dysgammaglobulinemia, uncontrolled diabetes mellitus, nephrotic syndrome, pancreatitis, and steroid therapy<br>◆ Incidence: rare | ◆ Premature CAD<br>◆ Abdominal pain<br>◆ Lipemia retinalis<br>◆ Eruptive xanthomas<br>◆ Hepatosplenomegaly | ◆ Increased VLDL, total cholesterol, and triglyceride levels<br>◆ Chylomicrons present<br>◆ Cholesterol-triglyceride ratio < 0.6 |

# PLAC TEST

The PLAC test, a new blood test that can help determine who might be at risk for coronary artery disease (CAD), was recently approved by the U.S. Food and Drug Administration (FDA). The FDA's decision was based on a recent study of more than 1,300 patients, which was a part of a large multicenter study sponsored by the National Heart, Lung, and Blood Institute.

The PLAC test works by measuring lipoprotein-associated phospholipase $A_2$, an enzyme produced by macrophages, a type of white blood cell. When heart disease is present, macrophages increase production of the enzyme. According to the FDA, an elevated PLAC test result, in conjunction with a low-density-lipoprotein (LDL) cholesterol level of less than 130 mg/dl, generally indicates that a patient has two to three times the risk of CAD compared with similar patients with lower PLAC test results. The study also found that those people with the highest PLAC test results and LDL cholesterol levels lower than 130 mg/dl had the greatest risk of heart disease.

(SI, < 3.36 mmol/L) in individuals who don't have CAD. Borderline high levels are greater than 160 mg/dl (SI, > 4.1 mmol/L).

The American College of Cardiology recommends an HDL of 40 mg/dl or higher with women maintaining an HDL cholesterol of at least 45 mg/dl. HDL levels greater than 60 mg/dl are considered heart healthy. LDL levels should optimally be less than 100 mg/dl, with levels of 60 mg/dl or more considered high.

## ABNORMAL FINDINGS

High LDL levels increase the risk of CAD. Elevated HDL levels generally reflect a healthy state but can also indicate chronic hepatitis, early-stage primary biliary cirrhosis, and alcohol consumption. Increased HDL levels can occur as a result of long-term aerobic and vigorous exercise. Rarely, a sharp rise (to as high as 100 mg/dl [SI, 2.58 mmol/L]) in a second type of HDL (alpha$_2$-HDL) may signal CAD. (See *PLAC test*.)

The types of hyperlipoproteinemias and hypolipoproteinemias are identified by characteristic electrophoretic patterns.

Familial lipoprotein disorders are classified as either hyperlipoproteinemias or hypolipoproteinemias. There are six types of hyperlipoproteinemias: I, IIa, IIb, III, IV, and V. Types IIa, IIb, and IV are relatively common. All hypolipoproteinemias are rare, including hypobetalipoproteinemia, betalipoproteinemia, and alpha-lipoprotein deficiency.

## INTERFERING FACTORS

● Concurrent illness, especially if accompanied by fever, recent surgery, or myocardial infarction
● Administration of heparin (which activates the enzyme lipase, producing fatty acids from triglycerides) or collection of sample in a heparinized tube (possible false-high due to activation of the enzyme lipase, which causes release of fatty acids from triglycerides)
● Antilipemic medications, such as cholestyramine (Questran), gemfibrozil, and niacin (decrease)
● Alcohol, disulfiram, hormonal contraceptives, miconazole, and high doses of phenothiazines (possible increase in fractionation)
● Estrogens (possible increase or decrease in fractionation)
● Presence of bilirubin, hemoglobin, iodine, salicylates, and vitamins A and D (altered fractionation results)

# Liver-spleen scanning

In liver-spleen scanning, a gamma camera records the distribution of radioactivity within the liver and spleen after I.V. injection of a radioactive colloid. The colloid most commonly used, technetium 99m ($^{99m}$Tc) sulfide, concentrates in the reticuloendothelial cells through phagocytosis. About 80% to 90% of the injected colloid is taken up by Kupffer's cells in the liver, 5% to 10% by the spleen, and 3% to 5% by bone marrow. The gamma camera images either organ instantaneously without moving.

Although the indications for this test include the detection of focal disease, such as tumors, cysts, and abscesses, liver-spleen scanning demonstrates focal disease non-specifically as a "cold spot" (a defect that fails to take up the colloid) and may fail to detect focal lesions smaller than $3/4"$ (2 cm) in diameter. Although clinical signs and symptoms may aid diagnosis, liver-spleen scanning usually requires confirmation by ultrasonography, computed tomography (CT) scan, gallium scanning, or biopsy. CT scan is the fastest method of evaluating liver or splenic injury in abdominal trauma and is preferred to other scans.

## PURPOSE
- To screen for hepatic metastasis and hepatocellular disease, such as cirrhosis and hepatitis
- To detect focal disease, such as tumors, cysts, and abscesses, in the liver and spleen
- To demonstrate hepatomegaly or splenomegaly (in patients with palpable abdominal masses)
- To assess the condition of the liver and spleen after abdominal trauma

## PATIENT PREPARATION
- Explain to the patient that liver-spleen scanning permits examination of the liver and spleen through scintigrams or scans taken after I.V. injection of a radioactive substance.
- Inform the patient that he need not restrict food and fluids.
- Tell the patient who will perform the test and where it will take place.
- Explain to the patient that he may experience transient discomfort from the needle puncture.
- Make sure the patient isn't scheduled for more than one radionuclide scan on the same day.
- Assure the patient that the injection isn't dangerous because the test substance contains only trace amounts of radioactivity and allergic reactions to it are rare.
- Explain to the patient that the detector head of the gamma camera may touch his abdomen (if appropriate) and reassure him that this isn't dangerous.
- Advise the patient that he'll be asked to lie still and to breathe quietly during the procedure to ensure good quality images; he may also be asked to hold his breath briefly. Explain that this technique helps to evaluate liver mobility and pliability.

- Make sure that the patient or a responsible family member has signed an informed consent form.

## PROCEDURE AND POSTTEST CARE
- The $^{99m}$Tc sulfide is injected I.V.; after 10 to 15 minutes, the patient's abdomen is scanned with the patient placed in supine, left and right lateral, left and right anterior oblique, and prone positions to ensure optimal visualization of the liver and spleen.
- The left anterior oblique position provides the best view of the spleen separate from the left lobe of the liver. With the patient supine, liver mobility and pliability may be evaluated by marking the costal margin and scanning as the patient breathes deeply (fixation suggests disease).
- The scintigrams are reviewed for clarity before the patient is allowed to leave. If necessary, additional views are obtained.

⊛ **Alert** *During liver-spleen scanning, watch for anaphylactoid reactions (shortness of breath, chest tightness, itching, headache) or pyrogenic (fever-producing) reactions, which may result from a stabilizer, such as dextran or gelatin, added to $^{99m}$Tc sulfide.*

- Inform the patient that the radioactive substance is eliminated from the body within 6 to 24 hours. Urge him to increase his fluid intake (unless contraindicated) to encourage this process.
- Instruct the patient to flush the toilet immediately after urinating to reduce exposure to radiation in the urine.

## PRECAUTIONS
- Be aware that liver-spleen scanning is usually contraindicated in a child and in the pregnant or lactating patient.

## NORMAL FINDINGS
Because the liver and spleen contain equal numbers of reticuloendothelial cells, both organs normally appear equally bright on the image. However, distribution of radioactive colloid is generally more uniform and homogeneous in the spleen than in the liver. The liver has various normal indentations and impressions, such as the gallbladder fossa and falciform ligament, that may mimic focal disease. (See *Identifying liver indentations in nuclear imaging,* page 264.)

# IDENTIFYING LIVER INDENTATIONS IN NUCLEAR IMAGING

In nuclear imaging, normal indentations and impressions may be mistaken for focal lesions. These drawings of the liver—anterior and posterior view—identify the contours and impressions that may be misread.

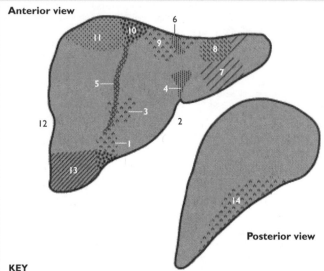

**Anterior view**

**Posterior view**

**KEY**

1. Gallbladder fossa
2. Ligamentum teres and falciform ligament
3. Hilum, main branching of the portal vein
4. Pars umbilicalis portion, left portal vein
5. Variable stripe of lobar fissure between right and left lobes
6. Variable stripe of semental fissure, left lobe
7. Thinning of left lobe
8. Impression of pectus excavatum
9. Cardiac impression
10. Hepatic veins and inferior vena cava
11. Shielding from right female breast
12. Harrison's groove or costal impression
13. Impression of hepatic flexure of colon
14. Right renal impression

## ABNORMAL FINDINGS

Although liver-spleen scanning may fail to detect early hepatocellular disease, it shows characteristic, distinct patterns as disease progresses. The most prominent sign of hepatocellular disease is a shift of the radioactive colloid that's caused by reduced hepatic blood flow and impaired Kupffer's cell function. This inhibits distribution of the colloid in the liver, causing the liver colloid distribution to appear uniformly decreased or patchy. The spleen and bone marrow then take up the abnormally large amounts of the colloid unabsorbed by the liver, thus concentrating more radioactivity than in the liver, and appear brighter on the scan. This same distribution pattern (colloid shift) also accompanies portal hypertension due to extrahepatic causes.

Hepatitis and cirrhosis are associated with hepatomegaly and a colloid shift, but certain characteristics help distinguish them. In hepatitis, colloid distribution is usually uniformly decreased; in cirrhosis, it's patchy. Splenomegaly is typical in cirrhosis, but not in hepatitis.

Metastasis to the liver or spleen may appear on the scan as a focal defect and requires biopsy to confirm the diagnosis. Liver metastasis usually originates in the GI or genitourinary tract, the breasts, or the lungs and is more common than metastasis to the spleen. After metastasis is confirmed, serial liver-spleen studies are useful in evaluating the effectiveness of therapy.

Because cysts, abscesses, and tumors fail to take up the radioactive colloid, they appear on the scan as solitary or multiple focal defects. Hepatic cysts may appear as solitary defects; polycystic hepatic disease, as multiple defects. Splenic cysts are less common than hepatic cysts and may have a parasitic or nonparasitic origin. Ultrasonography can confirm hepatic or splenic cysts.

Intrahepatic abscesses are usually pyogenic or amebic. Subphrenic abscesses, located beneath the diaphragm, may distort the dome of the right lobe. Splenic abscesses are characteristic in bacterial endocarditis. All abscesses require gallium scanning or ultrasonography to confirm diagnosis.

Benign hepatic tumors—such as hemangiomas, adenomas, and hamartomas—require confirming biopsy or flow studies. Primary malignant tumors, such as hepatomas, also require biopsy. Benign splenic tumors are rare and include hemangiomas, fibromas, myomas, and hamartomas. Primary malignant splenic tumors are also rare except in lymphoreticular malignancies such as Hodgkin's disease. Splenic tumors also require biopsy to confirm diagnosis. Although focal disease usually inhibits the uptake of the radioactive colloid, obstruction of the superior vena cava and Budd-Chiari syndrome cause markedly increased uptake.

Liver-spleen scanning can verify palpable abdominal masses and differentiate between splenomegaly and hepatomegaly. A left upper quadrant mass may result from splenomegaly or, if the liver is grossly extended across the abdomen, from hepatomegaly. A right upper quadrant mass may result from hepatomegaly; a right lower quadrant mass may be a Riedel's lobe or a large dependent gallbladder. Splenic infarcts, commonly associated with bacterial endocarditis and massive splenomegaly, appear as peripheral defects, with decreased and irregular colloid distribution.

Scanning can assess hepatic injury after abdominal trauma. An intrahepatic hematoma appears as a focal defect; subcapsular hematoma, as a lentiform defect on the periphery of the liver; hepatic laceration, as a linear defect.

Scanning can also detect splenic injury after abdominal trauma. An intrahepatic hema-

toma appears as a focal defect; hepatic laceration appears as a linear defect. A splenic hematoma appears as a focal defect in or next to the spleen and may transect it. A subcapsular hematoma appears as a lentiform defect on the spleen's periphery.

## INTERFERING FACTORS
● Radionuclides administered in other studies on the same day (possible poor imaging)
● Inability of patient to remain still during the procedure

# Loop electrosurgical excision procedure

Loop electrosurgical excision procedure (LEEP) is a method for obtaining tissue specimens of the cervix for biopsy and removing abnormal tissue from the cervix and high in the endocervical canal. This procedure is usually done after a Papanicolaou (Pap) smear and colposcopy as follow-up to ensure the accuracy of results and for further investigation of abnormal tissue as a means to exclude the diagnosis of invasive cancer and to determine the extent of noninvasive lesions. Complications associated with LEEP include heavy bleeding, severe cramping, infection, and accidental cutting or burning of normal tissue. Cervical stenosis is also a possible risk.

## PURPOSE
● To confirm results of colposcopy and Pap smear
● To identify lesions as benign or cancerous, invasive or noninvasive
● To remove cervical dysplasia and noninvasive cervical cancers

## PATIENT PREPARATION
● Describe the LEEP to the patient, and explain that it provides a cervical tissue specimen for microscopic study and treats abnormal tissue growth.
● Help allay the patient's anxiety about a possible diagnosis of cervical cancer.
● Tell the patient who will perform the procedure and where it will be done.
● Tell the patient that she may experience mild discomfort during and after the proce-

dure and that she may have some vaginal drainage afterward.

- Advise the outpatient to have someone accompany her home after the procedure.
- Make sure the patient or a responsible family member has signed an informed consent form.

## PROCEDURE AND POSTTEST CARE

- Place the patient in the lithotomy position, and encourage her to relax.
- The examiner inserts a vaginal speculum and applies a local anesthetic to the area.
- The cervix is cleaned with a mild vinegar solution (3% acetic acid solution) or iodine to remove any debris or mucus. The solution also aids in identifying normal and abnormal tissues.
- The examiner inserts a thin wire loop attached to a high-frequency current, uses the loop to remove the suspected tissue, and sends the tissue to the laboratory.
- The examiner applies a cervical paste to the area where tissue was removed to reduce bleeding.
- Inform the patient that she may experience some vaginal bleeding and mild cramping after the procedure; inform her that she may experience brown-black vaginal discharge or a white watery discharge for about 1 week after the procedure, with possible spotting for up to 4 weeks. Encourage her to wear a perineal pad and change it frequently.
- Instruct the patient to notify her health care provider if she experiences fever, bleeding greater than a normal menstrual flow, increasing pelvic pain or severe abdominal pain, or a foul-smelling or malodorous vaginal discharge.
- Advise the patient not to douche, use tampons or bubble baths, or engage in sexual intercourse for approximately 3 to 4 weeks.
- Urge the patient to return for follow-up with health care provider as indicated for information about results.

## PRECAUTIONS

- Be aware that LEEP is contraindicated in patients with active menstrual bleeding and pregnant patients.

## NORMAL FINDINGS

Normal squamous cells of the cervix that flatten as they grow.

## ABNORMAL FINDINGS

Abnormal findings include evidence of dysplastic cervical cells or more extensive invasion of the cancerous cells deeper into the cervix.

## INTERFERING FACTORS

- Inability to obtain full specimen for removal

# Lower limb venography

Lower limb venography, or ascending contrast phlebography, is the radiographic examination of a vein. Commonly used to assess the condition of the deep leg veins after injection of a contrast medium, it's the definitive test for deep vein thrombosis (DVT), an acute condition marked by inflammation and thrombus formation in the deep veins of the legs. Such thrombi usually develop in valve pockets — venous junctions or sinuses of the calf muscle — then travel to the deep calf veins; if untreated, they may occlude the popliteal, femoral, and iliac vein systems, which may lead to pulmonary embolism, a potentially lethal complication.

Predisposing factors to DVT include vein wall injury, prolonged bed rest, coagulation abnormalities, surgery, childbirth, and use of hormonal contraceptives. Venography shouldn't be used for routine screening because it exposes the patient to relatively high doses of radiation and can cause complications, such as phlebitis, local tissue damage and, occasionally, DVT itself.

Venography is also expensive and not easily repeated. A combination of three non-invasive tests — Doppler ultrasonography, impedance plethysmography, and $^{125}$I fibrinogen scan — is an acceptable though less accurate alternative to venography. Radionuclide tests, such as the $^{125}$I fibrinogen scan, are used to screen for DVT or to attempt to detect the disorder in a patient who's too ill for venography or is hypersensitive to the contrast medium.

## PURPOSE

- To confirm a diagnosis of DVT
- To distinguish clot formation from venous obstruction (for example, a large tumor

of the pelvis impinging on the venous system)
- To evaluate congenital venous abnormalities
- To assess deep vein valvular competence (especially helpful in identifying underlying causes of leg edema)
- To locate a suitable vein for arterial bypass grafting

## PATIENT PREPARATION
- Explain to the patient that lower limb venography helps detect abnormal conditions in the veins of the legs.
- Instruct the patient to restrict food and to drink only clear liquids for 4 hours before the test.
- Describe the test, including who will perform it and where it will take place. Tell the patient pretest blood work for coagulation and kidney function may be needed.
- Warn the patient that he may feel a burning sensation in his leg on injection of the contrast medium and some discomfort during the procedure.
- Make sure that the patient or a responsible family member has signed an informed consent form.
- Check the patient's history for hypersensitivity to iodine or iodine-containing foods or to contrast media. Mark any sensitivities on the chart and notify the physician.
- Reassure the patient that contrast media complications are rare, but tell him to report nausea, severe burning or itching, constriction in the throat or chest, or dyspnea immediately. Restrict anticoagulant therapy, if ordered.
- Just before the test, instruct the patient to void, to remove all clothing below the waist, and to put on a gown.
- If ordered, administer a prescribed sedative to an anxious or uncooperative patient.

## PROCEDURE AND POSTTEST CARE
- The patient is positioned on a tilting radiographic table inclined 40 to 60 degrees so that the leg being tested doesn't bear any weight. He's instructed to relax this leg and keep it still; a tourniquet may be tied around the ankle to expedite venous filling.
- A superficial vein in the dorsum of the patient's foot is injected with normal saline solution.

- When needle placement is correct, 100 to 150 ml of the contrast medium is slowly injected over 90 seconds to 3 minutes and the presence of extravasation is checked.
- If a suitable superficial vein can't be found (due to edema), a surgical cutdown of the vein may be performed.
- Using a fluoroscope, the distribution of the contrast medium is monitored, and spot films are taken from the anteroposterior and oblique projections and over the thigh and femoroiliac regions. Then, overhead films are taken of the calf, knee, thigh, and femoral area.
- After filming, the patient is repositioned horizontally, the leg is quickly elevated, and normal saline solution is infused to flush the contrast medium from the veins.
- The fluoroscope is checked to confirm complete emptying. Then the needle is removed.
- Apply an adhesive bandage to the injection site.
- Monitor the patient's vital signs until he's stable; check his pulse rate and quality on the dorsalis pedis, popliteal, and femoral arteries.
- Administer prescribed analgesics, as ordered, to counteract the irritating effects of the contrast medium.
- **Alert** *Watch the patient for an allergic reaction to the contrast medium, hematoma, redness, bleeding, or infection (especially if a vein cutdown was performed) at the puncture site. Replace the dressing when necessary. Notify the physician if complications develop.*
- If the venogram indicates DVT, initiate the prescribed therapy (heparin infusion, bed rest, leg elevation or support, or blood chemistry tests).
- Tell the patient that he may resume his usual diet and medications, as ordered.
- Observe the patient for signs and symptoms of a latent reaction to the dye. Encourage fluids to flush the dye from the kidneys.

## PRECAUTIONS
**Alert** *Most allergic reactions to the contrast medium occur within 30 minutes of injection. Carefully observe the patient for signs of anaphylaxis (flushing, urticaria, laryngeal stridor).*

## NORMAL FINDINGS
A normal venogram shows steady opacification of the superficial and deep vasculature with no filling defects.

## ABNORMAL FINDINGS

A venogram that shows consistent filling defects on repeat views, abrupt termination of a column of contrast material, unfilled major deep veins, or diversion of flow (for example, through collateral veins) is diagnostic of DVT.

## INTERFERING FACTORS

● The patient placing weight on the leg being tested (possible filling of leg veins with contrast medium)
● Movement of the leg being tested
● Excessive tourniquet constriction
● Insufficient injection or dilution of contrast medium
● Delay between injection and radiography
● Previous thrombosis, severe edema or obesity, or cellulitis (may limit visualization of the deep venous system)

# Lung biopsy

In lung biopsy, a specimen of pulmonary tissue is excised by closed or open technique for histologic examination. Closed technique, performed under local anesthesia, includes needle and transbronchial biopsies, transcatheter bronchial brushing, and video-assisted thoracotomy. Open technique, performed under general anesthesia in the operating room, includes limited and standard thoracotomies. Needle biopsy is appropriate when the lesion is readily accessible, originates in the lung parenchyma and is confined to it, or is affixed to the chest wall; it provides a much smaller specimen than the open technique. Transbronchial biopsy, the removal of multiple tissue specimens through a fiber-optic bronchoscope, may be used in patients with diffuse infiltrative pulmonary disease or tumors or when severe debilitation contraindicates open biopsy. Open biopsy is appropriate for the study of a well-circumscribed lesion that may require resection.

Generally, a lung biopsy is recommended after chest X-rays, computed tomography scan, and bronchoscopy have failed to identify the cause of diffuse parenchymal pulmonary disease or a pulmonary lesion. Complications of lung biopsy include bleeding, infection, and pneumothorax.

## PURPOSE

● To confirm a diagnosis of diffuse parenchymal pulmonary disease and pulmonary lesions

## PATIENT PREPARATION

● Explain to the patient that the lung biopsy is used to confirm or rule out a diagnostic finding in the lung.
● Describe the procedure to the patient, and answer his questions.
● Tell the patient that a chest X-ray and blood studies (prothrombin time, partial thromboplastin time, and platelet count) will be performed before the biopsy.
● Tell the patient who will perform the biopsy and where it will be done.
● Instruct the patient to fast after midnight before the procedure. (Sometimes the patient is permitted to have clear liquids the morning of the test.)
● Make sure the patient or a responsible family member has signed an informed consent form.
● Check the patient's history for hypersensitivity to the local anesthetic.
● Administer a mild sedative, as ordered, 30 minutes before the biopsy to help the patient relax. Tell him that he'll receive a local anesthetic, but he may experience a sharp, transient pain when the biopsy needle touches the lung.
● Reinforce that the patient needs to lie still during the procedure because any movement or coughing can result in laceration of lung tissue by the biopsy needle.

## PROCEDURE AND POSTTEST CARE

● After the biopsy site is selected, lead markers are placed on the patient's skin, and X-rays are ordered to verify their correct placement.
● Position the patient in a sitting position with his arms folded on a table in front of him; instruct him to maintain this position, remaining as still as possible, and to refrain from coughing.
● Prepare the skin over the biopsy site and drape the appropriate area.
● With a 25G needle, the local anesthetic is injected just above the rib below the selected site to prevent damage to the intercostal nerves and vessels.
● Using a 22G needle, the examiner anesthetizes the intercostal muscles and parietal

pleura, makes a small incision (2 to 3 mm) with a scalpel, and introduces the biopsy needle through the incision, chest wall, and pleura into the tumor or pulmonary tissue.

● If the intercostal space at the incision site is wide, the needle is inserted at a 90-degree angle; if the ribs overlap and the intercostal space is narrow, the needle is inserted at a 45-degree angle. When the needle is in the tumor or pulmonary tissue, the specimen is obtained and the needle is withdrawn.

● The specimen is divided immediately: The tissue for histology is placed in a properly labeled bottle containing 10% neutral buffered formalin solution; the tissue for microbiology is placed in a sterile container.

● Immediately following the procedure, apply pressure on the biopsy site to stop bleeding and apply a small bandage.

*Alert* *Check the patient's vital signs every 15 minutes for 1 hour, every 30 minutes for 2 hours, every hour for 4 hours, and then every 4 hours until the patient is stable or until discharge. Watch for bleeding, dyspnea, elevated pulse rate, diminished breath sounds on the biopsy side and, eventually, cyanosis. Complications include pneumothorax and bleeding. Make sure the chest X-ray is repeated as soon as the biopsy has been completed.*

● Inform the patient that he may resume his usual diet, as ordered.

## PRECAUTIONS

● Needle biopsy is contraindicated in the patient with a lesion that's separated from the chest wall or accompanied by emphysematous bullae, cysts, or gross emphysema and in the patient with coagulopathy, hypoxia, pulmonary hypertension, or cardiac disease with cor pulmonale.

● During biopsy, observe for signs of respiratory distress — shortness of breath, elevated pulse rate, and cyanosis (late sign). If such signs develop, report them immediately.

● Because coughing and movement during biopsy can cause lung tearing by the biopsy needle, keep the patient calm and still.

## NORMAL FINDINGS

Normal pulmonary tissue shows uniform texture of the alveolar ducts, alveolar walls, bronchioles, and small vessels.

## ABNORMAL FINDINGS

Histologic examination of a pulmonary tissue specimen can reveal squamous cell or oat cell carcinoma and adenocarcinoma and supplements the results of microbiologic cultures, deep-cough sputum specimens, chest X-rays, bronchoscopy, and the patient's physical history in confirming cancer or parenchymal pulmonary disease.

## INTERFERING FACTORS

● Inability to obtain a representative tissue specimen

# Lung perfusion and ventilation scan

A lung perfusion scan produces an image of pulmonary blood flow after I.V. injection of a radiopharmaceutical, either human serum albumin microspheres or macroaggregated albumin bonded to technetium.

The lung ventilation scan is performed after the patient inhales a mixture of air and radioactive gas that delineates areas of the lung ventilated during respiration. The scan records gas distribution during three phases: the buildup of radioactive gas (wash-in phase), the time after rebreathing when radioactivity reaches a steady level (equilibrium phase), and after removal of the radioactive gas from the lungs (wash-out phase).

## PURPOSE

● To assess arterial perfusion of the lungs
● To detect pulmonary emboli
● To evaluate pulmonary function before lung resection
● To identify areas of the lung capable of ventilation, evaluate regional respiratory function and locate regional hypoventilation, which may indicate atelectasis, obstructing tumors, or chronic obstructive pulmonary disease (COPD) (ventilation scan)

## PATIENT PREPARATION

● Tell the patient that the lung perfusion and ventilation scan helps evaluate respiratory function.
● Explain to the patient that he need not restrict food and fluids.
● Describe the test to the patient, including who will perform it and where it will take place.
● On the test request, note if the patient has conditions, such as COPD, vasculitis,

pulmonary edema, tumor, sickle cell disease, or parasitic disease.

● Ensure that the patient or a responsible family member has signed an informed consent form, if required.

## Lung perfusion scan

● Tell the patient that a radiopharmaceutical will be injected into a vein in his arm and that he'll then sit in front of a camera or lie under it. Explain that neither the camera nor the uptake probe emits radiation and that the amount of radioactivity in the radiopharmaceutical is minimal.

● Assure the patient that he'll be comfortable during the test and that he doesn't have to remain perfectly still.

## Lung ventilation scan

● Ask the patient to remove all jewelry and metal objects from the scanning field.

● Explain to the patient that he'll be asked to hold his breath for a short time after inhaling a gas and to remain still while a machine scans his chest.

● Reassure the patient that a minimal amount of radioactive gas is used.

## PROCEDURE AND POSTTEST CARE
### Lung perfusion scan

● With the patient supine and taking moderately deep breaths, the radiopharmaceutical is injected I.V. slowly over 5 to 10 seconds to allow more even distribution of pulmonary blood flow.

● After the injection, the gamma camera takes a series of single stationary images in the anterior, posterior, oblique, and both lateral chest views.

● Images, which are projected on an oscilloscope screen, show the distribution of radioactive particles.

● If a hematoma develops at the injection site, apply pressure.

## Lung ventilation scan

● After the patient inhales air mixed with a small amount of radioactive gas through a mask, its distribution in the lungs is monitored on a nuclear scanner.

● The patient's chest is scanned as he exhales.

## PRECAUTIONS

● A lung perfusion scan is contraindicated in the patient who's hypersensitive to the radiopharmaceutical.

● With a ventilation scan, watch for leaks in the closed system of radioactive gas, such as through the mask, which can contaminate the surrounding atmosphere.

## NORMAL FINDINGS

Areas with normal blood perfusion, called hot spots, show a high uptake of the radioactive substance; a normal lung shows a uniform uptake pattern. For the ventilation scan, normal findings include an equal distribution of gas in both lungs and normal wash-in and wash-out phases.

## ABNORMAL FINDINGS

Areas of low radioactive uptake, called cold spots, indicate poor perfusion, suggesting an embolism; however, a ventilation scan is necessary to confirm diagnosis. Decreased regional blood flow that occurs without vessel obstruction may indicate pneumonitis.

Unequal gas distribution in both lungs indicates poor ventilation or airway obstruction in areas with low radioactivity. When compared with a lung scan (perfusion scan), in vascular obstructions — such as pulmonary embolism — the perfusion to the embolized area is decreased, but the ventilation to this area is maintained; in parenchymal disease, such as pneumonia, ventilation is abnormal within the areas of consolidation.

## INTERFERING FACTORS

● Scheduling more than one radionuclide test per day, especially if using different tracing substances (may hinder diffusion of tracer isotope in second test)

● Administering all the radiopharmaceutical while the patient is sitting (possible poor imaging due to settling of tracer isotope in lung bases)

● Conditions, such as COPD, vasculitis, pulmonary edema, tumor, sickle cell disease, and parasitic disease (possible poor imaging)

● Failure to remove jewelry and other metal objects from the scanning field (possible poor imaging)

# Lupus erythematosus cell preparation

Lupus erythematosus (LE) cell preparation is an in vitro procedure used in diagnosing systemic lupus erythematosus (SLE). Although this test is less sensitive and reliable than either the antinuclear antibody (ANA) or the antideoxyribonucleic acid (DNA) antibody test, it's commonly used because it requires minimal equipment and reagents.

In this test, a blood sample is mixed with laboratory-treated nucleoprotein (the antigen). If the sample contains ANAs, they react with the nucleoprotein, causing swelling and rupture. Phagocytes from the serum then engulf the extruded nuclei, forming LE cells, which are then detected by microscopic examination of the sample.

## PURPOSE
● To aid in the diagnosis of SLE
● To monitor treatment of SLE (About 60% of successfully treated patients fail to show LE cells after 4 to 6 weeks of therapy.)

## PATIENT PREPARATION
● Explain to the patient that the LE cell preparation test helps detect antibodies to his own tissue.
● If appropriate, inform the patient that the test will be repeated to monitor his response to therapy.
● Inform the patient that he need not restrict food and fluids.
● Tell the patient that the test requires a blood sample. Explain who will perform the venipuncture and when.
● Explain to the patient that he may experience slight discomfort from the tourniquet and needle puncture.
● Check the patient's medication history for drugs that may affect test results, such as isoniazid, hydralazine, and procainamide. If such drugs must be continued, be sure to note this on the laboratory request.

## PROCEDURE AND POSTTEST CARE
● Perform a venipuncture and collect the sample in a 7-ml red-top tube.
● Because the patient with SLE may have a compromised immune system, keep a clean, dry bandage over the venipuncture site for at least 24 hours and check for infection.
● Apply direct pressure to the venipuncture site until bleeding stops.
● If a hematoma develops at the venipuncture site, apply pressure.
● If test results indicate SLE, tell the patient further tests may be required to monitor treatment.

## PRECAUTIONS
● Handle the sample gently to prevent hemolysis.

## NORMAL FINDINGS
No LE cells are normally present in serum.

## ABNORMAL FINDINGS
The presence of at least two LE cells may indicate SLE. Although these cells occur primarily in SLE, they may also appear in chronic active hepatitis, rheumatoid arthritis, scleroderma, and certain drug reactions. Also, up to 25% of patients with SLE demonstrate no LE cells.

Apart from supportive clinical signs, a definitive diagnosis of SLE may require a confirming ANA or anti-DNA test. The ANA test detects autoantibodies in the serum of many patients with SLE who have negative LE cell tests. Anti-DNA antibodies appear in two-thirds of all patients with SLE, but are rare in other conditions; thus, the presence of these antibodies is strong evidence of SLE.

## INTERFERING FACTORS
● Hydralazine, isoniazid, and procainamide (may produce a syndrome resembling SLE)
● Chlorpromazine (Thorazine), ethosuximide (Zarontin), gold salts, hormonal contraceptives, methyldopa (Aldoril), penicillin, phenytoin (Dilantin), primidone (Mysoline), propylthiouracil, quinidine, streptomycin, sulfonamides, and tetracyclines

# Lyme disease serology

Lyme disease is a multisystem disorder characterized by dermatologic, neurologic, cardiac, and rheumatic manifestations in various stages. Epidemiologic and serologic studies implicate a common tick-borne spirochete, Borrelia burgdorferi, as the causative agent.

Serologic tests for Lyme disease, both indirect immunofluorescent and enzyme-linked immunosorbent assays, measure antibody response to this spirochete and indicate current infection or past exposure. Serologic tests can identify 50% of patients with early-stage Lyme disease and all patients with later complications of carditis, neuritis, and arthritis or patients in remission.

In an indirect immunofluorescent assay, B. burgdorferi is grown in culture, fixed to a microscope slide, and then incubated with a human serum sample. A fluorescein-labeled antiglobulin is then introduced into the antigen-antibody complex. Any human antibody that binds to the spirochete is detected by viewing (under an ultraviolet microscope) the fluorescent antiglobulin that attaches to it.

## PURPOSE
● To confirm a diagnosis of Lyme disease

## PATIENT PREPARATION
● Explain to the patient that the Lyme disease serology test helps determine whether his symptoms are caused by Lyme disease.
● Instruct the patient to fast for 12 hours before the sample is drawn but to drink fluids as usual.
● Tell the patient that the test requires a blood sample. Explain who will perform the venipuncture and when.
● Explain to the patient that he may experience slight discomfort from the tourniquet and needle puncture.

## PROCEDURE AND POSTTEST CARE
● Perform a venipuncture, and collect the sample in a 7-ml clot-activator tube.
● Apply direct pressure to the venipuncture site until bleeding stops.
● If a hematoma develops at the venipuncture site, apply pressure.
● Inform the patient that he may resume his usual diet, as ordered.

## PRECAUTIONS
● Handle the sample gently to prevent hemolysis.
● Send the sample to the laboratory immediately.

## REFERENCE VALUES
Normal serum values are nonreactive.

## ABNORMAL FINDINGS
A positive result can help confirm the diagnosis, but it isn't definitive. Other treponemal diseases and high rheumatoid factor titers can cause false-positive results. More than 15% of patients with Lyme disease fail to develop antibodies.

## INTERFERING FACTORS
● High serum lipid levels (possible inaccurate results, requiring a repeat test after a period of restricted fat intake)
● Samples contaminated with other bacteria (possible false-positive)
● Measurement too early in disease
● Antibiotic treatment

# Lymphangiography

Lymphangiography (or lymphography) is the radiographic examination of the lymphatic system after the injection of an oil-based contrast medium into a lymphatic vessel in each foot or, less commonly, in each hand. This test is no longer used widely.

Injection into the foot allows visualization of the lymphatics of the leg, inguinal and iliac regions, and the retroperitoneum up to the thoracic duct.

Injection into the hand allows visualization of the axillary and supraclavicular nodes. This procedure may also be used to study the cervical region (retroauricular area), but this is less useful and less common.

X-ray films are taken immediately after injection to demonstrate the filling of the lymphatic system and then again 24 hours later to visualize the lymph nodes. Because the contrast medium remains in the nodes for up to 2 years, subsequent X-ray films can assess progression of disease and monitor effectiveness of treatment.

## PURPOSE
● To detect and stage lymphomas and to identify metastatic involvement of the lymph nodes (Computed tomography [CT] is used more commonly for staging.)
● To distinguish primary from secondary lymphedema
● To suggest surgical treatment or evaluate the effectiveness of chemotherapy and radiation therapy in controlling malignancy

To investigate enlarged lymph nodes detected by CT or ultrasonography

## PATIENT PREPARATION

- Explain to the patient that lymphangiography permits examination of the lymphatic system through X-rays taken after the injection of a contrast medium.
- Inform the patient that he need not restrict food and fluids.
- Tell the patient who will perform the procedure and where it will take place.
- Mention to the patient that additional X-rays are also taken the following day, but that these take less than 30 minutes.
- Inform the patient that blue contrast medium will be injected into each foot to outline the lymphatic vessels, that the injection causes transient discomfort, and that the contrast medium discolors urine and stools for 48 hours and may give his skin and vision a bluish tinge for 48 hours.
- Tell the patient that a local anesthetic will be injected before a small incision is made in each foot.
- Inform the patient that the contrast medium is then injected for the next 1¼ hours using a catheter inserted into a lymphatic vessel.
- Advise the patient that he must remain as still as possible during injection of the contrast medium and that he may experience some discomfort in the popliteal or inguinal areas at the beginning of the injection.
- If this test is performed on an outpatient basis, advise the patient to have a friend or relative accompany him.
- Warn the patient that the incision site may be sore for several days after lymphangiography.
- Make sure that the patient or a responsible family member has signed an informed consent form.
- Check the patient's history to determine if he's hypersensitive to iodine, seafood, or the contrast media used in other diagnostic tests such as excretory urography. Alert the physician to any sensitivities.
- Just before the procedure, instruct the patient to void. Check his vital signs for a baseline. If prescribed, administer a sedative and an oral antihistamine (if hypersensitivity to the contrast medium is suspected).

## PROCEDURE AND POSTTEST CARE

- A preliminary X-ray of the chest is taken with the patient in an erect or a supine position.
- The skin over the dorsum of each foot is cleaned with antiseptics.
- Blue contrast dye is injected intradermally into the area between the toes, usually the first and fourth toe webs.
- The contrast medium infiltrates the lymphatic system, and within 15 to 30 minutes, the lymphatic vessels appear as small blue lines on the upper surface of the instep of each foot.
- A local anesthetic is then injected into the dorsum of each foot and a transverse incision is made to expose the lymphatic vessel.
- Each vessel is cannulated with a 30G needle attached to polyethylene tubing and a syringe filled with ethiodized oil.
- After the needles are positioned, the patient is instructed to remain still throughout the injection period to avoid dislodging the needles.
- The syringe is then placed within an infusion pump that injects the contrast medium at a constant rate of 0.1 to 0.2 ml/minute for about 1½ hours to avoid injury to delicate lymphatic vessels.
- Fluoroscopy may be used to monitor filling of the lymphatic system.
- The needles are removed, the incisions are sutured, and sterile dressings are applied.
- X-rays of the legs, pelvis, abdomen, and chest are taken.
- The patient is then taken to his room, but must return 24 hours later for additional X-rays.
- Check the patient's vital signs every 4 hours for 48 hours.

*Alert* Watch the patient for pulmonary complications, such as shortness of breath, pleuritic pain, hypotension, low-grade fever, and cyanosis caused by embolization of the contrast medium.

- Enforce bed rest for 24 hours, with the patient's feet elevated to help reduce swelling.
- Apply ice packs to the incision sites to help reduce swelling and administer prescribed analgesics.
- Check the incision sites for infection and leave the dressings in place for 2 days, making sure the wounds remain dry. Tell the pa-

tient that the sutures will be removed in 7 to 10 days.

- Prepare the patient for follow-up X-rays, as needed.

## PRECAUTIONS

- Be aware that lymphangiography is contraindicated in the patient with hypersensitivity to iodine, pulmonary insufficiencies, cardiac diseases, or severe renal or hepatic disease.

## NORMAL FINDINGS

The lymphatic system normally demonstrates homogeneous and complete filling with contrast medium on the initial films. On the 24-hour films, the lymph nodes are fully opacified and well circumscribed; the lymphatic channels are emptied a few hours after injection of the contrast medium.

## ABNORMAL FINDINGS

Enlarged, foamy-looking nodes indicate Hodgkin's disease or malignant lymphoma. Filling defects or lack of opacification indicates metastatic involvement of the lymph nodes. The number of nodes affected, unilateral or bilateral involvement, and the extent of extranodal involvement help determine staging of lymphoma. However, definitive staging may require additional diagnostic tests, such as CT, ultrasonography, selective biopsy, and laparotomy.

In differential diagnosis of primary and secondary lymphedema, shortened lymphatic vessels and a deficient number of vessels indicate primary lymphedema. Abruptly terminating lymphatic vessels, caused by retroperitoneal tumors impinging on the vessels, inflammation, filariasis, and trauma resulting from surgery or radiation, indicate secondary lymphedema.

## INTERFERING FACTORS

- Inability to cannulate the lymphatic vessels (precludes use of this test)

## *Lymph node biopsy*

Lymph node biopsy is the surgical excision of an active lymph node or the needle aspiration of a nodal specimen for histologic examination. Both techniques usually use a local anesthetic and sample the superficial nodes in the cervical, supraclavicular, axillary, or inguinal region. Excision is preferred because it yields a larger specimen.

Although lymph nodes swell during infection, biopsy is indicated when nodal enlargement is prolonged and accompanied by backache, leg edema, breathing and swallowing difficulties and, later, weight loss, weakness, severe itching, fever, night sweats, cough, hemoptysis, and hoarseness. Generalized or localized lymph node enlargement is typical of such diseases as chronic lymphatic leukemia, Hodgkin's disease, infectious mononucleosis, and rheumatoid arthritis.

Complete blood count, liver function studies, liver and spleen scans, and X-rays should precede this test.

## PURPOSE

- To determine the cause of lymph node enlargement
- To distinguish between benign and malignant lymph node processes
- To stage metastatic cancer

## PATIENT PREPARATION

- Explain to the patient that the lymph node biopsy allows microscopic study of lymph node tissue.
- Describe the procedure to the patient, and answer his questions.
- For excisional biopsy, instruct the patient to restrict food after midnight and to drink only clear liquids on the morning of the test (if general anesthesia is needed for deeper nodes, he must also restrict fluids).
- For needle biopsy, inform him that he need not restrict food and fluids. Tell him who will perform the biopsy and where it will be done.
- Make sure the patient or a responsible family member has signed an informed consent form.
- Check the patient's history for hypersensitivity to the anesthetic.
- If the patient is to receive a local anesthetic, explain that he may experience slight discomfort during the injection.
- Record the patient's baseline vital signs just before the biopsy.

## PROCEDURE AND POSTTEST CARE
### Excisional biopsy
● After the skin over the biopsy site is prepared and draped, the local anesthetic is administered.
● The examiner makes an incision, removes an entire node, and places it in a properly labeled bottle containing normal saline solution.
● The wound is sutured, and a sterile dressing is applied.

### Needle biopsy
● After preparing the biopsy site and administering a local anesthetic, the examiner grasps the node between his thumb and forefinger, inserts the needle directly into the node, and obtains a small core specimen.
● The needle is removed, and the specimen is placed in a properly labeled bottle containing normal saline solution.
● Pressure is exerted at the biopsy site to control bleeding, and an adhesive bandage is applied.

### Both procedures
● Check the patient's vital signs, and watch for bleeding, tenderness, and redness at the biopsy site.
● Inform the patient that he may resume his usual diet, as ordered.

## PRECAUTIONS
● Storing the tissue specimen in normal saline solution instead of 10% formalin solution allows part of the specimen to be used for cytologic impression smears, which are studied along with the biopsy specimen.

## NORMAL FINDINGS
The normal lymph node is encapsulated by collagenous connective tissue and divided into smaller lobes by tissue strands called *trabeculae*. It has an outer cortex, composed of lymphoid cells and nodules or follicles containing lymphocytes, and an inner medulla, composed of reticular phagocytic cells that collect and drain fluid.

## ABNORMAL FINDINGS
Histologic examination of the tissue specimen distinguishes between malignant and nonmalignant causes of lymph node enlargement. Lymphatic cancer accounts for up to 5% of all cancers and is slightly more preva-

lent in males than in females. Hodgkin's disease, a lymphoma affecting the entire lymph system, is the leading cancer affecting adolescents and young adults. Lymph node cancer may also result from metastatic cancer.

When histologic results aren't clear or nodular material isn't involved, mediastinoscopy or laparotomy can provide another nodal specimen. Occasionally, lymphangiography can furnish additional diagnostic information.

## INTERFERING FACTORS
● Inability to obtain a representative tissue specimen
● Inability to differentiate nodal disorder

# Lymphocyte transformation tests

Transformation tests evaluate lymphocyte competency without injection of antigens into the patient's skin. These in vitro tests eliminate the risk of adverse effects but can still accurately assess the ability of lymphocytes to proliferate and to recognize and respond to antigens.

The mitogen assay evaluates the mitotic response of T and B lymphocytes to a foreign antigen. The antigen assay uses specific substances, such as purified protein derivative, Candida, mumps, tetanus toxoid, and streptokinase, to stimulate lymphocyte transformation. The mixed lymphocyte culture (MLC) assay is useful in matching transplant recipients and donors and in testing immunocompetence. (See *Lymphocyte marker assays,* page 276.)

The neutrophils' ability to engulf and destroy bacteria and foreign particles can also be determined. (See *Neutrophil function tests,* page 277.)

## PURPOSE
● To assess and monitor genetic and acquired immunodeficiency states
● To provide histocompatibility typing of tissue transplant recipients and donors
● To detect if a patient has been exposed to various pathogens such as those that cause malaria, hepatitis, and mycoplasmal pneumonia

# LYMPHOCYTE MARKER ASSAYS

A normal immune response requires a balance between the regulatory activities of several interacting cell types, most notably T-helper and T-suppressor cells. By using highly specific monoclonal antibodies, levels of lymphocyte differentiation can be defined, and normal and malignant cell populations can be analyzed. Direct and indirect immunofluorescence, microcytotoxicity, and immunoperoxidase immunoassay techniques are the most commonly used: They use an anticoagulated blood sample combined with monoclonal antibodies that react with specific T- and B-cell markers. The chart below lists some commonly ordered lymphocyte marker assays and their indications.

| LYMPHOCYTE MARKER | PURPOSE |
|---|---|
| Pan T-cell marker (CD3) | ◆ To measure mature T cells in immune dysfunction |
| T-helper/inducer subset marker (CD4) | ◆ To identify and characterize the proportion of T-helper cells in autoimmune or immunoregulatory disorders<br>◆ To detect immunodeficiency disorders such as acquired immunodeficiency syndrome<br>◆ To differentiate T-cell acute lymphoblastic leukemia from T-cell lymphomas and other lymphoproliferative disorders |
| T-suppressor/cytotoxic subset marker (CD8) | ◆ To identify and characterize the proportion of T-suppressor cells in autoimmune and immunoregulatory disorders<br>◆ To characterize lymphoproliferative disorders |
| T-cell/E-Rosette receptor (CD2) | ◆ To differentiate lymphoproliferative disorders of T-cell origin, such as T-cell lymphocytic leukemia and lymphoblastic lymphoma, from those of non–T-cell origin |
| Pan-B (B-1) marker (CD20) | ◆ To differentiate lymphoproliferative disorders of B-cell origin, such as B-cell chronic lymphocytic leukemia, from those of T-cell origin |
| Pan-B (BA-1) marker (CD19) | ◆ To identify B-cell lymphoproliferative disorders such as B-cell chronic lymphocytic leukemia |
| CALLA (common acute lymphocytic leukemia antigen) marker, CD10 | ◆ To identify bone marrow regeneration<br>◆ To identify non–T-cell acute lymphocytic leukemia |
| Lymphocyte subset panel (CD3/CD4/CD8/CD19) | ◆ To evaluate immunodeficiencies<br>◆ To identify immunoregulation associated with autoimmune disorders<br>◆ To characterize lymphoid neoplasms |
| Lymphocytic leukemia marker panel (CD3/CD4/CD8/CD19/CD10) | ◆ To characterize lymphocytic leukemias as T, B, non-T, or non-B, regardless of the stage of differentiation of the malignant cells |

## PATIENT PREPARATION

● Explain to the patient that the lymphocyte transformation test evaluates lymphocyte function, which is crucial to the immune system.

● Inform the patient that the test monitors his response to therapy, if appropriate.

● For histocompatibility typing, explain that this test helps determine the best match for a transplant.

● Inform the patient that he need not restrict food and fluids.

# Neutrophil function tests

Neutrophil function tests may reveal the inability of neutrophils to kill a target bacteria or to migrate to the bacterial site (chemotaxis). The killing ability can be evaluated by the nitroblue tetrazolium (NBT) test, which relies on neutrophil generation of bactericidal enzymes and toxins during killing. This action results in increased oxygen consumption and glucose metabolism, which reduces colorless NBT to blue formazan. The reduced dye is then extracted with pyridine and measured photometrically; the level of reduction indicates phagocytic activity.

Neutrophil killing activity can also be evaluated by noting the neutrophil's chemiluminescence, its ability to emit light. After a neutrophil phagocytizes a microorganism, oxygen-containing substances form within phagocytic vacuoles. As the cell is stimulated, it emits light in proportion to the amount of oxygen-containing substances that are formed, providing an indirect measurement of phagocytosis.

Chemotaxis can be assessed in vitro by placing bacteria in the lower half of a two-part chamber and phagocytic neutrophils in the upper half. After incubation, migrating cells are counted microscopically and compared with standard values.

---

- Tell the patient that the test requires a blood sample. Explain who will perform the venipuncture and when.
- Explain to the patient that he may experience slight discomfort from the tourniquet and needle puncture.
- If a radioisotope scan is scheduled, make sure the serum sample for this test is drawn first.

## PROCEDURE AND POSTTEST CARE

- Perform a venipuncture. If the patient is an adult, collect the sample in a 7-ml heparinized tube.

  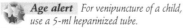 **Age alert** *For venipuncture of a child, use a 5-ml heparinized tube.*

- Because the patient may have a compromised immune system, take special care to keep the venipuncture site clean and dry.
- Apply direct pressure to the venipuncture site until bleeding stops.
- If a hematoma develops at the venipuncture site, apply pressure.

## PRECAUTIONS

- Completely fill the collection tube and invert it gently several times to mix the sample and the anticoagulant.
- Send the sample to the laboratory immediately.
- Don't refrigerate or freeze the sample.

## REFERENCE VALUES

Results depend on the mitogens used. Reference ranges accompany test results. In general, a positive test is normal; a negative test indicates a deficiency.

## ABNORMAL FINDINGS

In the mitogen and antigen assays, a low stimulation index or unresponsiveness indicates a depressed or defective immune system. Serial testing can be performed to monitor the effectiveness of therapy in a patient with an immunodeficiency disease.

In the MLC test, the stimulation index is a measure of compatibility. A high index indicates poor compatibility. Conversely, a low stimulation index indicates good compatibility.

A high stimulation index, in response to the relevant pathogen, can also demonstrate exposure to malaria, hepatitis, mycoplasmal pneumonia, periodontal disease, and certain viral infections in a patient who no longer has detectable serum antibodies.

## INTERFERING FACTORS

- Pregnancy or use of hormonal contraceptives, depressing lymphocyte response to phytohemagglutinin (low stimulation index)
- Chemotherapy (unless pretherapy baseline values are available for comparison)
- Radioisotope scan within 1 week before the test

## Magnesium, serum

The magnesium test is used to measure serum levels of magnesium, an electrolyte that's vital to neuromuscular function. It also helps in intracellular metabolism, activates many essential enzymes, and affects the metabolism of nucleic acids and proteins. Magnesium also helps transport sodium and potassium across cell membranes and influences intracellular calcium levels. Most magnesium is found in bone and intracellular fluid; a small amount is found in extracellular fluid. Magnesium is absorbed by the small intestine and excreted in urine and stools.

### PURPOSE
● To evaluate electrolyte status
● To assess neuromuscular and renal function

### PATIENT PREPARATION
● Explain to the patient that the serum magnesium test is used to determine the magnesium content of the blood.
● Instruct the patient not to use magnesium salts (such as milk of magnesia or Epsom salt) for at least 3 days before the test, but tell him that he need not restrict food and fluids.
● Tell the patient that the test requires a blood sample. Explain who will perform the venipuncture and when.
● Explain to the patient that he may experience slight discomfort from the tourniquet and needle puncture.

### PROCEDURE AND POSTTEST CARE
● Perform a venipuncture without a tourniquet, if possible, and collect the sample in a 3- or 4-ml clot-activator tube.
● Apply pressure to the venipuncture site until bleeding stops.
● If a hematoma develops at the venipuncture site, apply pressure.

### PRECAUTIONS
● Handle the sample gently to prevent hemolysis.

### REFERENCE VALUES
Serum magnesium levels range from 1.3 to 2.1 mg/dl (SI, 0.65 to 1.05 mmol/L).

### ABNORMAL FINDINGS
Elevated serum magnesium levels (hypermagnesemia) most commonly occur in renal failure, when the kidneys excrete inadequate amounts of magnesium, and by magnesium administration or ingestion. Adrenal insufficiency (Addison's disease) can also increase serum magnesium levels.

In suspected or confirmed hypermagnesemia, observe the patient for lethargy; flushing; diaphoresis; decreased blood pressure; slow, weak pulse; muscle weakness; diminished deep tendon reflexes; slow, shallow respiration, and electrocardiogram (ECG) changes (prolonged PR interval, wide QRS complex, elevated T waves, atrioventricular block, premature ventricular contractions [PVCs]).

Decreased serum magnesium levels (hypomagnesemia) most commonly result from chronic alcoholism. Other causes include malabsorption syndrome, diarrhea, faulty absorption after bowel resection, prolonged bowel or gastric aspiration, acute pancreatitis, primary aldosteronism, severe burns, hypercalcemic conditions (including hyperparathyroidism), malnutrition, and certain diuretic therapy.

In hypomagnesemia, watch for leg and foot cramps, hyperactive deep tendon reflexes, arrhythmias, muscle weakness, seizures, twitching, tetany, tremors, and ECG changes (PVCs and ventricular fibrillation).

## INTERFERING FACTORS

- Venous stasis due to tourniquet use
- Obtaining a sample above an I.V. site that's receiving a solution containing magnesium
- Excessive use of antacids or cathartics or excessive infusion of magnesium sulfate (increase)
- Prolonged I.V. infusions without magnesium; excessive use of diuretics (decrease)
- I.V. administration of calcium gluconate (possible false-low if measured using the Titan yellow method)
- Lithium (increase)
- Alcohol, aminoglycosides, amphotericin B, calcium salts, cardiac glycosides, cisplatin (Platinol-AQ), and loop and thiazide diuretics (decrease)

# Magnetic resonance imaging, intracranial

Intracranial magnetic resonance imaging (MRI) produces highly detailed, cross-sectional images of the brain and spine in multiple planes. The primary advantage of MRI is its ability to "see through" bone and to delineate fluid-filled soft tissue. It has proved useful in the diagnosis of cerebral infarction, tumors, abscesses, edema, hemorrhage, nerve fiber demyelination (as in multiple sclerosis), and other disorders that increase the fluid content of affected tissues. It can also show irregularities of the spinal cord with a resolution and detail previously unobtainable. It can also produce images of organs and vessels in motion.

Exposed to an external magnetic field, positively charged atomic nuclei and their negatively charged electrons align uniformly in the field. Radiofrequency energy is then directed at the atoms, knocking them out of this magnetic alignment and causing them to precess, or spin. When the radiofrequency pulse is discontinued, the atoms realign themselves with the magnetic field, emitting radiofrequency energy as a tissue-specific signal based on the relative density of nuclei and the realignment time. These signals are monitored by the MRI computer, which processes them and displays the information on a video monitor as a high-resolution image.

MRI technology makes use of magnetic fields and radio-frequency waves, which are imperceptible by the patient; no harmful effects have been documented. Research continues on the optimal magnetic fields and radio-frequency waves for each type of tissue. (See *New methods of monitoring cerebral function,* page 280, and *MRI techniques,* page 281.)

## PURPOSE

- To aid in the diagnosis of intracranial and spinal lesions and soft-tissue abnormalities

## PATIENT PREPARATION

- Explain to the patient that intracranial MRI assesses bone and soft tissue. Tell him who will perform the test and where it will take place.
- Explain to the patient that MRI is painless and involves no exposure to radiation from the scanner. A radioactive contrast dye may be used, depending on the type of tissue being studied.
- Advise the patient that he'll have to remain still for the entire procedure.
- Inform the patient that the opening for the head and body is quite small and deep. Tell him that he'll hear the scanner clicking, whirring, and thumping as it moves inside its housing.
- Explain to the patient that sedation may be administered if he suffers from claustrophobia or if extensive time is required for scanning. As an alternative, an open MRI scanner may be used, which delivers accurate results, but may take longer to complete.
- Reassure the patient that he'll be able to communicate with the technician at all times.
- Instruct the patient to remove all metallic objects, including jewelry, hairpins, and a watch. Also ask him if he has any surgically implanted joints, pins, clips, valves, pumps,

# New Methods of Monitoring Cerebral Function

## Optical Imaging

Optical imaging uses fiber-optic light and a camera to produce visual images of the brain as it responds to stimulation. This technique produces higher-resolution pictures of the brain than magnetic resonance imaging (MRI) or positron emission tomography scans. Researchers believe it may be valuable during neurosurgery to minimize damage to crucial areas of the brain that control speech, movement, and other activities. Because the procedure scans only the brain's surface, it's meant to be used in combination with other diagnostic techniques.

## Fast MRI

Fast MRI produces pictures less than a second apart. These images display blood flow through the brain and the changes that occur in blood flow when the patient performs different tasks. Neuroscientists believe that active areas of the brain must consume more oxygen and that areas of the brain that are currently working become laden with oxygen. Fast MRI can distinguish between oxygen-laden and oxygen-depleted blood. Thus, this test may be used to help identify which areas of the normal brain are involved in certain activities and emotions. Possible applications for fast MRI include guiding neurosurgeons during surgery and helping researchers better understand epilepsy, brain tumors, and even psychiatric illnesses.

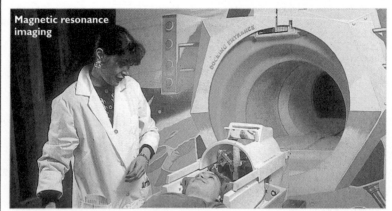

Magnetic resonance imaging

Photo from Timby, B.K. *Fundamental Nursing Skills and Concepts*, 8e. Philadelphia, Lippincott Williams & Wilkins, 2005

or pacemakers containing metal that could be attracted to the strong MRI magnet. If he does, he won't be able to undergo the test.

● Make sure that the patient or a responsible family member has signed an informed consent form, if required.

## Procedure and Posttest Care

● The patient is placed in a supine position on a narrow bed, which then slides him to the desired position inside the scanner, where radio-frequency energy is directed at his head or spine.

● The resulting images are displayed on a monitor and recorded on film or magnetic tape for permanent storage.

● The radiologist may vary radio-frequency waves and use the computer to manipulate and enhance the images.

● During the procedure, the patient must remain still.

● Tell the patient that he may resume his usual activity after the test.

● If the patient was sedated, make sure that a responsible person drives him home.

# MRI TECHNIQUES

Magnetic resonance imaging (MRI) is used to provide clear images of parts of the brain, such as the brain stem and cerebellum, that are difficult to image by other methods. Four MRI techniques are available to examine other aspects of the brain.

## MAGNETIC RESONANCE ANGIOGRAPHY

Magnetic resonance angiography allows the visualization of blood flowing through the cerebral vessels. Images of blood vessels done with magnetic resonance angiography aren't as clear as those obtained by angiography, but this technique is less invasive.

## MAGNETIC RESONANCE SPECTROSCOPY

Magnetic resonance spectroscopy creates images over time that show the metabolism of certain chemical markers in a specific area of the brain. Some researchers have dubbed this test a "metabolic biopsy" because it reveals pathologic neurochemistry over time.

## DIFFUSION-PERFUSION IMAGING

Diffusion-perfusion imaging uses a stronger-than-normal magnetic gradient to reveal areas of focal cerebral ischemia within minutes. Currently used in stroke research, this MRI technique may be used by diagnosticians to distinguish permanent from reversible ischemia.

## NEUROGRAPHY

Neurograms provide a three-dimensional image of nerves. They may be used to find the exact location of nerves that are damaged, crimped, or in disarray.

---

● If the test took a long time and the patient was lying flat for an extended period, observe him for orthostatic hypotension.

## PRECAUTIONS

● Because MRI works through a powerful magnetic field, be aware that it can't be performed on the patient with a pacemaker, an intracranial aneurysm clip, or other ferrous metal implants or on a patient with gunshot wounds to the head.
● Because of the strong magnetic field, know that metallic or computer-based equipment (for example, ventilators and I.V. pumps) can't enter the MRI area.

## NORMAL FINDINGS

MRI can show normal anatomic details of the central nervous system in any plane, without bone interference. Brain and spinal cord structures should appear distinct and sharply defined. Tissue color and shading will vary, depending on the radio-frequency energy, magnetic strength, and degree of computer enhancement.

## ABNORMAL FINDINGS

Because MRI depicts the density (water content) of tissue, it clearly shows structural changes resulting from disorders that in-crease tissue water content, such as cerebral edema, demyelinating disease, and pontine and cerebellar tumors. Edematous fluid, for example, generally appears cloudy or gray, whereas blood generally appears dark. Lesions of multiple sclerosis appear as areas of demyelination (curdlike, gray or gray-white areas) around the edges of ventricles. Tumors appear as changes in normal anatomy, which computer enhancement may further delineate.

## INTERFERING FACTORS

● Excessive patient movement (possible poor imaging)

## Magnetic resonance imaging of the urinary tract

Magnetic resonance imaging (MRI) is becoming more commonly used for diagnosing urinary tract disorders. It's unclear at present whether MRI is better than computed tomography or ultrasound for imaging the urinary system. In most cases, MRI is used when these alternative tests fail to produce a clear image. MRI uses radio-frequency waves and magnetic fields to visualize specific structures (kidney or prostate), which are then converted to computer-generated images.

## PURPOSE
- To evaluate genitourinary tumors and abdominal or pelvic masses
- To detect prostate stones and cysts
- To detect cancer invasion into seminal vesicles and pelvic lymph nodes

## PATIENT PREPARATION
- Explain to the patient that MRI of the urinary tract helps evaluate abnormalities in the urinary system.
- Advise the patient to avoid alcohol, caffeine-containing beverages, and smoking for at least 2 hours and food for at least 1 hour before the test.
- Tell the patient who will perform the test, where it will take place, and that it takes about 30 to 90 minutes.
- Explain to the patient that he can continue taking medications, except for iron, which interferes with the imaging.
- Before the test, tell the patient that he'll need to remove all clothing, jewelry, and metallic objects and wear a special hospital gown without snaps or closures.
- Inform the patient that he won't feel pain but may feel claustrophobic while lying supine in the tubular MRI chamber. If so, the physician may order an antianxiety medication.
- Tell the patient that he'll hear loud, crushing noises throughout the test. However, he'll probably receive a headset with a choice of music to decrease the loud noise.
- If contrast media will be used, obtain a history of allergies or hypersensitivity to these agents. Mark any sensitivities on the chart and notify the physician.
- Ask the patient if he has any implanted metal devices or prostheses, such as vascular clips, shrapnel, pacemakers, joint implants, filters, and intrauterine devices. If so, he may not be able to have the test.
- Make sure that the patient or a responsible family member has signed an informed consent form.
- Just before the procedure, have the patient urinate.

## PROCEDURE AND POSTTEST CARE
- If a contrast medium is used, start an I.V. line so that the medium is administered before the procedure.
- The patient is placed in the supine position on a narrow, flat table, and the table is then moved into the enclosed cylindrical scanner.
- Varying radio-frequency waves are directed at the area being scanned.
- The patient is told to lie completely still in the scanner while the images are being produced.
- Although his face remains uncovered to allow him to see out, the patient is advised to keep his eyes closed to promote relaxation and prevent a closed-in feeling.
- If nausea occurs because of claustrophobia, the patient is encouraged to take deep breaths.
- If sedatives were given, monitor the patient's vital signs until he's awake and responsive.
- Advise the patient that he may resume his usual diet, fluids, and medications, as ordered.
- Monitor the patient for adverse reactions to the contrast medium (flushing, nausea, urticaria, and sneezing).
- Watch the I.V. site for a hematoma, if applicable. If a hematoma occurs, apply pressure.

## PRECAUTIONS
- Be aware that MRI of the urinary tract is contraindicated in the patient with metal implants, rods, or screws or prosthetic devices.
- Know that this test is contraindicated in the pregnant patient unless its benefits greatly outweigh the possible risks to the fetus.
- Keep in mind that the scanner can't be used with an extremely obese patient.
- Make sure that all metal objects, such as jewelry, hairpins, and dentures, are removed before the test.

## NORMAL FINDINGS
In visualizing the soft-tissue structures of the kidneys, MRI can determine blood vessel size and anatomy. However, this test hasn't proved useful for detecting calculi or calcified tumors.

## ABNORMAL FINDINGS

MRI can reveal tumors, strictures, stenosis, thrombosis, malformations, abscess, inflammation, edema, fluid collection, bleeding, hemorrhage, and organ atrophy.

## INTERFERING FACTORS

- Uncooperative behavior, unstable medical conditions (confusion, combativeness), or inability to remain still during the procedure
- Use of I.V. pumps or assistive life-support equipment

# Mammography

Mammography is used as a screening test for breast cancer. It helps to detect breast cysts or tumors, especially those not palpable on physical examination. Biopsy of suspicious areas may be required to confirm malignancy. Mammography may follow screening procedures, such as ultrasonography or thermography. (See *Using ultrasonography to detect breast cancer*.)

Although mammography can detect 90% to 95% of breast cancers, this test produces many false-positive results. The American College of Radiologists and the American Cancer Society have established separate guidelines for the use and potential risks of mammography. Both groups agree that despite low radiation levels, the test is contraindicated during pregnancy. Magnetic resonance imaging, which is highly sensitive, is becoming a more popular method of breast imaging; however, it isn't very specific and leads to biopsies of many benign lesions. A new digital image approved by the U.S. Food and Drug Administration is similar in use as with mammography. (See *Digital mammography,* page 284.)

For the patient at high risk for breast cancer, a newer test, ductal lavage, may identify abnormal cells before they're large enough to form a tumor (see pages 143 and 144 for more information).

## PURPOSE

- To screen for malignant breast tumors
- To investigate palpable and unpalpable breast masses, breast pain, or nipple discharge

---

## USING ULTRASONOGRAPHY TO DETECT BREAST CANCER

Ultrasonography is especially usedful for diagnosing tumors less than ¼" (0.6 cm) in diameter and in distinguishing cysts from solid tumors in dense breast tissue. As in other ultrasound techniques, a transducer sends a beam of high-frequency sound waves through the patient's skin and into the breast. The sound waves are then processed and displayed for interpretation.

A benefit to ultrasonography is that it can show all areas of the breast, including the area close to the chest wall, which is difficult to study with X-rays. When used as an adjunct to mammography, ultrasound increases diagnostic accuracy; when used alone, it's more accurate than mammography in examining the denser breast tissue of a young patient.

---

- To help differentiate between benign breast disease and breast cancer
- To monitor the patient with breast cancer who has been treated with breast-conserving surgery and radiation

## PATIENT PREPARATION

- Assess the patient's understanding of the mammogram, answer her questions, and correct any misconceptions.
- Tell the patient who will perform the test and where it will take place.
- Tell the patient not to use underarm deodorant or powder on the day of the examination.
- If the patient has breast implants, tell her to inform the staff when she schedules the mammogram so that a technologist familiar with imaging implants is on duty.
- Inform the patient that although the test takes only about 15 minutes to perform, she may be asked to wait while the films are checked to make sure they're readable. Advise her that there's a high rate of false-positive results.
- Just before the test, give the patient a gown to wear that opens in the front, and ask her to remove all jewelry and clothing above the waist.

## DIGITAL MAMMOGRAPHY

Digital mammography produces pictures of the breast using X-rays. Instead of film, this process uses detectors that change the X-rays into electrical signals, which are then converted to an image. Digital mammography is used for screening and diagnosis. For the patient, the procedure is the same as with ordinary mammography.

Digital mammography may offer the following advantages over conventional mammography:

◆ The images can be stored and retrieved electronically, which makes long-distance consultations with other mammography specialists easier.

◆ Because the images can be adjusted by the radiologist, subtle differences between tissues may be noted.

◆ The number of follow-up procedures that are necessary may be reduced.

◆ The need for fewer exposures with digital mammography can reduce the already low levels of radiation.

The U.S. Food and Drug Administration has recently approved the Lorad Digital Breast Imager to be used in conjunction with the Lorad M-IV Mammography X-ray System for this digital procedure.

Digital mammography has been shown to be effective in the detection of breast cancer and other abnormalities.

## PROCEDURE AND POSTTEST CARE

● The patient stands and is asked to rest one of her breasts on a table above an X-ray cassette.

● The compression plate is placed on the breast and the patient is told to hold her breath. A radiograph is taken of the craniocaudal view. The machine is rotated, the breast is compressed again, and a radiograph of the lateral view is taken.

● The procedure is repeated on the other breast.

● After the films are developed, they're checked to make sure they're readable.

## PRECAUTIONS

● None.

## NORMAL FINDINGS

A normal mammogram reveals normal duct, glandular tissue, and fat architecture. No abnormal masses or calcifications should be seen.

## ABNORMAL FINDINGS

Well-outlined, regular, and clear spots suggest benign cysts; irregular, poorly outlined, and opaque areas suggest a malignant tumor. Malignant tumors are generally solitary and unilateral; benign cysts tend to occur bilaterally. Findings that suggest cancer require further tests, such as biopsy, for confirmation.

## INTERFERING FACTORS

● Powders or salves on the breasts (possible false-positive results)

● Failure to remove jewelry and clothing (possible false-positive results or poor imaging)

● Glandular breasts (common under age 30), active lactation, and previous breast surgery (possible poor imaging)

● Breast implants (may hinder detection of masses)

# Mediastinoscopy

Using an exploring speculum with built-in fiber light and side slit, mediastinoscopy allows direct viewing of mediastinal structures. It also permits palpation and biopsy of paratracheal and carinal lymph nodes. This surgical procedure is indicated when other tests, such as sputum cytology, lung scans, radiography, and bronchoscopic biopsy, fail to confirm the diagnosis. Scarring of the area from previous mediastinoscopy contraindicates this procedure.

## PURPOSE

● To diagnose bronchogenic carcinoma, lymphoma (including Hodgkin's disease), and sarcoidosis

● To determine stages of lung cancer

## PATIENT PREPARATION

● Explain to the patient that mediastinoscopy is used to evaluate the lymph nodes and other structures in the chest. Review his history for previous mediastinoscopy because scarring from a previous mediastinoscopy contraindicates the test.

● Describe the procedure to the patient, and answer his questions.

● Instruct the patient to fast after midnight before the test.

● Tell the patient who will perform the procedure, where it will be done, that he'll be given general anesthesia, and that the procedure takes about 1 hour.

● Tell the patient that he may have temporary chest pain, tenderness at the incision site, or a sore throat (from intubation).

● Reassure the patient that complications are rare.

● Make sure that the patient or a responsible family member has signed an informed consent form.

● Check the patient's history for hypersensitivity to the anesthetic.

● Give a sedative the night before the test and again before the procedure, as ordered.

## PROCEDURE AND POSTTEST CARE

● After the endotracheal tube is in place, a small transverse suprasternal incision is made.

● Using finger dissection, the surgeon forms a channel and palpates the lymph nodes.

● The mediastinoscope is inserted, and tissue specimens are collected and sent to the laboratory for frozen section examination.

● If analysis confirms malignancy of a resectable tumor, thoracotomy and pneumonectomy may follow immediately.

● Monitor the patient's postoperative vital signs and check his dressings for bleeding and fluid drainage.

⭐ *Alert Observe the patient for the following complications: fever (a sign of mediastinitis); crepitus (a sign of subcutaneous emphysema); dyspnea, cyanosis, and diminished breath sounds on the affected side (signs of pneumothorax); and tachycardia and hypotension (signs of hemorrhage).*

● Administer the prescribed analgesic, as needed.

## PRECAUTIONS

● Immediately send collected specimens to the laboratory.

## NORMAL FINDINGS

Lymph nodes appear as small, smooth, flat oval bodies of lymphoid tissue.

## ABNORMAL FINDINGS

Malignant lymph nodes usually indicate inoperable, but not always untreatable, lung or esophageal cancer or lymphomas (such as Hodgkin's disease). Staging of lung cancer helps determine the therapeutic regimen. (For example, multiple nodular involvement can contraindicate surgery.)

## INTERFERING FACTORS

● Previous mediastinoscopy with scarring (makes lymph node dissection difficult or impossible)

# *Myelography*

Myelography uses fluoroscopy and radiography to evaluate the spinal subarachnoid space after injection of a contrast medium. Because the contrast medium is heavier than cerebrospinal fluid (CSF), it flows through the subarachnoid space to the dependent area when the patient, lying prone on a fluoroscopic table, is tilted up or down. The fluoroscope allows the physician to see the flow of the contrast medium and the outline of the subarachnoid space. X-rays are taken to provide a permanent record.

Myelography can help locate a spinal lesion, a ruptured disk, spinal stenosis, or an abscess. Sometimes it's performed to confirm the need for surgery; in such cases, a neurosurgeon may stand by. If this test confirms a spinal tumor, the patient may be taken directly to the operating room. Immediate surgery may also be necessary when the contrast medium causes a total block of the subarachnoid space.

## PURPOSE

● To evaluate and determine the cause of neurologic symptoms (numbness, pain, weakness)

● To identify lesions, such as tumors and herniated intervertebral disks that partially or

totally block the flow of CSF in the sub-arachnoid space
● To help detect arachnoiditis, spinal nerve root injury, or tumors in the posterior fossa of the skull

## PATIENT PREPARATION
● Explain to the patient that myelography reveals obstructions in the spinal cord.
● Tell the patient that his food and fluid intake will be restricted for 8 hours before the test. If the test is scheduled for the afternoon and facility policy permits, the patient may have clear liquids before the test.
● Describe the test, including who will administer it and where it will take place.
● Explain to the patient that he may feel a transient burning sensation as the contrast medium is injected; a warm, flushed feeling; transient headache; a salty taste; or nausea and vomiting after the dye is injected. Explain that he may feel some pain caused by his positioning, needle insertion and, in some cases, removal of the contrast medium.
● Make sure that the patient or a responsible family member has signed an informed consent form.

**Alert** *Check the patient's history for hypersensitivity to iodine and iodine-containing substances (for example, shellfish), radiographic contrast media, and associated medications. Notify the radiologist if the patient has a history of epilepsy or phenothiazine use. If metrizamide is to be used as a contrast medium, discontinue phenothiazine 48 hours before the test.*

● Tell the patient to remove all jewelry and other metallic objects in the X-ray field.
● Tell the patient that the head of his bed must be elevated for 6 to 8 hours after the test and that he'll remain on bed rest for an additional 6 to 8 hours. If an oil-based contrast agent is used, inform the patient that it will be manually removed after the test and that he'll need to remain flat in bed for 6 to 24 hours.
● Perform pretest procedures and administer prescribed medications. If the puncture is to be performed in the lumbar region, an enema may be prescribed. A sedative and anticholinergic (such as atropine sulfate) may be prescribed to reduce swallowing during the procedure. Make sure that pretest laboratory work (may include coagulation and kidney function studies) is present in the chart.

## PROCEDURE AND POSTTEST CARE
● Position the patient on his side at the edge of the table with his chin on his chest and his knees drawn up to his abdomen. (If the patient has a lumbar deformity or an infection at the puncture site, a cisternal puncture may be done.)
● After the lumbar puncture is performed, the fluoroscope is used to verify proper positioning of the needle in the subarachnoid space. Some CSF may be removed for routine laboratory analysis.
● Turn the patient to the prone position and secure him with straps across his upper back, under his arms, and across his ankles. Hyperextend his chin to prevent the contrast medium from flowing into the cranium; place a towel under his chin for comfort.
● If the patient complains of a headache or difficulty swallowing or reports that he isn't breathing deeply enough, provide reassurance and explain that he can rest periodically during the procedure.
● The contrast medium is injected and the table tilted so that the dye flows through the subarachnoid space. (In rare circumstances, air is used as a negative contrast medium; however, this is typically reserved for a patient with suspected congenital abnormalities such as syringomyelia.)
● The contrast medium flow is observed by fluoroscope, and X-rays are taken. If an obstruction in the subarachnoid space blocks the upward flow of the contrast medium, a cisternal puncture may be performed.
● The contrast medium is withdrawn, if necessary, after satisfactory X-rays are obtained and the needle is removed. Clean the puncture site with povidone-iodine solution and apply a small adhesive bandage.
● Based on the contrast medium used during the test, position the patient as follows: If metrizamide was used, tell him to stay in bed for the next 12 to 16 hours. Keep the head of his bed elevated for at least 8 hours. If an oil-based contrast medium was used, tell him to remain flat in bed for 24 hours.
● Monitor the patient's vital signs and neurologic status at least every 15 minutes for the first hour, every 30 minutes for the next 2 hours, and then every 4 hours for 24 hours. The patient may be discharged the same day.
● Encourage the patient to drink extra fluids. He should void within 8 hours after returning to his room.

- If there are no complications or adverse reactions, tell the patient that he may resume his usual diet and activities the day after the test, as ordered.
- Monitor the patient for radicular pain, fever, back pain, or signs of meningeal irritation, such as headache, irritability, or stiff neck. If these signs or symptoms occur, keep the room quiet and dark and administer an analgesic or antipyretic, as needed.

## PRECAUTIONS
- Be aware that, generally, myelography is contraindicated in the patient with increased intracranial pressure, hypersensitivity to iodine or contrast media, or an infection at the puncture site.
- Know that improper positioning after the test may affect recovery.

## NORMAL FINDINGS
Normally, the contrast medium flows freely through the subarachnoid space, showing no obstruction or structural abnormalities.

## ABNORMAL FINDINGS
Myelography can identify and localize lesions within or surrounding the spinal cord or subarachnoid space. Examples of common extradural lesions include herniated intervertebral disks and metastatic tumors. Neurofibromas and meningiomas are common lesions within the subarachnoid space, and ependymomas and astrocytomas are common within the spinal cord.

If the test confirms a spinal tumor, the patient may be taken directly to the operating room. Immediate surgery may also be necessary if the contrast medium causes a total block of the subarachnoid space.

Myelography may help locate or confirm a ruptured or herniated disk, spinal stenosis, or abscess and, occasionally, confirm the need for surgery. This test may also detect syringomyelia (a congenital abnormality marked by fluid-filled cavities within the spinal cord and widening of the cord itself), arachnoiditis, spinal nerve root injury, and tumors in the posterior fossa of the skull. Other findings may include fractures, dislocations, thinning of bones (osteoporosis), deformities in the curvature of the spine, bone spurs, and vertebral degeneration. Test results must be correlated with the patient's history and clinical status.

## INTERFERING FACTORS
- Incorrect needle placement
- An uncooperative patient

# Myoglobins

Myoglobin, which is usually found in skeletal and cardiac muscle, functions as an oxygen-binding muscle protein. It's released into the bloodstream in ischemia, trauma, and inflammation of the muscle.

The release of myoglobin into the bloodstream is especially important when trying to determine damaged cardiac muscle. Creatine kinase (CK) and its isoform CK-MB are released more slowly than myoglobin during a myocardial infarction (MI). Therefore, myoglobin, which can be detected as soon as 2 hours after the onset of chest pain and peaks in 4 hours, can be useful as an early indicator of an MI.

## PURPOSE
- As a nonspecific test, to estimate damage to skeletal or cardiac muscle tissue
- To predict flare-ups of polymyositis
- Specifically, to determine if an MI has occurred

## PATIENT PREPARATION
- Explain the purpose of the myoglobins test to the patient.
- Obtain a patient history, including disorders that may be associated with increased myoglobin levels.
- Tell the patient that the test requires a blood sample. Explain who will be performing the venipuncture and when.
- Explain to the patient that he may experience slight discomfort from the tourniquet and needle puncture.
- Inform the patient that the results need to be correlated with other tests for a definitive diagnosis.

## PROCEDURE AND POSTTEST CARE
- Perform a venipuncture, and collect the sample in a 4-ml tube with no additives.
- Apply direct pressure to the venipuncture site until bleeding stops.
- If a hematoma develops at the venipuncture site, apply pressure.

## PRECAUTIONS

- Expect to collect blood samples 4 to 8 hours after the onset of an acute MI.
- Handle the sample gently to avoid hemolysis.
- Send the sample to the laboratory immediately.

## REFERENCE VALUES

Normal myoglobin values are 0 to 0.09 µg/ml (SI, 5 to 70 µ/L).

## ABNORMAL FINDINGS

Besides MI, increased myoglobin levels may occur in acute alcohol intoxication, dermatomyositis, hypothermia (with prolonged shivering), muscular dystrophy, polymyositis, rhabdomyelitis, severe burns, trauma, severe renal failure, and systemic lupus erythematosus.

## INTERFERING FACTORS

- Radioactive scans performed within 1 week of the test
- Recent angina, cardioversion, or improper timing of the test (possible increase)
- I.M. injection (possible false-positive)

## *Myoglobin, urine*

The myoglobin test detects the presence of myoglobin — a red pigment found in the cytoplasm of cardiac and skeletal muscle cells — in the urine. When muscle cells are extensively damaged, as by disease or severe crushing trauma, myoglobin is released into the blood, quickly cleared by renal glomerular filtration, and eliminated in the urine (myoglobinuria). For example, myoglobin appears in the urine within 24 hours after a myocardial infarction (MI).

Urine myoglobin must be differentiated from urine hemoglobin because of their marked structural similarities. The most commonly used test method is the differential precipitation test. Hemoglobin — bound to haptoglobin — precipitates when urine is mixed with ammonium sulfate. Myoglobin, however, remains soluble and can be measured.

## PURPOSE

- To aid in the diagnosis of muscular disease of rhabdomyolysis
- To detect extensive infarction of muscle tissue
- To assess the extent of muscular damage from crushing trauma

## PATIENT PREPARATION

- Explain to the patient that the urine myoglobin test detects a red pigment found in muscle cells and helps evaluate muscle injury or disease.
- Inform the patient that he need not restrict food and fluids.
- Tell the patient that this test requires a random urine specimen, and teach him the proper collection technique.

## PROCEDURE AND POSTTEST CARE

- Collect a random urine specimen.

## PRECAUTIONS

- Send the specimen to the laboratory immediately after collection.

## NORMAL FINDINGS

Normally, myoglobin doesn't appear in urine.

## ABNORMAL FINDINGS

Myoglobinuria occurs in acute or chronic muscular disease, alcoholic polymyopathy, familial myoglobinuria, extensive MI, and in severe trauma to the skeletal muscles (which may result from a crush injury, extreme hyperthermia, or severe burns). It also occurs in strenuous or prolonged exercise, but disappears after rest.

## INTERFERING FACTORS

- Extremely dilute urine (reduces sensitivity)
- Contamination with iodine during surgery (positive results)
- Recent ingestion of large amounts of vitamin C (inhibits reaction if testing is performed with Chemstrip or other reagent strips)

## Nasopharyngeal culture

A nasopharyngeal culture is used to evaluate nasopharyngeal secretions for the presence of pathogenic organisms. It requires direct microscopic examination of a Gram-stained smear of the specimen. Preliminary identification of organisms may be used to guide clinical management and determine the need for additional testing. Cultured pathogens may then require susceptibility testing to determine appropriate antimicrobial therapy.

Nasopharyngeal cultures are typically useful for identifying *Bordetella pertussis* and *Neisseria meningitidis,* especially in very young, elderly, or debilitated patients. They can also be used to isolate viruses, especially carriers of influenza virus A and B. However, because the laboratory procedure required for such testing is complex, time-consuming, and costly, this culture is performed infrequently.

### PURPOSE
● To identify pathogens causing upper respiratory tract symptoms
● To identify proliferation of normal nasopharyngeal flora, which may be pathogenic in debilitated and other immunocompromised patients
● To identify *B. pertussis* and *N. meningitidis,* especially in very young, elderly, or debilitated patients and asymptomatic carriers
● Rarely, to isolate viruses, especially to identify carriers of influenza virus A and B

### PATIENT PREPARATION
● Explain to the patient that the nasopharyngeal culture is used to isolate the cause of nasopharyngeal infection.
● Describe the procedure to the patient; tell him that secretions will be obtained from the back of the nose and the throat, using a cotton-tipped swab, and who will collect the specimen.
● Warn the patient that he may experience slight discomfort and gagging, but reassure him that obtaining the specimen takes less than 15 seconds.

### PROCEDURE AND POSTTEST CARE
● Put on gloves.
● Moisten the swab with sterile water or saline.
● Ask the patient to cough before you begin collecting the specimen.
● Position the patient with his head tilted back.
● Using a penlight and a tongue blade, inspect the nasopharyngeal area.
● Gently pass the swab through the nostril and into the nasopharynx, keeping the swab near the septum and floor of the nose. Rotate the swab quickly and remove it.
● Alternatively, place the glass tube in the patient's nostril, and carefully pass the swab through the tube into the nasopharynx. (See *Obtaining a nasopharyngeal specimen,* page 290.) Rotate the swab for 5 seconds and then place it in the culture tube with transport medium. Remove the glass tube.
● Label the specimen with the patient's name, physician's name, date and time of

# OBTAINING A NASOPHARYNGEAL SPECIMEN

When the swab passes into the nasopharynx, gently but quickly rotate it to collect a specimen. Then remove the swab, taking care not to injure the nasal mucous membrane.

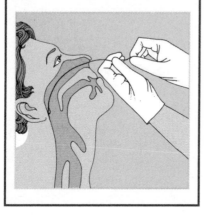

collection, origin of the material, and the suspected organism.

● Ideally, specimens for *B. pertussis* should be inoculated to fresh culture medium at the patient's bedside because of the organism's susceptibility to environmental changes.

● If the purpose of specimen collection is to isolate a virus, follow the laboratory's recommended collection technique.

## PRECAUTIONS

● Wear gloves when performing the procedure and handling the specimen.

● Don't let the swab touch the sides of the patient's nostril or his tongue to prevent specimen contamination.

● ⊛ **Alert** *Laryngospasm may occur after the culture is obtained if the patient has epiglottiditis or diphtheria. Keep resuscitation equipment nearby.*

● Note antimicrobial therapy or chemotherapy on the laboratory request.

● Keep the container upright.

● Tell the laboratory if the suspected organism is *Corynebacterium diphtheriae* or *B. pertussis* because these need special growth media.

● Refrigerate a viral specimen according to your laboratory's procedure.

● If *B. pertussis* is suspected, use Dacron or calcium alginate mini-tipped swabs for collection.

● Know that when specimens can't be directly placed onto growth media, the best media-based transport is one supplemented with antibiotics to reduce the growth of normal flora.

## NORMAL FINDINGS

Flora commonly found in the nasopharynx include nonhemolytic streptococci, alpha-hemolytic streptococci, *Neisseria* species (except *N. meningitidis* and *N. gonorrhoeae*), coagulase-negative staphylococci, such as *Staphylococcus epidermidis* and, occasionally, the coagulase-positive *S. aureus.*

## ABNORMAL FINDINGS

Pathogens include group A beta-hemolytic streptococci; occasionally groups B, C, and G beta-hemolytic streptococci; *B. pertussis, C. diphtheriae,* and *S. aureus;* large numbers of pneumococci; *Haemophilus influenzae; Myxovirus influenzae;* paramyxoviruses; *Candida albicans;* mycoplasma species; and *Mycobacterium tuberculosis.*

## INTERFERING FACTORS

● Recent antimicrobial therapy (decrease in bacterial growth)

# Neonatal thyroid-stimulating hormone

The neonatal thyroid-stimulating hormone (TSH) test is an immunoassay that confirms congenital hypothyroidism after an initial screening test detects low thyroxine ($T_4$) levels. Normally, TSH levels surge after birth, triggering a rise in thyroid hormone that's essential for neurologic development. In primary congenital hypothyroidism, the thyroid gland doesn't respond to TSH stimulation, resulting in diminished thyroid hormone levels and elevated TSH levels. Early detection and treatment of congenital hypothyroidism is critical to prevent mental retardation and cretinism.

## PURPOSE
● To confirm diagnosis of congenital hypothyroidism

## PATIENT PREPARATION
● Explain to the infant's parents that the neonatal TSH test helps confirm the diagnosis of congenital hypothyroidism.
● Emphasize the importance of detecting the disorder early so that prompt therapy can prevent irreversible brain damage.

## PROCEDURE AND POSTTEST CARE
### Filter paper sample
● Assemble the necessary equipment, wash your hands thoroughly, and put on gloves.
● Wipe the infant's heel with an alcohol or povidone-iodine swab, and then dry it thoroughly with a gauze pad.
● Perform a heelstick.
● Squeezing the infant's heel gently, fill the circles on the filter paper with blood. Make sure that the blood saturates the paper.
● Gently apply pressure with a gauze pad to ensure hemostasis at the puncture site.
● Allow the filter paper to dry, label it appropriately, and send it to the laboratory.

### Serum sample
● Perform a venipuncture, and collect the sample in a 3-ml clot-activator tube. Label the sample and send it to the laboratory immediately.
● Apply direct pressure to the venipuncture or heelstick site until bleeding stops.
● If a hematoma develops at the venipuncture site, apply pressure.

## PRECAUTIONS
● Handle the samples carefully to prevent hemolysis.

## REFERENCE VALUES
At age 1 to 2 days, TSH levels are normally 25 to 30 µIU/ml (SI, 25 to 30 mU/L). Thereafter, levels are normally less than 25 µIU/ml (SI, < 25 mU/L).

## ABNORMAL FINDINGS
Neonatal TSH levels must be interpreted in light of the $T_4$ concentration. Elevated TSH levels accompanied by decreased $T_4$ levels indicate primary congenital hypothyroidism (thyroid gland dysfunction). Low TSH and $T_4$ levels may be present in secondary congenital hypothyroidism (pituitary or hypothalamic dysfunction). Normal TSH levels accompanied by low $T_4$ levels may indicate hypothyroidism due to a congenital defect in $T_4$-binding globulin or transient congenital hypothyroidism due to prematurity or prenatal hypoxia. A complete thyroid workup must be done to confirm the cause of hypothyroidism before treatment can begin.

## INTERFERING FACTORS
● Corticosteroids, triiodothyronine, and $T_4$ (decrease)
● Lithium carbonate, potassium iodide, excessive topical resorcinol, and TSH injection (increase)

# *Nephrotomography*

In nephrotomography, special films are exposed before and after opacification of the renal arterial network and parenchyma with contrast medium. The resulting tomographic slices clearly delineate various linear layers of the kidneys, while blurring structures in front of and behind these selected planes.

Nephrotomography can be performed as a separate procedure or as an adjunct to excretory urography. Nephrotomography is particularly helpful in visualizing space-occupying lesions suggested by excretory urography or retrograde ureteropyelography. Additional films are exposed to define the wall thickness of the mass and its interior. Other tests that may resolve nephrotomographic findings include renal angiography and radionuclide renal imaging.

## PURPOSE
● To differentiate between a simple renal cyst and a solid neoplasm
● To assess renal lacerations as well as posttraumatic nonperfused areas of the kidneys
● To localize adrenal tumors when laboratory tests indicate their presence

## PATIENT PREPARATION
● Explain to the patient that nephrotomography provides images of sections or layers of the kidney tissues and blood vessels.

- Instruct the patient to fast for 8 hours before the test. Tell him who will perform the test and where it will take place.
- Tell the patient that he'll be positioned on an X-ray table and that he may hear loud, clacking sounds as the films are exposed. Tell him that he may experience transient adverse effects from the contrast medium injection — usually a burning or stinging sensation at the injection site, flushing, and a metallic taste.
- Make sure that the patient or a responsible family member has signed an informed consent form.

**Alert** *Check the patient's history for hypersensitivity to iodine or iodine-containing foods or to contrast media used in other diagnostic tests. If he has a history of sensitivity, provide antiallergenic prophylaxis (such as diphenhydramine) or use a non-iodine-containing contrast medium, as necessary.*

**Age alert** *An elderly or a dehydrated patient is at increased risk for contrast-induced renal failure. Check serum creatinine levels and inform the physician if they're elevated. I.V. fluids may be ordered before the test to ensure hydration and decrease nephrotoxic potential.*

## PROCEDURE AND POSTTEST CARE

- The test may be performed using either the infusion method or bolus method. Complications resulting from either technique are minor and infrequent.
- A plain film of the kidneys is exposed to provide general information about their position, size, and shape, and preliminary anteroposterior tomograms are made to determine tomographic levels. Posterior oblique tomograms are made to rule out the presence of radiopaque renal calculi, which would be masked by the contrast medium.

### Infusion method

- After test tomograms are reviewed, five vertical slices of renal parenchyma ⅜″ (1 cm) apart are selected for filming.
- Contrast medium is then administered through the antecubital vein — the first half in 4 to 5 minutes (rapid phase) and the second half in the following 8 to 10 minutes (slow phase). Serial tomograms are made as soon as the slow phase begins.

### Bolus method

- After test tomograms are reviewed, circulation time from arm to tongue is determined

by injecting a bolus of a bitter-tasting agent (dehydrocholic acid or sodium dehydrocholate) into the antecubital vein. Arm-to-tongue circulation time is close to arm-to-kidney circulation time.
- With the needle still in place, a loading dose of a conventional urographic contrast medium is injected to perform excretory urography.
- Five minutes after this injection, a loading dose of a contrast medium is quickly injected to ensure a high concentration of the contrast medium in the kidneys. A multifilm tomographic cassette, exposed at the predetermined arm-to-kidney circulation time, visualizes the main renal vessels and possible vessels within tumors.
- A series of individual tomograms measuring ⅜″ (1 cm) are then made in rapid succession through the opacified kidneys.
- If the exposures are poor, this method requires a second infusion of contrast medium because normal kidneys quickly clear the substance.

### Both methods

- If a hematoma develops at the injection site, apply pressure.
- Monitor the patient's vital signs and urine output for 24 hours after the test.
- Ensure adequate hydration (unless contraindicated) and monitor serum creatinine levels because of the risk of contrast-induced renal failure.

**Alert** *Observe the patient for signs of a posttest allergic reaction (flushing, nausea, urticaria, and sneezing). Have epinephrine (1:1,000) and an antihistamine readily available to counter allergic reactions.*

## PRECAUTIONS

- Know that nephrotomography should be performed with extreme caution in the patient with hypersensitivity to iodine-based compounds, cardiovascular disease, or multiple myeloma and in an elderly or a dehydrated patient with impaired renal function, as evidenced by elevated serum creatinine.

## NORMAL FINDINGS

The size, shape, and position of the kidneys appear within normal range, with no space-occupying lesions or other abnormalities.

## SIMPLE CYST OR SOLID TUMOR: DIFFERENTIAL DIAGNOSIS IN NEPHROTOMOGRAPHY

| FEATURE | CYST | TUMOR |
|---------|------|-------|
| Consistency | Homogeneous | Irregular |
| Contact with healthy renal tissue | Sharply distinct | Poorly resolved |
| Density | Radiolucent | Variable radiolucent patches (or same as normal renal parenchyma) |
| Shape | Spheric | Variable |
| Wall of lesion | Thin and well defined | Thick and irregular |

### ABNORMAL FINDINGS
Among the abnormalities detectable through nephrotomography are simple cysts and solid tumors, renal sinus-related lesions, ectopic renal lobes, adrenal tumors, areas of nonperfusion, and renal lacerations following trauma. (See *Simple cyst or solid tumor: Differential diagnosis in nephrotomography*.)

### INTERFERING FACTORS
* Residual barium from a recent enema or other GI studies (possible poor imaging)

# Ocular ultrasonography

Ocular ultrasonography involves the transmission of high-frequency sound waves through the eye and the measurement of their reflection from ocular structures. An A-scan converts the resulting echoes into waveforms whose crests represent the positions of different structures, providing a linear dimensional picture. The B-scan converts the echoes into patterns of dots that form a two-dimensional, cross-sectional image of the ocular structure.

Because the B-scan is easier to interpret than the A-scan, it's used more commonly to evaluate the structures of the eye and to diagnose abnormalities. However, the A-scan is more valuable in measuring the eye's axial length and characterizing the tissue texture of abnormal lesions. Thus, a combination of A- and B-scans produces the most useful test results.

Illustrating the eyes' structures through ultrasound is especially helpful in evaluating a fundus clouded by an opaque medium such as a cataract. In such a patient, this test can identify pathologies that are normally undetectable through ophthalmoscopy.

Ophthalmologists may also perform this test before surgery—for example, cataract removal—to ensure the integrity of the retina. If an intraocular lens is to be implanted, ultrasound may be used preoperatively to measure the length of the eye and the curvature of the cornea as a guide for the surgeon. Unlike computed tomography, ocular ultrasonography is readily available and provides information immediately.

In addition to its diagnostic capabilities, ocular ultrasonography can also identify intraocular foreign bodies and determine their position in relation to ocular structures as well as assess the severity of resulting ocular damage.

## PURPOSE
● To aid in evaluating the fundus in an eye with an opaque medium such as a cataract
● To aid in the diagnosis of vitreous disorders and retinal detachment
● To diagnose and differentiate between intraocular and orbital lesions and to follow their progression through serial examinations
● To locate intraocular foreign bodies

## PATIENT PREPARATION
● Describe the procedure to the patient and explain that ocular ultrasonography evaluates the eye's structures.
● Inform the patient that he need not restrict food and fluids.
● Tell the patient who will be performing the test and where it will be done.
● Reassure the patient that the procedure is safe and painless and takes about 5 minutes to perform.
● Tell the patient that a small transducer will be placed on his closed eyelid and that the transducer transmits high-frequency sound waves that are reflected by the structures in the eye.
● Inform the patient that he may be asked to move his eyes or change his gaze during the procedure and that his cooperation is required to ensure accurate test results.

# Normal B-scan

This is a normal B-scan using the lid contact method. The posterior lens capsule is visible, but the cornea and iris aren't because of obscuring echoes from the eyelid.

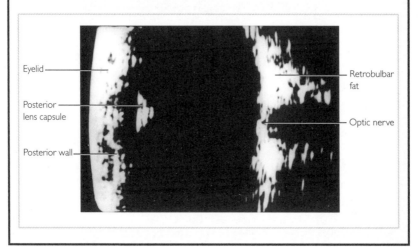

Eyelid

Posterior lens capsule

Posterior wall

Retrobulbar fat

Optic nerve

## Procedure and Posttest Care

● The patient is placed in the supine position on an X-ray table.

● For the B-scan, the patient is asked to close his eyes, and a water-soluble gel (such as Goniosol) is applied to his eyelid. The transducer is then placed on the eyelid.

● For the A-scan, the patient's eye is numbed with anesthetizing drops and a clear plastic eye cup is placed directly on the eyeball. A water-soluble gel is then applied to the eye cup, and the transducer is positioned on the medium.

● The transducer then transmits high-frequency sound waves into the patient's eye, and the resulting echoes are transformed into images or waveforms on the oscilloscope screen.

● After the test, the water-soluble gel is removed from the patient's eyelid.

## Precautions

● None

## Normal findings

The optic nerve and the posterior lens capsule produce echoes that take on characteristic forms on A- and B-scan images. The pos-

terior wall of the eye appears as a smooth, concave curve; retrobulbar fat can also be identified, as can the lens and vitreous humor, which don't produce echoes. Normal orbital echo patterns depend on the position of the transducer and the position of the patient's gaze during the procedure. (See *Normal B-scan*.)

## Abnormal findings

In eyes clouded by a vitreous hemorrhage, the organization of the hemorrhage can be identified by the degree of density that appears on the image. In some instances, the cause of the hemorrhage, the prognosis, and associated abnormalities can also be determined.

Other vitreous abnormalities, such as massive vitreous organization and vitreous bands, may also be detected by ultrasonography. Retinal detachment, commonly found in a patient with an opaque medium, characteristically produces a dense, sheetlike echo on a B-scan. The extent of retinal or choroidal detachment can be defined by transmitting ultrasound waves through the quadrants of the patient's eye.

Ocular ultrasonography can be used to diagnose and differentiate intraocular tumors according to size, shape, location, and texture. The most common tumors identified are melanomas, metastatic tumors, and hemangiomas. This test can also identify retinoblastomas and measure the dimensions of other tumors detectable by ophthalmoscopy.

Hemangiomas and cystic lesions produce characteristic ultrasound patterns. Other orbital lesions detectable by ultrasound include meningiomas, neurofibromas, gliomas, neurilemomas, and the inflammatory changes associated with Graves' disease.

## INTERFERING FACTORS
● None

# Oculoplethysmography

An important cerebrovascular test, oculoplethysmography (OPG) is a noninvasive procedure that indirectly measures blood flow in the ophthalmic artery. Because the ophthalmic artery is the first major branch of the internal carotid artery, its blood flow accurately reflects carotid blood flow and ultimately that of cerebral circulation. Two techniques are used for this test. In OPG, pulse arrival times in the eyes and ears are measured and compared to detect carotid occlusive disease. In ocular pneumoplethysmography (OPG-Gee), ophthalmic artery pressures are measured indirectly and compared with the higher brachial pressure and with each other.

Indications for both of these tests include symptoms of transient ischemic attacks, asymptomatic carotid bruits, and nonhemispheric neurologic symptoms, such as dizziness, ataxia, or syncope. This test may also be performed as a follow-up procedure after carotid endarterectomy or with transcranial Doppler studies or carotid imaging. If indicated, it may be followed by cerebral angiography. Carotid phonoangiography is commonly a valuable complement to OPG. (See *Carotid phonoangiography*.)

## PURPOSE
● To aid in the detection and evaluation of carotid occlusive disease

## PATIENT PREPARATION
● Explain to the patient that the OPG test evaluates carotid artery function.
● Inform the patient that he need not restrict food and fluids.
● Tell the patient who will perform the test, where it will take place, and that the procedure takes only a few minutes.
● Warn the patient that his eyes may burn slightly after the eyedrops are instilled.
● If OPG-Gee is scheduled, warn the patient that he may experience transient loss of vision when suction is applied to the eyes.
● Instruct the patient not to blink or move during the procedure.
● If the patient wears contact lenses, tell him to remove them before the test.
● The patient with glaucoma may take his usual medications and eyedrops.

## PROCEDURE AND POSTTEST CARE
### For OPG
● Anesthetic eyedrops are instilled to minimize patient discomfort during the test.
● Small photoelectric cells are attached to the earlobes; these cells can detect blood flow to the ear through the external carotid artery. Tracings for both ears are taken and compared, but only right ear tracings are compared with the eyes. (Tracings for the ears should be the same; if they aren't, this discrepancy is considered during interpretation of test results.)
● Eyecups resembling contact lenses are applied to the corneas and held in place with light suction (40 to 50 mm Hg). Tracings of the pulsations within each eye are compared with each other and with tracings for the right ear.

### For OPG-Gee
● Anesthetic eyedrops are instilled, and eyecups like those used in OPG are attached to the scleras of the eyes.
● A vacuum of 300 mm Hg is applied to each eye, corresponding to a mean pressure of 100 mm Hg in the ophthalmic artery, and then is gradually released.
● When suction is applied, the pulse in both eyes disappears; when suction is gradually released, pulses should return simultaneously. Pulse arrival times are converted to ophthalmic artery pressures and then compared.

# CAROTID PHONOANGIOGRAPHY

Carotid phonoangiography graphically records the intensity of carotid bruits during systolic and diastolic phases. Thus, it helps identify the presence, site, and severity of carotid artery occlusive disease.

For this test, the patient assumes a supine position and holds his breath while a transducer is placed at several sites along the carotid artery. Soundings are made directly over the clavicle (common carotid artery), midway up the neck (carotid bifurcation), and directly below the mandible (internal carotid artery). Oscillographic recordings are obtained and stored on Polaroid film and magnetic tape for later study.

Absence of bruits generally indicates an absence of significant carotid artery disease.

However, bruits may also be absent when stenosis nears total occlusion. Bruits heard at all three sites, but loudest over the clavicle, usually originate in the aortic arch or in the heart. Blood flow in the carotid artery itself is unobstructed. Bruits heard over the carotid bifurcation and internal carotid sites, but louder over the latter, indicate turbulent blood flow in the internal carotid artery and the probability of more than 40% occlusion.

Carotid phonoangiography is a quick test and relatively simple to perform, but it's less sensitive and less specific than other noninvasive techniques such as carotid imaging with Doppler ultrasound. Nevertheless, this test is approximately 85% accurate in detecting carotid artery stenosis of more than 40%.

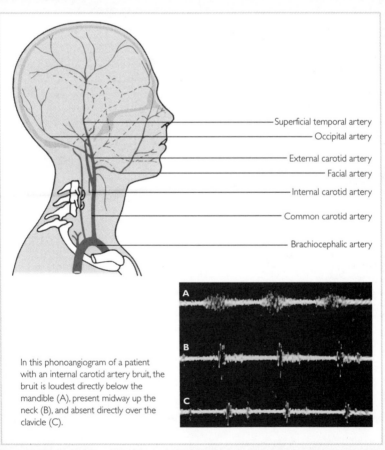

Superficial temporal artery
Occipital artery
External carotid artery
Facial artery
Internal carotid artery
Common carotid artery
Brachiocephalic artery

A

B

C

In this phonoangiogram of a patient with an internal carotid artery bruit, the bruit is loudest directly below the mandible (A), present midway up the neck (B), and absent directly over the clavicle (C).

# OPG EXAMINATION AND TRACINGS

The patient shown here is undergoing oculoplethysmography (OPG). The eyecups on the patient's corneas detect ocular pulsations, which are compared with each other and with the blood flow in the ear. Blood flow in the ear is detected by a small photoelectric cell (not shown).

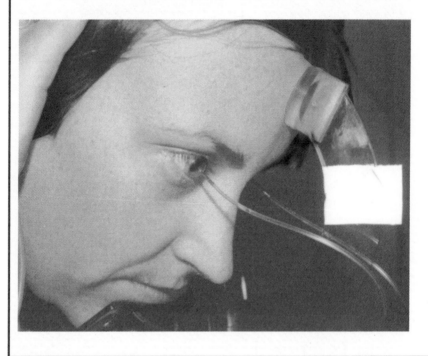

● Both brachial pressures are taken. The higher systolic pressure is then compared with the ophthalmic artery pressures. (See *OPG examination and tracings*.)
● To prevent corneal abrasion, instruct the patient not to rub his eyes for 2 hours after the test. Observe for symptoms of corneal abrasion, such as pain or photophobia, and report them to the physician.
● Advise the patient that mild burning as the eyedrops wear off is normal. Tell him to report severe burning.
● If the patient wears contact lenses, instruct him not to reinsert them for about 2 hours after OPG; this will allow the effect of the anesthetic drops to wear off.

## PRECAUTIONS
● Know that OPG is contraindicated in the patient who has had recent eye surgery (within 2 to 6 months), enucleation, or a history of retinal detachment or lens implantation and in the patient who's hypersensitive to the local anesthetic. Because of the risk of scleral hematoma or erythema, OPG-Gee is contraindicated in the patient receiving anticoagulants.
● To limit the risk of corneal abrasions, both techniques must be performed by specially trained personnel.

## NORMAL FINDINGS
### For OPG
All pulses should occur simultaneously.

The OPG tracing at right is normal, showing simultaneous pulsations in the right and left eyes and in the right ear. The differential waveform of ocular pulses (horizontal waveform), which amplifies pulse differences, and the vertical lines drawn on valleys and peaks of pulses, to indicate pulse delays, confirm simultaneous pulsation.

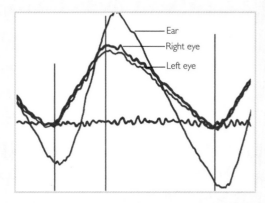

The OPG tracing at right is abnormal; the left-eye pulsation (vertical lines) arrives later than the other two pulsations, indicating left internal carotid artery stenosis. Note the elevation of the differential waveform.

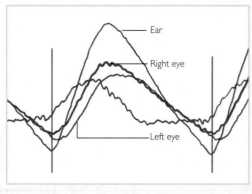

### For OPG-Gee

The difference between ophthalmic artery pressures should be less than 5 mm Hg. Ophthalmic artery pressure divided by the higher brachial systolic pressure should be greater than 0.67.

### ABNORMAL FINDINGS
### For OPG

Carotid occlusive disease reduces the rate of blood flow during systole and delays the arrival of a pulse in the ipsilateral eye or ear. When all pulses are compared, any delay can be measured and the degree of carotid artery stenosis estimated as mild, moderate, or severe. This test only estimates the extent of stenosis; it can't provide an exact percentage. (See *Understanding carotid imaging,* pages 300 and 301.) .

### For OPG-Gee

A difference between ophthalmic artery pressures of more than 5 mm Hg suggests the presence of carotid occlusive disease on the side with the lower pressure. A ratio between the ophthalmic artery pressure and the higher brachial systolic pressure of less than 0.67 reinforces this finding. In other words, the ratio is related to the degree of stenosis: The lower the ratio, the more severe the stenosis. As with OPG, OPG-Gee only estimates the degree of stenosis present; angiography may be necessary to provide a precise evaluation.

### INTERFERING FACTORS
● Hypertension due to elevated ophthalmic artery pressures

# Understanding carotid imaging

Carotid imaging is a diagnostic test that assesses the carotid arteries for occlusive disease. In this test, a pulsed Doppler ultrasonic flow transducer or a real-time imager produces images of the carotid artery and records them.

*Real-time imaging* (photo below) uses the echo technique to visualize the carotid artery. In this technique, a Doppler signal can be directed to specific points along the vessel. The audio signal is then evaluated.

*Pulsed Doppler technique* (photos at right) uses a transducer with a range-gating system that allows alternate transmission and reception of ultrasonic signals. The sound reflected from moving red blood cells within the lumen is then collected and stored in a computer for subsequent image reconstruction.

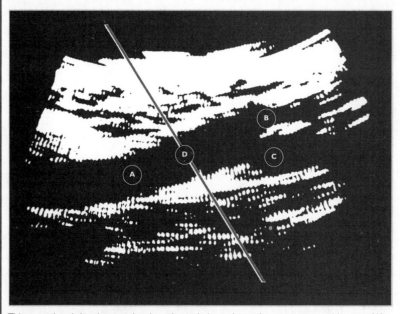

This normal, real-time image, taken by echo technique, shows the common carotid artery (A), external carotid artery (B), internal carotid artery (C), and Doppler beam (D).

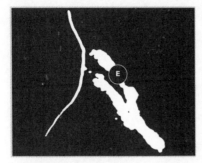

The abnormal pulsed Doppler image above shows total occlusion (E) of the internal carotid artery. Compare this to the normal pulsed Doppler image below.

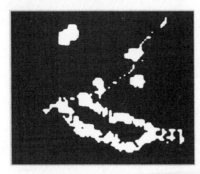

## PROCEDURE

The patient is placed in the supine position, and the probe is placed on his neck and moved slowly from the vicinity of the common carotid artery to that of the bifurcation and then to the site of the internal and external carotid arteries.

## ADVANTAGES AND DISADVANTAGES

Carotid imaging detects ulcerating plaques that can't be detected by other methods; it can also differentiate between total and near-total arterial occlusion.

Intramural calcification prevents sound penetration and may lead to false-positive results.

- Constant blinking or nystagmus causing an artifact
- Severe cardiac arrhythmias

# *Oral cholecystography*

Oral cholecystography is the radiographic examination of the gallbladder after administration of a contrast medium. This test is now commonly replaced by nuclear medicine 99 technetium-labeled scan, ultrasound, and computerized tomography. It's indicated in patients with symptoms of biliary tract disease, such as right-upper-quadrant epigastric pain, fat intolerance, and jaundice, and is most commonly performed to confirm gallbladder disease.

After the contrast medium is ingested, it's absorbed by the small intestine, filtered by the liver, excreted in the bile, and then concentrated and stored in the gallbladder. Full gallbladder opacification usually occurs 12 to 14 hours after ingestion, and a series of X-ray films then records gallbladder appearance. Additional information is obtained by giving the patient a fat stimulus, causing the gallbladder to contract and empty the contrast-laden bile into the common bile duct and small intestine. Films are then taken to record this emptying and to evaluate common bile duct patency.

Oral cholecystography should precede barium studies because retained barium may cloud subsequent X-ray films.

## PURPOSE
- To detect gallstones
- To aid in the diagnosis of inflammatory disease and gallbladder tumors

## PATIENT PREPARATION
- Explain to the patient that oral cholecystography permits examination of the gallbladder through X-ray films taken after ingestion of a contrast medium.
- Describe the test, including who will perform it and when and where it will take place.
- Instruct the patient to eat a normal meal at noon the day before the test and a fat-free meal in the evening. The former stimulates release of bile from the gallbladder, preparing

it to receive the contrast-laden bile; the latter inhibits gallbladder contraction, promoting bile accumulation.

● Instruct the patient to restrict food and fluids (except water) after the evening meal.

● Give the patient 6 tablets (3 g) of iopanoic acid 2 or 3 hours after the evening meal, as necessary. (Other commercial contrast agents are available, such as sodium ipodate, but iopanoic acid is most commonly used.) Have the patient swallow the tablets one at a time at 5-minute intervals, with one or two mouthfuls of water for a total of 8 oz (236.6 ml) of water. Thereafter, withhold water, cigarettes, and gum.

● Tell the patient that he'll be placed on an X-ray table and that films will be taken of his gallbladder.

● Check the patient's history for hypersensitivity to iodine, seafood, or contrast media used for other diagnostic tests.

● Inform the patient that the possible adverse effects of dye ingestion include diarrhea (common) and, rarely, nausea, vomiting, abdominal cramps, and dysuria. Tell him to report such symptoms immediately if they develop.

● Examine any vomitus or diarrhea for undigested tablets. If tablets were expelled, notify the X-ray department.

● Administer an enema the morning of the test, if prescribed, to clear the GI tract of interfering shadows that may obscure the gallbladder.

## PROCEDURE AND POSTTEST CARE

● After the patient is in a prone position on the radiographic table, the abdomen is examined fluoroscopically to evaluate gallbladder opacification, and films are taken of significant findings.

● The patient is then examined while in the left lateral decubitus and erect positions to detect possible layering or mobility of any filling defects, and additional films are taken.

● The patient may then be given a fat stimulus, such as a high-fat meal or a synthetic fat-containing agent (such as sincalide [Kinevac]).

● Fluoroscopy is used to observe gallbladder emptying in response to the fat stimulus, and spot films are taken at 15- and 30-minute intervals to visualize the common bile duct. If the gallbladder empties slowly

or not at all, these films are also taken at 60 minutes.

● If the test results are normal, tell the patient he may resume his usual diet.

● If gallstones are discovered during opacification, the patient will need an appropriate diet — usually one that restricts fat intake — to help prevent acute attacks.

● Nonopacification and repeat cholecystography require continuation of a low-fat diet until definitive diagnosis can be made.

## PRECAUTIONS

● Know that oral cholecystography is contraindicated in the patient with severe renal or hepatic damage and in the patient with hypersensitivity to iodine, seafood, or contrast media.

● Be aware that this test is also contraindicated in the pregnant patient because of radiation's possible teratogenic effects.

## NORMAL FINDINGS

The gallbladder is normally opacified and appears pear-shaped, with smooth, thin walls. Although its size is variable, its basic structure — neck, infundibulum, body, and fundus — is clearly outlined on film.

## ABNORMAL FINDINGS

When the gallbladder is opacified, filling defects (typically appearing within the lumen as negative shadows that show mobility) indicate the presence of gallstones. Fixed defects, on the other hand, may indicate the presence of cholesterol polyps or a benign tumor such as an adenomyoma.

When the gallbladder fails to opacify or when only faint opacification occurs, inflammatory disease such as cholecystitis — with or without gallstone formation — may be present. Gallstones may obstruct the cystic duct and prevent the contrast medium from entering the gallbladder; inflammation may impair the concentrating ability of the gallbladder mucosa and prevent or diminish opacification.

When the gallbladder fails to contract following stimulation by a fatty meal, cholecystitis or common bile duct obstruction may be present. If the X-ray films are inconclusive, oral cholecystography is repeated the following day.

## INTERFERING FACTORS

● Inability of the patient to remain still

- The patient's inability to ingest the full dose of contrast medium or partial loss of contrast medium through emesis or diarrhea (may invalidate test results)
- Inadequate absorption of the contrast medium in the small intestine or barium retained from previous studies (may invalidate test results)
- Decreased excretion of the contrast medium into the bile duct to impaired hepatic function and moderate jaundice (possible poor imaging)

# Oral glucose tolerance test

The oral glucose tolerance test (OGTT) is the most sensitive method of evaluating borderline cases of diabetes mellitus. Plasma and urine glucose levels are monitored for 3 hours after ingestion of a challenge dose of glucose to assess insulin secretion and the body's ability to metabolize glucose.

The OGTT isn't generally used in patients with fasting plasma glucose values greater than 140 mg/dl (SI, > 7.7 mmol/L) or postprandial plasma glucose values greater than 200 mg/dl (SI, > 11 mmol/L).

## PURPOSE
- To confirm diabetes mellitus in selected patients
- To aid in the diagnosis of hypoglycemia and malabsorption syndrome

## PATIENT PREPARATION
- Explain to the patient that the OGTT is used to evaluate glucose metabolism.
- Instruct the patient to maintain a high-carbohydrate diet for 3 days and then to fast for 12 to 14 hours before the test, as instructed by the physician.
- Tell the patient not to smoke, drink coffee or alcohol, or exercise strenuously for 8 hours before or during the test.
- Tell the patient that this test requires five blood samples and, usually, five urine samples. Explain who will perform the venipunctures and when and that the patient may experience slight discomfort from the needle punctures and the tourniquet.
- Suggest to the patient that he bring a book or other quiet diversion with him to

the test. The procedure usually takes 3 hours, but can last as long as 6 hours.
- Notify the laboratory and physician of medications the patient is taking that may affect test results; they may need to be restricted.
- Alert the patient to the symptoms of hypoglycemia (weakness, restlessness, nervousness, hunger, and sweating) and tell him to report such symptoms immediately.

## PROCEDURE AND POSTTEST CARE
- Between 7 a.m. and 9 a.m., perform a venipuncture to obtain a fasting blood sample. Draw this sample into a 7-ml clot-activator tube. A saline lock may be inserted and used to collect the multiple blood samples needed, as per facility protocol.
- Collect a urine sample at the same time if your facility includes this as part of the test.
- After collecting these samples, administer the test load of oral glucose and record the time of ingestion. Encourage the patient to drink the entire glucose solution within 5 minutes.
- Draw blood samples 30 minutes, 1 hour, 2 hours, and 3 hours after giving the loading dose using 7-ml clot-activator tubes.
- Collect urine samples at the same intervals.
- Tell the patient to lie down if he feels faint from the numerous venipunctures.
- Encourage the patient to drink water throughout the test to promote adequate urine excretion.
- Apply direct pressure to the venipuncture site until bleeding stops.
- If a hematoma develops at the venipuncture site, apply pressure.
- Provide a balanced meal or a snack, but observe for a hypoglycemic reaction.
- Instruct the patient that he may resume his usual medications discontinued before the test, as ordered.

## PRECAUTIONS
- Send blood and urine samples to the laboratory immediately or refrigerate them.
- Specify when the patient last ate and the blood and urine sample collection times.
- As appropriate, record the time the patient received his last pretest dose of insulin or oral antidiabetic drug.
- If the patient develops severe hypoglycemia, notify the physician. Draw a blood

sample, record the time on the laboratory request, and discontinue the test. Have the patient drink a glass of orange juice with sugar added or administer I.V. glucose to reverse the reaction.

## REFERENCE VALUES

Normal plasma glucose levels peak at 160 to 180 mg/dl (SI, 8.8 to 9.9 mmol/L) within 30 minutes to 1 hour after administration of an oral glucose test dose and return to fasting levels or lower within 2 to 3 hours. Urine glucose tests remain negative throughout.

## ABNORMAL FINDINGS

Decreased glucose tolerance, in which levels peak sharply before falling slowly to fasting levels, may confirm diabetes mellitus or may result from Cushing's disease, hemochromatosis, pheochromocytoma, or central nervous system lesions.

Increased glucose tolerance, in which levels may peak at less than normal levels, may indicate insulinoma, malabsorption syndrome, adrenocortical insufficiency (Addison's disease), hypothyroidism, or hypopituitarism.

## INTERFERING FACTORS

● Acute illness, such as myocardial infarction, fever, pregnancy, or recent infection (possible increase)
● Carbohydrate deprivation before the test (causing a diabetic response [abnormal increase with a delayed decrease] because the pancreas is unaccustomed to responding to high-carbohydrate load)
● Arginine, benzodiazepines, caffeine, epinephrine, chlorthalidone (Hygroton), corticosteroids, diazoxide (Hyperstat I.V.), furosemide (Lasix), hormonal contraceptives, recent I.V. glucose infusions, lithium, large doses of nicotinic acid, phenothiazines, phenytoin (Dilantin), thiazide diuretics, and triamterene (Dyrenium) (possible increase)
● Amphetamines, beta-adrenergic blockers, clofibrate, ethanol, insulin, monoamine oxidase inhibitors, and oral antidiabetic drugs (possible decrease)

*Age alert* Patients age 50 or older experience decreasing carbohydrate tolerance, which causes increasing glucose tolerance to upper limits of about 1 mg/dl for every year over age 50.

# Oral lactose tolerance test

The oral lactose tolerance test is used to measure plasma glucose levels after ingestion of a challenge dose of lactose. It's used to screen for lactose intolerance due to lactase deficiency.

Absence or deficiency of lactase causes undigested lactose to remain in the intestinal lumen, producing such symptoms as abdominal cramps and watery diarrhea. True congenital lactase deficiency is rare. Usually, lactose intolerance is acquired because lactase levels generally decrease with age.

## PURPOSE

● To detect lactose intolerance

## PATIENT PREPARATION

● Explain to the patient that the oral lactose tolerance test is used to determine if his symptoms are due to an inability to digest lactose.
● Instruct the patient to fast and to avoid strenuous activity for 8 hours before the test.
● Inform the patient that this test requires four blood samples. Tell the patient who will be performing the venipunctures and when and where the test will take place.
● Explain to the patient that he may experience slight discomfort from the needle punctures and the tourniquet. Tell the patient that the entire procedure may take up to 2 hours.
● Notify the laboratory and physician of medications the patient is taking that may affect test results; they may need to be restricted.

## PROCEDURE AND POSTTEST CARE

● After the patient has fasted for 8 hours, perform a venipuncture and collect a blood sample in a 4-ml tube with sodium fluoride and potassium oxalate added.
● Administer the test load of lactose: for an adult, 50 g of lactose dissolved in 400 ml of water.

*Age alert* For a child, administer 50 g/m² of body surface area. Record the time of ingestion.
● Draw a blood sample 30, 60, and 120 minutes after giving the loading dose.

Use a 4-ml tube with sodium fluoride and potassium oxalate added.

● If ordered, collect a stool sample 5 hours after giving the loading dose.

● Apply direct pressure to the venipuncture site until bleeding stops.

● If a hematoma develops at the venipuncture site, apply pressure.

● Instruct the patient to resume his usual diet, medications, and activity discontinued before the test, as ordered.

## PRECAUTIONS

● Send blood and stool samples to the laboratory immediately or refrigerate them if transport is delayed.

● Specify the collection time on the laboratory requests.

● Watch for symptoms of lactose intolerance — abdominal cramps, nausea, bloating, flatulence, and watery diarrhea — caused by the loading dose.

## REFERENCE VALUES

Normally, plasma glucose levels rise over 20 mg/dl (SI, > 1.1 mmol/L) over fasting levels within 15 to 60 minutes after ingestion of the lactose loading dose.

## ABNORMAL FINDINGS

A rise in plasma glucose of less than 20 mg/dl (SI, <1.1 mmol/L) indicates lactose intolerance, as does stool acidity (pH of 5.5 or less) and high glucose content (more than 1+ on the dipstick). Accompanying signs and symptoms provoked by the test also suggest, but don't confirm, the diagnosis because such symptoms may appear in the patient with normal lactase activity after a loading dose of lactose. Small-bowel biopsy with lactase assay may be performed to confirm the diagnosis. Abnormal levels may be seen in patients with Crohn's disease, small bowel resections, *Giardia* infections, and cystic fibrosis.

## INTERFERING FACTORS

● Benzodiazepines, hormonal contraceptives, insulin, propranolol, and thiazide diuretics (possible false-low)

● Delayed emptying of stomach contents (possible decrease)

● Glycolysis (possible false-negative)

# Orbital computed tomography

Orbital computed tomography (CT) allows visualization of abnormalities not readily seen on standard radiographs, delineating their size, position, and relationship to adjoining structures. A series of tomograms reconstructed by a computer and displayed as anatomic slices on a monitor, the orbital CT scan identifies space-occupying lesions earlier and more accurately than do other radiographic techniques and provides three-dimensional images of orbital structures, especially the ocular muscles and the optic nerve.

## PURPOSE

● To evaluate pathologies of the orbit and eye — especially expanding lesions and bone destruction

● To evaluate fractures of the orbit and adjoining structures

● To determine the cause of unilateral exophthalmos

## PATIENT PREPARATION

● Describe the procedure to the patient, and explain that the orbital CT scan visualizes the anatomy of the eye and its surrounding structures.

● If contrast enhancement isn't scheduled, inform the patient that he need not restrict food and fluids. If contrast enhancement is scheduled, withhold food and fluids from the patient for 4 hours before the test.

● Tell the patient that a series of X-ray films will be taken of his eye and explain who will perform the test and when and where it will take place.

● Reassure the patient that the test will cause him no discomfort.

● Tell the patient that he'll be positioned on an X-ray table and that the head of the table will be moved into the scanner, which will rotate around his head and make loud, clacking sounds.

● If a contrast medium will be used for the procedure, tell the patient that he may feel flushed and warm and may experience a transient headache, a salty or metallic taste, and nausea or vomiting after the contrast medium is injected. Reassure him that these reactions are normal.

● Make sure that the patient or a responsible family member has signed an informed consent form, if required.

● Check the patient's history for hypersensitivity reactions to iodine, shellfish, or contrast media, and notify the physician of these sensitivities.

● Instruct the patient to remove jewelry, hairpins, or other metal objects in the X-ray field to allow for precise imaging of the orbital structures.

## PROCEDURE AND POSTTEST CARE

● The patient is placed in a supine position on the X-ray table with his head immobilized by straps, if required. Ask him to lie still.

● The head of the table is moved into the scanner, which rotates around the patient's head, taking radiographs.

● Information obtained is stored on magnetic tapes, and the images are displayed on a monitor. Photographs may be made if a permanent record is desired.

● When this series of radiographs has been taken, contrast enhancement is performed. The contrast medium is injected intravenously, and a second series of scans is recorded.

● If a contrast medium was used, watch for its residual adverse effects, including headache, nausea, or vomiting. After the procedure, advise the patient that he may resume his usual diet.

## PRECAUTIONS

**Alert** *Be aware that use of contrast enhancement is contraindicated in the patient with known hypersensitivity reactions to iodine, shellfish, or contrast media used in other tests.*

## NORMAL FINDINGS

Orbital structures are evaluated for size, shape, and position. Dense orbital bone provides a marked contrast to less dense periocular fat. The optic nerve and the medial and lateral rectus muscles are clearly defined. The rectus muscles appear as thin, dense bands on each side, behind the eye. The optic canals should be equal in size.

## ABNORMAL FINDINGS

Orbital CT scans can identify intraorbital and extraorbital space-occupying lesions that ob-

scure the normal structures or cause orbital enlargement, indentation of the orbital walls, or bone destruction. This test can also help determine the type of lesion. For example, infiltrative lesions, such as lymphomas and metastatic carcinomas, appear as irregular areas of density. However, encapsulated tumors, such as benign hemangiomas and meningiomas, appear as clearly defined masses of consistent density. CT scans can also visualize intracranial tumors that invade the orbit, thickening of the optic nerve that may occur with gliomas, meningiomas, and secondary tumors that may cause enlargement of the optic canal.

In evaluating fractures, CT scans allow a complete three-dimensional view of the affected structures. In determining the cause of unilateral exophthalmos, CT scans can show early erosion or expansion of the medial orbital wall that may arise from lesions in the ethmoidal cells. They can also detect space-occupying lesions in the orbit or paranasal sinuses that cause exophthalmos. Additionally, they can show thickening of the medial and lateral rectus muscles in proptosis resulting from Graves' disease.

Enhancement with a contrast medium may provide information about the circulation through abnormal ocular tissues.

## INTERFERING FACTORS

● Head movement

● Failure to remove metallic objects from examination field (possible poor imaging)

# Orbital radiography

Orbital radiography evaluates the orbit, the bony cavity that houses the eye and the lacrimal glands, as well as blood vessels, nerves, muscles, and fat. Because portions of the orbit are composed of thin bone that fractures easily, X-rays are commonly taken following facial trauma. They're also useful in diagnosing ocular and orbital pathologies. Special radiographic techniques can reveal foreign bodies in the orbit or eye that are invisible to an ophthalmoscope. In some cases, radiography is used in conjunction with computed tomography scans and ultrasonography to better define an abnormality.

## PURPOSE

- To aid in the diagnosis of orbital fractures and pathologies
- To help locate intraorbital or intraocular foreign bodies

## PATIENT PREPARATION

- Explain that orbital radiography involves taking several X-rays to assess the condition of the bones around the eye.
- Describe the test, including who will perform it and when and where it will take place.
- Reassure the patient that the procedure is usually painless unless he has suffered facial trauma, in which case positioning may cause some discomfort. Explain that he'll be asked to turn his head from side to side and to flex or extend his neck.
- Instruct the patient to remove all jewelry and other metallic objects from the X-ray field.

## PROCEDURE AND POSTTEST CARE

- Have the patient recline on the X-ray table or sit in a chair.
- Instruct the patient to remain still while the X-rays are taken.
- Remember that a series of orbital X-rays usually includes a lateral view, posteroanterior view, submentovertical (base) view, stereo Waters' views (views from both sides), Towne's (half-axial) projection, and optic canal projections. If enlargement of the superior orbital fissure is suspected, apical views are obtained.
- The films are developed and inspected by the radiography department before the patient is released.

## PRECAUTIONS

- None

## NORMAL FINDINGS

Each orbit is composed of a roof, a floor, and medial and lateral walls. The bones of the roof and floor are very thin (the floor can be less than 1 mm thick). The medial walls, which parallel each other, are slightly thicker, except for the portion formed by the ethmoid bone. The lateral walls are the thickest part of the orbit and are strongest at the orbital rim.

The superior orbital fissure, at the back of the orbit between the lateral wall and the roof, is actually a gap between the greater and lesser wings of the sphenoid bone. The optic canal, which carries the optic nerve and ophthalmic artery, is an opening in the lesser wing of the sphenoid bone located at the apex of the orbit.

## ABNORMAL FINDINGS

Orbital fractures associated with facial trauma are most common in the thin structures of the floor and ethmoid bone. Abnormalities are detected by comparing the size and shape of orbital structures on the affected side with those on the opposite side.

Generally, orbit enlargement indicates the presence of a lesion that has caused proptosis due to increased intraorbital pressure. Any growing tumor can produce these changes. Superior orbital fissure enlargement can result from orbital meningioma, from intracranial conditions, such as pituitary tumors or, more characteristically, from vascular anomalies.

*Age alert* *Optic canal enlargement may result from extraocular extension of a retinoblastoma or, in children, from an optic nerve glioma. In adults, only prolonged pathology can increase orbital size; however, in children, even a rapidly growing lesion can cause orbital enlargement because orbital bones aren't fully developed. A decrease in the size of the orbit may follow childhood enucleation of the eye or conditions such as congenital microphthalmia.*

Destruction of the orbital walls may indicate a malignant neoplasm or an infection. A benign tumor or cyst produces a clear-cut local indentation of the orbital wall. Lesions of adjacent structures may also produce radiographic changes due to enlargement and erosion of the orbit.

Increased bone density may be seen in such conditions as osteoblastic metastasis, sphenoid ridge meningioma, or Paget's disease. To confirm orbital pathology, however, radiographic findings must be supplemented with results from other appropriate tests and procedures.

## INTERFERING FACTORS

- None significant

# Osmolality, urine

The kidneys normally concentrate or dilute urine according to fluid intake. When intake is excessive, the kidneys excrete more water in the urine; when intake is limited, they excrete less. To make such variation possible, the distal segment of the tubule varies its permeability to water in response to antidiuretic hormone, which, with renal blood flow, determines urine concentration or dilution.

This test measures the concentrating ability of the kidneys in acute and chronic renal failure. Osmolality is a more sensitive index of renal function than are dilution techniques that measure specific gravity. It measures the number of osmotically active ions or particles present per kilogram of water. Osmolality is high in concentrated urine and low in dilute urine. It's determined by the effect of solute particles on the freezing point of the fluid.

## PURPOSE
- To evaluate renal tubular function
- To detect renal impairment

## PATIENT PREPARATION
- Explain to the patient that the urine osmolality test evaluates kidney function.
- Tell the patient that the test requires a urine specimen and collection of blood within 1 hour before or after the urine is collected. Withhold diuretics, as ordered.
- Emphasize to the patient that his cooperation is necessary to obtain accurate results.

## PROCEDURE AND POSTTEST CARE
- Collect a random urine specimen and draw a blood sample within 1 hour of urine collection.
- If a 24-hour urine collection is ordered, record the total urine volume on the laboratory request. (Preservatives aren't required for a 24-hour container.)
- After collecting the final specimen, provide the patient with a balanced meal or snack.
- Make sure the patient voids within 8 to 10 hours after the catheter has been removed.

## PRECAUTIONS
- Send each specimen to the laboratory immediately after collection.
- If the patient is unable to urinate into the specimen containers, provide him with a clean bedpan, urinal, or toilet specimen pan. Rinse the collection device after each use.
- If the patient is catheterized, empty the drainage bag before the test. Obtain the specimen from the catheter.

## REFERENCE VALUES
For a random urine specimen, osmolality normally ranges from 50 to 1,400 mOsm/kg; for a 24-hour urine specimen, osmolality ranges from 300 to 900 mOsm/kg.

## ABNORMAL FINDINGS
Decreased renal capacity to concentrate urine in response to fluid deprivation, or to dilute urine in response to fluid overload, may indicate tubular epithelial damage, decreased renal blood flow, loss of functional nephrons, or pituitary or cardiac dysfunction.

## INTERFERING FACTORS
- Diuretics (increase urine volume and dilution, thereby lowering specific gravity)
- Nephrotoxic drugs (cause tubular epithelial damage, thereby decreasing renal concentrating ability)
- Patients who have been markedly overhydrated for several days before the test (may have depressed concentration values)
- Patients who are dehydrated or have electrolyte imbalances (may retain fluids, leading to inaccurate results)

# Otoacoustic emissions testing

Otoacoustic emissions testing is a rapid method of screening that assesses the function of outer hair cells of the cochlea. Because outer hair cells almost invariably are lost before damage to inner hair cells, this technique screens for cochlear hearing loss. Otoacoustic emissions are absent when more than a slight to mild hearing loss is present. Subtle changes in otoacoustic emissions are sometimes present in normal hearing carriers of recessive hearing loss genes.

Abnormalities of otoacoustic emissions may precede hearing loss.

Commercially available since 1988, this test has provided a cost-effective method of neonatal screening because patient participation isn't necessary. It provides a measure of outer hair cell function, assists in patient triage during diagnostic testing, and provides a rapid indication of whether the outer hair cells are intact. It can assist in detecting nonorganic hearing loss. However, hearing loss developing after birth, such as from maternal cytomegalovirus infection, and some genetic hearing losses may not be identified with neonatal screening. Moreover, slight (minimal) hearing loss may go undetected.

## PURPOSE
- To screen and assess the health of the outer hair cells of the cochlea
- To screen hearing of neonates

## PATIENT PREPARATION
- Inform the patient (if appropriate) that the otoacoustic emissions test is rapidly administered, requiring approximately 1 minute per ear (if the patient is quiet and has normal hearing) or just slightly longer (if findings aren't immediately normal).
- Remove significant cerumen accumulation from the patient's ear canals.

## PROCEDURE AND POSTTEST CARE
- In screening, the technician places the probe in the patient's ear after having cleared it of debris, such as vernix, which is present in the neonate's ear.
- The audiologist adjusts signal levels, and in the case of distortion-product otoacoustic emissions, the frequency characteristics.
- The emission level is monitored and compared to the background noise level.

## PRECAUTIONS
- None

## NORMAL FINDINGS
Otoacoustic emissions are normally present at 500 to 6,000 Hz, with signal-to-noise ratios of at least 5 dB. Emissions sufficiently above the background physiologic and ambient noise provide evidence of functional outer hair cells in the cochlea, typically associated with normal or near-normal hearing. Results are frequency specific.

## ABNORMAL FINDINGS
An absence of otoacoustic emissions at any test frequency suggests outer hair cell dysfunction and hearing loss of at least 25 dB HL. The presence of otoacoustic emissions at traditional screening levels indicates no more than a slight cochlear hearing disorder. Significant conductive hearing loss can reduce or eliminate the size of the otoacoustic emission.

## INTERFERING FACTORS
- Screening by inexperienced technicians in the technique, possibly leading to high false-positive rates (Retesting is typically incorporated into screening programs.)
- Significant conductive hearing loss, which can create a failure during diagnostic testing or a "refer to" during screening (While this test allows most congenital conductive losses to be discovered, it means that some children with transient conductive loss will fail to pass the screening or diagnostic version of otoacoustic emissions testing.)
- Presence of cerumen obstruction
- Auditory dyssynchrony, sometimes called auditory neuropathy, such as from hyperbilirubinemia or kernicterus, undetected with this procedure (If outer hair cells function, but the disorder is such that a neural signal isn't transmitted to the brain, otoacoustic emissions will be normal and the hearing deficit won't be discovered.)

## Papanicolaou test

The Papanicolaou (Pap) test is a widely known cytologic test for early detection of cervical cancer. A physician or specially trained nurse scrapes secretions from the patient's cervix and spreads them on a slide, which is sent to the laboratory for cytologic analysis. The test relies on the ready exfoliation of malignant cells from the cervix and shows cell maturity, metabolic activity, and morphology variations.

Although cervical scrapings are the most common test specimen, the test may involve cytologic evaluation of the vaginal pool, prostatic secretions, urine, gastric secretions, cavity fluids, bronchial aspirations, sputum, or solid tumor cells obtained by fine needle aspiration. The American Cancer Society recommends a Pap test every 3 years for women between ages 20 and 40 who aren't in a high-risk category and who have had negative results from three previous Pap tests. Yearly tests (or tests at physician-recommended intervals) are advised for women over age 40, for those in a high-risk category, and for those who have had a positive test previously. If a Pap test is positive or suggests malignancy, cervical biopsy can confirm the diagnosis.

### PURPOSE
- To detect malignant cells
- To detect inflammatory tissue changes
- To assess the patient's response to chemotherapy and radiation therapy
- To detect viral, fungal and, occasionally, parasitic invasion

### PATIENT PREPARATION
- Explain to the patient that the Pap test allows for the study of cervical cells.
- Stress its importance as an aid for detection of cancer at a stage when the disease is commonly asymptomatic and still curable.
- The test shouldn't be scheduled during the menstrual period; the best time is midcycle.
- Instruct the patient to avoid having intercourse for 24 hours, not to douche for 48 hours, and not to insert vaginal medications for 1 week before the test because doing so can wash away cellular deposits and change the vaginal pH.
- Tell the patient that the test requires that the cervix be scraped, who will perform the procedure and when, and that she may experience slight discomfort but no pain from the speculum (but may feel some pain when the cervix is scraped).
- Inform her that the procedure takes 5 to 10 minutes or slightly longer if the vagina, pelvic cavity, and rectum are examined bimanually.
- Obtain an accurate patient history, and ask these questions: When did you last have a Pap test? Have you ever had an abnormal Pap test? When was your last menstrual period? Are your periods regular? How many days do they last? Is bleeding heavy or light? Have you taken or are you presently taking hormones or oral contraceptives? Do you use an intrauterine device? Do you have any vaginal discharge, pain, or itching? Which, if any, gynecologic disorders have occurred in your family? Have you ever had gynecologic surgery, chemotherapy, or radiation therapy? If so, describe it fully. Note the pertinent patient history data on the laboratory request.

- Provide emotional support if the patient is anxious; tell her that test results should be available in a few weeks.
- Ask the patient to empty her bladder before the test is performed.

## PROCEDURE AND POSTTEST CARE

- Instruct the patient to disrobe from the waist down and to drape herself.
- Ask the patient to lie on the examining table and to place her heels in the stirrups. (She may be more comfortable if she keeps her shoes or socks on.) Tell her to slide her buttocks to the edge of the table. Adjust the drape to minimize exposure.
- To avoid startling the patient, tell her when the examination will begin.
- The examiner puts on gloves and inserts an unlubricated speculum into the vagina. To make insertion easier, the speculum may be moistened with saline solution or warm water.
- After the examiner locates the cervix, he collects secretions from the cervix and material from the endocervical canal. He places the endocervical brush inside the endocervix and rolls it firmly inside the canal. If using a Pap stick (wooden spatula), it's placed against the cervix with the longest protrusion in the cervical canal, then rotates the stick clockwise 360 degrees firmly against the cervix.
- He then spreads the specimen on the slide according to laboratory recommendations and immediately immerses the slide in (or sprays it with) a fixative.
- Alternatively, posterior vaginal pool secretions and pancervical material may be collected and smeared on a single slide, which must be fixed immediately according to laboratory instructions.
- Label the specimen appropriately, including the date, the patient's name, age, the date of her last menstrual period, and the collection site and method.
- A bimanual examination may follow after the removal of the speculum. Help the patient up and ask her to dress when the examination is completed.
- Supply the patient with a sanitary napkin if cervical bleeding occurs.
- Tell the patient when to return for her next Pap test.

## PRECAUTIONS

- Make sure the cervical specimen is aspirated and scraped from the cervix. A vaginal pool sample isn't recommended for cervical or endometrial cancer screening.
- Know that the specimen should be thick enough that it isn't transparent.
- Be aware that scrapings taken directly from the lesion are preferred if vaginal or vulval lesions are present.
- Use a small pipette, if necessary, in a patient whose uterus is involuting or atrophying from age, to aspirate cells from the squamocolumnar junction and the cervical canal.
- Preserve the slides immediately after the specimen is collected.

## NORMAL FINDINGS

Normally, no malignant cells or other abnormalities are present.

## ABNORMAL FINDINGS

Malignant cells usually have relatively large nuclei and only small amounts of cytoplasm. They show abnormal nuclear chromatin patterns and marked variation in size, shape, and staining properties and may have prominent nucleoli.

A Pap smear may be graded in different ways, so check your laboratory's reporting format. In the Bethesda system, the current standardized method, potentially premalignant squamous lesions fall into three categories: atypical squamous cells of undetermined significance, low-grade squamous intraepithelial lesions, and high-grade squamous intraepithelial lesions. The low-grade category includes mild dysplasia and the changes of the human papillomavirus. The high-grade category includes moderate to severe dysplasia and carcinoma in situ.

Human papillomavirus (HPV) has been identified as a major risk factor for cervical cancer. Currently there's a test available that detects the types of HPV via their deoxyribonucleic acid. In addition, to confirm a suggestive or positive cytology report, the test may be repeated or followed by a biopsy. (See *Testing for cervical cancer,* page 312.)

## INTERFERING FACTORS

- Douching within 48 hours or having intercourse within 24 hours before the test (can wash away cellular deposits)

# TESTING FOR CERVICAL CANCER

## THINPREP TEST

Cervical cells for ThinPrep test analysis may be collected in the same manner as those of a Papanicolaou (Pap) test, using a cytobrush and plastic spatula. The specimens are deposited in a bottle provided with a fixative and sent to the laboratory. A filter is then inserted into the bottle and excess mucus, blood, and inflammatory cells are filtered out by centrifuge. Remaining cells are then placed on a slide in a uniform, thin layer and read as a Pap test. This procedure causes fewer slides to be classified as unreadable, significantly reducing the incidence of false negatives and the need for repeat tests.

## HPV DNA TEST

When using the ThinPrep test, screening can also be easily done for the human papillomavirus (HPV), of which certain strains have been identified as the primary cause of cervical cancer. The Digene hc2 HPV deoxyribonucleic acid (DNA) test has been approved by the U.S. Food and Drug Administration to determine if those identified at high risk for developing cervical cancer have been exposed to HPV. The specimen is collected as a Pap smear, but is dispersed with ThinPrep solution. Separate aliquots are used for each test, from brushings of the endocervix. The brush is then inserted into the specialized tube, snapped off at the shaft, and capped securely. The target solution in the tube disrupts the virus and releases target DNA, which combines with specific ribonucleic acid (RNA) probes creating RNA:DNA hybrids. The hybrids are captured, bound, and magnified and measured using a luminometer.

If the patient is found to be positive for HPV, she has been infected with the virus. Depending on the type of HPV found through DNA testing, the patient harboring high-risk HPV strains has a higher risk of developing cervical cancer. It's recommended that the patient undergo colposcopy, in which the cervix is viewed under microscope and a biopsy is taken from the tissue sample.

---

- Excessive use of lubricating jelly on the speculum (false-negative)
- Collection of the specimen during menstruation
- Exclusive use of a specimen collected from the vaginal fornix (possible false-negative)
- Delay in fixing the specimen (difficult cytologic interpretation due to dehydration of cells)
- Too thin or thick a specimen

# Paranasal sinus radiography

The paranasal sinuses — air-filled cavities lined with mucous membranes — lie within the maxillary, ethmoid, sphenoid, and frontal bones. Sinus abnormalities resulting from inflammation, trauma, cysts, mucoceles, granulomatosis, and other conditions may include distorted bony sinus walls, altered mucous membranes, and fluid or masses within the cavities. In paranasal sinus radiography, X-rays or electromagnetic waves penetrate the paranasal sinuses and react on specially sensitized film, forming a film image that differentiates sinus structures.

When surrounding facial structures that are superimposed on the paranasal sinuses interfere with visualization of relevant areas, computed tomography scanning may be performed to provide further information.

## PURPOSE

- To detect unilateral or bilateral abnormalities, possibly indicating trauma or disease
- To confirm diagnosis of neoplastic or inflammatory paranasal sinus disease
- To determine the location and size of a malignant neoplasm

## PATIENT PREPARATION

- Explain to the patient that paranasal sinus radiography helps evaluate abnormalities of the paranasal sinuses.
- Describe the test, including who will perform it and when and where it will take place.

## Abnormal findings in paranasal sinus radiography

| DISORDER | ABNORMAL FINDINGS |
|---|---|
| Paranasal sinus trauma or fracture | ◆ Edema or hemorrhage in mucous membrane lining or sinus cavity<br>◆ Clouded sinus air cells<br>◆ Air-fluid level<br>◆ Radiolucent, linear bone defects<br>◆ Irregular, overriding bone edges<br>◆ Depression or displacement of bone fragments<br>◆ Foreign bodies |
| Acute sinusitis | ◆ Swollen, inflamed mucous membrane<br>◆ Inflammatory exudate<br>◆ Hazy to opaque sinus air cells<br>◆ Air-fluid level |
| Chronic sinusitis | ◆ Thickening or sclerosis of bony wall of affected sinus |
| Wegener's granulomatosis | ◆ Clouded to opaque sinus air cells<br>◆ Destruction of bony sinus wall |
| Malignant neoplasm | ◆ Rounded or lobulated soft-tissue mass, projecting into sinus<br>◆ Destruction of bony sinus wall |
| Benign bone tumor | ◆ Distortion of bony sinus wall in specific patterns |
| Cyst, polyp, or benign tumor | ◆ Rounded or lobulated soft-tissue mass, projecting into sinus |
| Mucocele | ◆ Clouded sinus air cells<br>◆ Destruction of bony sinus wall resulting in various degrees of radiolucency |

● Tell the patient that his head may be immobilized in a foam vise during the test to help him maintain the correct position, but that the vise doesn't hurt.

● Explain to the patient that he'll be asked to sit upright and avoid moving while the X-rays are being taken to prevent blurring of the image and to allow visualization of air-fluid levels, if present. Emphasize the importance of his cooperation.

● Instruct the patient to remove dentures, all jewelry, and metallic objects in the X-ray field.

## PROCEDURE AND POSTTEST CARE

● Have the patient sit upright (his head may be placed in a foam vise) between the X-ray tube and a film cassette.

● During the test, the X-ray tube is positioned at specific angles and the patient's head is placed in various standard positions while his paranasal sinuses are filmed from different angles. If necessary, assist with positioning the patient.

## PRECAUTIONS

● Be aware that paranasal sinus radiography is usually contraindicated during pregnancy; however, when it's absolutely necessary, a lead-lined apron placed over the patient's abdomen can shield the fetus.

● To avoid exposure to radiation, leave the room or the immediate area during the test; if you must stay in the area, wear a lead-lined apron.

## NORMAL FINDINGS

Normal paranasal sinuses are radiolucent and filled with air, which appears black on films.

## ABNORMAL FINDINGS

See *Abnormal findings in paranasal sinus radiography,* page 313.

## INTERFERING FACTORS

● The presence of dentures, jewelry, or other metallic objects in the X-ray field or the presence of numerous metallic foreign bodies around the paranasal sinuses (possible poor imaging)
● Patient movement (possible poor imaging)
● Patient unable to sit upright (may require supine position, reducing diagnostic value of test)
● Superimposition of the surrounding facial structures on the film (obscures paranasal sinuses)

# Parathyroid hormone

Parathyroid hormone (PTH), also known as *parathormone,* regulates plasma concentration of calcium and phosphorus. Normally, PTH release is regulated by a negative feedback mechanism involving serum calcium. Normal or elevated circulating calcium levels (especially the ionized form) inhibit PTH release; decreased levels stimulate PTH release. The overall effect of PTH is to raise plasma levels of calcium while lowering phosphorus levels.

Circulating PTH exists in three distinct molecular forms: the intact PTH molecule, which originates in the parathyroid glands, and two smaller circulating forms, N-terminal fragments and C-terminal fragments. Two radioimmunoassays are available to detect intact PTH and the N- and C-terminal fragments. Both tests can be used to confirm diagnosis of hyperparathyroidism and hypoparathyroidism.

Each test has other specific applications as well. The C-terminal PTH assay is more useful in diagnosing chronic disturbances in PTH metabolism, such as secondary and tertiary hyperparathyroidism; it also better differentiates ectopic from primary hyperparathyroidism. The assay for intact PTH and the N-terminal fragment (both forms are measured concomitantly) more accurately reflects acute changes in PTH metabolism and thus is useful in monitoring a patient's response to PTH therapy.

The clinical and diagnostic effects of PTH excess or deficiency are directly related to the effects of PTH on bone and the renal tubules and to its interaction with ionized calcium and biologically active vitamin D. Therefore, measuring serum calcium, phosphorus, and creatinine levels with serum PTH is helpful when trying to understand the causes and effects of pathologic parathyroid function. Suppression or stimulation tests may help confirm findings.

## PURPOSE

● To aid the differential diagnosis of parathyroid disorders

## PATIENT PREPARATION

● Explain to the patient that the PTH test helps evaluate parathyroid function.
● Instruct the patient to observe an overnight fast because food may affect PTH levels and interfere with results.
● Tell the patient that the test requires a blood sample. Explain who will perform the venipuncture and when and where it will take place.
● Explain to the patient that he may experience slight discomfort from the needle puncture and the tourniquet.

## PROCEDURE AND POSTTEST CARE

● Perform a venipuncture and collect 3 ml of blood into two separate 7-ml clot-activator tubes.
● Apply direct pressure to the venipuncture site until bleeding stops.
● If a hematoma develops at the venipuncture site, apply pressure.
● Instruct the patient that he may resume his usual diet.

## PRECAUTIONS

● Handle the sample gently to prevent hemolysis.
● Send the sample to the laboratory immediately so the serum can be separated and frozen for assay.

## CLINICAL IMPLICATIONS OF ABNORMAL PARATHYROID SECRETION

| CONDITIONS | CAUSES | PTH LEVELS | IONIZED CALCIUM LEVELS |
|---|---|---|---|
| Primary hyperparathyroidism | ◆ Parathyroid adenoma or carcinoma | High | High to Low |
| Secondary hyperparathyroidism | ◆ Chronic renal disease<br>◆ Severe vitamin D deficiency<br>◆ Calcium malabsorption<br>◆ Pregnancy and lactation | High | Low |
| Tertiary hyperparathyroidism | ◆ Progressive secondary hyperparathyroidism | High | High to Low |
| Hypoparathyroidism | ◆ Accidental removal of the parathyroid glands<br>◆ Autoimmune disease | Low | Low |
| Malignant tumors | ◆ Squamous-cell carcinoma of the lung<br>◆ Renal, pancreatic, or ovarian carcinoma | High to Normal | High |

**KEY**
High ● Normal ◑ Low ○

### REFERENCE VALUES

Normal serum PTH levels vary, depending on the laboratory, and must be interpreted in association with serum calcium levels. Typical values for intact PTH range from 10 to 50 pg/ml (SI, 1.1 to 5.3 pmol/L); N-terminal fraction is 8 to 24 pg/ml (SI, 0.8 to 2.5 pmol/L); C-terminal fraction, 0 to 340 pg/ml (SI, 0 to 35.8 pmol/L).

### ABNORMAL FINDINGS

Measured concomitantly with serum calcium levels, abnormally elevated PTH values may indicate primary, secondary, or tertiary hyperparathyroidism. Abnormally low PTH levels may result from hypoparathyroidism and from certain malignant diseases. (See *Clinical implications of abnormal parathyroid secretion*.)

### INTERFERING FACTORS

● Failure to fast overnight before the test

## *Partial thromboplastin time*

The partial thromboplastin time (PTT) test is used to evaluate all the clotting factors of the intrinsic pathway — except platelets — by measuring the time required for formation of a fibrin clot after the addition of calcium and phospholipid emulsion to a plasma sample. An activator, such as kaolin, is used to shorten clotting time.

### PURPOSE

● To screen for deficiencies of the clotting factors in the intrinsic pathways
● To monitor response to heparin therapy

### PATIENT PREPARATION

● Explain to the patient that the PTT test is used to determine if blood clots normally.

- Tell the patient that a blood sample will be taken. Explain who will perform the venipuncture and when and where the test will take place.
- Explain to the patient that he may feel slight discomfort from the needle puncture and the tourniquet.
- When appropriate, tell the patient receiving heparin therapy that this test may be repeated at regular intervals to assess his response to treatment.
- Inform the patient that he need not restrict food and fluids.

## PROCEDURE AND POSTTEST CARE
- Perform a venipuncture and collect the sample in a 7-ml tube with sodium citrate added.
- If a hematoma develops at the venipuncture site, apply pressure. If the hematoma is large, monitor pulses distal to the venipuncture site.
- Make sure subdermal bleeding has stopped before removing pressure.

## PRECAUTIONS
- Completely fill the collection tube, invert it gently several times, and send it to the laboratory on ice.
- To prevent hemolysis, avoid excessive probing at the venipuncture site and handle the sample gently.
- For a patient on anticoagulant therapy, apply additional pressure at the venipuncture site to control bleeding.

## REFERENCE VALUES
Normally, a fibrin clot forms 21 to 35 seconds (SI, 21 to 35 s) after adding reagents. For a patient on anticoagulant therapy, ask the physician to specify the reference values for the therapy being delivered.

## ABNORMAL FINDINGS
A prolonged PTT may indicate a deficiency of certain plasma clotting factors, the presence of heparin, or the presence of fibrin split products, fibrinolysins, or circulating anticoagulants that are antibodies to specific clotting factors.

## INTERFERING FACTORS
- Anticoagulant therapy

## Parvovirus B-19 antibodies

Parvovirus B-19, a small, single-stranded deoxyribonucleic acid virus belonging to the family *Parvoviridae,* destroys red blood cell (RBC) precursors and interferes with normal RBC production. It's also associated with erythema infectiosum (a self-limiting, low-grade fever and rash in young children) and aplastic crisis (in patients with chronic hemolytic anemia and immunodeficient patients with bone marrow failure). Immunoglobulin (Ig) G and IgM antibodies can be detected by enzyme-linked immunosorbent assay and immunofluorescence.

## PURPOSE
- To detect parvovirus B-19 antibody, especially in prospective organ donors
- To diagnose erythema infectiosum, parvovirus B-19 aplastic crisis, and related parvovirus B-19 diseases

## PATIENT PREPARATION
- Explain the parovirus B-19 antibody test purpose and procedure to the patient. To a potential organ donor, explain that the test is part of a panel of tests performed before organ donation to protect the organ recipient from potential infection.
- Tell the patient that the test requires a blood sample. Explain who will perform the venipuncture and when and where the test will take place.
- Explain to the patient that he may experience slight discomfort from the needle puncture and the tourniquet.

## PROCEDURE AND POSTTEST CARE
- Perform a venipuncture, collect the blood sample in a 5-ml clot-activator tube, and store it on ice.
- Apply direct pressure to the venipuncture site until bleeding stops.
- If a hematoma develops at the venipuncture site, apply pressure.

## PRECAUTIONS
- Handle the sample gently to prevent hemolysis.

## NORMAL FINDINGS

Normally, results are negative for IgM- and IgG-specific antibodies to parvovirus B-19.

## ABNORMAL FINDINGS

About 50% of all adults lack immunity to parvovirus B-19, with as many as 20% of susceptible adults becoming infected after exposure. Positive results have been associated with joint arthralgia, hydrops fetalis, fetal loss, transient aplastic anemia, chronic anemia in immunocompromised patients, and bone marrow failure.

Abnormal findings for parvovirus B-19 should be confirmed using the Western blot test.

## INTERFERING FACTORS

● None significant

# Pelvic ultrasonography

In pelvic ultrasonography, high-frequency sound waves are reflected to a transducer to provide images of the interior pelvic area on a monitor. Techniques of sound imaging include A-mode (amplitude modulation, recorded as spikes), B-mode (brightness modulation), gray scale (a representation of organ texture in shades of gray), and real-time imaging (instantaneous images of the tissues in motion, similar to fluoroscopic examination). Selected views may be photographed for later examination and a permanent record of the test.

## PURPOSE

● To detect foreign bodies and distinguish between cystic and solid masses (tumors)
● To measure organ size
● To evaluate fetal viability, position, gestational age, and growth rate
● To detect multiple pregnancy
● To confirm fetal and maternal abnormalities
● To guide amniocentesis by determining placental location and fetal position

## PATIENT PREPARATION

● Describe pelvic ultrasonography to the patient and tell her the reason it's being performed.

● Assure the patient that this procedure is safe, noninvasive, and painless.
● Because this test requires a full bladder as a landmark to define pelvic organs, instruct the patient to drink liquids and not to void before the test.
● Tell the patient who will perform the procedure and when and where it will take place.
● Explain that a water enema may be necessary to produce a better outline of the large intestine.
● Reassure the patient that the test won't harm the fetus and provide emotional support throughout.

## PROCEDURE AND POSTTEST CARE

● With the patient in a supine position, the pelvic area is coated with mineral oil or water-soluble conductive gel to increase sound wave conduction.
● The transducer is guided over the area, images are observed on the monitor, and good images are photographed.
● Allow the patient to immediately empty her bladder after the test.

## PRECAUTIONS

● None.

## NORMAL FINDINGS

The uterus is normal in size and shape. The ovaries' size, shape, and sonographic density are normal. The body of the uterus lies on the superior surface of the bladder; the uterine tubes are attached laterally. The ovaries are located on the lateral pelvic walls, with the external iliac vessels above the ureter posteroinferiorly and covered by the fimbria of the uterine tubes medially. No other masses are visible. If the patient is pregnant, the gestational sac and fetus are of normal size in relation to gestational age.

## ABNORMAL FINDINGS

Cystic and solid masses have homogeneous densities, but solid masses (such as fibroids) appear denser. Inappropriate fetal size may indicate miscalculated conception or delivery date, fetal anomalies, or a dead fetus.

Abnormal echo patterns may indicate foreign bodies (such as an intrauterine device), multiple pregnancy, maternal abnormalities (such as placenta previa or abruptio placentae), fetal abnormalities (such as molar pregnancy or abnormalities of the arms and legs, spine, heart, head, kidneys, and abdomen), fetal malpresentation (such as breech or shoulder presentation), and cephalopelvic disproportion.

## INTERFERING FACTORS
- Empty bladder
- Obesity, or fetal head deep in the pelvis (possible poor imaging)

# *Percutaneous liver biopsy*

Percutaneous biopsy of the liver is the needle aspiration of a core of liver tissue for histologic analysis. This procedure is performed under local or general anesthesia using a special needle. (See *Using a Menghini needle.*)

Findings may help to identify hepatic disorders after ultrasonography, computed tomography scan, and radionuclide studies have failed to detect them. Because many patients with hepatic disorders have clotting defects, testing for hemostasis should precede liver biopsy.

## PURPOSE
- To diagnose hepatic parenchymal disease, malignant tumors, and granulomatous infections

## PATIENT PREPARATION
- Explain to the patient that the percutaneous biopsy of the liver is used to diagnose liver disorders.
- Describe the procedure to the patient, and answer his questions.
- Instruct the patient to restrict food and fluids for 4 to 8 hours before the test.
- Tell the patient who will perform the biopsy and where it will be done.
- Make sure the patient or a responsible family member has signed an informed consent form.
- Check the patient's history for hypersensitivity to the local anesthetic.
- Make sure coagulation studies (prothrombin [PT] time, partial thromboplastin time, and platelet counts) have been performed and that the results are recorded on the patient's chart.

- A blood sample is usually drawn for baseline hematocrit assessment.
- Just before the biopsy, tell the patient to void, and then record his vital signs.
- Inform the patient that he'll receive a local anesthetic but may experience pain similar to that of a punch in his right shoulder as the biopsy needle passes the phrenic nerve.

## PROCEDURE AND POSTTEST CARE
- For aspiration biopsy using the Menghini needle, place the patient in a supine position with his right hand under his head. Instruct him to maintain this position and remain as still as possible during the procedure.
- The liver is palpated, the biopsy site is selected and marked, and the local anesthetic is then injected.
- The needle flange is set to control the depth of penetration, and 2 ml of sterile normal saline solution are drawn into the syringe.
- The syringe is attached to the biopsy needle, and the needle is introduced into the subcutaneous tissue through the right eighth or ninth intercostal space at the midaxillary line and advanced up to the pleura.
- Next, 1 ml of normal saline solution is injected to clear the needle and the plunger, and then the plunger is drawn back to the 4-ml mark to create negative pressure.
- At this point in the procedure, ask the patient to take a deep breath, exhale, and hold his breath at the end of expiration to prevent movement of the chest wall.
- As the patient holds his breath, the biopsy needle is quickly inserted into the liver and withdrawn in 1 second.
- For the patient who can't hold his breath, the biopsy needle is quickly inserted and withdrawn at the end of expiration.
- After the needle is withdrawn, tell the patient to resume normal respirations.
- The tissue specimen is then placed in a properly labeled specimen cup containing 10% formalin solution. This placement is done by releasing negative pressure while the point of the needle is in the formalin solution. Send the specimen to the laboratory immediately.
- Again, 1 ml of normal saline solution is injected to clear the needle of the tissue specimen.
- Apply pressure to the biopsy site to stop bleeding.

# Using a Menghini needle

In percutaneous liver biopsy, a Menghini needle attached to a 5-ml syringe containing normal saline solution is introduced through the chest wall and intercostal space (1). Negative pressure is created in the syringe. Then the needle is pushed rapidly into the liver (2) and pulled out of the body entirely (3) to obtain a tissue specimen.

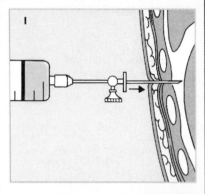

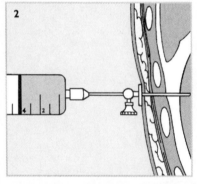

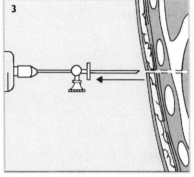

• Position the patient on his right side for 2 to 4 hours, with a small pillow or sandbag under the costal margin to provide extra pressure. Advise bed rest for at least 24 hours.

• Check the patient's vital signs every 15 minutes for 1 hour, every 30 minutes for 4 hours, and every 4 hours thereafter for 24 hours. Throughout, observe him carefully for signs of shock.

*Alert* *Immediately report bleeding or signs of bile peritonitis, such as tenderness and rigidity around the biopsy site. Be alert for symptoms of pneumothorax, such as rising respiratory rate, depressed breath sounds, dyspnea, persistent shoulder pain, and pleuritic chest pain. Report such complications promptly.*

• If the patient experiences pain, which may persist for several hours after the test, administer an analgesic.

• Inform the patient that he may resume his usual diet, as ordered.

## PRECAUTIONS

• Be aware that percutaneous liver biopsy is contraindicated in a patient with a platelet count below 100,000/µl; PT time longer than 15 seconds; empyema of the lungs, pleurae, peritoneum, biliary tract, or liver; vascular tumor; hepatic angiomas; hydatid cyst; or tense ascites. If extrahepatic obstruction is suspected, ultrasonography or subcutaneous transhepatic cholangiography should rule out this condition before the biopsy is considered.

• Know that pain in the abdomen or dyspnea after the biopsy may indicate perforation of an abdominal organ or pneumothorax, respectively. In such cases, complete a thorough assessment and notify the physician at once.

- Instruct the patient to hold his breath while the needle is in place.

## NORMAL FINDINGS

The normal liver consists of sheets of hepatocytes supported by a reticulin framework.

## ABNORMAL FINDINGS

Examination of the hepatic tissue may reveal diffuse hepatic disease, such as cirrhosis or hepatitis, or granulomatous infections such as tuberculosis. Primary malignant tumors include hepatocellular carcinoma, cholangiocellular carcinoma, and angiosarcoma, but hepatic metastasis is more common.

Nonmalignant findings with a known focal lesion require further studies, such as laparotomy or laparoscopy with biopsy.

## INTERFERING FACTORS

- Inability to obtain a representative specimen
- Hemorrhage caused by inadvertent puncture of a liver blood vessel

---

# Percutaneous transhepatic cholangiography

---

Percutaneous transhepatic cholangiography is the fluoroscopic examination of the biliary ducts after injection of an iodinated contrast medium directly into a biliary radicle. This test is especially useful for evaluating patients with persistent upper abdominal pain after cholecystectomy or severe jaundice.

Although a computed tomography scan or ultrasonography is usually performed first when obstructive jaundice is suspected, percutaneous transhepatic cholangiography may provide the most detailed view of the obstruction; however, this invasive procedure carries a potential risk of complications that include bleeding, septicemia, bile peritonitis, extravasation of the contrast medium into the peritoneal cavity, and subcapsular injection.

## PURPOSE

- To determine the cause of upper abdominal pain following cholecystectomy

- To distinguish between obstructive and nonobstructive jaundice
- To determine the location, the extent and, commonly, the cause of mechanical obstruction

## PATIENT PREPARATION

- Explain to the patient that percutaneous transhepatic cholangiography allows examination of the biliary ducts through X-ray films taken after a contrast medium is injected into the liver.
- Instruct the patient to fast for 8 hours before the test.
- Describe the test, including who will perform it and when and where it will take place.
- Inform the patient that he may receive a laxative the night before and an enema the morning of the test.
- Inform the patient that he'll be placed on a tilting X-ray table that rotates into vertical and horizontal positions during the procedure.
- Assure the patient that he'll be adequately secured to the table and assisted to supine and side-lying positions throughout the procedure.
- Warn the patient that injection of the local anesthetic may sting the skin and produce transient pain when it punctures the liver capsule.
- Advise the patient that injection of the contrast medium may produce a sensation of pressure and epigastric fullness and may cause transient upper-back pain on his right side.
- Tell the patient that he must rest for at least 6 hours after the procedure.
- Make sure that the patient or a responsible family member has signed an informed consent form.
- Check the patient's history for hypersensitivity to iodine, seafood, contrast media used in other diagnostic tests, and the local anesthetic. Advise him of possible adverse effects of contrast medium administration, such as nausea, vomiting, excessive salivation, flushing, urticaria, sweating and, rarely, anaphylaxis; tachycardia and fever may accompany intraductal injection.
- Check the patient's history for normal bleeding, clotting, and prothrombin times and a normal platelet count. If prescribed, administer 1 g of I.V. ampicillin every 4 to 6 hours for 24 hours before the procedure.

- Just before the procedure, administer a sedative, if prescribed.

## PROCEDURE AND POSTTEST CARE

- After the patient is placed in a supine position on the X-ray table and is adequately secured, the right upper quadrant of the abdomen is cleaned and draped; the skin, subcutaneous tissue, and liver capsule are infiltrated with a local anesthetic.
- While the patient holds his breath at the end of expiration, the flexible needle is inserted under fluoroscopic guidance through the 10th or 11th intercostal space at the right midclavicular line.
- The needle is aimed toward the xiphoid process and is advanced through the liver parenchyma. It's then slowly withdrawn, injecting the contrast medium to locate a biliary radicle. When fluoroscopy reveals placement in a radicle, the needle is held in position and the remaining contrast medium is injected.
- Using a fluoroscope and television monitor, biliary duct opacification is observed, and spot films of significant findings are taken with the patient in supine and lateral recumbent positions. When the required films have been taken, the needle is removed.
- Apply a sterile dressing to the puncture site.
- Check the patient's vital signs until they're stable.
- Enforce bed rest for at least 6 hours after the test, preferably with the patient lying on his right side, to help prevent hemorrhage.
- Check the injection site for bleeding, swelling, and tenderness. Watch for signs of peritonitis: chills, temperature of 102° to 103° F (38.8° to 39.4° C), and abdominal pain, tenderness, and distention. Notify the physician immediately if such complications develop.
- Tell the patient that he may resume his usual diet.

## PRECAUTIONS

- Be aware that percutaneous transhepatic cholangiography is contraindicated in the patient with cholangitis, massive ascites, uncorrectable coagulopathy, or hypersensitivity to iodine, as well as in the pregnant patient because of radiation's possible teratogenic effects.

## NORMAL FINDINGS

The biliary ducts are of normal diameter and appear as regular channels homogeneously filled with contrast medium.

## ABNORMAL FINDINGS

Distinguishing between obstructive and nonobstructive jaundice hinges on whether biliary ducts are dilated or of normal size. Obstructive jaundice is associated with dilated ducts; nonobstructive jaundice, with normal-sized ducts. When ducts are dilated, the obstruction site may be defined. Obstruction may result from cholelithiasis, biliary tract carcinoma, or carcinoma of the pancreas or papilla of Vater that impinges on the common bile duct, causing deviation or stricture.

When ducts are of normal size and intrahepatic cholestasis is indicated, liver biopsy may be performed to distinguish among hepatitis, cirrhosis, and granulomatous disease. If ducts are dilated as a result of obstruction, a drainage tube may be inserted to allow percutaneous drainage of bile into a collection bag.

## INTERFERING FACTORS

- Marked obesity or gas overlying the biliary ducts (possible poor imaging)

# *Pericardial fluid analysis*

Analysis of the fluid inside the pericardial sac of the heart is usually done for the patient with pericardial effusion (an accumulation of excess pericardial fluid), which may result from inflammation (as in pericarditis), rupture, or penetrating trauma.

Obtaining a specimen for analysis requires needle aspiration of pericardial fluid, a procedure called pericardiocentesis. This procedure must be performed cautiously because of the risk of potentially fatal complications, such as myocardial or coronary artery laceration, ventricular fibrillation or vasovagal arrest, pleural infection, or accidental puncture of the lung, liver, or stomach. If possible, echocardiography should determine the effusion site before pericardiocentesis is performed to minimize the risk of complications. (See *Aspirating pericardial fluid,* page 322.)

# Aspirating pericardial fluid

In pericardiocentesis, a needle and syringe assembly is inserted through the chest wall into the pericardial sac, as illustrated here. Electrocardiographic (ECG) monitoring with a leadwire attached to the needle and electrodes placed on the limbs (right arm [RA], right leg [RL], left arm [LA], and left leg [LL]) helps to ensure proper needle placement and to avoid damage to the heart.

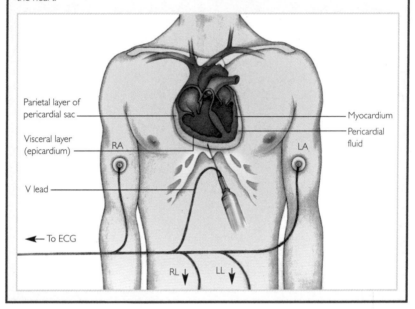

Parietal layer of pericardial sac

Visceral layer (epicardium)

RA

V lead

← To ECG

RL ↓   LL ↓

Myocardium

Pericardial fluid

LA

## Purpose
● To assist in identifying the cause of pericardial effusion and to help determine appropriate therapy

## Patient preparation
● Explain to the patient that pericardial fluid analysis detects excessive fluid around the heart, determines its cause, and helps determine appropriate therapy.
● Inform him that he need not restrict food and fluids.
● Tell him who will perform the test and where and when it will take place.
● Inform the patient that a local anesthetic will be injected before the aspiration needle is inserted.
● Warn him that although fluid aspiration isn't painful, he may experience pressure upon needle insertion into the pericardial sac.

● Advise him that he may be asked to briefly hold his breath to aid needle insertion and placement.
● Tell the patient that an I.V. line will be started at a slow rate in case medications need to be administered.
● Assure him that someone will remain with him during the test and that his pulse and blood pressure will be monitored after the procedure.
● Check the patient's history for current antimicrobial usage and record such usage on the test request form.
● Make sure that the patient or a responsible family member has signed an informed consent form.
● Explain the test to the family if pericardiocentesis is performed to relieve cardiac tamponade and the patient is in shock.

## Procedure and Posttest Care

● Place the patient in the supine position with the thorax elevated 60 degrees.

● When the patient is comfortable and well supported, instruct him to remain still during the procedure.

● A local anesthetic is administered at the insertion site after the skin is prepared with alcohol or povidone-iodine solution from the left costal margin to the xiphoid process.

● With the three-way stopcock open, a 50-ml syringe is aseptically attached to one end and the cardiac needle to the other end.

● The electrocardiogram (ECG) leadwire is attached to the needle hub with an alligator clip. The ECG is set to lead $V_1$ and turned on (or the patient is connected to a bedside monitor).

● The needle is inserted through the chest wall into the pericardial sac, maintaining gentle aspiration until fluid appears in the syringe.

● The needle is angled 35 to 45 degrees toward the tip of the right scapula between the left costal margin and the xiphoid process. A Kelly clamp is attached at the skin surface after the needle is properly positioned so it won't advance further.

● While the fluid is being aspirated, label and number the specimen tubes.

● When the needle is withdrawn, apply pressure to the site immediately with sterile gauze pads for 3 to 5 minutes. Then apply a bandage.

● Check blood pressure readings, pulse, respiration, and heart sounds every 15 minutes until stable, every 1/2 hour for 2 hours, every hour for 4 hours, and then every 4 hours thereafter. Reassure the patient that such monitoring is routine.

*Alert Be alert for respiratory or cardiac distress. Watch especially for signs of cardiac tamponade: muffled and distant heart sounds, distended neck veins, paradoxical pulse, and shock. Cardiac tamponade may result from rapid reaccumulation of pericardial fluid or puncture of a coronary vessel, causing bleeding into the pericardial sac.*

## Precautions

● Be sure to carefully observe the ECG tracing during insertion of the cardiac needle; an ST-segment elevation indicates that the needle has reached the epicardial surface and should be retracted slightly; an abnormally shaped QRS complex may indicate perforation of the myocardium. Also, know that premature ventricular contractions usually indicate that the needle has touched the ventricular wall.

● Watch for grossly bloody aspirate — a sign of inadvertent puncture of a cardiac chamber.

● Be sure to use specimen tubes with the proper additives. Although fibrin isn't a normal component of pericardial fluid, it does appear in fluid in some pericardial diseases and in carcinoma, and clotting is possible.

● Clean the top of the culture and sensitivity tube with povidone-iodine solution or according to facility policy to reduce the risk of extrinsic contamination.

● If bacterial culture and sensitivity tests are scheduled, record any antimicrobial therapy the patient is receiving on the laboratory request.

● If anaerobic organisms are suspected, consult the laboratory concerning the proper collection technique to avoid exposing the aspirate to air. The aspirate may be placed in an anaerobic collection tube, or the syringe may be filled completely, displacing all air, and the collection tube capped tightly with a sterile rubber tip.

● Send all specimens to the laboratory immediately after collection.

● Have resuscitation equipment on hand.

## Normal Findings

Normally, 10 to 50 ml of sterile fluid is present in the pericardium. Pericardial fluid is clear and straw-colored, without evidence of pathogens, blood, or malignant cells. It normally contains fewer than 1,000/µl (SI, $< 1.0 \times 10^9$/L) white blood cells (WBCs). Its glucose concentration approximately equals the levels in whole blood.

## Abnormal Findings

Generally, pericardial effusions are classified as transudates or exudates. Transudates are protein-poor effusions that usually arise from mechanical factors altering fluid formation or resorption, such as increased hydrostatic pressure, decreased plasma oncotic pressure, or obstruction of the pericardial lymphatic drainage system by a tumor.

Most exudates result from inflammation and contain large amounts of protein. In these effusions, inflammation damages the capillary membrane, allowing protein molecules to leak into the pericardial fluid. Exudate effusions may occur in pericarditis, neoplasms, acute myocardial infarction, tuberculosis (TB), rheumatoid disease, and systemic lupus erythematosus.

An elevated WBC count or neutrophil fraction may also accompany inflammatory conditions such as bacterial pericarditis; a high lymphocyte fraction may indicate fungal or tuberculous pericarditis. Turbid or milky effusions may result from lymph or pus accumulation in the pericardial sac or from TB or rheumatoid disease.

Bloody pericardial fluid may indicate hemopericardium, hemorrhagic pericarditis, or a traumatic tap. Hemopericardium, the accumulation of blood in the pericardium, may result from myocardial rupture after infarction or aortic rupture secondary to a dissecting aortic aneurysm or thoracic trauma. In hemopericardium, the fluid has a hematocrit level similar to that of whole blood; in hemorrhagic pericarditis, it has a relatively low hematocrit and doesn't clot on standing.

Hemorrhagic effusions may indicate a malignant tumor, closed chest trauma, Dressler's syndrome, or postcardiotomy syndrome. A traumatic tap is easily distinguished from hemopericardium or hemorrhagic pericarditis because the fluid becomes progressively clearer.

Glucose concentrations below whole blood levels may reflect increased local metabolism due to malignancy, inflammation, or infection. Possible causes of bacterial pericarditis include *Staphylococcus aureus, Haemophilus influenzae,* and various gram-negative organisms; possible causes of granulomatous pericarditis include *Mycobacterium tuberculosis* or various fungal agents; and possible causes of viral pericarditis include coxsackieviruses, echoviruses, and others.

## INTERFERING FACTORS
● Failure to use aseptic collection technique, allowing skin contaminants to be mistaken for the causative organism
● Antimicrobial therapy (can prevent isolation of the causative organisms)

# Peritoneal fluid analysis

Peritoneal fluid analysis assesses a specimen of peritoneal fluid obtained by paracentesis. This procedure requires inserting a trocar and cannula through the abdominal wall while the patient receives a local anesthetic. If the fluid specimen is removed for therapeutic purposes, the trocar may be connected to a drainage system. However, if only a small amount of fluid is removed for diagnostic purposes, an 18G needle may be used in place of the trocar and cannula. In a four-quadrant tap, fluid is aspirated from each quadrant of the abdomen to verify abdominal trauma and confirm the need for surgery.

## PURPOSE
● To determine the cause of ascites
● To detect abdominal trauma

## PATIENT PREPARATION
● Explain to the patient that peritoneal fluid analysis helps determine the cause of ascites or detects abdominal trauma.
● Inform the patient that he need not restrict food and fluids.
● Tell the patient that the test requires a peritoneal fluid specimen, that he'll receive a local anesthetic to minimize discomfort, and that the procedure takes about 45 minutes to perform.
● Provide psychological support to decrease the patient's anxiety and assure him that complications are rare.
● If the patient has severe ascites, inform him that the procedure will relieve his discomfort and allow him to breathe more easily.
● Make sure that the patient or a responsible family member has signed an informed consent form.
● Record the patient's baseline vital signs, weight, and abdominal girth.
● Tell the patient that a blood sample may be taken for analysis.
● Tell the patient to void just before the test; doing so helps to prevent accidental bladder injury during needle insertion.
● X-rays may be performed before peritoneal analysis to ensure reliability.

## PROCEDURE AND POSTTEST CARE

• Have the patient sit on a bed or in a chair with his feet flat on the floor and his back well supported. If he can't tolerate being out of bed, place him in high Fowler's position and make him as comfortable as possible.

• Except for at the puncture site, keep the patient covered to keep him warm.

• Provide a plastic sheet or absorbent pad to collect spillage and to protect the patient and bed linens.

• The puncture site is shaved, the skin prepared, and the area draped.

• The local anesthetic is injected.

• The examiner inserts the needle or trocar and cannula 1″ to 2″ (2.5 to 5 cm) below the umbilicus. (However, it may also be inserted through the flank, the iliac fossa, the border of the rectus, or at each quadrant of the abdomen.)

• If a trocar and cannula are used, a small incision is made to facilitate insertion. When the needle pierces the peritoneum, it "gives" with an audible sound. The trocar is removed and a sample of fluid is aspirated with a 50-ml luer-lock syringe.

• If additional fluid is to be drained, assist in attaching one end of an I.V. tube to the cannula and the other end to a collection bag. The fluid is then aspirated (no more than 1,500 ml). If aspirating is difficult, reposition the patient as ordered.

• After aspiration, the trocar needle is removed and a pressure dressing is applied. Occasionally, the wound may be sutured first.

• Label the specimens in the order they were drawn. If the patient has received antibiotic therapy, note this on the laboratory request.

• Carefully and properly dispose of needles and contaminated articles according to the Centers for Disease Control and Prevention guidelines; incinerate disposable items and return reusable ones to the central supply area.

• Apply a gauze dressing to the puncture site. Make sure it's thick enough to absorb all drainage. Check the dressing frequently (for example, whenever you check vital signs) and reinforce or apply a pressure dressing if needed.

• Monitor the patient's vital signs until they're stable. If his recovery is poor, check his vital signs every 15 minutes. Weigh him and measure his abdominal girth; compare these with his baseline values.

• Allow the patient to rest and, if possible, withhold treatment or procedures that may cause undue stress such as linen changes.

• Monitor the patient's urine output for at least 24 hours, and watch for hematuria, which may indicate bladder trauma.

⚙ **Alert** *Watch the patient for signs of hemorrhage or shock and for increasing pain or abdominal tenderness. These signs may indicate a perforated intestine or, depending on the site of the tap, puncture of the inferior epigastric artery, hematoma of the anterior cecal wall, or rupture of the iliac vein or bladder.*

• If a large amount of fluid was aspirated, watch the patient for signs of vascular collapse (color change, elevated pulse and respiratory rates, decreased blood pressure and central venous pressure, mental changes, and dizziness). Administer fluids orally if the patient is alert and can accept them.

⚙ **Alert** *Observe the patient with severe hepatic disease for signs of hepatic coma, which may result from sodium and potassium loss accompanying hypovolemia. Watch him for mental changes, drowsiness, and stupor. Such a patient is also prone to uremia, infection, hemorrhage, and protein depletion.*

• As ordered, administer I.V. infusions and albumin. Check the laboratory report for electrolyte (especially sodium) and serum protein levels.

## PRECAUTIONS

• Know that peritoneal fluid analysis should be performed cautiously in a pregnant patient and in the patient with bleeding tendencies or unstable vital signs.

• Check the patient's vital signs every 15 minutes during the procedure. Watch for deviations from baseline findings. Observe for dizziness, pallor, perspiration, and increased anxiety.

• If rapid fluid aspiration induces hypovolemia and shock, reduce the vertical distance between the trocar and the collection bag to slow the drainage rate. If necessary, stop the drainage by turning off the stopcock or clamping the tubing.

• Avoid contamination of the specimens, which alters their bacterial content. Send them to the laboratory immediately after collection.

## NORMAL FINDINGS IN PERITONEAL FLUID ANALYSIS

Use the below chart to determine the normal findings in peritoneal fluid.

| ELEMENT | NORMAL VALUE OR FINDING |
|---|---|
| Gross appearance | Sterile, odorless, clear to pale yellow color; scant amount (< 50 ml) |
| Red blood cells | None |
| White blood cells | < 300/µl (SI, < 300 × 10⁹/L) |
| Protein | 0.3 to 4.1 g/dl (SI, 3 to 41 g/L) |
| Glucose | 70 to 100 mg/dl (SI, 3.5 to 5 mmol/L) |
| Amylase | 138 to 404 U/L (SI, 138 to 404 U/L) |
| Ammonia | < 50 mcg/dl (SI, < 29 µmol/L) |
| Alkaline phosphatase | Males > age 18: 90 to 239 U/L (SI, 90 to 239 U/L)<br>Females < age 45: 76 to 196 U/L (SI, 76 to 196 U/L)<br>Females > age 45: 87 to 250 U/L (SI, 87 to 250 U/L) |
| Cytology | No malignant cells present |
| Bacteria | None |
| Fungi | None |

### REFERENCE VALUES

For normal peritoneal fluid values, see *Normal findings in peritoneal fluid analysis.*

### ABNORMAL FINDINGS

Milk-colored peritoneal fluid may result from chyle or lymph fluid escaping from a thoracic duct that's damaged or blocked by a malignant tumor, lymphoma, tuberculosis, parasitic infestation, adhesion, or hepatic cirrhosis; a pseudochylous condition may result from the presence of leukocytes or tumor cells. Differential diagnosis of true chylous ascites depends on the presence of elevated triglyceride levels (greater than 400 mg/dl [SI, ≥ 4.36 mmol/L]) and microscopic fat globules.

Cloudy or turbid fluid may indicate peritonitis due to primary bacterial infection, a ruptured bowel (after trauma), pancreatitis, a strangulated or an infarcted intestine, or appendicitis. Bloody fluid may result from a benign or malignant tumor, hemorrhagic

pancreatitis, or a traumatic tap; however, if the fluid fails to clear on continued aspiration, a traumatic tap isn't the cause. Bile-stained, green fluid may indicate a ruptured gallbladder, acute pancreatitis, or a perforated intestine or duodenal ulcer.

A red blood cell count over 100/µl (SI, > 100/L) indicates neoplasm or tuberculosis; a count over 100,000/µl (SI, > 100,000/L) indicates intra-abdominal trauma. An elevated white blood cell count with more than 25% neutrophils occurs in 90% of patients with spontaneous bacterial peritonitis and in 50% of those with cirrhosis. A high percentage of lymphocytes suggests tuberculous peritonitis or chylous ascites. Numerous mesothelial cells indicate tuberculous peritonitis.

Protein levels rise above 3 g/dl in malignancy (SI, > 3 g/L) and above 4 g/dl (SI, > 4 g/L) in tuberculosis. Peritoneal fluid glucose levels fall in the patient with tuberculous peritonitis or peritoneal carcinomatosis.

Amylase levels rise with pancreatic trauma, pancreatic pseudocyst, or acute pancreatitis and may also rise in intestinal necrosis or strangulation.

Peritoneal alkaline phosphatase levels rise to more than twice the normal serum levels in the patient with ruptured or strangulated small intestines. Peritoneal ammonia levels also exceed twice the normal serum levels in ruptured or strangulated large and small intestines and in a ruptured ulcer or an appendix.

A protein ascitic fluid to serum ratio of 0.5 or greater may suggest a malignancy or tuberculous or pancreatic ascites. The presence of this finding indicates a nonhepatic cause; its absence suggests uncomplicated hepatic disease. An albumin gradient between ascitic fluid and serum greater than 1 g/dl (SI, > 1 g/L) indicates chronic hepatic disease; a lesser value suggests malignancy.

Cytologic examination of peritoneal fluid accurately detects malignant cells. Microbiological examination can reveal coliforms, anaerobes, and enterococci, which can enter the peritoneum from a ruptured organ or from infections accompanying appendicitis, pancreatitis, tuberculosis, or ovarian disease. Gram-positive cocci commonly indicate primary peritonitis; gram-negative organisms, secondary peritonitis. The presence of fungi may indicate histoplasmosis, candidiasis, or coccidioidomycosis.

## INTERFERING FACTORS
- Unsterile collection technique or failure to send the specimen to the laboratory immediately after collection
- Contamination of the specimen with blood, bile, urine, or stool due to injury to underlying structures during paracentesis

# Persantine-thallium imaging

Persantine-thallium imaging is an alternative method of assessing coronary vessel function for the patient who can't tolerate exercise or stress electrocardiography (ECG). Dipyridamole (Persantine) infusion simulates the effects of exercise by increasing blood flow to the collateral circulation and away from the coronary arteries, thereby inducing ischemia.

Thallium infusion allows the examiner to evaluate the cardiac vessels' response. The heart is scanned immediately after the thallium infusion and again 2 to 4 hours later. Diseased vessels can't deliver thallium to the heart, and thallium lingers in diseased areas of the myocardium.

## PURPOSE
- To identify exercise- or stress-induced arrhythmias
- To assess the presence and degree of cardiac ischemia

## PATIENT PREPARATION
- Tell the patient that a painless, 5- to 10-minute baseline ECG will precede Persantine-thallium imaging.
- Explain to the patient that he'll need to restrict food and fluids before the test. Tell him to avoid caffeine and other stimulants (which may cause arrhythmias).
- Instruct the patient to continue to take all his regular medications, with the possible exception of beta-adrenergic blockers as prescribed.
- Explain to the patient that an I.V. line infuses the medications for the study. Tell him who will start the I.V., when and where the test will take place, and that he may experience slight discomfort from the needle insertion and the tourniquet.
- Inform the patient that he may experience mild nausea, headache, dizziness, or flushing after Persantine administration. Reassure him that these adverse reactions are usually temporary and rarely need treatment.
- Make sure that the patient or a responsible family member has signed an informed consent form.

## PROCEDURE AND POSTTEST CARE
- The patient reclines or sits while a resting ECG is performed. Then Persantine is given either orally or I.V. over 4 minutes. Blood pressure, pulse rate, and cardiac rhythm are monitored continuously.
- After Persantine administration, the patient is asked to get up and walk. After it takes effect, thallium is injected.
- The patient is placed in a supine position for about 40 minutes while the scan is performed. Then the scan is reviewed. If necessary, a second scan is performed.

- If the patient must return for further scanning, tell him to rest and to restrict food and fluids in the interim.

## PRECAUTIONS
- Be aware that the patient may experience arrhythmias, angina, ST-segment depression, or bronchospasm. Make sure resuscitation equipment is readily available.
- Know that more common adverse reactions are nausea, headache, flushing, dizziness, and epigastric pain.

## NORMAL FINDINGS
Imaging should reveal characteristic distribution of the isotope throughout the left ventricle and no visible defects.

## ABNORMAL FINDINGS
The presence of ST-segment depression, angina, and arrhythmias strongly suggests coronary artery disease (CAD). Persistent ST-segment depression generally indicates a myocardial infarction. In contrast, transient ST-segment depression indicates ischemia from CAD.

Cold spots usually indicate CAD, but may result from sarcoidosis, myocardial fibrosis, cardiac contusion, attenuation due to soft tissue (for example, breast and diaphragm), apical cleft, and coronary spasm. The absence of cold spots in the presence of CAD may result from insignificant obstruction, single-vessel disease, or collateral circulation.

## INTERFERING FACTORS
- Artifacts, such as implants and electrodes (possible false-positive)
- Absence of cold spots with CAD (possible delay in imaging)

## *Phosphates, serum*

The phosphate test is used to measure serum levels of phosphates, the primary anion in intracellular fluid. Phosphates are essential in the storage and utilization of energy, calcium regulation, red blood cell function, acid-base balance, formation of bone, and the metabolism of carbohydrates, protein, and fat. The intestines absorb most phosphates from dietary sources; the kidneys excrete phosphates and serve as a regulatory mechanism. Abnormal concentrations of serum phosphates usually result from improper excretion rather than faulty ingestion or absorption from dietary sources.

Normally, calcium and phosphates have an inverse relationship; if one is increased, the other is decreased.

## PURPOSE
- To aid diagnosis of renal disorders and acid-base imbalance
- To detect endocrine, skeletal, and calcium disorders

## PATIENT PREPARATION
- Explain to the patient that the serum phosphate test is used to measure phosphate levels in the blood.
- Tell the patient that the test requires a blood sample. Explain who will perform the venipuncture and when and where the test will take place.
- Explain to the patient that he may experience slight discomfort from the needle puncture and the tourniquet.
- Inform the patient that he need not restrict food and fluids.
- Notify the laboratory and physician of medications the patient is taking that may affect test results; they may need to be restricted.

## PROCEDURE AND POSTTEST CARE
- Perform a venipuncture without using a tourniquet, if possible, and collect the sample in 3- or 4-ml clot-activator tube.
- Apply pressure to the venipuncture site until bleeding stops.
- If a hematoma develops at the venipuncture site, apply pressure.
- Instruct the patient that he may resume medications discontinued before the test, as ordered.

## PRECAUTIONS
- Handle the sample gently to prevent hemolysis.

## REFERENCE VALUES
Normally, serum phosphate levels in adults range from 2.7 to 4.5 mg/dl (SI, 0.87 to 1.45 mmol/L).

**Age alert** *In children, the normal serum phosphate level range is 4.5 to 6.7 mg/dl (SI, 1.45 to 1.78 mmol/L).*

## ABNORMAL FINDINGS

Decreased phosphate levels (hypophosphatemia) may result from malnutrition, malabsorption syndromes, hyperparathyroidism, renal tubular acidosis, and treatment of diabetic ketoacidosis (DKA). In children, hypophosphatemia can suppress normal growth. Symptoms of hypophosphatemia include anemia, prolonged bleeding, bone demineralization, decreased white blood cell count, and anorexia.

Increased levels (hyperphosphatemia) may result from skeletal disease, healing fractures, hypoparathyroidism, acromegaly, DKA, high intestinal obstruction, lactic acidosis (due to hepatic impairment), and renal failure. Hyperphosphatemia is seldom clinically significant, but it can alter bone metabolism in prolonged cases. Symptoms of hyperphosphatemia include tachycardia, muscular weakness, diarrhea, cramping, and hyperreflexia.

## INTERFERING FACTORS

- Venous stasis due to tourniquet use
- Sample obtained above an I.V. site that's receiving a solution containing phosphate
- Excessive vitamin D intake or therapy with anabolic steroids or androgens (possible increase)
- Use of acetazolamide, epinephrine, insulin, or phosphate-binding antacids; excessive excretion due to prolonged vomiting or diarrhea; vitamin D deficiency; and extended I.V. infusion of dextrose 5% in water (possible decrease)

## *Phospholipids*

The phospholipid test is a quantitative analysis of phospholipids, the major form of lipids in cell membranes. Phospholipids are involved in cellular membrane composition and permeability and help control enzyme activity within the membrane. They aid the transport of fatty acids and lipids across the intestinal barrier and from the liver and other fat stores to other body tissues. Phospho-

lipids are essential for pulmonary gas exchange.

## PURPOSE

- To aid in the evaluation of fat metabolism
- To aid in the diagnosis of hypothyroidism, diabetes mellitus, nephrotic syndrome, chronic pancreatitis, obstructive jaundice, and hypolipoproteinemia

## PATIENT PREPARATION

- Explain to the patient that the phospholipid test is used to determine how the body metabolizes fats.
- Tell the patient that the test requires a blood sample. Explain who will perform the venipuncture and when and where the test will take place.
- Explain to the patient that he may experience slight discomfort from the needle puncture and the tourniquet.
- Instruct the patient to abstain from drinking alcohol for 24 hours before the test and not to eat or drink anything after midnight before the test.
- Notify the laboratory and physician of medications the patient is taking that may affect test results; they may need to be restricted.

## PROCEDURE AND POSTTEST CARE

- Perform a venipuncture and collect the sample in a 10- to 15-ml tube without additives.
- Apply direct pressure to the venipuncture site until bleeding stops.
- If a hematoma develops at the venipuncture site, apply pressure.
- Instruct the patient that he may resume his usual diet and medications discontinued before the test, as ordered.

## PRECAUTIONS

- Send the sample to the laboratory immediately because spontaneous redistribution may occur among plasma lipids.

## REFERENCE VALUES

Normal phospholipid levels range from 180 to 320 mg/dl (SI, 1.8 to 3.2 g/L). Although men usually have higher levels than women, values in pregnant women exceed those of men.

## ABNORMAL FINDINGS

Elevated phospholipid levels may indicate hypothyroidism, diabetes mellitus, nephrotic syndrome, chronic pancreatitis, or obstructive jaundice. Decreased levels may indicate primary hypolipoproteinemia.

## INTERFERING FACTORS

- Antilipemics (possible decrease)
- Epinephrine, estrogens, and some phenothiazines (increase)

## *Plasma thrombin time*

Plasma thrombin time, or thrombin clotting time, measures how quickly a clot forms when a standard amount of bovine thrombin is added to a platelet-poor plasma sample from the patient and to a normal plasma control sample. After thrombin is added, the clotting time for each sample is compared and recorded. This test allows a quick but imprecise estimation of plasma fibrinogen levels, which are a function of clotting time. (See *Understanding the antithrombin III test*, for information about another test that helps determine the cause of coagulation disorders.)

## PURPOSE

- To detect a fibrinogen deficiency or defect
- To aid the diagnosis of disseminated intravascular coagulation (DIC) and hepatic disease

- To monitor the effectiveness of treatment with heparin or thrombolytic agents

## PATIENT PREPARATION

- Explain to the patient that the plasma thrombin time test is used to determine if blood clots normally.
- Notify the laboratory and physician of medications the patient is taking that may affect test results; they may need to be restricted.
- Tell the patient that a blood sample will be taken. Explain who will perform the venipuncture and when and where the test will take place.
- Explain to the patient that he may feel slight discomfort from the needle puncture and the tourniquet.
- Inform the patient that he need not restrict food and fluids.

## PROCEDURE AND POSTTEST CARE

- Perform a venipuncture and collect the sample in a 3- to 4.5-ml siliconized tube.
- If a hematoma develops at the venipuncture site, apply pressure. If the hematoma is large, monitor pulses distal to the phlebotomy site.
- Make sure bleeding has stopped before removing pressure.
- Instruct the patient that he may resume any medications discontinued before the test, as ordered.

## PRECAUTIONS

- Be aware that if the tube isn't filled to the correct volume, an excess of citrate appears

---

## UNDERSTANDING THE ANTITHROMBIN III TEST

The antithrombin III test helps detect the cause of impaired coagulation, especially hypercoagulation, by measuring levels of antithrombin III (AT III), a protein that inactivates thrombin and inhibits coagulation. AT III may be evaluated by a functional clotting assay or synthetic substrates. Exogenous heparin is added to a fresh, citrated blood sample to accelerate activity, then excess thrombin (factor Xa) is added to the plasma. The amount of factor Xa not activated by AT III is quantitated

and compared to a normal control sample. Reference values may vary for each laboratory, but should lie between 80% and 120% of normal.

Decreased AT III levels can indicate disseminated intravascular coagulation, fibrinolytic disorders, thrombophlebitis, or hepatic disorders. Slightly decreased levels can result from hormonal contraceptives. Elevated levels can result from kidney transplantation and the use of oral anticoagulants or anabolic steroids.

in the sample. Completely fill the collection tube and invert it gently several times to mix the sample and the anticoagulant thoroughly.
● To prevent hemolysis, avoid excessive probing during venipuncture and rough handling of the sample.
● Immediately put the sample on ice and send it to the laboratory.

## REFERENCE VALUES
Normal thrombin times range from 10 to 15 seconds (SI, 10 to 15 s). Test results are usually reported with a normal control value.

## ABNORMAL FINDINGS
A prolonged thrombin time may indicate heparin therapy, hepatic disease, DIC, hypofibrinogenemia, or dysfibrinogenemia. The patient with a prolonged thrombin time may require measurement of fibrinogen levels; in suspected DIC, the test for fibrin split products is also necessary.

## INTERFERING FACTORS
● Fibrin degradation products, fibrinogen, or heparin (possible increase)

## *Plasminogen, plasma*

Plasma plasminogen testing is used to assess plasminogen levels in a plasma sample. During fibrinolysis, plasmin dissolves fibrin clots to prevent excessive coagulation and impaired blood flow. Plasmin doesn't circulate in active form, however, so it can't be directly measured. Its circulating precursor, plasminogen, can be measured and used to evaluate the fibrinolytic system.

## PURPOSE
● To assess fibrinolysis
● To detect congenital and acquired fibrinolytic disorders

## PATIENT PREPARATION
● Explain to the patient that the plasma plasminogen test is used to evaluate blood clotting.
● Tell the patient that a blood sample will be taken. Explain who will perform the venipuncture and when and where the test will take place.

● Explain to the patient that he may feel slight discomfort from the needle puncture and the tourniquet.
● Notify the laboratory and physician of medications the patient is taking that may affect test results; they may need to be restricted.
● Inform the patient that he need not restrict food and fluids.

## PROCEDURE AND POSTTEST CARE
● Perform a venipuncture and collect the sample in a 4.5-ml siliconized tube.
● If a hematoma develops at the venipuncture site, apply pressure. If the hematoma is large, monitor pulses distal to the venipuncture site.
● Make sure bleeding has stopped before removing pressure.
● Instruct the patient that he may resume medications discontinued before the test, as ordered.

## PRECAUTIONS
● Collect the sample as quickly as possible to prevent stasis, which can slow blood flow, causing coagulation and plasminogen activation.
● To prevent hemolysis, avoid excessive probing during venipuncture and rough handling of the sample.
● Invert the tube gently several times and immediately send the sample to the laboratory. If testing must be delayed, plasma must be separated and frozen at –94° F (–67.8° C).

## REFERENCE VALUES
Normal plasminogen levels range from 10 to 20 mg/dl (0.1 to 0.2 g/L) by immunologic methods.

## ABNORMAL FINDINGS
Diminished plasminogen levels can result from disseminated intravascular coagulation, tumors, preeclampsia, and eclampsia, which accelerate plasminogen conversion to plasmin and increase fibrinolysis. Some liver diseases prevent formation of sufficient plasminogen, decreasing fibrinolysis.

## INTERFERING FACTORS
● Failure to use the proper collection tube, to adequately mix the sample and citrate, to send the sample to the laboratory immedi-

ately, or to have the sample separated and frozen

- Hemolysis due to excessive probing during venipuncture or to rough handling of the sample
- Hemoconcentration due to prolonged tourniquet use before venipuncture (possible false-low)
- Hormonal contraceptives (possible slight increase)
- Thrombolytic drugs, such as streptokinase and urokinase (possible decrease)

# Platelet aggregation test

After vascular injury, platelets gather at the injury site and clump together to form an aggregate or plug that helps maintain hemostasis and promotes healing. The platelet aggregation test, an in vitro procedure, is used to measure the rate at which the platelets in a plasma sample form a clump after the addition of an aggregating reagent.

## PURPOSE
- To assess platelet aggregation
- To detect congenital and acquired platelet bleeding disorders

## PATIENT PREPARATION
- Explain to the patient that the platelet aggregation test is used to determine if blood clots properly.
- Tell the patient that the test requires a blood sample. Explain who will perform the venipuncture and when and where the test will take place. (See *Aspirin and platelet aggregation*.)
- Explain to the patient that he may feel slight discomfort from the needle puncture and the tourniquet.
- Instruct the patient to fast or to maintain a nonfat diet for 8 hours before the test because lipemia can affect the test results.
- Notify the laboratory and physician of medications the patient is taking that may affect test results; they may need to be restricted.

## PROCEDURE AND POSTTEST CARE
- Perform a venipuncture and collect the sample in a 4.5-ml siliconized tube.
- Completely fill the collection tube and invert it gently several times to mix the sample and the anticoagulant thoroughly.
- Apply pressure to the venipuncture site for 5 minutes or until bleeding stops.
- If a hematoma develops at the venipuncture site, apply pressure.
- Instruct the patient that he may resume his usual diet and medications discontinued before the test, as ordered.

## PRECAUTIONS
- Be aware that because the list of medications known to alter the results of this test is long and continually growing, the patient should be as drug-free as possible before the test.
- Be sure to check if the patient has taken aspirin within the past 14 days. The test can't be postponed if the patient has used aspirin. Ask the laboratory to verify the presence of aspirin in the plasma. If test results are abnormal for such a sample, the use of aspirin must be discontinued and the test repeated in 2 weeks.
- Avoid excessive probing at the venipuncture site.
- Remove the tourniquet promptly to avoid bruising.
- Handle the sample gently to prevent hemolysis and keep it between 71.6° F and 98.6° F (22° C and 37° C) to prevent aggregation.

## REFERENCE VALUES
Normal aggregation occurs in 3 to 5 minutes (SI, 3 to 5 min), but findings are temperature-dependent and vary with the laboratory. Aggregation curves obtained by using different reagents help to distinguish various qualitative platelet defects.

## ABNORMAL FINDINGS
Abnormal findings may indicate von Willebrand's disease, Bernard-Soulier syndrome, storage pool disease, Glanzmann's thrombasthenia, polycythemia vera, severe liver disease, or uremia.

## INTERFERING FACTORS
- Antihistamines, anti-inflammatory drugs, aspirin and aspirin compounds, phenothia-

# ASPIRIN AND PLATELET AGGREGATION

Unlike other salicylates, aspirin inhibits platelet aggregation. This inhibition occurs in the second phase of platelet aggregation, when it prevents the release of adenosine diphosphate from platelets. Mean bleeding time may double in healthy individuals after ingestion of aspirin. In children or in patients with bleeding disorders, such as hemophilia, bleeding time may be even more prolonged.

## EFFECT ON PLATELETS

The effect of aspirin on platelets seems to result from the inhibition of prostaglandin synthesis. A single 325-mg oral dose of aspirin results in about 90% inhibition of the enzyme cyclooxygenase in circulating platelets, preventing the synthesis of compounds that induce platelet aggregation. The inhibition of cyclooxygenase is irreversible; thus, its effect lasts for 4 to 6 days—the life span of platelets. Bleeding time peaks within 12 hours. Altered hemostasis persists about 36 hours after the last dose of aspirin, sometimes longer for the patient receiving long-term therapy.

## EFFECT ON BLOOD VESSELS

Aspirin's action on blood vessels may oppose that seen in platelets because cyclooxygenase plays a different role in the vascular endothelium. Here, the enzyme produces prostacyclin, a compound that inhibits platelet aggregation and causes vasodilation. Inhibition of cyclooxygenase in the vascular endothelium, in effect, reverses aspirin's antithrombotic effect on platelets. However, studies suggest that cyclooxygenase in the platelets is more sensitive than that in the vascular endothelium; therefore, a low aspirin dosage (for example, 80 mg daily or 325 mg every other day) may prove more effective in preventing thrombosis than do higher dosages.

---

zines, phenylbutazone, tricyclic antidepressants, and sulfinpyrazone (Anturane) (decrease)
● Ingestion of large amounts of garlic (inhibits platelet aggregation)

# *Platelet count*

Platelets, or thrombocytes, are the smallest formed elements in blood. They promote coagulation and the formation of a hemostatic plug in vascular injury.

Platelet count is one of the most important screening tests of platelet function. Accurate counts are vital.

## PURPOSE

● To evaluate platelet production
● To assess the effects of chemotherapy or radiation therapy on platelet production
● To diagnose and monitor severe thrombocytosis or thrombocytopenia
● To confirm a visual estimate of platelet number and morphology from a stained blood film

## PATIENT PREPARATION

● Explain to the patient that the platelet count test is used to determine if the patient's blood clots normally.
● Tell the patient that a blood sample will be taken. Explain who will perform the venipuncture and when and where the test will take place.
● Inform the patient that he need not restrict food and fluids.
● Explain to the patient that he may feel slight discomfort from the needle puncture and the tourniquet.
● Notify the laboratory and physician of medications the patient is taking that may affect test results; they may need to be restricted.

## PROCEDURE AND POSTTEST CARE

● Perform a venipuncture and collect the sample in a 3- or 4.5-ml EDTA tube.
● If a hematoma develops at the venipuncture site, apply pressure. If the hematoma is large, monitor pulses distal to the venipuncture site.
● Make sure subdermal bleeding has stopped before removing pressure.

- Instruct the patient that he may resume any medications discontinued before the test, as ordered.

## PRECAUTIONS

- To prevent hemolysis, avoid excessive probing at the venipuncture site and handle the sample gently.
- Completely fill the collection tube and invert it gently several times to mix the sample and the anticoagulant thoroughly.

## REFERENCE VALUES

Normal platelet counts range from 140,000 to 400,000/µl (SI, 140 to 400 × 10⁹/L) in adults.

*Age alert In children, normal platelet counts range from 150,000 to 450,000/µl (SI, 150 to 450 × 10⁹/L).*

## ABNORMAL FINDINGS

A platelet count below 50,000/µl can cause spontaneous bleeding; when the count is below 5,000/µl, fatal central nervous system bleeding or massive GI hemorrhage is possible. A decreased platelet count (thrombocytopenia) can result from aplastic or hypoplastic bone marrow; infiltrative bone marrow disease, such as leukemia, or disseminated infection; megakaryocytic hypoplasia; ineffective thrombopoiesis due to folic acid or vitamin B₁₂ deficiency; pooling of platelets in an enlarged spleen; increased platelet destruction due to drugs or immune disorders; disseminated intravascular coagulation; Bernard-Soulier syndrome; or mechanical injury to platelets.

An increased platelet count (thrombocytosis) can result from hemorrhage, infectious disorders, iron deficiency anemia, recent surgery, pregnancy, splenectomy, or inflammatory disorders. In such cases, the platelet count returns to normal after the patient recovers from the primary disorder.

However, the count remains elevated in primary thrombocythemia, myelofibrosis with myeloid metaplasia, polycythemia vera, and chronic myelogenous leukemia.

When the platelet count is abnormal, diagnosis usually requires further studies, such as complete blood count, bone marrow biopsy, direct antiglobulin test (direct Coombs' test), and serum protein electrophoresis.

## INTERFERING FACTORS

- Heparin (decrease)
- Acetazolamide (Dazamide), acetohexamide (Dymelor), antineoplastics, brompheniramine maleate, carbamazepine (Tegretol), chloramphenicol, ethacrynic acid (Edecrin), furosemide (Lasix), gold salts, hydroxychloroquine (Plaquenil), indomethacin (Indocin), isoniazid (INH), mefenamic acid, methazolamide (Glauctabs), methimazole (Tapazole), methyldopa (Aldomet), oral diazoxide (Proglycem), penicillamine (Cuprimine), penicillin, phenylbutazone, phenytoin (Dilantin), quinidine sulfate, quinine, salicylates, streptomycin, sulfonamides, thiazide and thiazide-like diuretics, and tricyclic antidepressants (possible decrease)
- Excitement, high altitudes, persistent cold temperatures, or strenuous exercise (increase)

# Pleural fluid aspiration

The pleura, a two-layer membrane that covers the lungs and lines the thoracic cavity, maintains a small amount of lubricating fluid between its layers to minimize friction during respiration. Increased fluid in this space may result from such diseases as cancer or tuberculosis or from blood or lymphatic disorders and can cause respiratory difficulty.

In pleural fluid aspiration (thoracentesis), the thoracic wall is punctured to obtain a specimen of pleural fluid for analysis or to relieve pulmonary (and possibly cardiac) compression and resultant respiratory distress.

## PURPOSE

- To determine the cause and nature of pleural effusion
- To permit better radiographic visualization of a lung with large effusions
- To obtain samples for cytologic, microbial, and pathologic examination

## PATIENT PREPARATION

- Explain to the patient that pleural fluid analysis assesses the space around the lungs for fluid.
- Inform the patient that he need not restrict food and fluids.
- Tell the patient who will perform the test and when and where it will be done.

- Explain that chest X-rays or an ultrasound study may precede the test to help locate the fluid.
- Check the patient's history for hypersensitivity to local anesthetics.
- Warn the patient that he may feel a stinging sensation on injection of the anesthetic and some pressure during withdrawal of the fluid.
- Advise the patient not to cough, breathe deeply, or move during the test to minimize the risk of injury to the lung.

## PROCEDURE AND POSTTEST CARE
- Record the patient's baseline vital signs.
- If necessary, shave the area around the needle insertion site.
- Position the patient to widen intercostal spaces and to allow easier access to the pleural cavity. He must be well supported and comfortable, preferably seated at the edge of the bed with a chair or stool supporting his feet and his head and arms resting on a padded overbed table. If the patient can't sit up, he may be positioned on his unaffected side, with the arm on the affected side elevated above his head.
- Remind the patient not to cough, breathe deeply, or move suddenly during the procedure.
- After positioning, the physician disinfects the skin, drapes the area, injects a local anesthetic into the subcutaneous tissue, and inserts the thoracentesis needle above the rib to avoid lacerating intercostal vessels. When the needle reaches the pocket of fluid, the 50-ml syringe is attached and the stopcock and clamps are opened on the tubing to aspirate the fluid into the container.
- During aspiration, observe the patient for signs of respiratory distress, such as weakness, dyspnea, pallor, cyanosis, changes in heart rate, tachypnea, diaphoresis, blood-tinged frothy mucus, and hypotension.
- After the needle is withdrawn, apply slight pressure and a small adhesive bandage to the puncture site.
- Label the specimen container and record the date and time of the test and the amount, color, and character of the fluid (clear, frothy, purulent, bloody) on the laboratory request.
- Note any signs of distress exhibited during the procedure.
- Record the exact location from which the fluid was removed to aid diagnosis.

- Reposition the patient comfortably on the affected side. Tell him to remain on this side for at least 1 hour to seal the puncture site. Elevate the head of the bed to facilitate breathing.
- Monitor the patient's vital signs every 30 minutes for 2 hours and then every 4 hours until they're stable.
- Tell the patient to call a nurse immediately if he experiences difficulty breathing.

*Alert* Watch the patient for signs of pneumothorax, tension pneumothorax, fluid reaccumulation and, if a large amount of fluid was withdrawn, pulmonary edema or cardiac distress due to mediastinal shift. Usually, a posttest X-ray is ordered to detect these complications before clinical symptoms appear.

- Check the puncture site for fluid leakage. A large amount of leakage is abnormal. Also check the site and surrounding area for subcutaneous emphysema.

## PRECAUTIONS
- Keep in mind that thoracentesis is contraindicated in the patient who has a history of bleeding disorders or anticoagulant therapy.
- Use strict aseptic technique.
- Note the patient's temperature and whether he's receiving antimicrobial therapy on the laboratory request.
- Send the specimen to the laboratory immediately after collection.

## NORMAL FINDINGS
Normally, the pleural cavity maintains negative pressure and contains less than 20 ml of serous fluid.

## ABNORMAL FINDINGS
Pleural effusion results from the abnormal formation or reabsorption of pleural fluid. Certain characteristics classify pleural fluid as either a transudate (a low-protein fluid leaked from normal blood vessels) or an exudate (a protein-rich fluid leaked from blood vessels with increased permeability).

Pleural fluid may contain blood (hemothorax), chyle (chylothorax), or pus (empyema) and necrotic tissue. Blood-tinged fluid may indicate a traumatic tap; if so, the fluid should clear as aspiration progresses.

Transudative effusion generally results from diminished colloidal pressure, increased negative pressure within the pleural cavity, ascites, systemic and pulmonary venous hypertension, heart failure, hepatic cirrhosis, and nephritis.

Exudative effusion results from disorders that increase pleural capillary permeability (possibly with changes in hydrostatic or colloid osmotic pressures), lymphatic drainage interference, infections, pulmonary infarctions, and neoplasms. Exudative effusion associated with depressed glucose levels, elevated lactate dehydrogenase (LD) isoenzymes, rheumatoid arthritis cells, and negative smears, cultures, and cytologic examination may indicate pleurisy associated with rheumatoid arthritis.

The most common pathogens that appear in pleural fluid culture studies are *Mycobacterium tuberculosis, Staphylococcus aureus, Streptococcus pneumoniae* and other streptococci, *Haemophilus influenzae* and, in the case of a ruptured pulmonary abscess, anaerobes such as *Bacteroides*.

Cultures are usually positive during the early stages of infection; however, antibiotic therapy may produce a negative culture despite a positive Gram stain and grossly purulent fluid. Empyema may result from complications of pneumonia, pulmonary abscess, perforation of the esophagus, or penetration from mediastinitis. A high percentage of neutrophils suggests septic inflammation; predominating lymphocytes suggest tuberculosis or fungal or viral effusions.

Serosanguineous fluid may indicate pleural extension of a malignant tumor. Elevated LD in a nonpurulent, nonhemolyzed, nonbloody effusion may also suggest malignancy. Pleural fluid glucose levels 30 to 40 mg/dl lower than blood glucose levels may indicate a malignant tumor, a bacterial infection, nonseptic inflammation, or metastasis. Increased amylase levels occur in pleural effusions associated with pancreatitis.

## INTERFERING FACTORS
- Failure to use aseptic technique
- Antimicrobial therapy before fluid aspiration for culture (possible decrease in numbers of bacteria, making it difficult to isolate the infecting organism)

# Pleural tissue biopsy

Pleural tissue biopsy is the removal of pleural tissue by needle biopsy or open biopsy for histologic examination. Needle pleural biopsy is performed under local anesthesia. It generally follows or is done in conjunction with thoracentesis (aspiration of pleural fluid), which is performed when the cause of an effusion is unknown, but it can be performed separately.

Open pleural biopsy, performed in the absence of pleural effusion, permits direct visualization of the pleura and the underlying lung. It's performed in the operating room.

## PURPOSE
- To differentiate between nonmalignant and malignant disease
- To diagnose viral, fungal, or parasitic disease and collagen vascular disease of the pleura

## PATIENT PREPARATION
- Explain to the patient that the pleural tissue biopsy permits microscopic examination of pleural tissue.
- Describe the procedure to the patient, and answer his questions.
- Tell the patient who will perform the biopsy, when and where it will be done, and that no fasting is required.
- Explain that blood studies will precede the biopsy, and chest X-rays will be taken before and after the biopsy.
- Make sure the patient or a responsible family member has signed an informed consent form.
- Check the patient's history for hypersensitivity to the local anesthetic.
- Tell the patient that he'll receive a local anesthetic and should experience minimal pain.
- Record the patient's vital signs just before the procedure.

## PROCEDURE AND POSTTEST CARE
- Seat the patient on the side of the bed, with his feet resting on a stool and his arms on the overbed table or supported by his upper body. Tell him to hold this position and remain still during the procedure.

## Using Cope's Needle

Cope's needle, which is used to obtain a pleural biopsy specimen, consists of three parts: a sharp obturator (A) and a cannula (B), which when fitted together are called a *trocar*, and a blunt-ended, hooked stylet (C). The trocar is used to gain access to the pleural cavity. The obturator is then removed, leaving the cannula in place. The stylet is passed through the cannula to excise a tissue specimen, as shown below.

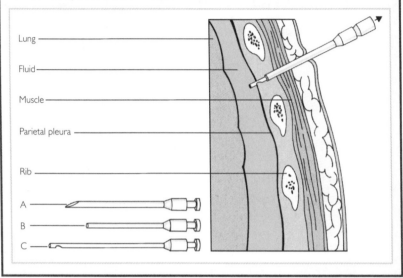

- Prepare the skin and drape the area.
- The local anesthetic is then administered.
- In a Vim-Silverman needle biopsy, a needle is inserted through the appropriate intercostal space into the biopsy site, with the outer tip distal to the pleura and the central portion pushed in deeper and held in place. The outer case is inserted about ⅜" (1 cm), the entire assembly is rotated 360 degrees, and the needle and tissue specimen are withdrawn. In Cope's needle biopsy, a trocar is introduced through the appropriate intercostal space into the biopsy site. To obtain the specimen, a hooked stylet is inserted through the trocar. While the outer tube is held stationary, the inner tube is twisted to cut off the tissue specimen, and the assembly is withdrawn. (See *Using Cope's needle*.)
- After the specimens are obtained, additional parietal fluid may be removed to treat the effusion.
- Immediately put the specimen into a 10% neutral buffered formalin solution in a labeled specimen bottle and send it to the laboratory.
- Clean the skin around the biopsy site, and apply an adhesive bandage.
- Make sure the chest X-ray is repeated immediately after the biopsy.
- Check the patient's vital signs every 15 minutes for 1 hour and then every hour for 4 hours or until stable.

*Alert* *Watch the patient for signs of respiratory distress (dyspnea), shoulder pain, and such complications as pneumothorax (immediate), pneumonia (delayed), and hemorrhage.*

- Instruct the patient to lie on his unaffected side to promote healing of the biopsy site, as indicated.

## PRECAUTIONS
- Know that pleural biopsy is contraindicated in the patient with a severe bleeding disorder.

## NORMAL FINDINGS

The normal pleura consists primarily of mesothelial cells that are flattened in a uniform layer. Layers of areolar connective tissue that contain blood vessels, nerves, and lymphatics lie below.

## ABNORMAL FINDINGS

Histologic examination of the tissue specimen can reveal malignant disease, tuberculosis, and viral, fungal, parasitic, or collagen vascular disease. Primary neoplasms of the pleura are generally fibrous and epithelial.

## INTERFERING FACTORS

● The patient's inability to remain still, keep from coughing, or follow instructions, such as "Hold your breath," during the procedure

# Postoperative cholangiography

During cholecystectomy or common bile duct exploration, a T-shaped rubber tube may be inserted into the common bile duct to facilitate drainage. Postoperative cholangiography — radiographic and fluoroscopic examination of the biliary ducts — may be performed 7 to 10 days after surgery.

This procedure requires injection of contrast medium through the T tube. The contrast medium flows through the biliary ducts and outlines the size and patency of the ducts, revealing any obstruction overlooked during surgery.

## PURPOSE

● To detect calculi, strictures, neoplasms, and fistulae in the biliary ducts

## PATIENT PREPARATION

● Explain to the patient that postoperative cholangiography permits examination of the biliary ducts through X-ray films taken after the injection of a contrast medium.
● Describe the test, including who will perform it and when and where it will take place.
● Warn the patient that he may feel a bloating sensation (not pain) in the right upper quadrant as the contrast medium is injected.

● Clamp the T tube the day before the procedure, if necessary. Because bile fills the tube after clamping, this helps prevent air bubbles from entering the ducts.
● Withhold the meal just before the test and administer an enema about 1 hour before the procedure.
● Make sure that the patient or a responsible family member has signed an informed consent form.
● Check the patient's history for hypersensitivity to iodine, seafood, or contrast media used in other diagnostic tests. Tell the patient that the adverse effects of intraductal administration may include nausea, vomiting, excessive salivation, flushing, urticaria, sweating and, rarely, anaphylaxis.

## PROCEDURE AND POSTTEST CARE

● After the patient is in a supine position on the X-ray table, the injection area of the T tube is cleaned with sponges soaked with povidone-iodine solution. The T tube is held in a vertical position, which allows trapped air to surface, and a needle attached to a long transparent catheter is carefully inserted into the end of the T tube. Care must be taken to avoid injecting air into the biliary tree because air bubbles may affect the clarity of the X-ray films.
● Approximately 5 ml of contrast medium is injected under fluoroscopic guidance, and a spot film is taken in the anteroposterior position. Additional injections are then administered, and spot films and plain films are taken with the patient in supine and right lateral decubitus positions.
● The T tube is then clamped and the patient is assisted to an erect position for additional films; in this position, air bubbles may be distinguished from calculi or other pathology.
● A final film is taken 15 minutes after contrast injection to record the emptying of contrast-laden bile into the duodenum. If emptying is delayed, additional films may be taken at 15- or 30-minute intervals until this action is demonstrated.
● If a sterile dressing is applied after T-tube removal, observe and record any drainage. Change the dressing, as necessary.
● If the T tube is left in place, attach it to the drainage system.
● Tell the patient that he may resume his usual diet and activity as directed.

## PRECAUTIONS

● Know that postoperative cholangiography is contraindicated in the patient who's hypersensitive to iodine, seafood, or contrast media used in other tests.

## NORMAL FINDINGS

Biliary ducts demonstrate homogeneous filling with contrast medium and are normal in diameter. When Oddi's sphincter is functioning properly and the ducts are patent, the contrast flows unimpeded into the duodenum.

## ABNORMAL FINDINGS

Negative shadows or filling defects within the biliary ducts associated with dilation may indicate calculi or neoplasms overlooked during surgery. Abnormal channels of contrast medium departing from the biliary ducts indicate fistulae.

## INTERFERING FACTORS

● Marked obesity or gas overlying the biliary ducts (possible poor imaging)

# Potassium, serum

The potassium test is used to measure serum levels of potassium, the major intracellular cation. Potassium helps to maintain cellular osmotic equilibrium and to regulate muscle activity, enzyme activity, and acid-base balance. It also influences renal function. The body has no efficient method for conserving potassium; the kidneys excrete nearly all ingested potassium, even when the body's supply is depleted.

Potassium levels are affected by variations in the secretions of adrenal steroid hormones and by fluctuations in pH, serum glucose levels, and serum sodium levels. A reciprocal relationship appears to exist between potassium and sodium; a substantial intake of one element causes a corresponding decrease in the other. Although it readily conserves sodium, the body has no efficient method for conserving potassium. Even in potassium depletion, the kidneys continue to excrete potassium; therefore, potassium deficiency can develop rapidly and is quite common.

Because the kidneys excrete nearly all ingested potassium daily, a dietary intake of at least 40 mEq/day is essential. A normal diet usually includes 60 to 100 mEq of potassium. (See *Dietary sources of potassium,* page 340. See also *Treating potassium imbalance*, page 341.)

## PURPOSE

● To evaluate clinical signs of potassium excess (hyperkalemia) or potassium depletion (hypokalemia)
● To monitor renal function, acid-base balance, and glucose metabolism
● To evaluate neuromuscular and endocrine disorders
● To detect the origin of arrhythmias

## PATIENT PREPARATION

● Explain to the patient that the serum potassium test is used to determine the potassium content of blood.
● Tell the patient that the test requires a blood sample. Explain who will perform the venipuncture and when and where it will take place.
● Explain to the patient that he may experience slight discomfort from the needle puncture and the tourniquet.
● Inform the patient that he need not restrict food and fluids.
● Notify the laboratory and physician of medications the patient is taking that may affect test results; they may need to be restricted.

## PROCEDURE AND POSTTEST CARE

● Perform a venipuncture and collect the sample in a 3- or 4-ml clot-activator tube.
● Apply direct pressure to the venipuncture site until bleeding stops.
● If a hematoma develops at the venipuncture site, apply pressure.
● Instruct the patient to resume medications discontinued before the test, as ordered.

## PRECAUTIONS

● Draw the sample immediately after applying the tourniquet because a delay may increase the potassium level by allowing intracellular potassium to leak into the serum.
● Handle the sample gently to avoid hemolysis.

# DIETARY SOURCES OF POTASSIUM

A healthy person needs to consume at least 40 mEq of potassium daily. The chart here highlights foods and beverages, their serving sizes, and the amount of potassium each contains.

| FOODS AND BEVERAGES | SERVING SIZE | AMOUNT OF POTASSIUM (mEq) |
|---|---|---|
| **MEATS** | | |
| Beef | 4 oz (112 g) | 11.2 |
| Chicken | 4 oz | 12 |
| Scallops | 5 large | 30 |
| Veal | 4 oz | 15.2 |
| **VEGETABLES** | | |
| Artichokes | 1 large bud | 7.7 |
| Asparagus (frozen, cooked) | ½ cup (120 g) | 5.5 |
| Asparagus (raw) | 6 spears | 7.7 |
| Beans (dried, cooked) | ½ cup | 10 |
| Beans (lima) | ½ cup | 9.5 |
| Broccoli (cooked) | ½ cup | 7 |
| Carrots (cooked) | ½ cup | 5.7 |
| Carrots (raw) | 1 large | 8.8 |
| Mushrooms (raw) | 4 large | 10.6 |
| Potatoes (baked) | 1 small | 15.4 |
| Spinach (raw or cooked) | ½ cup | 8.5 |
| Squash (winter, baked) | ½ cup | 12 |
| Tomatoes (raw) | 1 medium | 10.4 |
| **FRUITS** | | |
| Apricots (dried) | 4 halves | 5 |
| Apricots (raw) | 3 small | 8 |
| Bananas | 1 medium | 12.8 |
| Cantaloupe | 6 oz | 13 |
| Figs (dried) | 7 small | 17.5 |
| Peaches (raw) | 1 medium | 6.2 |
| Pears (raw) | 1 medium | 6.2 |
| **BEVERAGES** | | |
| Apricot nectar | 1 cup (240 ml) | 9 |
| Grapefruit juice | 1 cup | 8.2 |
| Orange juice | 1 cup | 11.4 |
| Pineapple juice | 1 cup | 9 |
| Prune juice | 1 cup | 14.4 |
| Tomato juice | 1 cup | 11.6 |
| Milk (whole or skim) | 1 cup | 8.8 |

## REFERENCE VALUES
Normally, serum potassium levels range from 3.5 to 5 mEq/L (SI, 3.5 to 5 mmol/L).

## ABNORMAL FINDINGS
Abnormally high serum potassium levels are common in conditions in which excess cellular potassium enters the blood, such as burn injuries, crush injuries, diabetic ketoacidosis, transfusions of large amounts of blood, and

myocardial infarction. Hyperkalemia may also indicate reduced sodium excretion, possibly due to renal failure (preventing normal exchange of sodium and potassium) or Addison's disease (due to potassium buildup and sodium depletion).

**Alert**  *Observe the patient with hyperkalemia for weakness, malaise, nausea, diarrhea, colicky pain, muscle irritability progressing to flaccid paralysis, oliguria, and bradycardia. The electrocardiogram (ECG) reveals flattened P waves; a prolonged PR interval; a wide QRS complex; tall, tented T waves; and ST-segment depression. Cardiac arrest may occur without warning.*

Below-normal potassium values commonly result from aldosteronism or Cushing's syndrome, loss of body fluids (such as long-term diuretic therapy, vomiting, or diarrhea), and excessive licorice ingestion. Although serum values and clinical symptoms can indicate a potassium imbalance, an ECG allows a definitive diagnosis.

**Alert**  *Observe the patient with hypokalemia for decreased reflexes; a rapid, weak, irregular pulse; mental confusion; hypotension; anorexia; muscle weakness; and paresthesia. The ECG shows a flattened T wave, ST-segment depression, and U-wave elevation. In severe cases, ventricular fibrillation, respiratory paralysis, and cardiac arrest can develop.*

## INTERFERING FACTORS

● Repeated clenching of the fist before venipuncture (possible increase)

● Excessive or rapid potassium infusion, spironolactone or penicillin G potassium therapy, and renal toxicity from administration of amphotericin B, methicillin, or tetracycline (increase)

● Insulin and glucose administration; diuretic therapy (especially with thiazides but not with triamterene [Dyrenium], amiloride [Midamor], or spironolactone [Aldactone]); and I.V. infusions without potassium (decrease)

# Pregnanediol, urine

Using gas chromatography or radioimmunoassay, this test measures urine levels of pregnanediol, the chief metabolite of progesterone. Although biologically inert, pregnanediol has diagnostic significance because it reflects about 10% of the endogenous production of its parent hormone.

Progesterone is produced in nonpregnant females by the corpus luteum during the latter half of each menstrual cycle, preparing the uterus for implantation of a fertilized ovum. If implantation doesn't occur, progesterone secretion drops sharply; if implantation does occur, the corpus luteum secretes more progesterone to further prepare the uterus for pregnancy and to begin development of the placenta. Toward the end of the first trimester, the placenta becomes the primary source of progesterone secretion, producing the progressively larger amounts needed to maintain pregnancy.

Normally, urine levels of pregnanediol reflect variations in progesterone secretion during the menstrual cycle and during pregnancy. Direct measurement of plasma progesterone levels by radioimmunoassay may also be done.

## PURPOSE
- To evaluate placental function in pregnant patients
- To evaluate ovarian function in nonpregnant patients
- To aid in the diagnosis of menstrual disorders

## PATIENT PREPARATION
- Explain to the patient that the urine pregnanediol test evaluates placental or ovarian function.
- Inform the patient that she need not restrict food and fluids.
- Tell the patient that the test requires collection of urine over a 24-hour period, and teach her the proper collection technique.
- Advise the pregnant patient that this test may be repeated several times to obtain serial measurements.
- Notify the laboratory and physician of medications the patient is taking that may affect test results; they may need to be restricted.

## PROCEDURE AND POSTTEST CARE
- Collect the patient's urine over a 24-hour period, discarding the first specimen and retaining the last.
- Instruct the patient that she may resume her usual medications, as ordered.

## PRECAUTIONS
- Refrigerate the specimen or keep it on ice during the collection period.

- If the patient is pregnant, note the approximate week of gestation on the laboratory request.
- For premenopausal women who aren't pregnant, note the stage of the menstrual cycle on the laboratory request.

## NORMAL FINDINGS
In nonpregnant females, urine pregnanediol values normally range from 0.5 to 1.5 mg/24 hours during the follicular phase of the menstrual cycle. In pregnant females, the values are:
- first trimester — 10 to 30 mg/24 hours
- second trimester — 35 to 70 mg/24 hours
- third trimester — 70 to 100 mg/24 hours.
  Normal postmenopausal values range from 0.2 to 1 mg/24 hours. In males, urine pregnanediol levels are 0 to 1 mg/24 hours.

## ABNORMAL FINDINGS
During pregnancy, a marked decrease in urine pregnanediol levels based on a single 24-hour urine specimen or a steady decrease in pregnanediol levels in serial measurements may indicate placental insufficiency and requires immediate investigation. A precipitous drop in pregnanediol values may suggest fetal distress — for example, threatened abortion or preeclampsia — or fetal death. However, pregnanediol measurements aren't reliable indicators of fetal viability because levels can remain normal even after fetal death, as long as maternal circulation to the placenta remains adequate.

In nonpregnant females, abnormally low urine pregnanediol levels may occur with anovulation, amenorrhea, or other menstrual abnormalities. Low to normal pregnanediol levels may be associated with hydatidiform mole. Elevations may indicate luteinized granulosa or theca cell tumors, diffuse thecal luteinization, or metastatic ovarian cancer.

Adrenal hyperplasia or biliary tract obstruction may elevate urine pregnanediol values in males or females. Some forms of primary hepatic disease produce abnormally low levels in both sexes.

## INTERFERING FACTORS
- Combination hormonal contraceptives, drugs containing corticotropin, methenamine hippurate, methenamine mandelate, and progestogens (possible increase or decrease)

# *Proctosigmoidoscopy*

Proctosigmoidoscopy uses a proctoscope, sigmoidoscope, and digital examination to evaluate the lining of the distal sigmoid colon, rectum, and anal canal. It's indicated in patients with recent changes in bowel habits, lower abdominal and perineal pain, prolapse on defecation, pruritus, and passage of mucus, blood, or pus in the stool. Specimens may be obtained from suspicious areas of the mucosa by biopsy, lavage or cytology brush, or culture swab.

Possible complications of this procedure include rectal bleeding and, rarely, bowel perforation.

## PURPOSE

- To aid in the diagnosis of inflammatory, infectious, and ulcerative bowel disease
- To detect hemorrhoids, hypertrophic anal papilla, polyps, fissures, fistulas, and abscesses in the rectum and anal canal

## PATIENT PREPARATION

- Explain to the patient that proctosigmoidoscopy allows visual examination of the lining of the distal sigmoid colon, rectum, and anal canal.
- Tell the patient that the test requires passage of two special instruments through the anus, who will perform the procedure, and when and where it will take place.
- Check the patient's history for allergies, medications, and information pertinent to the current complaint. Find out if he has had a barium test within the past week because barium in the colon hinders accurate examination.
- Because dietary and bowel preparations for this procedure vary according to the physician's preference, follow the orders carefully. If a special bowel preparation is ordered, explain to the patient that this preparation clears the intestine to ensure a better view.
- Instruct the patient to maintain a clear liquid diet for 24 to 48 hours before the test, to avoid eating fruits and vegetables before the procedure, and to fast the morning of the procedure, according to the physician's preference.

- Describe the position the patient will be asked to assume and assure him that he'll be adequately draped.
- As ordered, administer a warm tap water or sodium biphosphate enema 3 to 4 hours before the procedure. The procedure may be started without bowel preparation because enemas can alter intestinal markings and traumatize mucous membranes. For this reason, irritating soapsuds enemas are inappropriate before this test. If the examination is hindered by excessive fecal matter, an enema may be ordered before the examination proceeds.
- Tell the patient that he may be secured to a tilting table that rotates into horizontal and vertical positions.
- Tell the patient that the examiner's finger and the instrument are well lubricated to ease insertion, that the instrument initially feels cool, and that he may experience the urge to defecate when the instrument is inserted and advanced.
- Inform the patient that the instrument may stretch the intestinal wall and cause transient muscle spasms or colicky lower abdominal pain.
- Instruct the patient to breathe deeply and slowly through his mouth to relax the abdominal muscles; this relaxation reduces the urge to defecate and eases discomfort.
- Explain to the patient that air may be introduced through the endoscope into the intestine to distend its walls. Tell him that this distension causes flatus to escape around the endoscope and that he shouldn't attempt to control it.
- Inform the patient that a suction machine may remove blood, mucus, or liquid stool that obscures vision, but that it won't cause discomfort.
- Inform the patient that an I.V. line may be started if an I.V. sedative is to be used. If the procedure is being done on an outpatient basis, advise him to arrange for someone to drive him home.
- Make sure that the patient or a responsible family member has signed an informed consent form.
- If the patient has rectal inflammation, provide a local anesthetic about 15 to 20 minutes before the procedure to minimize discomfort.

## PROCEDURE AND POSTTEST CARE

● Obtain the patient's baseline vital signs and monitor him throughout the procedure.

● Place the patient in a knee-chest or left lateral position with his knees flexed and drape him.

● If a left lateral position is used, a sandbag may be placed under the patient's left hip so that the buttocks project over the edge of the table. The right buttock is gently raised, and the anus and perianal region are examined under good lighting.

● Instruct the patient to breathe deeply and slowly through his mouth as the examiner palpates the anal canal, rectum, and rectal mucosa for induration and tenderness; the examiner then withdraws his finger and checks for the presence of blood, mucus, or stool.

● The sigmoidoscope is lubricated, and the patient is told that the instrument is about to be inserted. The right buttock is raised, and the sigmoidoscope is inserted into the anus. As the scope is passed with steady pressure through the anal sphincters, instruct the patient to bear down as though defecating to aid its passage. The sigmoidoscope is advanced through the anal canal into the rectum.

● At the rectosigmoid junction, a small amount of air may be insufflated to open the bowel lumen. The scope is then gently advanced to its full length into the distal sigmoid colon.

● As the sigmoidoscope is slowly withdrawn, air is carefully insufflated, and the intestinal mucosa is thoroughly examined.

● If stool obscures vision, the eyepiece on the scope is removed, a cotton swab is inserted through the scope, and the bowel lumen is swabbed. A suction machine may remove blood, excessive secretions, or liquid stool.

● To obtain specimens from suspicious areas of the intestinal mucosa, a biopsy forceps, cytology brush, or culture swab is passed through the sigmoidoscope.

● Polyps may be removed for histologic examination by inserting an electrocautery snare through the sigmoidoscope.

● Specimens are collected in accordance with laboratory and pathology guidelines and immediately placed in a specimen bottle containing 10% formalin, cytology slides are placed in a Coplin jar containing 95% ethyl alcohol, and culture swabs are placed in a culture tube.

● After the sigmoidoscope is withdrawn, the proctoscope is lubricated and the patient is told that it's about to be inserted. Assure him that he'll experience less discomfort during passage of the proctoscope.

● The right buttock is raised, and the proctoscope is inserted through the anus and gently advanced to its full length.

● The obturator is removed, and the light source is inserted through the proctoscope handle.

● As the instrument is slowly withdrawn, the rectal and anal mucosa are carefully examined. Specimens may be obtained from suspicious areas of the intestinal mucosa.

● If a biopsy of the anal canal is required, a local anesthetic may be administered first.

● Withdraw the proctoscope after the examination is completed.

● If the patient has been examined in a knee-chest position, instruct him to rest in a supine position for several minutes before standing to prevent orthostatic hypotension.

● Observe the patient closely for signs of bowel perforation and for vasovagal attack due to emotional stress. Report such signs immediately.

● Allow the patient nothing by mouth until he's alert.

● Monitor the patient's vital signs as per facility protocol until he's alert.

● If air was introduced into the intestine, tell the patient that he may pass large amounts of flatus. Provide privacy while he rests after the test.

● If a biopsy or polypectomy was performed, inform the patient that a small amount of blood may appear in his stool.

## PRECAUTIONS

● If a tissue specimen or culture swab has been obtained, label it and send it to the appropriate laboratory immediately.

● Keep in mind that in general, anticoagulant therapy isn't contraindicated; however, it may increase the risk of bleeding.

● Know that if the patient received sedation, he should avoid alcohol for 24 hours and shouldn't drive for 12 hours, so make sure he has transportation home.

## NORMAL FINDINGS

The mucosa of the sigmoid colon appears light pink-orange and is marked by semilunar folds and deep tubular pits. The rectal mucosa is redder due to its rich vascular network, deepens to a purple hue at the pectinate line (the anatomic division between the rectum and anus), and has three distinct valves. The lower two-thirds of the anus (anoderm) is lined with smooth gray-tan skin and joins with the hair-fringed perianal skin.

## ABNORMAL FINDINGS

Visual examination and palpation demonstrate abnormalities of the anal canal and rectum, including internal and external hemorrhoids, hypertrophic anal papilla, anal fissures, anal fistulas, and anorectal abscesses. The examination may also reveal inflammatory bowel diseases, polyps, cancer, and other tumors. Biopsy, culture, and other laboratory tests are typically necessary to detect various disorders.

## INTERFERING FACTORS

● Barium in the intestine from previous diagnostic studies (hinders visualization)
● Large amounts of stool in the intestine (hinders visual examination and advancement of the endoscope)

# Progesterone, plasma

Progesterone, an ovarian steroid hormone secreted by the corpus luteum, causes thickening and secretory development of the endometrium in preparation for implantation of the fertilized ovum. Progesterone levels, therefore, peak during the midluteal phase of the menstrual cycle. If implantation doesn't occur, progesterone (and estrogen) levels drop sharply and menstruation begins about 2 days later.

During pregnancy, the placenta releases about 10 times the normal monthly amount of progesterone to maintain the pregnancy. Increased secretion begins toward the end of the first trimester and continues until delivery. Progesterone prevents abortion by decreasing uterine contractions. Along with estrogen, progesterone helps prepare the breasts for lactation.

This radioimmunoassay is a quantitative analysis of plasma progesterone levels and provides reliable information about corpus luteum function in fertility studies and placental function in pregnancy. Serial determinations are recommended. Although plasma levels provide accurate information, progesterone can also be monitored by measuring urine pregnanediol, a chief metabolite of progesterone.

## PURPOSE

● To assess corpus luteum function as part of infertility studies
● To evaluate placental function during pregnancy
● To aid in confirming ovulation; test results support basal body temperature readings

## PATIENT PREPARATION

● Explain to the patient that the plasma progesterone test helps determine if her female sex hormone secretion is normal.
● Inform the patient that she need not restrict food and fluids.
● Tell the patient that the test requires a blood sample. Explain who will perform the venipuncture and when and where the test will take place.
● Explain to the patient that she may experience slight discomfort from the needle puncture and the tourniquet.
● Inform the patient that the test may be repeated at specific times coinciding with phases of her menstrual cycle or with each prenatal visit.
● Check the patient's history to determine if she's taking drugs that may interfere with test results, including progesterone and estrogen. Note your findings on the laboratory request.

## PROCEDURE AND POSTTEST CARE

● Perform a venipuncture and collect the sample in a 7-ml heparinized tube.
● Apply direct pressure to the venipuncture site until bleeding stops.
● If a hematoma develops at the venipuncture site, apply pressure.

## PRECAUTIONS

● Handle the sample gently to prevent hemolysis.
● Completely fill the collection tube; then invert it gently at least 10 times to mix the sample and the anticoagulant adequately.
● Indicate the date of the patient's last menstrual period and the phase of her cycle

on the laboratory request. If the patient is pregnant, also indicate the month of gestation.

● Send the sample to the laboratory immediately.

## REFERENCE VALUES

During menstruation, normal progesterone values are:
● follicular phase—less than 150 ng/dl (SI, < 5 nmol/L)
● luteal phase—300 to 1,200 ng/dl (SI, 10 to 40 nmol/L).

During pregnancy, normal progesterone values are:
● first trimester—1,500 to 5,000 ng/dl (SI, 50 to 160 nmol/L)
● second and third trimester—8,000 to 20,000 ng/dl (SI, 250 to 650 nmol/L).

Normal values in menopausal women are 10 to 22 ng/dl (SI, 0 to 2 nmol/L).

## ABNORMAL FINDINGS

Elevated progesterone levels may indicate ovulation, luteinizing tumors, ovarian cysts that produce progesterone, or adrenocortical hyperplasia and tumors that produce progesterone along with other steroidal hormones.

Low progesterone levels are associated with amenorrhea due to several causes (such as panhypopituitarism and gonadal dysfunction), eclampsia, threatened abortion, and fetal death.

## INTERFERING FACTORS

● Progesterone or estrogen therapy
● Radioactive scans performed within 1 week of the test

## *Prolactin, serum*

Similar in molecular structure and biological activity to growth hormone (hGH), prolactin is a polypeptide hormone secreted by the anterior pituitary gland. Prolactin is essential for the development of the mammary glands for lactation during pregnancy and for stimulating and maintaining lactation postpartum. Like hGH, prolactin acts directly on tissues, and its levels rise in response to sleep and physical or emotional stress.

This radioimmunoassay is a quantitative analysis of serum prolactin levels, which normally rise 10- to 20-fold during pregnancy, corresponding to concomitant elevations in human placental lactogen levels. After delivery, prolactin secretion falls to basal levels in mothers who don't breast-feed. However, prolactin secretion increases during breast-feeding, apparently as a result of a stimulus triggered by suckling that curtails the release of prolactin-inhibiting factor by the hypothalamus. This release, in turn, allows transient elevations of prolactin secretion by the pituitary gland.

This test is considered useful for patients suspected of having pituitary tumors, which are known to secrete prolactin in excessive amounts. Another test used to evaluate hypothalamic dysfunction is the thyrotropin-releasing hormone (TRH) stimulation test. (See *TRH stimulation test.*)

## PURPOSE

● To facilitate diagnosis of pituitary dysfunction, possibly due to pituitary adenoma
● To aid in the diagnosis of hypothalamic dysfunction regardless of cause
● To evaluate secondary amenorrhea and galactorrhea

## PATIENT PREPARATION

● Tell the patient that the serum prolactin test helps evaluate hormonal secretion.
● Advise the patient to restrict food and fluids and limit physical activity for 12 hours before the test. Encourage her to relax for about 30 minutes before the test.
● Tell the patient the test requires a blood sample. Explain who will perform the venipuncture and when and where the test will take place.
● Explain to the patient that she may experience slight discomfort from the needle puncture and the tourniquet.
● Withhold drugs that may interfere with test results, as ordered. If they must be continued, note this on the laboratory request.

## PROCEDURE AND POSTTEST CARE

● Perform a venipuncture at least 3 hours after the patient wakes; samples collected earlier are likely to show sleep-induced peak levels. Collect the sample in a 7-ml clot-activator tube.

- Apply direct pressure to the venipuncture site until bleeding stops.
- If a hematoma develops at the venipuncture site, apply pressure.
- Instruct the patient that she may resume her usual diet, activities, and medications discontinued before the test, as ordered.

## PRECAUTIONS
- Handle the sample gently to prevent hemolysis.
- Confirm slight elevations with repeat measurements on two other occasions.

## REFERENCE VALUES
Normal values range from undetectable to 23 ng/ml (SI, undetectable to 23 µg/L) in nonlactating females. Levels normally rise ten- to twenty-fold during pregnancy and, after delivery, fall to basal levels in mothers who don't breast-feed. Prolactin secretion increases during breast-feeding.

## ABNORMAL FINDINGS
Abnormally high prolactin levels (100 to 300 ng/ml [SI, 100 to 300 µg/L]) suggest autonomous prolactin production by a pituitary adenoma, especially when amenorrhea or galactorrhea is present (Forbes-Albright syndrome). Rarely, hyperprolactinemia may also result from severe endocrine disorders such as hypothyroidism. Idiopathic hyperprolactinemia may be associated with anovulatory infertility. Confirm slight elevations with repeat measurements on two other occasions.

Decreased prolactin levels in a lactating patient cause failure of lactation and may be associated with postpartum pituitary infarction (Sheehan's syndrome). Abnormally low prolactin levels have also been found in the patient with empty-sella syndrome. In these cases, a flattened pituitary gland makes the pituitary fossa look empty.

## INTERFERING FACTORS
- Failure to take into account physiologic variations related to sleep or stress
- Estrogens, ethanol, methyldopa (Aldomet), and morphine (increase)
- Apomorphine, ergot alkaloids, and levodopa (decrease)
- Radioactive scan performed within 1 week before the test or recent surgery
- Breast stimulation

---

## TRH STIMULATION TEST

The thyrotropin-releasing hormone (TRH) test evaluates hypothalamic dysfunction and pituitary tumors by stimulating the release of prolactin. The procedure is as follows: perform a venipuncture in the basal state to obtain a baseline prolactin level, and then place the patient in the supine position. Administer an I.V. bolus dose (500 mcg) of synthetic TRH over 15 to 30 seconds. Take blood samples at 15- and 30-minute intervals to measure prolactin.

A baseline prolactin reading greater than 200 ng/ml (SI, 200 IU/L) indicates a pituitary tumor, but levels between 30 and 200 ng/ml (SI, 30 to 200 IU/L) are also consistent with this condition. Normally, patients show at least a twofold increase in prolactin after injection with TRH. If the prolactin level fails to rise, hypothalamic dysfunction or adenoma of the pituitary gland is likely.

---

# Prostate gland biopsy

Prostate gland biopsy is the needle excision of a prostate tissue specimen for histologic examination. Indications include potentially malignant prostatic hypertrophy and prostatic nodules. A perineal, transrectal, or transurethral approach may be used — the transrectal approach is used for high prostatic lesions.

## PURPOSE
- To confirm prostate cancer
- To determine the cause of prostatic hyperplasia

## PATIENT PREPARATION
- Describe the prostate gland biopsy to the patient, answer his questions, and tell him that the test provides a tissue specimen for microscopic study.
- Tell the patient who will perform the biopsy, when and where it will be done, and that he'll receive a local anesthetic.
- Make sure the patient or a responsible family member has signed an informed consent form.

- Check the patient's history for hypersensitivity to the anesthetic or other drugs.
- For a transrectal approach, administer enemas until the return is clear and administer an antibacterial agent to minimize the risk of infection. This approach may be performed on an outpatient without an anesthetic.
- Just before the biopsy, check the patient's vital signs and administer a sedative.
- Administer a prophylactic antibiotic, as ordered.
- Instruct the patient to remain still during the procedure and to follow instructions.

## PROCEDURE AND POSTTEST CARE
### Perineal approach
- Place the patient in the proper position (left lateral, knee-chest, or lithotomy), and clean the perineal skin.
- After the local anesthetic is administered, a 2-mm incision may be made into the perineum.
- The examiner immobilizes the prostate by inserting a finger into the rectum and introduces the biopsy needle into a prostate lobe. The needle is rotated gently, pulled out about 5 mm, and reinserted at another angle. The procedure is repeated at several areas.
- Pressure is exerted on the puncture site, which is then bandaged.

### Transrectal approach
- Place the patient in the left lateral position.
- A digital rectal examination is performed before an ultrasound probe is inserted. A curved needle guide is attached to the finger palpating the rectum. The biopsy needle is pushed along the guide into the prostate that was localized by ultrasonography.
- As the needle enters the prostate, the patient may experience pain. The needle is rotated to cut off the tissue and is then withdrawn.
- An alternative method of transrectal detection is the automated cone biopsy, in which the physician uses a spring-powered device with an inner trocar needle to cut through prostatic tissue. This technique is quick and reportedly painless.

### Transurethral approach
- An endoscopic instrument is passed through the urethra, permitting direct viewing of the prostate and passage of a cutting loop.
- The loop is rotated to obtain tissue and then withdrawn.

### All approaches
- The specimen is placed immediately in a labeled specimen bottle containing 10% formalin solution and sent to the laboratory for analysis.
- Check the patient's vital signs immediately after the procedure, every 2 hours for 4 hours, and then every 4 hours.
- Observe the biopsy site for hematoma and for signs and symptoms of infection, such as redness, swelling, and pain. Watch for urine retention, urinary frequency, and hematuria.

## PRECAUTIONS
- Be aware that complications may include transient, painless hematuria and bleeding into the prostatic urethra and bladder.

## NORMAL FINDINGS
Normally, the prostate gland consists of a thin, fibrous capsule surrounding the stroma, which is made up of elastic and connective tissues and smooth-muscle fibers. The epithelial glands found in these tissues and muscle fibers drain into the chief excreting ducts.

## ABNORMAL FINDINGS
Histologic examination can confirm cancer. Further tests — bone scans, bone marrow biopsy, tests for prostate-specific antigen, and serum acid phosphatase and prostatic acid phosphatase determinations — identify the extent of the cancer. Acid phosphatase levels usually rise in metastatic prostatic carcinoma; they tend to be low in carcinoma that's confined to the prostatic capsule.

Histologic examination can also be used to detect benign prostatic hyperplasia, prostatitis, tuberculosis, lymphomas, and rectal or bladder cancer.

## INTERFERING FACTORS
- Inability to obtain an adequate tissue specimen

## Prostate-specific antigen

Until recently, digital rectal examination (DRE) and measurement of prostatic acid phosphatase were the primary methods of monitoring the progression of prostate cancer. Now measurement of prostate-specific antigen (PSA) helps track the course of this disease and evaluate the patient's response to treatment.

PSA appears in normal, benign hyperplastic, and malignant prostatic tissue as well as metastatic prostatic carcinoma. Serum PSA levels are used to monitor the spread or recurrence of prostate cancer and to evaluate the patient's response to treatment. Measurement of serum PSA levels along with a DRE is now recommended as a screening test for prostate cancer in men over age 50. (See *Controversy over PSA screening*.) It's also useful in assessing response to treatment in a patient with stage B3 to D1 prostate cancer and in detecting tumor spread or recurrence.

## PURPOSE
- To screen for prostate cancer in men over age 50
- To monitor prostate cancer's course and evaluate treatment

## PATIENT PREPARATION
- Explain to the patient that the PSA test is used to screen for prostate cancer or, if appropriate, to monitor the course of treatment.
- Tell the patient that the test requires a blood sample. Explain who will perform the venipuncture and when and where the test will take place.
- Explain to the patient that he may experience slight discomfort from the needle puncture and the tourniquet.
- Inform the patient that he need not restrict food and fluids.

## PROCEDURE AND POSTTEST CARE
- Perform a venipuncture and collect the sample in a 7-ml clot-activator tube.
- Apply direct pressure to the venipuncture site until bleeding stops.

---

## CONTROVERSY OVER PSA SCREENING

Measurement of prostate-specific antigen (PSA) allows earlier detection of prostate cancer than does digital rectal examination (DRE) alone. Accordingly, the American Cancer Society and the American Urological Association currently recommend that PSA screening begin at age 40 (in combination with DRE) in black men and any man who has a father or brother with prostate cancer, and at age 50 in all other men.

But, does this test actually reduce mortality from prostate cancer? The answer to that question remains unknown. Some specialists question the value of all prostate cancer screening tests because of the costs involved, the uncertain benefits, and the known risks associated with current treatments.

Before undergoing a PSA test, the patient should understand that controversy surrounds nearly every aspect of prostate cancer screening and treatment. Among the issues he'll face may include:
◆ Even if cancer is detected, treatment may not be advisable, either because of the patient's advanced age or because the physician believes the tumor is so slow-growing that it won't result in death.
◆ The current treatments for prostate cancer — surgery and radiation therapy — may not be as effective as experts formerly believed, and no effective chemotherapy protocol is currently available.
◆ Surgery and radiation therapy carry a high risk of impotence, incontinence, and other problems, which the patient must weigh against the uncertain benefits of therapy.
◆ Screening tests sometimes yield false-positive results, requiring transrectal ultrasonography or a biopsy to confirm the diagnosis.
◆ A mildly elevated PSA level may be the result of normal age-related increases. (Data from a study of more than 9,000 men showed that PSA levels increase about 30% per year in men under age 70 and more than 40% per year in men over age 70.)

In summary, the value of prostate cancer screening in general and PSA testing in particular won't be clearly established until studies show a definitive link between early treatment and reduced mortality.

- If a hematoma develops at the venipuncture site, apply pressure.

## PRECAUTIONS
- Collect the sample either before digital prostate examination or at least 48 hours after examination to avoid falsely elevated PSA levels.
- Handle the sample gently to prevent hemolysis.
- Immediately put the sample on ice and send it to the laboratory.

## REFERENCE VALUES
 *Age alert*
*Normal values are as follows:*
- *ages 40 to 50—2 to 2.8 ng/ml (SI, 2 to 2.8 µg/L)*
- *ages 51 to 60—2.9 to 3.8 ng/ml (SI, 2.9 to 3.8 µg/L)*
- *ages 61 to 70—4 to 5.3 ng/ml (SI, 4 to 5.3 µg/L)*
- *ages 71 and older—5.6 to 7.2 ng/ml (SI, 5.6 to 7.2 µg/L).*

## ABNORMAL FINDINGS
About 80% of patients with prostate cancer have pretreatment PSA values greater than 4 ng/ml. However, PSA results alone don't confirm a diagnosis of prostate cancer. About 20% of patients with benign prostatic hyperplasia also have levels greater than 4 ng/ml. Further assessment and testing, including tissue biopsy, are needed to confirm cancer.

## INTERFERING FACTORS
- Excessive doses of chemotherapeutic drugs, such as cyclophosphamide (Cytoxan), diethylstilbestrol (DES), and methotrexate (MTX) (possible increase or decrease)

# Protein electrophoresis

Protein electrophoresis is used to measure serum albumin and globulin, the major blood proteins, by separating the proteins into five distinct fractions: albumin and alpha$_1$, alpha$_2$, beta, and gamma globulin proteins.

## PURPOSE
- To aid in the diagnosis of hepatic disease, protein deficiency, renal disorders, and GI and neoplastic diseases

## PATIENT PREPARATION
- Explain to the patient that protein electrophoresis is used to determine the protein content of blood.
- Tell the patient that the test requires a blood sample. Explain who will perform the venipuncture and when and where the test will take place.
- Explain to the patient that he may experience slight discomfort from the needle puncture and the tourniquet.
- Inform the patient that he need not restrict food and fluids.
- Notify the laboratory and physician of medications the patient is taking that may affect test results; they may need to be restricted.

## PROCEDURE AND POSTTEST CARE
- Perform a venipuncture and collect the sample in a 7-ml clot-activator tube.
- Apply direct pressure to the venipuncture site until bleeding stops.
- If a hematoma develops at the venipuncture site, apply pressure.
- Inform the patient that he may resume his usual medications discontinued before the test, as ordered.

## PRECAUTIONS
- Know that protein electrophoresis must be performed on a serum sample to avoid measuring the fibrinogen fraction.

## REFERENCE VALUES
Normally, total serum protein levels range from 6.4 to 8.3 g/dl (SI, 64 to 83 g/L), and the albumin fraction ranges from 3.5 to 5 g/dl (SI, 35 to 50 g/L). The alpha$_1$-globulin fraction ranges from 0.1 to 0.3 g/dl (SI, 1 to 3 g/L); alpha$_2$-globulin ranges from 0.6 to 1 g/dl (SI, 6 to 10 g/L). Beta globulin ranges from 0.7 to 1.1 g/dl (SI, 7 to 11 g/L); gamma globulin ranges from 0.8 to 1.6 g/dl (SI, 8 to 16 g/L).

## ABNORMAL FINDINGS
For common abnormal findings, see *Clinical implications of abnormal protein levels.*

# CLINICAL IMPLICATIONS OF ABNORMAL PROTEIN LEVELS

## Increased levels

### TOTAL PROTEINS
- Chronic inflammatory disease (such as rheumatoid arthritis or early-stage Laënnec's cirrhosis)
- Dehydration
- Diabetic ketoacidosis
- Fulminating and chronic infections
- Multiple myeloma
- Monocytic leukemia
- Vomiting, diarrhea

### ALBUMIN
- Multiple myeloma

### GLOBULINS
- Chronic syphilis
- Collagen diseases
- Diabetes mellitus
- Hodgkin's disease
- Multiple myeloma
- Rheumatoid arthritis
- Subacute bacterial endocarditis
- SLE
- Tuberculosis

## Decreased levels

### TOTAL PROTEINS
- Benzene and carbon tetrachloride poisoning
- Blood dyscrasias
- Essential hypertension
- GI disease
- Heart failure
- Hepatic dysfunction
- Hemorrhage
- Hodgkin's disease
- Hyperthyroidism
- Malabsorption
- Malnutrition
- Nephrosis
- Severe burns
- Surgical and traumatic shock
- Toxemia of pregnancy
- Uncontrolled diabetes mellitus

### ALBUMIN
- Acute cholecystitis
- Collagen diseases
- Diarrhea
- Essential hypertension
- Hepatic disease
- Hodgkin's disease
- Hyperthyroidism
- Hypogammaglobulinemia
- Malnutrition
- Metastatic carcinoma
- Nephritis, nephrosis
- Peptic ulcer
- Plasma loss from burns
- Rheumatoid arthritis
- Sarcoidosis
- Systemic lupus erythematosus (SLE)

### GLOBULINS
- Benzene and carbon tetrachloride poisoning
- Blood dyscrasias
- Essential hypertension
- GI disease
- Heart failure
- Hepatic dysfunction
- Hemorrhage
- Hodgkin's disease
- Hyperthyroidism
- Malabsorption
- Malnutrition
- Nephrosis
- Severe burns
- Surgical and traumatic shock
- Toxemia of pregnancy
- Uncontrolled diabetes mellitus

## INTERFERING FACTORS
- Pretest administration of a contrast agent, such as sulfobromophthalein (false-high total protein)
- Cytotoxic drugs or pregnancy (possible decrease in serum albumin)
- Use of plasma instead of serum

## Protein, urine

A urine protein test is a quantitative test for proteinuria. Normally, the glomerular membrane allows only proteins of low molecular weight to enter the filtrate. The renal tubules then reabsorb most of these proteins, normally excreting a small amount that's undetectable by a screening test. A damaged glomerular capillary membrane and impaired tubular reabsorption allow excretion of proteins in the urine.

A qualitative screening commonly precedes this test. A positive result requires quantitative analysis of a 24-hour urine specimen by acid precipitation tests. Electrophoresis can detect Bence Jones proteins, hemoglobins, myoglobins, or albumin.

## PURPOSE
- To aid in the diagnosis of pathologic states characterized by proteinuria, primarily renal disease

## PATIENT PREPARATION
- Explain to the patient that the urine protein test detects proteins in the urine.
- Inform the patient that he need not restrict food and fluids.
- Tell the patient that the test usually requires urine collection over a 24-hour period; random collection can be done.
- Notify the laboratory and physician of medications the patient is taking that may affect test results; they may need to be restricted.

## PROCEDURE AND POSTTEST CARE
- Collect the patient's urine over a 24-hour period, discarding the first specimen and retaining the last. A special specimen container can be obtained from the laboratory.
- Instruct the patient that he may resume his usual medications, as ordered.

## PRECAUTIONS
- Tell the patient not to contaminate the urine with toilet tissue or stool.
- Refrigerate the specimen or place it on ice during the collection period.

## NORMAL FINDINGS
At rest, normal urine protein values range from 50 to 80 mg/24 hours (SI, 50 to 80 mg/d).

## ABNORMAL FINDINGS
Proteinuria is a chief characteristic of renal disease. When proteinuria is present in a single specimen, a 24-hour urine collection is required to identify specific renal abnormalities.

Proteinuria can result from glomerular leakage of plasma proteins (a major cause of protein excretion), from overflow of filtered proteins of low molecular weight (when these are present in excessive concentrations), from impaired tubular reabsorption of filtered proteins, and from the presence of renal proteins derived from the breakdown of kidney tissue.

Persistent proteinuria indicates renal disease resulting from increased glomerular permeability. Minimal proteinuria (less than 0.5 g/24 hours), however, is commonly associated with renal diseases in which glomerular involvement isn't a major factor, as in chronic pyelonephritis.

Moderate proteinuria (0.5 to 4 g/24 hours) occurs in several types of renal disease — acute or chronic glomerulonephritis, amyloidosis, or toxic nephropathies — or in diseases in which renal failure typically develops as a late complication (diabetes or heart failure, for example). Heavy proteinuria (greater than 4 g/24 hours) is commonly associated with nephrotic syndrome.

When accompanied by an elevated white blood cell count, proteinuria indicates urinary tract infection. When accompanied by hematuria, proteinuria indicates local or diffuse urinary tract disorders. Other pathologic states (infections and lesions of the central nervous system, for example) can also result in detectable amounts of proteins in the urine.

Many drugs (such as amphotericin B, gold preparations, aminoglycosides, and trimethadione) inflict renal damage, causing true proteinuria. This fact makes the routine evaluation of urine proteins essential during such treatment. In all forms of proteinuria, fractionation results obtained by electrophoresis provide more precise information than the screening test. For example, excessive hemoglobin in the urine indicates intravascular hemolysis; elevated myoglobin suggests muscle damage; albumin, increased glomerular permeability; and Bence Jones protein, multiple myeloma.

Not all forms of proteinuria have pathologic significance. Benign proteinuria can result from changes in body position. Functional proteinuria is associated with exercise as well as emotional or physiologic stress and is usually transient.

## INTERFERING FACTORS

- Contamination of the specimen with toilet tissue or stool
- Acetazolamide (Diamox), cephalosporins, iodine-containing contrast media, para-aminosalicylic acid, penicillin, sodium bicarbonate, sulfonamides, and tolbutamide (Orinase) (possible false-positive or false-negative)
- Very dilute urine, such as from forcing fluids, possibly depressing protein values and causing false-negative results

# *Prothrombin time*

Prothrombin time (PT) measures the time required for a fibrin clot to form in a citrated plasma sample after addition of calcium ions and tissue thromboplastin (factor III).

## PURPOSE

- To evaluate the extrinsic coagulation system (factors V, VII, and X and prothrombin and fibrinogen)
- To monitor response to oral anticoagulant therapy

## PATIENT PREPARATION

- Explain to the patient that the PT test is used to determine if the blood clots normally.
- Notify the laboratory and physician of medications the patient is taking that may affect test results; they may need to be restricted.
- Tell the patient that a blood sample will be taken. Explain who will perform the venipuncture and when and where the test will take place.
- Explain to the patient that he may feel slight discomfort from the needle puncture and the tourniquet.
- When appropriate, explain that this test is used to monitor the effects of oral anticoagulants; the test will be performed daily when therapy begins and will be repeated at longer intervals when medication levels stabilize.
- Inform the patient that he need not restrict food and fluids.

## PROCEDURE AND POSTTEST CARE

- Perform a venipuncture and collect the sample in a 3- or 4.5-ml siliconized tube.
- If a hematoma develops at the venipuncture site, apply pressure. If the hematoma is large, monitor pulses distal to the venipuncture site.
- Make sure subdermal bleeding has stopped before removing pressure.
- Instruct the patient that he may resume his usual diet and medications discontinued before the test, as ordered.

## PRECAUTIONS

- Completely fill the collection tube and invert it gently several times to mix the sample and the anticoagulant thoroughly. If the tube isn't filled to the correct volume, an excess of citrate appears in the sample.
- To prevent hemolysis, avoid excessive probing during venipuncture and handle the sample gently.

## REFERENCE VALUES

Normally, PT values range from 10 to 14 seconds (SI, 10 to 14 s). Values vary, however, depending on the source of tissue thromboplastin and the type of sensing devices used to measure clot formation. In a patient receiving oral anticoagulants, PT is usually maintained between 1 and $2^1/_2$ times the normal control value.

## ABNORMAL FINDINGS

Prolonged PT may indicate deficiencies in fibrinogen; prothrombin; factors V, VII, or X (specific assays can pinpoint such deficiencies); or vitamin K. It may also result from ongoing oral anticoagulant therapy. A prolonged PT that exceeds $2^1/_2$ times the control value is commonly associated with abnormal bleeding.

## INTERFERING FACTORS

- Salicylates, more than 1 g/day (increase)
- Fibrin or fibrin split products in the sample or plasma fibrinogen levels greater than 100 mg/dl (possible prolonged PT)
- Antihistamines, chloral hydrate, corticosteroids, digoxin (Lanoxin), diuretics, glutethimide, griseofulvin, progestin-estrogen combinations, pyrazinamide, vitamin K, and xanthines, such as caffeine and theophylline (TheoDur) (possible decrease)

- Anabolic steroids, cholestyramine resin, corticotropin, heparin I.V. (within 5 hours of sample collection), indomethacin (Indocin), mefenamic acid (Ponstel), methimazole (Tapazole), phenylbutazone, phenytoin (Dilantin), propylthiouracil (PTU), quinidine, quinine, thyroid hormones, vitamin A, or alcohol in excess (prolonged PT)
- Antibiotics, barbiturates, hydroxyzine (Vistaril), mineral oil, or sulfonamides (possible increase or decrease)

# Pulmonary angiography

Also called pulmonary arteriography, pulmonary angiography is the radiographic examination of the pulmonary circulation following injection of a radiopaque iodine contrast agent into the pulmonary artery or one of its branches.

Possible complications include arterial occlusion or rupture, myocardial perforation or rupture, ventricular arrhythmias from myocardial irritation, and acute renal failure from hypersensitivity to the contrast agent.

## PURPOSE
- To detect pulmonary embolism when less invasive studies are nondiagnostic
- To evaluate pulmonary circulation abnormalities
- To evaluate pulmonary circulation preoperatively in the patient with congenital heart disease
- To locate a large embolus before surgical removal

## PATIENT PREPARATION
- Describe the pulmonary angiography procedure to the patient. Explain that this test permits evaluation of the blood vessels to help identify the cause of his symptoms.
- Instruct the patient to fast for 8 hours before the test or as prescribed. Tell him who will perform the test, where it will take place, and that laboratory work for kidney function and coagulation may precede the test.
- Tell the patient that a small puncture will be made in the blood vessel of his right arm where blood samples are usually drawn, or in the right groin at the femoral vein, and that a local anesthetic will be used to numb

the area. Inform him that a small catheter will then be inserted into the blood vessel and passed into the right side of the heart to the pulmonary artery.
- Tell the patient the contrast medium will then be injected into this artery. Warn him that he may feel flushed, experience an urge to cough, or experience a salty taste for approximately 3 to 5 minutes after the injection.
- Inform the patient that his heart rate will be monitored continuously during the procedure and that he should tell the physician or nurse if he has concerns.
- Make sure that the patient or a responsible family member has signed an informed consent form. Check the patient's history for hypersensitivity to anesthetics, iodine, seafood, or radiographic contrast agents.
- Obtain or check laboratory tests (including prothrombin time, partial thromboplastin time, platelet count, and blood urea nitrogen [BUN] and serum creatinine levels), and notify the radiologist of any abnormal results. I.V. hydration may need to be considered depending on the patient's renal and cardiac status. The radiologist may want to discontinue a heparin drip 3 to 4 hours before the test.

## PROCEDURE AND POSTTEST CARE
- After the patient is placed in a supine position, the local anesthetic is injected and the cardiac monitor is attached to the patient. Blood pressure and pulse oximeter are monitored as per facility protocol.
- A puncture is made at the procedure site, and a catheter is introduced into the antecubital or femoral vein. As the catheter passes through the right atrium, the right ventricle, and the pulmonary artery, pressures are measured and blood samples are drawn from various regions of the pulmonary circulation.
- The contrast medium is injected and circulates through the pulmonary artery and lung capillaries while X-rays are taken.
- Apply pressure over the catheter insertion site for 15 to 20 minutes or until bleeding stops.
- Maintain bed rest for about 6 hours.
- Observe the site for bleeding and swelling. If either occur, maintain pressure at the insertion site for 10 minutes and notify the radiologist.

- Check the patient's blood pressure and pulse rate and the catheter insertion site (arm or groin) every 15 minutes for 1 hour, every hour for 4 hours, and then every 4 hours for 16 hours.
- Observe the patient for signs of myocardial perforation or rupture by monitoring vital signs.
- Be alert for signs of acute renal failure, such as sudden onset of oliguria, nausea, and vomiting. Check BUN and serum creatinine levels.
- Check the catheter insertion site for inflammation or hematoma formation and report symptoms of a delayed hypersensitivity response to the contrast agent or to the local anesthetic (dyspnea, itching, tachycardia, palpitations, hypotension or hypertension, excitation, or euphoria).
- Advise the patient about any restriction of activity. Tell him that he may resume his usual diet after the test (encourage him to drink lots of fluids), or administer I.V. fluids, as ordered, to flush the contrast agent from his body.

## PRECAUTIONS

- Know that pulmonary angiography is contraindicated during pregnancy.
- Monitor the patient for ventricular arrhythmias due to myocardial irritation from passage of the catheter through the heart chambers.
- **Alert** *Observe the patient for signs of hypersensitivity to the contrast agent, such as dyspnea, nausea, vomiting, sweating, increased heart rate, and numbness of extremities. Keep emergency equipment available in case of a hypersensitivity reaction to the contrast agent.*
- Measure pulmonary artery pressures. Right ventricular end-diastolic pressure is usually less than or equal to 20 mm Hg, and pulmonary artery systolic pressure is usually less than or equal to 70 mm Hg. Pressures greater than this increase the risk of mortality associated with this procedure.

## NORMAL FINDINGS

Normally, the contrast agent flows symmetrically and without interruption through the pulmonary circulatory system.

## ABNORMAL FINDINGS

Interruption of blood flow may result from emboli and from other types of pulmonary vascular abnormalities or tumors.

## INTERFERING FACTORS
- None significant

# Pulmonary artery catheterization

In pulmonary artery (PA) catheterization, also known as Swan-Ganz catheterization, a balloon-tipped, flow-directed catheter is threaded through the right atrium to provide intermittent occlusion of the pulmonary artery. PA catheterization permits measurement of pulmonary artery pressure (PAP) and pulmonary artery wedge pressure (PAWP).

The PAWP reading accurately reflects left atrial pressure (LAP) and left ventricular end-diastolic pressure, although the catheter itself never enters the left side of the heart. Obtaining this information is possible because the heart momentarily relaxes during diastole as it fills with blood from the pulmonary veins; at this instant, the pulmonary vasculature, left atrium, and left ventricle act as a single chamber, and all have identical pressures. Thus, changes in PAP and PAWP reflect changes in left ventricular filling pressure, permitting detection of left ventricular impairment.

The procedure is usually performed at bedside in an intensive or coronary care unit. The catheter is inserted through the cephalic vein in the antecubital fossa or the subclavian (sometimes femoral) vein. In addition to measuring atrial and PA pressures, this procedure evaluates pulmonary vascular resistance and tissue oxygenation, as indicated by mixed venous oxygen content. It should be performed cautiously in the patient with left bundle-branch block or an implanted pacemaker.

## PURPOSE
- To help assess right and left ventricular function
- To monitor therapy for myocardial infarction, cardiogenic shock, septic shock, pulmonary edema, fluid-related hypovolemia and hypotension, systolic murmur, unexplained sinus tachycardia, and various cardiac arrhythmias
- To monitor fluid status in the patient with serious burns, renal disease, noncardio-

genic pulmonary edema, or acute respiratory distress syndrome

● To monitor the effects of cardiovascular drugs, such as nitroglycerin and nitroprusside

● To establish baseline pressures preoperatively in the patient with existing cardiac disease and then adjust I.V. medications for optimal surgical success

● To differentiate between pulmonary and cardiac pulmonary edema

## PATIENT PREPARATION

● Explain to the patient that PA catheterization evaluates heart function and provides data necessary to determine appropriate therapy or manage fluid status.

● Tell the patient that he need not restrict food and fluids.

● Describe the test, including who will perform it and when and where it will take place.

● Tell the patient that he'll be conscious during catheterization and that he may experience discomfort from administration of the local anesthetic.

● Explain that catheter insertion takes about 30 minutes, but that the catheter will remain in place, causing little or no discomfort.

● Instruct the patient to report any discomfort immediately.

● Explain that after insertion, he'll need to have a portable chest X-ray to confirm proper placement of the PA catheter.

● Make sure that the patient or a responsible family member has signed an informed consent form.

## PROCEDURE AND POSTTEST CARE

● Choose an appropriate flexible PA catheter. Catheters used in this test come in 2- to 5-lumen modes and in various lengths. In the 2-lumen catheter, one lumen contains the balloon, 1 mm behind the catheter tip; the other lumen, which opens at the tip, measures pressure in front of the balloon. The 2-lumen catheter measures PAP and PAWP and can be used to sample mixed venous blood and infuse I.V. solutions. The 3-lumen catheter has another proximal lumen that opens 12" (30.5 cm) behind the tip; when the tip is in the main pulmonary artery, the proximal lumen lies in the right atrium, permitting fluid administration or right atrial

pressure ([RAP]; central venous pressure) monitoring. The 4-lumen type includes a transistorized thermistor for monitoring blood temperature and allows for cardiac output measurement. A 4-lumen catheter with thermodilution and pacer port mode is used in critical care settings to allow for pacing, if necessary. The introducer part of the system may also be used to infuse large amounts of fluids.

● Before catheterization, set up the equipment according to the manufacturer's directions and your facility's protocol.

● If the insertion site is being prepared for a cutdown procedure, prepare the patient's skin and cover it with a sterile drape.

● Assist the patient to the supine position. For antecubital insertion, his arm is abducted with the palm upward on an overbed table for support; for subclavian insertion, the patient is placed in the supine position with his head and shoulders slightly lower than his trunk to make the vein more accessible. If the patient can't tolerate the supine position, assist him to semi-Fowler's position. During the test, monitor all pressures with the patient in the same position.

● Check the catheter balloon for defects, using sterile technique, and flush all ports to ensure patency.

● The catheter introducer is inserted into the vein percutaneously or by cutdown. Then the catheter is inserted through the introducer and directed to the right atrium, and the catheter balloon is partially inflated so that venous flow carries the catheter tip through the right atrium and tricuspid valve into the right ventricle and the pulmonary artery.

● Observe the monitor for characteristic waveform changes. Obtain a printout of each stage of catheter insertion. (See *PA catheterization: Insertion sites and associated waveforms.*)

● Instruct the patient to extend the appropriate arm (or leg, if the catheter is inserted into the femoral vein).

● *Alert During PA catheterization—as the catheter is passed into the chambers of the right side of the heart—observe the monitor and the patient for frequent premature ventricular contractions or tachycardia (including ventricular tachycardia), which may result from right ventricular catheter irritation. If irritation occurs, the catheter may be partially withdrawn or medication administered to*

# PA CATHETERIZATION: INSERTION SITES AND ASSOCIATED WAVEFORMS

As the pulmonary artery (PA) catheter is directed through the chambers on the right side of the heart to its wedge position, it produces distinctive waveforms on the oscilloscope screen that are important indicators of the catheter's position in the heart.

### RIGHT ATRIAL PRESSURE

When the catheter tip reaches the right atrium from the superior vena cava, the waveform on the oscilloscope screen or readout strip resembles the one shown at right. When this waveform appears, the physician inflates the catheter balloon, which floats the tip through the tricuspid valve into the right ventricle.

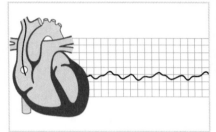

### RIGHT VENTRICULAR PRESSURE

When the catheter tip reaches the right ventricle, the waveform looks like the one shown at right.

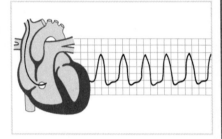

### PULMONARY ARTERY PRESSURE

A waveform that resembles the one shown at right indicates that the balloon has floated the catheter tip through the pulmonic valve into the pulmonary artery. A dicrotic notch (see arrow) should be visible in the waveform, indicating the closing of the pulmonic valve.

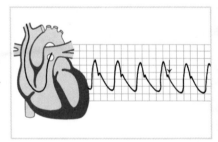

### PULMONARY ARTERY WEDGE PRESSURE

Blood flow in the pulmonary artery then carries the catheter balloon into one of the pulmonary artery's many smaller branches. When the vessel becomes too narrow for the balloon to pass through, the balloon wedges in the vessel, occluding it. The monitor then displays a pulmonary artery wedge pressure waveform such as the one shown at right.

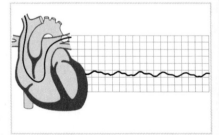

suppress the arrhythmia or right bundle-branch block.

● To record the PAWP, carefully inflate the catheter balloon with the specified amount of air; the catheter tip will float into the wedge position, as indicated by an altered waveform on the monitor. If a PAWP waveform occurs with less than the recommended inflation volume, don't inflate the balloon further.

● After the balloon is inflated, record the PAWP. Then allow the balloon to deflate passively. This allows the catheter to float back into the pulmonary artery. Observe the monitor for a PA waveform.

● The 1.5-ml syringe that comes in the introducer kit has an indentation along the barrel that won't allow you to inject more than 1.5 cc of air, to prevent overinflation. The stopcock should be turned so that it's perpendicular to the insertion port to prevent air from the syringe from accidentally inflating the balloon.

● **Alert** Don't overinflate the balloon catheter. Overinflation could distend the pulmonary artery, causing vessel rupture.

● If the balloon can't be fully deflated after recording the PAWP, don't reinflate it unless the physician is present; balloon rupture may cause a life-threatening air embolism. Check all connections for air leaks that may have prevented balloon inflation, particularly if the patient is confused or uncooperative.

● When the catheter's correct positioning and function are established, it's sutured to the skin. An airtight dressing are applied to the insertion site according to your facility's policy.

● A chest X-ray is obtained, as ordered, to verify catheter placement.

● Set alarms on the electrocardiogram (ECG) and pressure monitors.

● Monitor the patient's vital signs, as ordered or per facility protocol.

● Document PAP waveforms at the beginning of each shift and monitor them frequently throughout each shift and with changes in treatment. Check PAWP and cardiac output, as ordered (usually every 6 to 8 hours).

● Take routine aseptic precautions to prevent infection.

● When the catheter is no longer needed, the dressing is removed and the catheter is slowly withdrawn after ensuring that the balloon is deflated. The ECG is monitored for

arrhythmias. In some facilities, the physician is required to remove the catheter.

● After the catheter is withdrawn, the catheter tip is usually sent to the laboratory for analysis.

● Apply a sterile dressing over the catheter introducer.

● Observe the site for signs of infection, such as redness, swelling, and discharge.

● Watch for complications, such as pulmonary emboli, PA perforation, heart murmurs, thrombi, and arrhythmias.

## PRECAUTIONS

● Before obtaining a PAWP reading, flush the monitoring system and recalibrate the system per facility protocol.

● After obtaining a PAWP reading, make sure the balloon is completely deflated.

● Maintain 300 mm Hg of pressure in the pressure bag to permit a fluid flow of 3 to 6 ml/hour. Instruct the patient to extend the appropriate arm (or leg, if the catheter is inserted in the femoral vein).

● Be aware that if a damped waveform occurs, the catheter may need to be adjusted. Pulmonary infarct may occur if the catheter is allowed to remain in a wedged position.

● Make sure that the stopcocks are properly positioned and the connections are secure. Loose connections may introduce air into the system or cause blood backup, leakage of deoxygenated blood, or inaccurate pressure readings.

● Make sure that the lumen hubs are properly identified to serve the appropriate catheter ports.

● **Alert** Don't add or remove fluids from the distal PA port; this could cause pulmonary extravasation or damage the artery.

● If the catheter hasn't been sutured to the skin, tape it securely to prevent dislodgment.

● If the patient shows signs of sepsis, treat the catheter as the source of infection and send it to the laboratory for culture when removed.

## REFERENCE VALUES

Normal pressures are as follows:
● RAP—1 to 6 mm Hg
● systolic right ventricular pressure—20 to 30 mm Hg
● end-diastolic right ventricular pressure—less than 5 mm Hg
● systolic PAP—20 to 30 mm Hg
● diastolic PAP—10 to 15 mm Hg

- mean PAP—less than 20 mm Hg
- PAWP—6 to 12 mm Hg
- LAP—about 10 mm Hg.

## ABNORMAL FINDINGS

An abnormally high RAP can indicate pulmonary disease, right-sided heart failure, fluid overload, cardiac tamponade, tricuspid stenosis and insufficiency, or pulmonary hypertension.

Elevated right ventricular pressure can result from pulmonary hypertension, pulmonary valvular stenosis, right-sided heart failure, pericardial effusion, constrictive pericarditis, chronic heart failure, or ventricular septal defects.

An abnormally high PAP is characteristic in increased pulmonary blood flow, as occurs in a left-to-right shunt secondary to atrial or ventricular septal defect; increased PA resistance, as occurs in pulmonary hypertension or mitral stenosis; chronic obstructive pulmonary disease; pulmonary edema or embolus; and left-sided heart failure from any cause. PA systolic pressure is the same as right ventricular systolic pressure. PA diastolic pressure is the same as LAP, except in the patient with severe pulmonary disease causing pulmonary hypertension; in such cases, catheterization is still important diagnostically.

An elevated PAWP can result from left-sided heart failure, mitral stenosis and insufficiency, cardiac tamponade, or cardiac insufficiency; a depressed PAWP can result from hypovolemia.

## INTERFERING FACTORS

- Malfunctioning monitoring and recording devices, loose connections, clot formation at the catheter tip, air in the fluid column, or a ruptured balloon
- Mechanical ventilation with positive pressure, causing increased intrathoracic pressure (increase in catheter pressure)
- Incorrect catheter placement, causing excessive movement called catheter fling (damped pressure tracing)
- Migration of the catheter against a vessel wall (possible constant occlusion, or wedging, of the pulmonary artery)
- Extreme patient agitation

# *Pulmonary function*

Pulmonary function tests (volume, capacity, and flow rate tests) are a series of measurements that evaluate ventilatory function through spirometric measurements; they're performed on patients with suspected pulmonary dysfunction.

Of the seven tests used to determine volume, tidal volume ($V_T$) and expiratory reserve volume (ERV) are direct spirographic measurements; minute volume, carbon dioxide response, inspiratory reserve volume, and residual volume are calculated from the results of other pulmonary function tests; and thoracic gas volume (TGV) is calculated from body plethysmography.

Of the pulmonary capacity tests, vital capacity (VC), inspiratory capacity (IC), functional residual capacity (FRC), total lung capacity, and forced expiratory flow may be measured directly or calculated from the results of other tests. Forced vital capacity (FVC), flow-volume curve, forced expiratory volume (FEV), peak expiratory flow rate, and maximal voluntary ventilation (MVV) are direct spirographic measurements. Diffusing capacity for carbon monoxide ($DL_{CO}$) is calculated from the amount of CO exhaled. (See *Interpreting pulmonary function tests,* pages 360 to 362.)

## PURPOSE

- To determine the cause of dyspnea
- To assess the effectiveness of specific therapeutic regimens
- To determine whether a functional abnormality is obstructive or restrictive
- To measure pulmonary dysfunction
- To evaluate a patient before surgery
- To evaluate a person as part of a job screening (firefighting, for example)

## PATIENT PREPARATION

- Explain to the patient that pulmonary function tests evaluate pulmonary function. Instruct him to eat only a light meal and not to smoke for 12 hours before the tests.
- Describe the tests and equipment. Explain who will perform the tests, where they will take place, and how long they will last.
- Describe the operation of a spirometer.

*(Text continues on page 362.)*

# INTERPRETING
## PULMONARY FUNCTION TESTS

| PULMONARY FUNCTION TEST | METHOD OF CALCULATION | IMPLICATIONS |
|---|---|---|
| **TIDAL VOLUME ($V_T$)** | | |
| Amount of air inhaled or exhaled during normal breathing | Determining the spirographic measurement for 10 breaths and then dividing by 10 | Decreased $V_T$ may indicate restrictive disease and requires further testing, such as full pulmonary function studies or chest X-rays. |
| **MINUTE VOLUME (MV)** | | |
| Total amount of air expired per minute | Multiplying $V_T$ by the respiratory rate | Normal MV can occur in emphysema; decreased MV may indicate other diseases such as pulmonary edema. Increased MV can occur with acidosis, increased $CO_2$, decreased partial pressure of arterial oxygen, exercise, and low compliance states. |
| **CARBON DIOXIDE ($CO_2$) RESPONSE** | | |
| Increase or decrease in MV after breathing various $CO_2$ concentrations | Plotting changes in MV against increasing inspired $CO_2$ concentrations | Reduced $CO_2$ response may occur in emphysema, myxedema, obesity, hypoventilation syndrome, and sleep apnea. |
| **INSPIRATORY RESERVE VOLUME (IRV)** | | |
| Amount of air inspired over above-normal inspiration | Subtracting $V_T$ from inspiratory capacity (IC) | Abnormal IRV alone doesn't indicate respiratory dysfunction; IRV decreases during normal exercise. |
| **EXPIRATORY RESERVE VOLUME (ERV)** | | |
| Amount of air exhaled after normal expiration | Direct spirographic measurement | ERV varies, even in healthy people, but usually decreases in obese people. |
| **RESIDUAL VOLUME (RV)** | | |
| Amount of air remaining in the lungs after forced expiration | Subtracting ERV from functional residual capacity (FRC) | RV > 35% of total lung capacity (TLC) after maximal expiratory effort may indicate obstructive disease. |
| **VITAL CAPACITY (VC)** | | |
| Total volume of air that can be exhaled after maximum inspiration | Direct spirographic measurement or adding $V_T$, IRV, and ERV | Normal or increased VC with decreased flow rates may indicate any condition that causes a reduction in functional pulmonary tissue such as pulmonary edema. Decreased VC with normal or increased flow rates may indicate decreased respiratory effort resulting from neuromuscular disease, drug overdose, or head injury; decreased thoracic expansion; or limited diaphragm movement. |

| PULMONARY FUNCTION TEST | METHOD OF CALCULATION | IMPLICATIONS |
|---|---|---|
| **INSPIRATORY CAPACITY (IC)** | | |
| Amount of air that can be inhaled after normal expiration | Direct spirographic measurement or adding IRV and $V_T$ | Decreased IC indicates restrictive disease. |
| **THORACIC GAS VOLUME (TGV)** | | |
| Total volume of gas in the lungs from ventilated and nonventilated airways | Body plethysmography | Increased TGV indicates air trapping, which may result from obstructive disease. |
| **FUNCTIONAL RESIDUAL CAPACITY (FRC)** | | |
| Amount of air remaining in the lungs after normal expiration | Nitrogen washout, helium dilution technique, or adding ERV and RV | Increased FRC indicates overdistention of the lungs, which may result from obstructive pulmonary disease. |
| **TOTAL LUNG CAPACITY (TLC)** | | |
| Total volume of the lungs when maximally inflated | Adding $V_T$, IRV, ERV, and RV; FRC and IC; or VC and RV | Low TLC indicates restrictive disease; high TLC indicates overdistended lungs caused by obstructive disease. |
| **FORCED VITAL CAPACITY (FVC)** | | |
| Amount of air exhaled forcefully and quickly after maximum inspiration | Direct spirographic measurement; expressed as a percentage of the total volume of gas exhaled | Decreased FVC indicates flow resistance in the respiratory system from obstructive disease such as chronic bronchitis or from restrictive disease such as pulmonary fibrosis. |
| **FLOW-VOLUME CURVE (ALSO CALLED FLOW-VOLUME LOOP)** | | |
| Greatest rate of flow ($V_{max}$) during FVC maneuvers versus lung volume change | Direct spirographic measurement at 1 second intervals; calculated from flow rates (expressed in L/second) and lung volume changes (expressed in liters) during maximal inspiratory and expiratory maneuvers | Decreased flow rates at all volumes during expiration indicate obstructive disease of the small airways such as emphysema. A plateau of expiratory flow near TLC, a plateau of inspiratory flow at mid-VC, and a square wave pattern through most of VC indicate obstructive disease of large airways. Normal or increased PEFR, decreased flow with decreasing lung volumes, and markedly decreased VC indicate restrictive disease. |
| **FORCED EXPIRATORY VOLUME (FEV)** | | |
| Volume of air expired in the first, second, or third second of an FVC maneuver | Direct spirographic measurement; expressed as a percentage of FVC | Decreased $FEV_1$ and increased $FEV_2$ and $FEV_3$ may indicate obstructive disease; decreased or normal $FEV_1$ may indicate restrictive disease. |

*(continued)*

| PULMONARY FUNCTION TEST | METHOD OF CALCULATION | IMPLICATIONS |
|---|---|---|
| **FORCED EXPIRATORY FLOW (FEF)** | | |
| Average rate of flow during the middle half of FVC | Calculated from the flow rate and the time needed for expiration of the middle 50% of FVC | Low FEF (25% to 75%) indicates obstructive disease of the small and medium-sized airways. |
| **PEAK EXPIRATORY FLOW RATE (PEFR)** | | |
| $V_{max}$ during forced expiration | Calculated from the flow-volume curve or by direct spirographic measurement using a pneumotachometer or electronic tachometer with a transducer to convert flow to electrical output display | Decreased PEFR may indicate a mechanical problem, such as upper airway obstruction, or obstructive disease. PEFR is usually normal in restrictive disease but decreases in severe cases. Because PEFR is effort dependent, it's also low in a person who has poor expiratory effort or doesn't understand the procedure. |
| **MAXIMAL VOLUNTARY VENTILATION (MVV) (ALSO CALLED MAXIMUM BREATHING CAPACITY)** | | |
| The greatest volume of air breathed per unit of time | Direct spirographic measurement | Decreased MVV may indicate obstructive disease; normal or decreased MVV may indicate restrictive disease such as myasthenia gravis. |
| **DIFFUSING CAPACITY FOR CARBON MONOXIDE ($DL_{CO}$)** | | |
| Milliliters of CO diffused per minute across the alveolocapillary membrane | Calculated from analysis of the amount of carbon monoxide exhaled compared with the amount inhaled | Decreased $DL_{CO}$ due to a thickened alveolocapillary membrane occurs in interstitial pulmonary diseases, such as pulmonary fibrosis, asbestosis, and sarcoidosis; $DL_{CO}$ is reduced in emphysema because of alveolocapillary membrane loss. |

● Advise the patient that the accuracy of the tests depends on his cooperation.

● Assure the patient that the procedures are painless and that he'll be able to rest between tests.

● Inform the laboratory if the patient is taking an analgesic that depresses respiration.

● As ordered, withhold bronchodilators for 4 to 8 hours.

● Just before the test, tell the patient to void and to loosen tight clothing. If he wears dentures, tell him to wear them during the test to help form a seal around the mouthpiece. Advise him to put on the noseclip so that he can adjust to it before the test.

## PROCEDURE AND POSTTEST CARE

● When measuring $V_T$, tell the patient to breathe normally into the mouthpiece 10 times.

● When measuring ERV, tell the patient to breathe normally for several breaths and then to exhale as completely as possible.

● When measuring VC, tell the patient to inhale as deeply as possible and to exhale into the mouthpiece as completely as possible. This procedure is repeated three times, and the test result showing the largest volume is used.

● When measuring IC, tell the patient to breathe normally for several breaths and then to inhale as deeply as possible.

● When measuring FRC, tell the patient to breathe normally into a spirometer that contains a known concentration of an insoluble gas (usually helium or nitrogen) in a known volume of air. After a few breaths, the concentrations of gas in the spirometer and in the lungs reach equilibrium. Then the point of equilibrium and the concentration of gas in the spirometer are recorded.

● When measuring TGV, be aware that the patient is put in an airtight box (or body plethysmograph) and told to breathe through a tube connected to a transducer. At end-expiration, the tube is occluded, the patient is told to pant, and changes in intrathoracic and plethysmographic pressures are measured. The results are used to calculate total TGV and FRC.

● When measuring FVC and FEV, tell the patient to inhale as slowly and deeply as possible and then exhale into the mouthpiece as quickly and completely as possible. This procedure is repeated three times, and the largest volume is recorded. The volume of air expired at 1 second ($FEV_1$), at 2 seconds ($FEV_2$), and at 3 seconds ($FEV_3$) during all three repetitions is also recorded.

● When measuring MVV, tell the patient to breathe into the mouthpiece as quickly and deeply as possible for 15 seconds.

● When measuring $DL_{CO}$, the patient inhales a gas mixture with a low concentration of carbon monoxide and then holds his breath for 10 seconds before exhaling.

● After the tests, instruct the patient to resume his usual activities, diet, and medications, as ordered.

## PRECAUTIONS

● Know that pulmonary function tests are contraindicated in the patient with acute coronary insufficiency, angina, or recent myocardial infarction.

● Watch the patient for respiratory distress, changes in pulse rate and blood pressure, and coughing or bronchospasm.

## REFERENCE VALUES

Normal values are predicted for each patient based on age, height, weight, and sex and are expressed as a percentage. Usually, results are considered abnormal if they're less than 80% of these values.

The following reference values can be calculated at bedside with a portable spirometer: $V_T$, 5 to 7 ml/kg of body weight; ERV, 25% of VC; IC, 75% of VC; $FEV_1$, 83% of VC (after 1 second); $FEV_2$, 94% of VC (after 2 seconds); and $FEV_3$, 97% of VC (after 3 seconds).

## ABNORMAL FINDINGS

See *Interpreting pulmonary function tests,* pages 360 to 362.

## INTERFERING FACTORS

● Hypoxia, metabolic disturbances, or lack of patient cooperation

● Gastric distention or pregnancy (possible lung volume displacement)

● Narcotic analgesics or sedatives (possible decrease in inspiratory and expiratory forces)

● Bronchodilators (possible temporary improvement in pulmonary function)

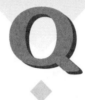

## Quantitative immunogl obulins G, A, and M

Immunoglobulins, proteins that can function as specific antibodies in response to antigen stimulation, are responsible for the humoral aspects of immunity. They are classified into five groups — immunoglobulin (Ig) G, IgA, IgM, IgD, and IgE — that are normally present in serum in predictable percentages.

IgG constitutes about 75% of serum immunoglobulins and includes the warm-temperature type; IgA, about 15% of the total; IgM, 5% to 7%, including cold agglutinins, rheumatoid factor, and ABO blood group isoagglutinins; and IgD and allergen-specific IgE, less than 2%.

Deviations from normal immunoglobulin percentages are characteristic in many immune disorders, including cancer, hepatic disorders, rheumatoid arthritis, and systemic lupus erythematosus. (See *Serum immunoglobulin levels in various disorders.*)

Immunoelectrophoresis identifies IgG, IgA, and IgM in a serum sample; the level of each is measured by radial immunodiffusion or nephelometry. Some laboratories detect immunoglobulin by indirect immunofluorescence and radioimmunoassay.

### Purpose
- To diagnose paraproteinemias, such as multiple myeloma and Waldenström's macroglobulinemia
- To detect hypogammaglobulinemia and hypergammaglobulinemia as well as nonim-

munologic diseases, such as cirrhosis and hepatitis, that are associated with abnormally high immunoglobulin levels
- To assess the effectiveness of chemotherapy and radiation therapy

### Patient preparation
- Explain to the patient that the IgG, IgA, and IgM tests measures antibody levels.
- If appropriate, tell the patient that the test evaluates the effectiveness of treatment.
- Instruct the patient to restrict food and fluids, except for water, for 12 to 14 hours before the test.
- Tell the patient that the test requires a blood sample. Explain who will perform the venipuncture and when and where the test will take place.
- Explain to the patient that he may experience slight discomfort from the needle puncture and the tourniquet.
- Check the patient's history for drugs that may affect test results.
- Be aware that alcohol or narcotic abuse may affect results.

### Procedure and posttest care
- Perform a venipuncture and collect the sample in a 7-ml clot-activator tube.
- Advise the patient with abnormally low immunoglobulin levels (especially IgG or IgM) to protect himself against bacterial infection. When caring for such a patient, watch for signs of infection, such as fever, chills, rash, and skin ulcers.
- Instruct the patient with abnormally high immunoglobulin levels and symptoms of monoclonal gammopathies to report bone pain and tenderness. Such a patient has nu-

# Serum immunoglobulin levels in various disorders

| Disorder | IgG | IgA | IgM |
| --- | --- | --- | --- |
| **Immunoglobulin disorders** | | | |
| Lymphoid aplasia | D | D | D |
| Agammaglobulinemia | D | D | D |
| Type I dysgammaglobulinemia (selective immuno-globulin [Ig] G and IgA deficiency) | D | D | N or I |
| Type II dysgammaglobulinemia (absent IgA and IgM) | N | D | D |
| IgA globulinemia | N | D | N |
| Ataxia-telangiectasia | N | D | N |
| **Multiple myeloma, macroglobulinemia, lymphomas** | | | |
| Heavy chain disease (Franklin's disease) | D | D | D |
| IgG myeloma | I | D | D |
| IgA myeloma | D | I | D |
| Macroglobulinemia | D | D | I |
| Acute lymphocytic leukemia | N | D | N |
| Chronic lymphocytic leukemia | D | D | D |
| Acute myelocytic leukemia | N | N | N |
| Chronic myelocytic leukemia | N | D | N |
| Hodgkin's disease | N | N | N |
| **Hepatic disorders** | | | |
| Hepatitis | I | I | I |
| Laënnec's cirrhosis | I | I | N |
| Biliary cirrhosis | N | N | I |
| Hepatoma | N | N | D |
| **Other disorders** | | | |
| Rheumatoid arthritis | I | I | I |
| Systemic lupus erythematosus | I | I | I |
| Nephrotic syndrome | D | D | N |
| Trypanosomiasis | N | N | I |
| Pulmonary tuberculosis | I | N | N |

KEY:
N = normal; I = increased; D = decreased

merous antibody-producing malignant plasma cells in bone marrow, which hamper production of other blood components. Watch for signs of hypercalcemia, renal failure, and spontaneous pathologic fractures.
● Apply direct pressure to the venipuncture site until bleeding stops.
● If a hematoma develops at the venipuncture site, apply pressure.

● Instruct the patient that he may resume his usual diet and medications discontinued before the test, as ordered.

## Precautions
● Send the sample to the laboratory immediately to prevent immunoglobulin deterioration.

## REFERENCE VALUES

When using nephelometry, serum immunoglobulin levels for adults range as follows:

- IgG — 800 to 1,800 mg/dl (SI, 8 to 18 g/L)
- IgA — 100 to 400 mg/dl (SI, 1 to 4 g/L)
- IgM — 55 to 150 mg/dl (SI, 0.55 to 1.5 g/L).

## ABNORMAL FINDINGS

The accompanying chart shows IgG, IgA, and IgM levels in various disorders. In congenital and acquired hypogammaglobulinemias, myelomas, and macroglobulinemia, the findings confirm the diagnosis. In hepatic and autoimmune diseases, leukemias, and lymphomas, such findings are less important, but they can support the diagnosis based on other tests, such as biopsies and white blood cell differential, and on the physical examination.

## INTERFERING FACTORS

- Chemotherapy or radiation therapy (possible decrease due to suppressive effects on bone marrow)
- Aminophenazone, anticonvulsants, asparaginase, hormonal contraceptives, hydralazine, hydantoin derivatives, and phenylbutazone (possible increase)
- Methotrexate and severe hypersensitivity to bacille Calmette-Guérin vaccine (possible decrease)
- Dextrans and methylprednisolone (decrease in IgM levels)
- Dextrans and high doses of methylprednisolone and phenytoin (decrease in IgG and IgA levels)
- Methadone (increase in IgA levels)

# Radioactive iodine uptake test

The radioactive iodine uptake (RAIU) test evaluates thyroid function by measuring the amount of orally ingested iodine 123 ($^{123}$I) or iodine 131 ($^{131}$I) that accumulates in the thyroid gland after 2, 6, and 24 hours. An external single counting probe measures the radioactivity in the thyroid as a percentage of the original dose, thus indicating its ability to trap and retain iodine. The RAIU test accurately diagnoses hyperthyroidism but is less accurate for hypothyroidism. When performed concurrently with radionuclide thyroid imaging and the triiodothyronine resin uptake test, the RAIU test helps differentiate Grave's disease from hyperfunctioning toxic adenoma. Indications for this test include abnormal results of chemical tests used to evaluate thyroid function.

Patients with suspected Hashimoto's disease may undergo the perchlorate suppression test in addition to the RAIU test. (See *Perchlorate suppression test,* page 368.)

## PURPOSE
- To evaluate thyroid function
- To help diagnose hyperthyroidism or hypothyroidism
- To help distinguish between primary and secondary thyroid disorders (in combination with other tests)

## PATIENT PREPARATION
- Tell the patient that the RAIU test assesses thyroid function.
- Instruct the patient to begin fasting at midnight the night before the test.
- Explain to the patient that he'll receive radioactive iodine (capsule or liquid) and that he'll then be scanned after 2 hours, 6 hours, and 24 hours.
- Assure the patient that the test is painless and that the small amount of radioactivity used is harmless.
- Check the patient's history for iodine exposure, which may interfere with test results. Note previous radiologic tests using contrast media, nuclear medicine procedures, or current use of iodine preparations or thyroid medications on the film request slip. Iodine hypersensitivity isn't considered a contraindication because the amount of iodine used is similar to that consumed in a normal diet.
- Make sure the patient or a responsible family member has signed an informed consent form, if required.

## PROCEDURE AND POSTTEST CARE
- After ingesting an oral dose of radioactive iodine, the patient's thyroid is scanned at 2, 6, and 24 hours by placing the anterior portion of his neck in front of an external single counting probe.
- The amount of radioactivity detected by the probe is compared with the amount of radioactivity contained in the original dose to determine the percentage of radioactive iodine retained by the thyroid.

● Instruct the patient to resume a light diet 2 hours after taking the oral dose of radioactive iodine. When the study is complete, the patient may resume his usual diet.

## PRECAUTIONS

● Know that RAIU testing is contraindicated during pregnancy and lactation because of possible teratogenic effects. It's also contraindicated in the patient who's allergic to iodine and shellfish.

## NORMAL FINDINGS

After 2 hours, 4% to 12% of the radioactive iodine should have accumulated in the thyroid; after 6 hours, 5% to 20%; at 24 hours, accumulation should be 8% to 29%. The remaining radioactive iodine is excreted in the urine. Local variations in the normal range of iodine uptake may occur due to regional differences in dietary iodine intake and procedural differences among laboratories.

## ABNORMAL FINDINGS

Below-normal iodine uptake may indicate hypothyroidism, subacute thyroiditis, or iodine overload. Above-normal uptake may indicate hyperthyroidism, early Hashimoto's disease, hypoalbuminemia, lithium ingestion, or iodine-deficient goiter. However, in hyperthyroidism, the rate of turnover may be so rapid that a false normal measurement occurs at 24 hours.

## INTERFERING FACTORS

● Diuresis; renal failure; severe diarrhea; X-ray contrast media studies; ingestion of iodine preparations, including cough syrups, iodized salt, and some multivitamins (decrease)

● Antihistamines, anticoagulants, corticosteroids, penicillins, phenylbutazone, salicylates, thyroid hormones, and thyroid hormone antagonists (decrease)

● Phenothiazines or an iodine-deficient diet (increase)

# Radionuclide renal imaging

Radionuclide renal imaging, which involves I.V. injection of a radionuclide followed by scintigraphy, provides a wealth of information for evaluating the kidneys. Observing the uptake concentration and transit of the radionuclide during this test allows assessment of renal blood flow, renal structure, and nephron and collecting system function. Depending on the patient's clinical presentation, this procedure may include dynamic scans to assess renal perfusion and function or static scans to assess structure.

The radioisotope injected depends on the specific information required and the examiner's preference. However, this procedure commonly includes double isotope technique to obtain a sequence of perfusion and function studies, followed by static images. This test may also be substituted for excretory urography in the patient with hypersensitivity to contrast agents.

## PURPOSE

- To detect and assess functional and structural renal abnormalities (such as lesions and renovascular hypertension) and acute or chronic disease (such as pyelonephritis or glomerulonephritis)
- To assess renal transplantation or renal injury due to trauma to the urinary tract or obstruction

## PATIENT PREPARATION

- Explain to the patient that radionuclide renal imaging permits the evaluation of the structure, blood flow, and function of the kidneys.
- Tell the patient who will perform the test and where. (If static scans are ordered, there will be a delay of several hours before the images are taken.)
- Inform the patient that he'll receive an injection of a radionuclide and that he may experience transient flushing and nausea.
- Emphasize to the patient that only a small amount of radionuclide is administered and that it's usually excreted within 24 hours.
- Tell the patient several series of films will be taken of his bladder.
- Make sure that the patient or a responsible family member has signed an informed consent form.
- Make sure that the patient isn't scheduled for other radionuclide scans on the same day as this test.
- If the patient receives antihypertensive medication, ask the physician if it should be withheld before the test.
- A pregnant patient or a young child may receive supersaturated solution of potassium iodide 1 to 3 hours before the test to block thyroid uptake of iodine.

## PROCEDURE AND POSTTEST CARE

- The patient is commonly placed in a prone position so that posterior views may be obtained. If the test is being performed to

evaluate transplantation, the patient is positioned supine for anterior views.
- Instruct the patient not to change his position.
- A perfusion study (radionuclide angiography) is performed first to evaluate renal blood flow. The technetium 99m ($^{99m}$Tc) is administered I.V., and rapid-sequence photographs (one per second) are taken for 1 minute.
- Next, a function study is performed to measure the transit time of the radionuclide through the kidneys' functional units. After Hippuran is administered intravenously, images are obtained at a rate of one per minute for 20 minutes. Alternatively, this entire procedure can be recorded on computer-compatible magnetic tape, and concurrent renogram curves can be plotted.
- Finally, static images are obtained 4 or more hours later, after the radionuclide has drained through the pelvicaliceal system.
- Instruct the patient to flush the toilet immediately after each voiding for 24 hours as a radiation precaution.
- If the patient is incontinent, change bed linens promptly and wear gloves to maintain standard precautions and prevent unnecessary skin contact.
- Monitor the infection site for signs of hematoma, infection, and discomfort. Apply warm compresses for comfort.
- Monitor the patient's intake and output and electrolyte, acid-base, blood urea nitrogen, and creatinine levels, as indicated.

## PRECAUTIONS

- Be aware that this test is contraindicated in a pregnant woman unless the benefits of the procedure outweigh the risk to the fetus.

## NORMAL FINDINGS

Because 25% of cardiac output goes directly to the kidneys, renal perfusion should be evident immediately following uptake of the $^{99m}$Tc in the abdominal aorta. Within 1 to 2 minutes, a normal pattern of renal circulation should appear. The radionuclide should delineate the kidneys simultaneously, symmetrically, and with equal intensity.

Hippuran administered for the function study rapidly outlines the kidneys — which should be normal in size, shape, and position — and also defines the collecting system and bladder. Maximum counts of the radionuclide in the kidneys occur within 5 minutes after injection (and within 1 minute of each other) and should fall to approximately one-third or less of the maximum counts in the same kidney within 25 minutes. Within this time, kidney function can be compared as the concentration of radionuclide shifts from the cortex to the pelvis and, finally, to the bladder.

Renal function is best evaluated by comparing these images with the renogram curves. Total function is considered normal when the effective renal plasma flow is 420 ml/minute or greater and the percentage of the dose excreted in the urine at 30 to 35 minutes is greater than 66%.

## ABNORMAL FINDINGS

Images from the perfusion study can identify impeded renal circulation, such as that caused by trauma and renal artery stenosis or renal infarction. These conditions may occur in the patient with renovascular hypertension or abdominal aortic disease. Because malignant renal tumors are usually vascular, these images can help differentiate tumors from cysts.

In evaluating a kidney transplant, abnormal perfusion may indicate obstruction of the vascular grafts. The function study can detect abnormalities of the collecting system and urine extravasation. Markedly decreased tubular function causes reduced radionuclide activity in the collecting system; outflow obstruction causes decreased radionuclide activity in the tubules, with increased activity in the collecting system.

This test can also define the level of ureteral obstruction.

Static images can demonstrate lesions, congenital abnormalities, and traumatic injury. These images also detect space-occupying lesions within or surrounding the kidney, such as tumors, infarcts, and inflammatory masses (abscesses, for example); they can also identify congenital disorders, such as horseshoe kidney and polycystic kidney disease. They can define regions of infarction, rupture, or hemorrhage after trauma.

A lower-than-normal total concentration of the radionuclide, as opposed to focal defects, suggests a diffuse renal disorder, such as acute tubular necrosis, severe infection, or ischemia. In a patient who has had a kidney

transplant, decreased radionuclide uptake generally indicates organ rejection. Failure of visualization may indicate congenital ectopia or aplasia.

Definitive diagnosis usually requires the combined analysis of static images, perfusion studies, and function studies.

## INTERFERING FACTORS

- Antihypertensives (possible masking of abnormalities)
- Scans of different organs performed on the same day (possible poor imaging

# *Radionuclide thyroid imaging*

In radionuclide thyroid imaging, the thyroid is studied by gamma camera after the patient receives a radioisotope (iodine 123 [$^{123}$I], technetium [$^{99m}$Tc] pertechnetate, or iodine 131 [$^{131}$I]). Thyroid imaging typically follows discovery of a palpable mass, an enlarged gland, or an asymmetrical goiter and is performed concurrently with thyroid uptake tests and measurements of serum triiodothyronine ($T_3$) and serum thyroxine ($T_4$) levels. Later, thyroid ultrasonography may be performed.

## PURPOSE

- To assess the size, structure, and position of the thyroid gland
- To evaluate thyroid function (in conjunction with other thyroid tests)

## PATIENT PREPARATION

- Tell the patient that radionuclide thyroid imaging helps determine the cause of thyroid dysfunction.
- If $^{123}$I or $^{131}$I will be used, tell the patient to fast after midnight the night before the test. Fasting isn't required if an I.V. injection of $^{99m}$Tc pertechnetate is used.
- Explain to the patient that after he receives the radiopharmaceutical, a gamma camera will be used to produce an image of his thyroid. Tell him that the imaging procedure will take about 30 minutes and assure him that his exposure to radiation is minimal.

Ask the patient if he has undergone tests that used radiographic contrast media within the past 60 days. Note previous radiographic contrast media exposure on the X-ray request.

Check the patient's diet and medication history. Medications, such as thyroid hormones, thyroid hormone antagonists, and iodine preparations (Lugol's solution, some multivitamins, and cough syrups) should be discontinued 2 to 3 weeks before the test, as ordered. Phenothiazines, corticosteroids, salicylates, anticoagulants, and antihistamines should be discontinued 1 week before the test, as ordered. Instruct the patient to stop consuming iodized salt, iodinated salt substitutes, and seafood for 14 to 21 days, as ordered. Liothyronine (Cytomel), propylthiouracil (PTU), and methimazole (Tapazole) should be discontinued 3 days before the test, and $T_4$ should be discontinued 10 days before the test, as ordered.

The patient receives $^{123}$I or $^{131}$I (oral) or $^{99m}$Tc pertechnetate (I.V.). Record the date and the time of administration.

The patient receiving an oral radioisotope should fast for another 2 hours after administration.

Just before the test, tell the patient to remove dentures, jewelry, and other materials that may interfere with the imaging process.

Make sure the patient or a responsible family member has signed an informed consent form, if required.

## PROCEDURE AND POSTTEST CARE

The test is performed 24 hours after oral administration of $^{123}$I or $^{131}$I or 20 to 30 minutes after I.V. injection of $^{99m}$Tc pertechnetate. Just before the test, tell the patient to remove his dentures and any jewelry that could interfere with visualization of the thyroid.

The patient is placed in a supine position with his neck extended; the thyroid gland is palpated. The gamma camera is positioned above the anterior portion of his neck.

Images of the patient's thyroid gland are projected on a monitor and are recorded on X-ray film. Three views of the thyroid are obtained: a straight-on anterior view and two bilateral oblique views.

Tell the patient that he may resume his usual diet and medications, as ordered.

## PRECAUTIONS

Be aware that radionuclide thyroid imaging is contraindicated during pregnancy and lactation and in the patient with a previous allergy to iodine, shellfish, or radioactive tracers.

## NORMAL FINDINGS

Normally, radionuclide thyroid imaging reveals a thyroid gland that's about 2″ (5 cm) long and 1″ (2.5 cm) wide, with a uniform uptake of the radioisotope and without tumors. The gland is butterfly-shaped, with the isthmus located at the midline. Occasionally, a third lobe called the pyramidal lobe may be present; this is a normal variant.

## ABNORMAL FINDINGS

During radionuclide thyroid imaging, hyperfunctioning nodules (areas of excessive iodine uptake) appear as black regions called *hot spots.* The presence of hot spots requires a follow-up $T_3$ thyroid suppression test to determine if the hyperfunctioning areas are autonomous. Hypofunctioning nodules (areas of little or no iodine uptake) appear as white or light gray regions called *cold spots.* If a cold spot appears, subsequent thyroid ultrasonography may be performed to rule out cysts; in addition, fine-needle aspiration and biopsy of such nodules may be performed to rule out malignancy. (See *Results of thyroid imaging in thyroid disorders,* page 372.)

## INTERFERING FACTORS

An iodine-deficient diet and phenothiazines (increase)

Decreased uptake of radioactive iodine due to renal disease; ingestion of iodized salt, iodine preparations, iodinated salt substitutes, or seafood; and use of aminosalicylic acid, corticosteroids, cough syrups containing inorganic iodine, multivitamins, thyroid hormones, or thyroid hormone antagonists (decrease)

Severe diarrhea and vomiting, impairing GI absorption of radioiodine (decrease)

# RESULTS OF THYROID IMAGING IN THYROID DISORDERS

This chart shows the characteristic findings in radionuclide imaging tests that are associated with various thyroid disorders as well as the possible causes of those disorders.

| CONDITION | FINDINGS | CAUSES |
|---|---|---|
| Hypothyroidism | ◆ Glandular damage or absent gland | ◆ Surgical removal of gland<br>◆ Inflammation<br>◆ Radiation<br>◆ Neoplasm (rare) |
| Hypothyroid goiter | ◆ Enlarged gland<br>◆ Decreased uptake (of radioactive iodine) if glandular destruction is present<br>◆ Increased uptake possible from congenital error in thyroxine synthesis | ◆ Insufficient iodine intake<br>◆ Hypersecretion of thyroid-stimulating hormone (TSH) caused by thyroid hormone deficiency |
| Myxedema (cretinismin in children) | ◆ Normal or slightly reduced gland size<br>◆ Uniform pattern<br>◆ Decreased uptake | ◆ Defective embryonic development, resulting in congenital absence or underdevelopment of thyroid gland<br>◆ Maternal iodine deficiency |
| Hyperthyroidism (Graves' disease) | ◆ Enlarged gland<br>◆ Uniform pattern<br>◆ Increased uptake | ◆ Unknown, but may be hereditary<br>◆ Production of thyroid-stimulating immunoglobulins |
| Toxic nodular goiter | ◆ Multiple hot spots | ◆ Long-standing simple goiter |
| Hyperfunctioning adenomas | ◆ Solitary hot spot | ◆ Adenomatous production of triiodothyronine and thyroxine, suppressing TSH secretion and producing atrophy of other thyroid tissue |
| Hypofunctioning adenomas | ◆ Solitary cold spot | ◆ Cyst or nonfunctioning nodule |
| Benign multinodular goiter | ◆ Multiple nodules with variable or no function | ◆ Local inflammation<br>◆ Degeneration |
| Thyroid carcinoma | ◆ Usually a solitary cold spot with occasional or no function | ◆ Neoplasm |

# Radiopharmaceutical myocardial perfusion imaging

Also known as *chemical stress imaging,* radiopharmaceutical myocardial perfusion imaging is an alternative method of assessing coronary vessel function in the patient who can't tolerate exercise electrocardiography (ECG).

In this test, I.V. infusion of a selected drug — for example, adenosine, dobutamine, or dipyridamole — is used to simulate the effects of exercise by increasing blood flow in the coronary arteries. Next, a radiopharmaceutical is injected I.V. to allow imaging that assists in evaluating the cardiac vessel's response to the drug-induced stress. Resting and stress images are obtained to evaluate coronary perfusion.

## PURPOSE

- To assess the presence and degree of coronary artery disease (CAD)
- To evaluate therapeutic procedures, such as bypass surgery or coronary angioplasty
- To evaluate myocardial perfusion

## PATIENT PREPARATION

- Describe to the patient what the radiopharmaceutical myocardial perfusion imaging test is, including who will perform it and where it will take place.
- Tell the patient that he'll need to arrive 1 hour before the test and that an I.V. line will be initiated before it begins.
- If the patient will receive adenosine or dipyridamole (Persantine), instruct him to avoid taking all theophylline medications for 24 to 36 hours and all caffeinated drinks for 12 hours before the test.
- If the patient will receive dobutamine (Dobutrex), instruct him to withhold beta-adrenergic blockers for 48 hours before the test. Also tell him not to eat for 3 to 4 hours before the test, although he may have water. Instruct him to take his other medications, as prescribed, with sips of water.
- Tell the patient to continue taking antihypertensive medications. If his systolic blood pressure is higher than 200 mm Hg, the dobutamine stress test can't be done until his blood pressure is under control.

**Alert** *Confirm that the female patient of childbearing age isn't pregnant before performing radiopharmaceutical myocardial perfusion imaging.*

- Tell the patient that a cardiologist, a nurse, an ECG technician, and a nuclear medicine technologist will be present for the medication infusion. Advise him that he'll be weighed first to determine the proper drug dose.
- Inform the patient that he may experience flushing, shortness of breath, dizziness, headache, chest pain, and increased heart rate during the infusion, but that these will end as soon as the infusion ends and that emergency equipment will be available, if needed.
- Screen the patient for bronchospastic lung disease or asthma. Adenosine and dipyridamole are contraindicated in these cases; use dobutamine instead. Weigh the patient to determine the appropriate dosage.
- Make sure that the patient or a responsible family member has signed an informed consent form.

## PROCEDURE AND POSTTEST CARE

- Place the patient on a bed or an examination table in the ECG or medical imaging department and start an I.V. line.
- Apply 12 ECG leadwires to appropriate sites and obtain baseline ECG and blood pressure readings.
- The selected chemical stress medication is infused, and blood pressure, pulse, and cardiac rhythm are monitored continuously.
- Tell the patient to report the symptoms he's feeling.
- At the appropriate time, the selected radiopharmaceutical is injected.
- Depending on which radiopharmaceutical is used, the patient either undergoes imaging immediately or is instructed to return for imaging 45 minutes to 2 hours later. Resting imaging may be done before stress imaging or 3 to 4 hours afterward, depending on the radiopharmaceutical used.
- Tell the patient when he needs to return and whether he should continue to fast.
- Remove the I.V. line after the images are completed.
- When all scans are completed, tell the patient that he may resume his usual diet.

- If the patient must return for further scanning, tell him to rest; he may also need to restrict foods and fluids in the interim.

## PRECAUTIONS
- Know that this test is usually contraindicated in a pregnant patient.
- Be aware that the use of adenosine or dipyridamole is contraindicated in the patient with bronchospastic lung disease or asthma.

  🌑 *Alert* *Keep resuscitation equipment available in case the patient experiences arrhythmias, angina, ST-segment depression, or bronchospasm.*

- Know that aminophylline, the reversal agent for adenosine and dipyridamole, can be administered to reverse severe adverse reactions.
- Keep in mind that contraindications include a myocardial infarction within 10 days of testing, acute myocarditis and pericarditis, unstable angina, arrhythmias, hypertension or hypotension, aortic or mitral stenosis, hyperthyroidism, and severe infection.
- Be aware that beta-adrenergic blockers, calcium channel blockers, and angiotensin-converting enzyme inhibitors should be withheld up to 36 hours before testing, as ordered. Nitrates should be withheld 6 hours before testing.

## NORMAL FINDINGS
Imaging should reveal characteristic distribution of the radiopharmaceutical throughout the left ventricle and show no visible defects.

## ABNORMAL FINDINGS
Cold spots are usually due to CAD, but may result from myocardial fibrosis, attenuation due to soft tissue (for example, breasts and diaphragm), or coronary spasm. The absence of cold spots in the presence of CAD may result from insignificant artifact obstruction, single-vessel disease, or collateral circulation.

## INTERFERING FACTORS
- Certain drugs such as digoxin (may produce a false-positive reading)
- Cold spots due to artifacts, such as implants and electrodes
- Delayed imaging (may cause absence of cold spots in the presence of CAD)

## *Rapid corticotropin test*
—◆—

The rapid corticotropin test (also known as the *cosyntropin test*) is gradually replacing the 8-hour corticotropin stimulation test as the most effective diagnostic tool for evaluating adrenal hypofunction. Using cosyntropin, the rapid corticotropin test provides faster results and causes fewer allergic reactions than does the 8-hour test, which uses natural corticotropin from animal sources.

This test requires prior determination of baseline cortisol levels to evaluate the effect of cosyntropin administration on cortisol secretion. An unequivocally high morning cortisol level rules out adrenal hypofunction and makes further testing unnecessary.

## PURPOSE
- To aid in identification of primary and secondary adrenal hypofunction

## PATIENT PREPARATION
- Explain to the patient that the rapid corticotropin test helps determine if his condition is due to a hormonal deficiency.
- Inform him that he may be required to fast for 10 to 12 hours before the test and must be relaxed and resting quietly for 30 minutes before the test.
- Tell him that the test takes at least 1 hour to perform.
- If the patient is an inpatient, withhold corticotropin and all steroid medications, as ordered. If he's an outpatient, tell him to refrain from taking these drugs, if instructed by his physician. If the drugs must be continued, note this on the laboratory request.
- Explain to the patient that he may experience slight discomfort from the tourniquet and needle puncture.

## PROCEDURE AND POSTTEST CARE
- Draw 5 ml of blood for a baseline value. Collect the sample in a 5-ml heparinized tube. Label this sample "preinjection" and send it to the laboratory.
- Inject 250 mcg (0.25 mg) of cosyntropin I.V. or I.M. (I.V. administration provides more accurate results because ineffective absorption after I.M. administration may cause

wide variations in response.) Direct I.V. injection should take about 2 minutes.

● Draw another 5 ml of blood at 30 and 60 minutes after the cosyntropin injection. Collect the samples in 5-ml heparinized tubes. Label the samples "30 minutes postinjection" and "60 minutes postinjection" and send them to the laboratory. Include the collection times on the laboratory request.

● Apply direct pressure to the venipuncture site until bleeding stops.

● If a hematoma develops at the venipuncture site, apply pressure.

● Observe the patient for signs of a rare allergic reaction to cosyntropin, such as hives, itching, and tachycardia.

● Instruct the patient that he may resume his usual diet, activities, and medications discontinued before the test, as ordered.

## PRECAUTIONS
● Handle the samples gently to prevent hemolysis. They require no special precautions other than avoiding stasis.

## REFERENCE VALUES
Normally, cortisol levels rise after 30 to 60 minutes to a peak of 18 mg/dl (SI, 500 mmol/L) or more 60 minutes after the cosyntropin injection. Generally, doubling the baseline value indicates a normal response.

## ABNORMAL FINDINGS
A normal result excludes adrenal hypofunction (insufficiency). In the patient with primary adrenal hypofunction (Addison's disease), cortisol levels remain low. Thus, the rapid corticotropin test provides an effective method of screening for adrenal hypofunction. If test results show subnormal increases in cortisol levels, prolonged stimulation of the adrenal cortex may be required to differentiate between primary and secondary adrenal hypofunction.

## INTERFERING FACTORS
● Amphetamines and estrogens (increase in plasma cortisol)
● Obesity and smoking  (possible increase in plasma cortisol)
● Lithium carbonate (decrease in plasma cortisol)
● Radioactive scan performed within 1 week before the test

# Rapid monoclonal test for cytomegalovirus

Cytomegalovirus (CMV), a member of the herpesvirus group, can cause systemic infection in congenitally infected infants and in immunocompromised patients, such as transplant recipients, patients receiving chemotherapy for neoplastic disease, and those with acquired immunodeficiency syndrome (AIDS).

In the past, CMV infections were detected in the laboratory by recognizing the distinctive cytopathic effects (CPE) that the virus produced in conventional tube cell cultures. In this slow method of detecting CMV, CPE cultures grow in about 9 days. The faster shell vial assay (rapid monoclonal test) is based on the availability of a monoclonal antibody specific for the 72 kd protein of CMV synthesized during the immediate early stage of viral replication.

Through indirect immunofluorescence, CMV-infected fibroblasts are recognized by their dense, homogeneous staining confined to the nucleus. Because of the smooth, regular shape of the nucleus and the surrounding nuclear membrane, infected cells are readily differentiated from nonspecific background fluorescence that may be present in some specimens.

## PURPOSE
● To obtain rapid laboratory diagnosis of CMV infection, especially in the immunocompromised patient who currently has, or is at risk for developing, systemic infections caused by this virus

## PATIENT PREPARATION
● Explain the purpose of the rapid monoclonal test for CMV, and describe the procedure for collecting the specimen, which will depend on the laboratory used.

## PROCEDURE AND POSTTEST CARE
● Specimens should be collected during the prodromal and acute stages of clinical infection to maximize the chances of detecting CMV.

● Each type of specimen requires a specific collection device, as listed below:

– for throat—microbiologic transport swab

– for urine or cerebrospinal fluid—sterile screw-capped tube or vial

– for bronchoalveolar lavage tissue—sterile screw-capped jar

– for blood—sterile tube with anticoagulant (heparin).

## PRECAUTIONS

● Transport the specimen to the laboratory as soon as possible after the collection. If the anticipated time between collection and inoculation into shell vial cell cultures is longer than 3 hours, store the specimen at 39.2° F (4° C). Don't freeze the specimen or allow it to become dry.

● Use gloves when obtaining and handling all specimens.

## NORMAL FINDINGS

CMV shouldn't appear in a culture specimen.

## ABNORMAL FINDINGS

CMV can be detected in urine and throat specimens from an asymptomatic patient. However, detection from these sites indicates active, asymptomatic infection, which may herald symptomatic involvement, especially in the immunocompromised patient. Detection of CMV in specimens of blood, tissue, and bronchoalveolar lavage generally indicates systemic infection and disease.

## INTERFERING FACTORS

● Administration of antiviral drugs before collecting the specimen

# Red blood cell count

The red blood cell (RBC) count, also called an *erythrocyte count,* is part of a complete blood count. It's used to detect the number of RBCs in a microliter (µl), or cubic millimeter (mm³), of whole blood. RBC count itself provides no qualitative information regarding the size, shape, or concentration of hemoglobin (Hb) within the corpuscles, but it may be used to calculate two erythrocyte indices: mean corpuscular volume (MCV) and mean corpuscular hemoglobin (MCH).

## PURPOSE

● To provide data for calculating MCV and MCH, which reveal RBC size and Hb content

● To support other hematologic tests for diagnosing anemia or polycythemia

## PATIENT PREPARATION

● Explain to the patient that the RBC count is used to evaluate the number of RBCs and to detect possible blood disorders.

● Tell the patient that a blood sample will be taken. Explain who will perform the venipuncture and when and where it will take place.

● Explain to the patient that he may feel slight discomfort from the tourniquet and needle puncture.

**Alert** *If the patient is a child, explain to him (if he's old enough) and his parents that a small amount of blood will be taken from his finger or earlobe.*

● Inform the patient that he need not restrict food and fluids.

## PROCEDURE AND POSTTEST CARE

● For adults and older children, draw venous blood into a 3- or 4.5-ml EDTA sodium metabisulfite solution tube.

**Alert** *For younger children, collect capillary blood in a microcollection device.*

● Make sure that subdermal bleeding has stopped before removing pressure.

● If a hematoma develops at the venipuncture site, apply pressure.

## PRECAUTIONS

● Fill the collection tube completely.

● Invert the tube gently several times to mix the sample and the anticoagulant.

● Handle the sample gently to prevent hemolysis.

## REFERENCE VALUES

Normal RBC values vary, depending on the type of sample and on the patient's age and sex, as follows:

● adult males—4.5 to 5.5 million RBCs/µl (SI, 4.5 to 5.5 × $10^{12}$/L) of venous blood

● adult females—4 to 5 million RBCs/µl (SI, 4 to 5 × $10^{12}$/L) of venous blood.

**Alert** *Reference values for infants and children also vary depending on age:*

● *full-term neonates—4.4 to 5.8 million/µl (SI, 4.4 to 5.8 × $10^{12}$/L) of capillary blood at birth,*

*decreasing to 3 to 3.8 million /µl (SI, 3 to 3.8 ×*
*10¹²/L) at age 2 months, and increasing slowly*
*thereafter*
- *children—4.6 to 4.8 million/µl (SI, 4.6 to 4.8*
*× 10¹²/L) of venous blood.*

Normal values may exceed these levels in patients living at high altitudes or those who are very active.

## ABNORMAL FINDINGS
An elevated RBC count may indicate absolute or relative polycythemia. A depressed count may indicate anemia, dilution due to fluid overload, or hemorrhage beyond 24 hours. Further tests, such as stained cell examination, hematocrit, Hb, red cell indices, and white cell studies, are needed to confirm the diagnosis.

## INTERFERING FACTORS
- Hemoconcentration due to prolonged tourniquet constriction
- Hemodilution due to drawing the sample from the same arm used for I.V. infusion of fluids
- High white blood cell count (false-high test results in semiautomated and automated counters)
- Diseases that cause RBCs to agglutinate or form rouleaux (false decrease)
- Hemolysis due to rough handling of the sample or drawing the blood through a small-gauge needle for venipuncture

# Red blood cell survival time

Normally, red blood cells (RBCs) are destroyed only when they reach senility. However, in hemolytic diseases, RBCs of all ages are randomly destroyed, resulting in anemia. The RBC survival time test measures the survival time of circulating RBCs and detects sites of abnormal RBC sequestration and destruction.

Survival time is measured by labeling a random sample of RBCs with radioactive chromium-51 sodium chromate (51Cr). This labeled group of RBCs is then injected back into the patient. Serial blood samples measure the percentage of labeled cells per unit volume over 3 to 4 weeks until 50% of the cells disappear. (The disappearance rate cor-

responds to destruction of a random cell population.)

A normal RBC survives about 120 days (half-life of 60 days); the 51Cr-labeled RBCs have a shorter half-life (25 to 30 days) because about 1% of senescent RBCs are removed from the circulation each day and about 1% of 51Cr is spontaneously eluted from the labeled RBCs each day.

During the test period, a gamma camera scans the body for sites of abnormally high radioactivity, which indicates sites of excessive RBC sequestration and destruction. Other tests performed with the RBC survival time test may include spot-checks of the stool to detect GI blood loss, hematocrit, blood volume studies, and radionuclide iron uptake and clearance tests to aid in the differential diagnosis of anemia.

## PURPOSE
- To help evaluate unexplained anemia, particularly hemolytic anemia
- To identify sites of abnormal RBC sequestration and destruction

## PATIENT PREPARATION
- Explain to the patient that the RBC survival time test helps identify the cause of his anemia.
- Advise the patient that he need not restrict food and fluids.
- Explain to the patient that the test involves labeling a blood sample with a radioactive substance and requires regular blood samples at 3-day intervals for 3 to 4 weeks. Tell him who will perform the test and when and where it will take place.
- Tell the patient that he may experience discomfort from the needle punctures and the tourniquet. Reassure him that collecting each sample takes less than 3 minutes and that the small amount of radioactive substance used is harmless.
- If stool collection is required to test for GI bleeding, teach the patient the proper collection technique.
- Make sure that the patient or a responsible family member has signed an informed consent form.

## PROCEDURE AND POSTTEST CARE
- A 30-ml blood sample is drawn and mixed with 100 microcuries of 51Cr for an adult.

• After an incubation period, the mixture is injected I.V. into the patient. A blood sample is drawn 30 minutes after injection to determine blood and RBC volumes.
• A 6-ml sample is collected in a heparinized tube after 24 hours; follow-up samples are collected at 3-day intervals for 3 to 4 weeks. (Intervals between samples may vary, depending on the laboratory.)
• To avoid error from physical decay of the 51Cr, each sample is measured with a scintillation well counter on the day it's drawn.
• Radioactivity per milliliter of RBCs is calculated, and the values are plotted to determine mean RBC survival time. Simultaneous gamma camera scans of the precordium, sacrum, liver, and spleen detect radioactivity at sites of excess RBC sequestration. A hematocrit test is done on a small portion of each blood sample to check for blood loss.
• At the end of the study, a sample is drawn to compare ending blood and RBC volumes with beginning volumes.
• If a hematoma develops at the venipuncture site, apply pressure.

## PRECAUTIONS
• Know that this test is contraindicated during pregnancy because it exposes the fetus to radiation.
• Be aware that because excess blood loss can invalidate test results, this test is usually contraindicated for a patient with active bleeding or poor clotting function. However, if the test is necessary for a patient with poor clotting function, observe the venipuncture sites carefully for signs of hemorrhage.
• Make sure that the patient doesn't receive blood transfusions during the test period and doesn't have blood samples drawn for other tests.

## NORMAL FINDINGS
The normal half-life for RBCs labeled with 51Cr is 25 to 30 days. Normal gamma camera scans reveal slight radioactivity in the spleen, liver, and sometimes the bone marrow.

## ABNORMAL FINDINGS
Decreased RBC survival time indicates a hemolytic disease, such as chronic lymphocytic leukemia, congenital nonspherocytic hemolytic anemia, hemoglobin C disease, hereditary spherocytosis, idiopathic acquired hemolytic anemia, paroxysmal nocturnal he-

moglobinuria, elliptocytosis, pernicious anemia, sickle cell anemia, sickle cell hemoglobin C disease, or hemolytic-uremic syndrome. If hemolytic anemia is diagnosed, additional tests using cross-transfusion of labeled RBCs can determine whether anemia results from an intrinsic RBC defect or an extrinsic factor.
A gamma camera scan that detects a site of excess RBC sequestration provides direction for treatment. For example, abnormally high RBC sequestration in the spleen may require a splenectomy.

## INTERFERING FACTORS
• Blood loss, dehydration, or overhydration (possible invalidation of results due to changed circulating RBC volume)
• Blood transfusions during the test period (alters proportion of labeled RBCs to total RBCs)

# Red cell indices

Using the results of the red blood cell (RBC) count, hematocrit (HCT), and total hemoglobin (Hb) tests, red cell indices (erythrocyte indices) provide important information about the size, Hb concentration, and Hb weight of an average RBC.

## PURPOSE
• To aid diagnosis and classification of anemias

## PATIENT PREPARATION
• Explain to the patient that red cell indices help determine if he has anemia.
• Tell the patient that a blood sample will be taken. Explain who will perform the venipuncture and when and where the test will take place.
• Explain to the patient that he may feel slight discomfort from the tourniquet and needle puncture.

## PROCEDURE AND POSTTEST CARE
• Perform a venipuncture and collect the sample in a 3- or 4.5-ml EDTA tube.
• Make sure subdermal bleeding has stopped before removing pressure.

## COMPARATIVE RED CELL INDICES IN ANEMIAS

|        | NORMAL VALUES (Normocytic, normochromic) | IRON DEFICIENCY (Microcytic, hypochromic) | PERNICIOUS ANEMIA (Macrocytic, normochromic) |
|--------|------------------------------------------|-------------------------------------------|----------------------------------------------|
| MCV    | 84 to 99 $\mu m^3$                       | 60 to 80 $\mu m^3$                        | 96 to 150 $\mu m^3$                          |
| MCH    | 26 to 32 pg/cell                         | 5 to 25 pg/cell                           | 33 to 53 pg/cell                             |
| MCHC   | 30 to 36 g/dl                            | 20 to 30 g/dl                             | 33 to 38 g/dl                                |

KEY: MCV = Mean corpuscular volume
MCH = Mean corpuscular hemoglobin
MCHC = Mean corpuscular hemoglobin concentration

● If a hematoma develops at the venipuncture site, apply pressure. If the hematoma is large, monitor pulses distal to the phlebotomy site.

## PRECAUTIONS
● Completely fill the collection tube and invert it gently several times to adequately mix the sample and the anticoagulant.
● Handle the sample gently to prevent hemolysis.

## REFERENCE VALUES
The indices tested include mean corpuscular volume (MCV), mean corpuscular hemoglobin (MCH), and mean corpuscular hemoglobin concentration (MCHC).

MCV, the ratio of HCT (packed cell volume) to the RBC count, expresses the average size of the erythrocytes and indicates whether they're undersized (microcytic), oversized (macrocytic), or normal (normocytic). MCH, the Hb-RBC ratio, gives the weight of Hb in an average red cell. MCHC, the ratio of Hb weight to HCT, defines the concentration of Hb in 100 ml of packed RBCs. It helps to distinguish normally colored (normochromic) RBCs from paler (hypochromic) RBCs.

The range of normal red cell indices is as follows:
● MCV—84 to 99 $\mu m^3$
● MCH—26 to 32 pg/cell
● MCHC—30 to 36 g/dl.

## ABNORMAL FINDINGS
Low MCV and MCHC indicate microcytic, hypochromic anemias caused by iron deficiency anemia, pyridoxine-responsive anemia, or thalassemia. A high MCV suggests macrocytic anemias caused by megaloblastic anemias, folic acid or vitamin $B_{12}$ deficiency, inherited disorders of deoxyribonucleic acid synthesis, or reticulocytosis. Because the MCV reflects the average volume of many cells, a value within the normal range can encompass RBCs of varying size, from microcytic to macrocytic. (See *Comparative red cell indices in anemias*.)

## INTERFERING FACTORS
● Hemoconcentration due to prolonged tourniquet constriction
● High white blood cell count (false-high RBC count in semiautomated and automated counters, invalidating MCV and MCHC results)
● Falsely elevated Hb values, invalidating MCH and MCHC results
● Diseases that cause RBCs to agglutinate or form rouleaux (false-low RBC count)

## Renal angiography

Renal angiography requires arterial injection of a contrast medium and permits radiographic examination of the renal vasculature and parenchyma. As the contrast pervades the renal vasculature, rapid-sequence radiographs show the vessels during three phases of filling: arterial, nephrographic, and venous.

This procedure usually follows standard bolus aortography, which shows individual variations in number, size, and condition of the main renal arteries, aberrant vessels, and the relationship of the renal arteries to the aorta.

## PURPOSE

- To demonstrate the configuration of total renal vasculature before surgical procedures
- To determine the cause of renovascular hypertension, such as from stenosis, thrombotic occlusions, emboli, and aneurysms
- To evaluate chronic renal disease or renal failure
- To investigate renal masses and renal trauma
- To detect complications following kidney transplantation, such as a nonfunctioning shunt or rejection of the donor organ
- To differentiate highly vascular tumors from avascular cysts

## PATIENT PREPARATION

- Explain to the patient that renal angiography permits visualization of the kidneys, blood vessels, and functional units and aids in diagnosing renal disease or masses.
- Instruct the patient to fast for 8 hours before the test and to drink extra fluids the day before the test and the day after the test to maintain adequate hydration (or to start an I.V. line, if needed). Oral medication may be continued; a special order is needed for the patient with diabetes.
- Tell the patient he may receive a laxative or an enema the evening before the test.
- Tell the patient who will perform the test and when and where it will take place.
- Describe the procedure to the patient and inform him that he may experience transient discomfort (flushing, burning sensation, and nausea) during injection of the contrast medium.
- Make sure that the patient or a responsible family member has signed an informed consent form.

*Alert  Check the patient's history for hypersensitivity to iodine-based contrast media or iodine-containing foods such as shellfish. Mark sensitivities on the chart and inform the physician because the patient may require prophylactic antiallergenics (corticosteroids or diphenhydramine).*

- Administer prescribed medications (usually a sedative and a narcotic analgesic) before the test.
- Instruct the patient to put on a gown and to remove all metallic objects that may interfere with test results.
- Ask the patient to void before leaving the unit.
- Record the patient's baseline vital signs. Make sure that recent laboratory test results (blood urea nitrogen and serum creatinine levels and bleeding studies) are documented on the patient's chart. Verification of adequate renal function and adequate clotting ability is vital.
- Evaluate peripheral pulse sites and mark them for easy access in postprocedure assessment.

## PROCEDURE AND POSTTEST CARE

- The patient is placed in a supine position, and a peripheral I.V. infusion is started. The skin over the arterial puncture site is cleaned with antiseptic solution, and a local anesthetic is injected.
- The femoral artery is punctured and, under fluoroscopic visualization, cannulated. (If a femoral pulse is absent or the artery is convoluted or plaque-ridden, percutaneous transaxillary, transbrachial, or translumbar catheterization may be performed instead.)
- After passing the flexible guide wire through the artery, the cannula is withdrawn, leaving several inches of wire in the lumen.
- A polyethylene catheter is passed over the wire and advanced, under fluoroscopic guidance, up the femoroiliac vessels to the aorta. The guide wire is removed, and the catheter is flushed with heparin flush solution.
- The contrast medium is injected, and screening aortograms are taken before proceeding.
- On completion of the aortographic study, a renal catheter is exchanged for the vascular catheter.
- To determine the position of the renal arteries and make sure that the tip of the catheter is in the lumen, a test bolus (3 to 5 ml) of contrast medium is injected immediately.
- If the patient has no adverse reaction to the contrast medium, 20 to 25 ml of the sub-

stance is injected just below the origin of the renal arteries.

- A series of rapid-sequence X-ray films of the filling of the renal vascular tree is exposed.
- If additional selective studies are required, the catheter remains in place while the films are examined. If the films are satisfactory, the catheter is removed.
- Apply a sterile pad firmly to the puncture site for 15 minutes.
- Before the patient is returned to his room, observe the puncture site for a hematoma.
- Keep the patient flat in bed and instruct him to keep the punctured leg straight for at least 6 hours or as otherwise ordered.
- Check the patient's vital signs every 15 minutes for 1 hour, every 30 minutes for 2 hours, and then every hour until they stabilize.
- Monitor popliteal and dorsalis pedis pulses for adequate perfusion at least every hour for 4 hours. Note the color and temperature of the involved extremity and compare with the uninvolved extremity. Watch for signs of pain or paresthesia in the involved limb.
- Watch for bleeding or hematomas at the injection site. Keep the pressure dressing in place and check for bleeding when you check the patient's vital signs. If bleeding occurs, promptly notify the physician and apply direct pressure or a sandbag to the site.
- Apply cold compresses to the puncture site to reduce edema and lessen pain.
- *Alert* Provide the patient with extra fluids (2,000 to 3,000 ml) in the 24-hour period after the test to prevent nephrotoxicity from the contrast medium. Also monitor for anaphylaxis from the contrast medium. (Signs include cardiorespiratory distress, renal failure, and shock.)
- Monitor the patient for atrial arrhythmias and evaluate aspartate aminotransferase and lactate dehydrogenase activity if renal stenosis is observed.

## PRECAUTIONS

- Know that renal angiography is contraindicated during pregnancy and in the patient with bleeding tendencies, allergy to contrast media, or renal failure caused by end-stage renal disease.

## NORMAL FINDINGS

Renal arteriographs show normal arborization of the vascular tree and normal architecture of the renal parenchyma.

## ABNORMAL FINDINGS

Renal tumors usually show hypervascularity; renal cysts typically appear as clearly delineated, radiolucent masses. Renal artery stenosis caused by arteriosclerosis produces a noticeable constriction in the blood vessels, usually within the proximal portion of its length; this is a crucial finding in confirming renovascular hypertension. Renal artery dysplasia, unlike renal artery stenosis, usually affects the middle and distal portions of the vessel. Alternating aneurysms and stenotic regions give this rare disorder a characteristic beads-on-a-string appearance.

In renal infarction, blood vessels may appear to be absent or cut off, with the normal tissue replaced by scar tissue. Another typical finding is the appearance of triangular areas of infarcted tissue near the periphery of the affected kidney. The kidney itself may appear shrunken due to tissue scarring.

Renal angiography may also detect renal artery aneurysms (saccular or fusiform) and renal arteriovenous fistula with abnormal widening of and direct passage between the renal artery and renal vein. Destruction, distortion, and fibrosis of renal tissue with areas of reduced and tortuous vascularity may be noted in severe or chronic pyelonephritis, and an increase in capsular vessels with abnormal intrarenal circulation may indicate renal abscesses or inflammatory masses.

When angiography is used to evaluate renal trauma, it may detect an intrarenal hematoma, a parenchymal laceration, shattered kidneys, and areas of infarction. Renal angiography may also be useful in distinguishing pseudotumors from tumors or cysts, in evaluating the volume of residual functioning renal tissue in hydronephrosis, and in evaluating donors and recipients before and after renal transplantation.

## INTERFERING FACTORS

- Patient movement
- Recent contrast studies, such as barium enema or an upper GI series (possible poor imaging)
- Presence of stool or gas in the GI tract (possible poor imaging)

# Renal computed tomography

Renal computed tomography (CT) provides a useful image of the kidneys made from a series of tomograms or cross-sectional slices, which are then translated by a computer and displayed on a monitor. The image density reflects the amount of radiation absorbed by renal tissue and permits identification of masses and other lesions. An I.V. contrast medium may be injected to accentuate the renal parenchyma's density and help differentiate renal masses. This highly accurate test is usually performed to investigate diseases found by other diagnostic procedures such as excretory urography.

## PURPOSE
● To detect and evaluate renal abnormalities, such as a tumor, an obstruction, calculi, polycystic kidney disease, congenital anomalies, and abnormal fluid accumulation around the kidneys
● To evaluate the retroperitoneum

## PATIENT PREPARATION
● Explain to the patient that renal CT permits examination of the kidneys.
● If contrast enhancement isn't scheduled, inform the patient that he need not restrict food and fluids. If contrast enhancement is scheduled, instruct him to fast for 4 hours before the test.
● Tell the patient who will perform the test and when and where it will take place.
● Inform the patient that he'll be positioned on an X-ray table and that a scanner will take films of his kidneys.
● Warn the patient that the scanner may make loud, clacking sounds as it rotates around his body.
● Tell the patient that he may experience transient adverse effects, such as flushing, a metallic taste, and headache, after contrast medium injection.
● Make sure that the patient or a responsible family member has signed an informed consent form.
  *Alert* Check the patient's history for hypersensitivity to shellfish, iodine, or contrast media. Mark any sensitivities in his chart.

● Just before the procedure, instruct the patient to put on a gown and to remove any metallic objects that could interfere with the scan.
● Administer prescribed sedatives.

## PROCEDURE AND POSTTEST CARE
● The patient is placed in a supine position on the X-ray table and secured with straps.
● The table is moved into the scanner.
● Instruct the patient to lie still.
● The scanner then rotates around the patient, taking multiple images at different angles within each cross-sectional slice.
● When one series of tomograms is complete, I.V. contrast enhancement may be performed. Another series of tomograms is then taken.
● After the I.V. contrast medium is administered, monitor the patient for allergic reactions, such as respiratory difficulty, urticaria, or skin eruptions.
● Information from the scan is stored on a disk or magnetic tape, fed into a computer, and converted into an image for display on a monitor. Radiographs and photographs are taken of selected views.
● If the procedure was performed with contrast enhancement, observe the patient for hypersensitivity to the contrast medium.
● After the test, tell the patient that he may resume his usual diet.
● If calculi are present, strain urine, hydrate the patient, and discuss nutritional adaptations as indicated.
● Support the patient and his family if surgery is indicated for a neoplasm.
● Monitor the patient's vital signs if a sedative was administered.

## PRECAUTIONS
● Watch for signs of hypersensitivity to the contrast medium if contrast enhancement is required.

## NORMAL FINDINGS
Normally, the density of the renal parenchyma is slightly higher than that of the liver, but is much less dense than bone, which appears white on a CT scan. The density of the collecting system is generally low (black), unless a contrast medium is used to enhance it to a higher (whiter) density. (See *Abnormal renal CT scan.*)

# ABNORMAL RENAL CT SCAN

This photograph of a renal computed tomography (CT) scan reveals a renal adenocarcinoma that has displaced and distorted the right kidney and that now exceeds the kidney in size. The left kidney appears normal, the spine is sharp and white in the center, and the stomach is equally clear at the top.

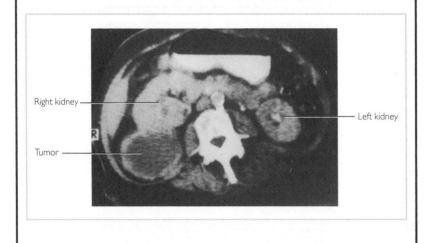

Right kidney

Left kidney

Tumor

The position of the kidneys is evaluated according to the surrounding structures; their size and shape are determined by counting cuts between the superior and inferior poles and following the contour of the kidneys' outline.

## ABNORMAL FINDINGS

Renal masses appear as areas of different density than do normal parenchyma, possibly altering the kidneys' shape or projecting beyond their margins. Renal cysts, for example, appear as smooth, sharply defined masses with thin walls and a lower density than do normal parenchyma.

Tumors, such as renal cell carcinoma, however, are usually not as well delineated; they tend to have thick walls and nonuniform density. With contrast enhancement, solid tumors show a higher density than renal cysts, but lower density than normal parenchyma. Tumors with hemorrhage, calcification, or necrosis show higher densities. Vascular tumors are more clearly defined with contrast enhancement. Adrenal tumors are confined masses, usually detached from

the kidneys and from other retroperitoneal organs.

Renal CT scanning may also identify other abnormalities, including obstructions, calculi, polycystic kidney disease, congenital anomalies, and abnormal accumulations of fluid around the kidneys, such as hematomas, lymphoceles, and abscesses. After nephrectomy, CT scanning can detect abnormal masses, such as recurrent tumors, in a renal fossa that should be empty.

## INTERFERING FACTORS
- Patient's inability to remain still
- Presence of contrast media from other recent tests or of foreign bodies, such as catheters or surgical clips (possible poor imaging)

## *Renal ultrasonography*

In renal ultrasonography, high-frequency sound waves are transmitted from a transducer to the kidneys and perirenal structures.

The resulting echoes are displayed on a monitor as anatomic images.

Renal ultrasonography can be used to detect abnormalities or clarify those detected by other tests. It's especially useful in cases in which excretory urography is ruled out. Unlike excretory urography, this test isn't dependent on renal function and, therefore, may be useful in the patient with renal failure. Ultrasonography of the ureter, bladder, and gonads also may be used to evaluate urologic disorders.

## PURPOSE

● To determine the size, shape, and position of the kidneys, their internal structures, and perirenal tissues
● To evaluate and localize urinary obstruction and abnormal fluid accumulation
● To assess and diagnose complications after kidney transplantation
● To detect renal or perirenal masses
● To differentiate between renal cysts and solid masses
● To verify placement of a nephrostomy tube

## PATIENT PREPARATION

● Explain to the patient that renal ultrasonography is used to detect kidney abnormalities.
● Inform the patient that he need not restrict food and fluids.
● Tell the patient who will perform the test, when and where it will take place, and that it's safe and painless.

## PROCEDURE AND POSTTEST CARE

● The patient is placed in the prone position, the area to be scanned is exposed, and conductive gel is applied.
● The longitudinal axis of the kidneys is located by using measurements from excretory urography or by performing transverse scans through the upper and lower renal poles.
● These points are marked on the skin and connected with straight lines. Sectional images $3/8''$ to $3/4''$ (1 to 2 cm) apart can then be obtained by moving the transducer longitudinally, transversely, or at any other angle required.
● During the test, the patient may be asked to breathe deeply to visualize upper portions of the kidney.

● After the test, remove the conductive gel from the patient's skin.
● If bladder abnormalities are found, prepare the patient for further testing.
● If rejection of a transplanted kidney is suspected or diagnosed, monitor the patient's intake and output, blood pressure, blood urea nitrogen and creatinine levels, and vital signs. In addition, monitor for adrenal dysfunction (hypotension, decreased urine output, and electrolyte imbalances) if a tumor is detected on the gland.
● If ultrasonography is used as a guide for nephrostomy tube placement or abscess drainage, monitor the amount and characteristics of drainage and tube patency.

## PRECAUTIONS

● None

## NORMAL FINDINGS

The kidneys are located between the superior iliac crests and the diaphragm. The renal capsule should be outlined sharply; the cortex should produce more echoes than does the medulla. In the center of each kidney, the renal collecting systems appear as irregular areas of higher density than surrounding tissue. The renal veins and, depending on the scanner, some internal structures can be visualized. If the bladder is also being evaluated, its size, shape, position, and urine content can be determined.

## ABNORMAL FINDINGS

Cysts are usually fluid-filled, circular structures that don't reflect sound waves. Tumors produce multiple echoes and appear as irregular shapes. Abscesses found within or around the kidneys usually echo sound waves poorly; their boundaries are slightly more irregular than those of cysts. A perirenal abscess may displace the kidney anteriorly.

Generally, acute pyelonephritis and glomerulonephritis aren't detectable unless the renal parenchyma is significantly scarred and atrophied. In such cases, the renal capsule appears irregular and the kidney may appear smaller than normal; also, an increased number of echoes may arise from the parenchyma due to fibrosis.

In the patient with hydronephrosis, renal ultrasonography may show a large, echo-free, central mass that compresses the renal cortex. Calyceal echoes are usually circularly diffused and the pelvis significantly enlarged. This test can also be used to detect congenital anomalies, such as horseshoe, ectopic, or duplicated kidneys. Ultrasonography clearly detects renal hypertrophy.

Following kidney transplantation, compensatory hypertrophy of the transplanted kidney is normal, but an acute increase in size indicates rejection.

This test allows identification of abnormal accumulations of fluid within or around the kidneys that sometimes arise from an obstruction. It also allows evaluation of perirenal structures and can identify abnormalities of the adrenal glands, such as tumors, cysts, and adrenal dysfunction. However, a normal adrenal gland is difficult to define ultrasonically because of its small size.

Renal ultrasonography can be used to detect changes in the shape of the bladder that result from masses and can assess urine volume. Increased urine volume or residual urine after voiding may indicate bladder outlet obstruction.

## INTERFERING FACTORS
- Retained barium from a previous test (possible poor imaging)
- An obese patient (possible poor imaging)

# Renal venography

Renal venography is a relatively simple procedure allowing radiographic examination of the main renal veins and their tributaries. In this test, contrast medium is injected by percutaneous catheter passed through the femoral vein and inferior vena cava into the renal vein. Indications for renal venography include renal vein thrombosis, a tumor, and venous anomalies.

## PURPOSE
- To detect renal vein thrombosis
- To evaluate renal vein compression due to extrinsic tumors or retroperitoneal fibrosis
- To assess renal tumors and detect invasion of the renal vein or inferior vena cava
- To detect venous anomalies and defects
- To differentiate renal agenesis from a small kidney
- To collect renal venous blood samples for evaluation of renovascular hypertension

## PATIENT PREPARATION
- Explain to the patient that renal venography permits radiographic study of the renal veins.
- If prescribed, instruct the patient to fast for 4 hours before the test.
- Tell the patient who will perform the test and when and where it will take place.
- Inform the patient that a catheter will be inserted into a vein in the groin area after he's given a sedative and a local anesthetic.
- Tell the patient that he may feel mild discomfort during injection of the local anesthetic and contrast medium and that he may also feel transient burning and flushing from the contrast medium.
- Warn the patient that the X-ray equipment may make loud, clacking noises as the films are taken.

  *Alert* Check the patient's history for hypersensitivity to contrast media, iodine, or iodine-containing foods such as shellfish. Mark sensitivities on the chart and report them to the physician.

- Check the patient's history and any coagulation studies for indications of bleeding disorders.
- If renin assays will be done, check the patient's diet and medications and consult with the health care team. As ordered, restrict the patient's salt intake and discontinue antihypertensive drugs, diuretics, estrogen, and hormonal contraceptives.
- Make sure that the patient or a responsible family member has signed an informed consent form.
- Administer a sedative, if necessary, just before the procedure.
- Record the patient's baseline vital signs. Make sure pretest blood urea nitrogen and urine creatinine levels are adequate because the kidneys clear contrast media.

## PROCEDURE AND POSTTEST CARE
- The patient is placed in a supine position on the X-ray table, with his abdomen centered over the film. The skin over the right femoral vein near the groin is cleaned with antiseptic solution and draped. (The left femoral vein or jugular veins may be used.)
- A local anesthetic is injected and the femoral vein is cannulated.
- Under fluoroscopic guidance, a guide wire is threaded a short distance through the cannula, which is then removed. A catheter

is passed over the wire into the inferior vena cava.

● When catheterization of the femoral vein is contraindicated, the right antecubital vein is punctured, and the catheter is inserted and advanced through the right atrium of the heart into the inferior vena cava.

● A test bolus of contrast medium is injected to determine that the vena cava is patent. If so, the catheter is advanced into the right renal vein and contrast medium (usually 20 to 40 ml) is injected.

● When studies of the right renal vasculature are completed, the catheter is withdrawn into the vena cava, rotated, and guided into the left renal vein.

● If visualization of the renal venous tributaries is indicated, epinephrine can be injected into the ipsilateral renal artery by catheter before contrast medium is injected into the renal vein. Epinephrine temporarily blocks arterial flow and allows filling of distal intrarenal veins. Obstructing the artery briefly with a balloon catheter produces the same effect.

● After anteroposterior films are made, the patient lies prone for posteroanterior films.

● For renin assays, blood samples are withdrawn under fluoroscopy within 15 minutes after venography. After catheter removal, apply pressure to the site for 15 minutes and put on a dressing.

● Check the patient's vital signs and distal pulses every 15 minutes for the first hour, every 30 minutes for the second hour, and then every 2 hours for 24 hours. Keep the patient on bed rest for 2 hours.

● Observe the puncture site for bleeding or a hematoma when checking the patient's vital signs; if bleeding occurs, apply pressure. Report bleeding as soon as possible.

⊛ *Alert Report signs of vein perforation, embolism, and extravasation of contrast medium. These include chills, fever, rapid pulse and respiration, hypotension, dyspnea, and chest, abdominal, or flank pain. Also report complaints of paresthesia or pain in the catheterized limb — symptoms of nerve irritation or vascular compromise.*

● Administer prescribed sedatives and antimicrobials.

● Prepare for further arteriography or surgery as ordered.

● As ordered, instruct the patient that he may resume his usual diet and medications.

● Instruct the patient to increase fluid intake (unless contraindicated) to help clear contrast media.

## PRECAUTIONS

● Know that renal venography is contraindicated in severe thrombosis of the inferior vena cava.

● Be aware that the guide wire and catheter should be advanced carefully if severe renal vein thrombosis is suspected.

● Watch the patient for signs of hypersensitivity to the contrast medium.

## NORMAL FINDINGS

After injection of the contrast medium, opacification of the renal vein and tributaries should occur immediately. Normal renin content of venous blood in an adult in a supine position is 1.5 to 1.6 ng/ml/ hour.

## ABNORMAL FINDINGS

Renal vein occlusion near the inferior vena cava or the kidney indicates renal vein thrombosis. If the clot is outlined by contrast medium, it may look like a filling defect. However, a clot can usually be identified because it's within the lumen and less sharply outlined than a filling defect.

Collateral venous channels, which opacify with retrograde filling during contrast injection, commonly surround the occlusion. Complete occlusion prolongs transit of the contrast medium through the renal veins.

A filling defect of the renal vein may indicate obstruction or compression by an extrinsic tumor or retroperitoneal fibrosis. A renal tumor that invades the renal vein or inferior vena cava usually produces a filling defect with a sharply defined border.

Venous anomalies are indicated by opacification of abnormally positioned or clustered vessels. Absence of a renal vein differentiates renal agenesis from a small kidney.

Elevated renin content in renal venous blood usually indicates essential renovascular hypertension when assay results correspond for both kidneys. Elevated renin levels in one kidney indicate a unilateral lesion and usually require further evaluation by arteriography.

## INTERFERING FACTORS

● Recent contrast studies or stool or gas in the bowel

- Failure to restrict antihypertensive drugs, diuretics, estrogen, hormonal contraceptives, and salt

# Renin activity, plasma

Renin secretion from the kidneys is the first stage of the renin-angiotensin-aldosterone cycle, which controls the body's sodium-potassium balance, fluid volume, and blood pressure. Renin is released into the renal veins in response to sodium depletion and blood loss. It catalyzes the conversion of angiotensinogen, an alpha$_2$-globulin plasma protein, to angiotensin I, which in turn is converted by hydrolysis into angiotensin II, a vasoconstrictor that stimulates aldosterone production in the adrenal cortex. (See *Renin-angiotensin feedback system,* page 388.) When present in excessive amounts, angiotensin II causes renal hypertension.

The plasma renin activity (PRA) test is a screening procedure for renovascular hypertension, but doesn't unequivocally confirm it. When supplemented by other special tests, the PRA test can help establish the cause of hypertension. For instance, sampling blood obtained from the renal veins by renal vein catheterization and analyzing the renal venous renin ratio can identify renovascular disorders. Indexing renin levels against urinary sodium excretion can help identify primary aldosteronism. A sodium-depleted PRA test can then confirm this disorder.

Some experts believe that the type of treatment chosen for essential hypertension should depend on whether renin levels are low, normal, or high; the PRA test can categorize the disease to allow for appropriate therapy.

PRA is measured by radioimmunoassay of a peripheral or renal blood sample; results are expressed as the rate of angiotensin I formation per unit of time. Patient preparation is crucial and may take up to 1 month.

## PURPOSE

- To screen for renal origin of hypertension
- To help plan treatment of essential hypertension, a genetic disease commonly aggravated by excess sodium intake
- To help identify hypertension linked to unilateral (sometimes bilateral) renovascular disease by renal vein catheterization
- To help identify primary aldosteronism (Conn's syndrome) resulting from an aldosterone-secreting adrenal adenoma
- To confirm primary aldosteronism (sodium-depleted plasma renin test)

## PATIENT PREPARATION

- Explain to the patient that the PRA test is used to determine the cause of hypertension.
- Notify the laboratory and physician of medications the patient is taking that may affect test results; they may need to be restricted.
- Tell the patient to maintain a normal sodium diet (3 g/day) during this period.
- For the sodium-depleted plasma renin test, tell the patient that he'll receive furosemide (Lasix) (or, if he has angina or cerebrovascular insufficiency, chlorthiazide [Diuril]) and will follow a specific low-sodium diet for 3 days.
- The patient shouldn't receive radioactive treatments for several days before the test.
- Tell the patient that the test requires a blood sample. Explain who will perform the venipuncture and when and where the test will take place.
- Explain to the patient that he may experience slight discomfort from the tourniquet and needle puncture. Collect a morning sample, if possible.
- If a recumbent sample is ordered, instruct the patient to remain in bed at least 2 hours before the sample is obtained. (Posture influences renin secretion.) If an upright sample is ordered, instruct him to stand or sit upright for 2 hours before the test is performed.
- If renal vein catheterization is ordered, make sure the patient has signed an informed consent form. Tell the patient that the procedure will be done in the X-ray department and that he'll receive a local anesthetic.

## PROCEDURE AND POSTTEST CARE
### Peripheral vein sample

- Perform a venipuncture and collect the sample in a 4-ml EDTA tube.
- Note on the laboratory request if the patient was fasting and whether he was upright or supine during sample collection.

# RENIN-ANGIOTENSIN FEEDBACK SYSTEM

The renin-angiotensin-aldosterone system, sometimes known as the *juxtaglomerular apparatus*, is an important homeostatic device for regulating the body's sodium and water levels and blood pressure. It works this way:

Juxtaglomerular cells (1) in each of the kidney's glomeruli secrete the enzyme renin into the blood. The rate of renin secretion depends on the rate of perfusion in the afferent renal arterioles (2) and on the amount of sodium in the serum. A low sodium load and low perfusion pressure (as in hypovolemia)

increase renin secretion; high sodium and high perfusion pressure decrease it.

Renin circulates throughout the body. In the liver, renin converts angiotensinogen to angiotensin I (3), which passes to the lungs. There it's converted by hydrolysis to angiotensin II (4), a potent vasoconstrictor that acts on the adrenal cortex to stimulate production of the hormone aldosterone (5). Aldosterone acts on the juxtaglomerular cells to stimulate or depress renin secretion, completing the feedback cycle that automatically readjusts homeostasis.

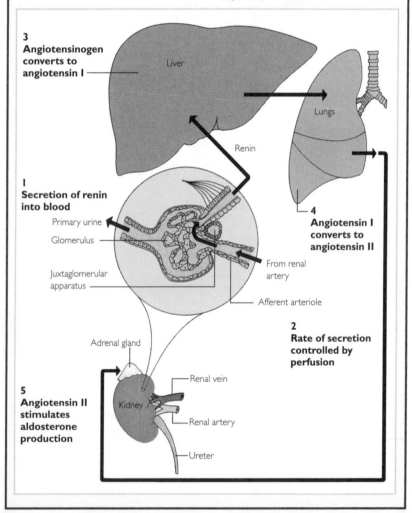

**3 Angiotensinogen converts to angiotensin I**

Liver

Lungs

Renin

**1 Secretion of renin into blood**

Primary urine

Glomerulus

Juxtaglomerular apparatus

From renal artery

Afferent arteriole

**4 Angiotensin I converts to angiotensin II**

**2 Rate of secretion controlled by perfusion**

Adrenal gland

Renal vein

Kidney

Renal artery

**5 Angiotensin II stimulates aldosterone production**

Ureter

- Apply direct pressure to the venipuncture site until bleeding stops.
- If a hematoma develops at the venipuncture site, apply pressure.

## Renal vein catheterization
- A catheter is advanced to the kidneys through the femoral vein under fluoroscopic control and samples are obtained from the renal veins and vena cava.
- After renal vein catheterization, apply pressure to the catheterization site for 10 to 20 minutes to prevent extravasation.
- Monitor vital signs and check the catheterization site every 30 minutes for 2 hours and then every hour for 4 hours to ensure that the bleeding has stopped. Check the patient's distal pulse for signs of thrombus formation and arterial occlusion (cyanosis, loss of pulse, cool skin).

## Both methods
- Instruct the patient that he may resume his usual diet and medications discontinued before the test, as ordered.

## PRECAUTIONS
- Because renin is unstable, be aware that the sample must be drawn into a chilled syringe and collection tube, placed on ice, and sent to the laboratory immediately.
- Completely fill the collection tube and invert it gently several times to mix the sample and the anticoagulant.

## REFERENCE VALUES
**Alert**  *PRA and aldosterone levels decrease with age.*
- *Sodium-depleted, upright, peripheral vein: For ages 18 to 39, the range is 2.9 to 24 ng/ml/hour; mean, 10.8 ng/ml/hour. For age 40 and over, the range is 2.9 to 10.8 ng/ml/hour; mean, 5.9 ng/ml/hour.0*
- *Sodium-replete, upright, peripheral vein: For ages 18 to 39, the range is less than or equal to 0.6 to 4.3 ng/ml/hour; mean, 1.9 ng/ml/hour. For age 40 and over, the range is less than or equal to 0.6 to 3.0 ng/ml/hour; mean, 1 ng/ml/hour.*
- *Renal vein catheterization: The renal venous renin ratio (the renin level in the renal vein compared to the level in the inferior vena cava) is less than 1.5 to 1.*

## ABNORMAL FINDINGS
Elevated renin levels may occur in essential hypertension (uncommon), malignant and renovascular hypertension, cirrhosis, hypokalemia, hypovolemia due to hemorrhage, renin-producing renal tumors (Bartter's syndrome), and adrenal hypofunction (Addison's disease). High renin levels may also be found in chronic renal failure with parenchymal disease, end-stage renal disease, and transplant rejection.

Decreased renin levels may indicate hypervolemia due to a high-sodium diet, salt-retaining steroids, primary aldosteronism, Cushing's syndrome, licorice ingestion syndrome, or essential hypertension with low renin levels.

High serum and urine aldosterone levels with low PRA help identify primary aldosteronism. In the sodium-depleted renin test, low plasma renin confirms this and differentiates it from secondary aldosteronism (characterized by increased renin).

## INTERFERING FACTORS
- Improper patient position
- Failure to use the proper anticoagulant in the collection tube, to completely fill it, or to adequately mix the sample and the anticoagulant (EDTA helps preserve angiotensin I; heparin doesn't.)
- Failure to chill the collection tube, syringe, and sample or to send the sample to the laboratory immediately
- Antihypertensives, hormonal contraceptives, licorice ingestion, pregnancy, and therapy with diuretics, salt intake, severe blood loss, or vasodilators (increase)
- Antidiuretic therapy and salt-retaining corticosteroid therapy (decrease)
- Radioisotope use within several days before the test

# Respiratory syncytial virus antibodies

Respiratory syncytial virus (RSV), a member of the paramyxovirus group, is the major viral cause of severe lower respiratory tract disease in infants, but may cause infections in people of any age. RSV infections are most common and produce the most severe disease during the first 6 months of life. Initial infection involves viral replication in epithelial cells of the upper respiratory tract, but in younger children especially, the infection spreads to the bronchi, the bronchioles, and even the parenchyma of the lungs.

In the RSV antibodies test, immunoglobulin (Ig) G and IgM class antibodies are quantified using indirect immunofluorescence.

## PURPOSE
- To diagnose infections caused by RSV

## PATIENT PREPARATION
- Explain the purpose of the RSV antibodies test to the patient (or, if the patient is a child, to his parents).
- Tell the patient or parents that the test requires a blood sample. Explain who will perform the venipuncture and when and where the test will take place.
- Tell the patient he may experience slight discomfort from the tourniquet and needle puncture.

## PROCEDURE AND POSTTEST CARE
- Perform a venipuncture and collect 5 ml of sterile blood in a clot-activator tube.
- Allow the blood to clot for at least 1 hour at room temperature.
- Apply direct pressure to the venipuncture site until bleeding stops.
- If a hematoma develops at the venipuncture site, apply pressure.

## PRECAUTIONS
- Handle the sample gently to prevent hemolysis.
- Transfer the serum to a sterile tube or vial and send it to the laboratory promptly.
- If transfer must be delayed, store the serum at 39.2° F (4° C) for 1 to 2 days or at –4° F (–20° C) for longer periods to avoid contamination.

## REFERENCE VALUES
Sera from patients who have never been infected with RSV have no detectable antibodies to the virus (less than 1:5).

## ABNORMAL FINDINGS
The qualitative presence of IgM or a fourfold or greater increase in IgG antibodies indicates active RSV infection. Note that, in infants, serologic diagnosis of RSV infections is difficult because of the presence of maternal IgG antibodies. Thus, the presence of IgM antibodies is most significant.

## INTERFERING FACTORS
- None significant

# Reticulocyte count

Reticulocytes are nonnucleated, immature red blood cells (RBCs) that remain in the peripheral blood for 24 to 48 hours while maturing. They're generally larger than mature RBCs. In the reticulocyte count test, reticulocytes in a whole blood sample are counted and expressed as a percentage of the total RBC count. Because the manual method of reticulocyte counting uses only a small sample, values may be imprecise and should be compared with the RBC count or hematocrit. The reticulocyte count is useful for evaluating anemia and is an index of effective erythropoiesis and bone marrow response to anemia.

## PURPOSE
- To aid in distinguishing between hypoproliferative and hyperproliferative anemias
- To help assess blood loss, bone marrow response to anemia, and therapy for anemia

## PATIENT PREPARATION
- Explain to the patient that the reticulocyte count is used to detect anemia or to monitor its treatment.
- Tell the patient that a blood sample will be taken. Explain who will perform the venipuncture and when and where it will take place.
- Explain to the patient that he may feel slight discomfort from the tourniquet and needle puncture.

  **Alert** *If the patient is an infant or child, explain to the parents that a small amount of blood will be taken from his finger or earlobe.*
- Notify the laboratory and physician of medications the patient is taking that may affect test results; they may need to be restricted.
- Inform the patient that he need not restrict food and fluids.

## PROCEDURE AND POSTTEST CARE
- Perform a venipuncture and collect the sample in a 3- or 4.5-ml EDTA tube.

- Make sure subdermal bleeding has stopped before removing pressure.
- If a hematoma develops at the venipuncture site, apply pressure. If the hematoma is large, monitor pulses distal to the phlebotomy site.
- Instruct the patient that he may resume medications discontinued before the test, as ordered.
- Monitor the patient with an abnormal reticulocyte count for trends or significant changes in repeated tests.

## PRECAUTIONS
- Completely fill the collection tube and invert it gently several times to mix the sample and the anticoagulant.
- Handle the sample gently.

## REFERENCE VALUES
Reticulocytes compose 0.5% to 2.5% (SI, 0.005 to 0.025) of the total RBC count.

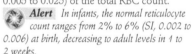 *Alert* *In infants, the normal reticulocyte count ranges from 2% to 6% (SI, 0.002 to 0.006) at birth, decreasing to adult levels in 1 to 2 weeks.*

## ABNORMAL FINDINGS
A low reticulocyte count indicates hypoproliferative bone marrow (hypoplastic anemia) or ineffective erythropoiesis (pernicious anemia).

A high reticulocyte count indicates a bone marrow response to anemia caused by hemolysis or blood loss. The reticulocyte count may also increase after therapy for iron deficiency anemia or pernicious anemia.

## INTERFERING FACTORS
- Prolonged tourniquet constriction
- Azathioprine (Imuran), chloramphenicol, dactinomycin (Cosmegen), and methotrexate (MTX) (possible false-low)
- Antimalarials, antipyretics, corticotropin, furazolidone (Furoxone) (in infants), and levodopa (possible false-high)
- Sulfonamides (possible false-low or false-high)
- Recent blood transfusion

# Retrograde cystography

Retrograde cystography involves the instillation of contrast medium into the bladder, followed by radiographic examination. This procedure is used to diagnose bladder rupture without urethral involvement because it can determine the location and extent of the rupture. Other indications for retrograde cystography include neurogenic bladder; recurrent urinary tract infections (UTIs), especially in children; suspected vesicoureteral reflux; and vesical fistulas, diverticula, and tumors. This test is also performed when cystoscopic examination is impractical, as in male infants, or when excretory urography hasn't adequately visualized the bladder. Voiding cystourethrography is commonly performed concomitantly.

## PURPOSE
- To evaluate the structure and integrity of the bladder

## PATIENT PREPARATION
- Explain to the patient that retrograde cystography permits radiographic examination of the bladder.
- Inform the patient that he need not restrict food and fluids.
- Tell the patient who will perform the test and when and where it will take place.
- Inform the patient that he may experience some discomfort when the catheter is inserted and when the contrast medium is instilled through the catheter.
- Tell the patient that he may hear loud, clacking sounds as the X-ray films are made.
- Make sure that the patient or a responsible family member has signed an informed consent form.
- Check the patient's history for hypersensitivity to contrast media, iodine, or shellfish; mark it on the chart and inform the physician.

## PROCEDURE AND POSTTEST CARE
- The patient is placed in a supine position on the X-ray table and a preliminary kidney-ureter-bladder radiograph is taken.

# NORMAL AND ABNORMAL RETROGRADE CYSTOGRAMS

A normal retrograde cystogram (left) contrasts sharply with one showing a ruptured bladder (right). In the photograph on the right, the bladder, usually smooth and rounded when filled, has collapsed downward on itself, against the pelvic floor, and contrast material has extravasated upward into the peritoneal cavity from the tear in the bladder wall.

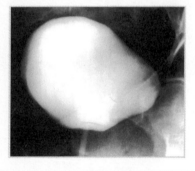 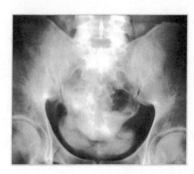

- The radiograph is developed immediately and scrutinized for renal shadows, calcifications, contours of the bone and psoas muscles, and gas patterns in the lumen of the GI tract.
- The bladder is catheterized and 200 to 300 ml of sterile contrast medium (50 to 100 ml for an infant) is instilled by gravity or gentle syringe injection. The catheter is then clamped.
- With the patient in a supine position, an anteroposterior film is taken. The patient is tilted first to one side, then the other, and two posterior oblique (and sometimes lateral) views are taken.
- If the patient's condition permits, he's placed in the jackknife position and a posteroanterior film is taken. A space-occupying vesical lesion may require additional exposures. Rarely, to enhance visualization, 100 to 300 ml of air may be insufflated into the bladder by syringe after removal of the contrast medium (double-contrast technique).
- The catheter is then unclamped, the bladder fluid is allowed to drain, and a radiograph is obtained to detect urethral diverticula, reflux into the ureters, fistulous tracts into the vagina, or intraperitoneal or extraperitoneal extravasation of the contrast medium.
- Monitor the patient's vital signs every 15 minutes for the first hour, every 30 min-

utes during the second hour, and then every 2 hours for up to 24 hours.
- Record the time of the patient's voidings and the color and volume of the urine. Observe for hematuria that persists after the third voiding and notify the physician.
- Watch for signs of urinary sepsis from UTIs (chills, fever, elevated pulse and respiration rates, and hypotension) or similar signs related to extravasation of contrast medium into the general circulation.
- Prepare the patient for surgery and urinary diversion, if indicated. Strain urine if calculi are detected.
- Monitor for retention or distention if neurogenic bladder is diagnosed and administer medication, as ordered (baclofen [Lioresal] for spasms; bethanechol [Duvoid] for hypotonic bladder).
- Discuss the use of a percutaneous stimulator if one is being contemplated. Teach self-catheterization, if indicated for neurogenic bladder.

## PRECAUTIONS
- Know that retrograde cystography is contraindicated during exacerbation of an acute UTI or in the patient with an obstruction that prevents passage of a urinary catheter.
- Be aware that this test shouldn't be performed in the patient with urethral evulsion

or transection, unless catheter passage and flow of contrast medium are monitored fluoroscopically.

## NORMAL FINDINGS

Retrograde cystography shows a bladder with normal contours, capacity, integrity, and urethrovesical angle and with no evidence of a tumor, diverticula, or a rupture. Vesicoureteral reflux should be absent. The bladder shouldn't be displaced or externally compressed; the bladder wall should be smooth, not thick. (See *Normal and abnormal retrograde cystograms.*)

## ABNORMAL FINDINGS

Retrograde cystography can identify vesical trabeculae or diverticula, space-occupying lesions (tumors), calculi or gravel, blood clots, high- or low-pressure vesicoureteral reflux, and a hypotonic or hypertonic bladder.

## INTERFERING FACTORS

● Gas, stool, or residual barium from recent diagnostic tests in the bowel (possible poor imaging)

---

# Retrograde ureteropyelography

Retrograde ureteropyelography allows radiographic examination of the renal collecting system after injection of a contrast medium through a ureteral catheter during cystoscopy. The contrast medium is usually iodine-based and although some of it may be absorbed through the mucous membranes, this test is preferred for the patient with hypersensitivity to iodine (in whom I.V. administration of an iodine-based contrast medium, as in excretory urography, is contraindicated). This test is also indicated when visualization of the renal collecting system by excretory urography is inadequate due to inferior films or marked renal insufficiency because retrograde ureteropyelography isn't influenced by impaired renal function.

## PURPOSE

● To assess the structure and integrity of the renal collecting system (calyces, renal pelvis, and ureter) (see *Sites and types of ob-*

*struction indicated by ureteropyelography,* page 394)

## PATIENT PREPARATION

● Explain to the patient that retrograde ureteropyelography permits visualization of the urinary collecting system.
● If a general anesthetic is to be used, instruct the patient to fast for 8 hours before the test. Generally, he should be well hydrated to ensure adequate urine flow.
● Tell the patient who will perform the test and when and where it will take place.
● Inform the patient that he'll be positioned on an examination table, with his legs in stirrups, and that the position may be tiring.
● If the patient will be awake throughout the procedure, tell him that he may feel pressure as the instrument is passed and a pressure sensation in the kidney area when the contrast medium is introduced. Also, he may feel an urgency to void.
● Make sure that the patient or a responsible family member has signed an informed consent form.
● Administer prescribed premedication just before the procedure.

## PROCEDURE AND POSTTEST CARE

● Place the patient in the lithotomy position. Care must be taken to avoid pressure points or impairment to circulation while his legs are in the stirrups.
● After the patient is anesthetized, the urologist first performs a cystoscopic examination.
● After visual inspection of the bladder, one or both ureters are catheterized with opaque catheters, depending on the condition or abnormality suspected. Radiographic monitoring allows correct positioning of the catheter tip in the renal pelvis.
● The renal pelvis is emptied by gravity drainage or aspiration. About 5 ml of contrast medium is then slowly injected through the catheter using the syringe with the special adapter.
● When adequate filling and opacification have occurred, anteroposterior radiographic films are taken and immediately developed. Lateral and oblique films can be taken, as needed, after the injection of more contrast medium.
● After the radiographs of the renal pelvis are examined, a few more milliliters of con-

## SITES AND TYPES OF OBSTRUCTION INDICATED BY URETEROPYELOGRAPHY

Ureteropyelography may detect a stricture, neoplasm, blood clot, or calculus that obstructs urine flow in the calyces, pelvis, or ureter. Small calculi may remain in the calyces and pelvis or pass down the ureter. A staghorn calculus (a cast of the calyceal and pelvic collecting system) may form from a calculus that stays in the kidney.

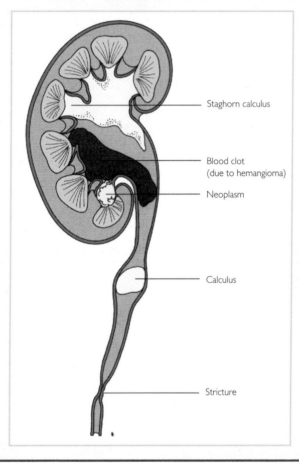

Staghorn calculus

Blood clot (due to hemangioma)

Neoplasm

Calculus

Stricture

trast medium are injected to outline the ureters as the catheter is slowly withdrawn.

● Delayed films (10 to 15 minutes after complete catheter removal) are then taken to check for contrast medium retention, indicating urinary stasis.

● If ureteral obstruction is present, the ureteral catheter may be kept in place and, together with an indwelling urinary catheter,

connected to a gravity drainage system until posttest urinary flow is corrected or returns to normal.

● Check the patient's vital signs every 15 minutes for the first hour, every 30 minutes for 1 hour, every hour for the next 2 hours, and then every 4 hours for 24 hours.

● Monitor the patient's fluid intake and urine output for 24 hours. Observe each specimen for hematuria. Gross hematuria or hematuria after the third voiding is abnormal and should be reported. If the patient doesn't void for 8 hours after the procedure or if the patient immediately feels distress and his bladder is distended, urethral catheterization may be necessary.

● Be especially attentive to catheter output if ureteral catheters have been left in place because inadequate output may reflect catheter obstruction, requiring irrigation. Protect ureteral catheters from dislodgment. Note output amounts for each catheter (indwelling, urinary, urethral) separately; this helps determine the location of an obstruction that's causing reduced output.

● Administer prescribed analgesics, tub baths, and increased fluid intake for dysuria, which commonly occurs after retrograde ureteropyelography.

🔎 *Alert* *Watch the patient for and report severe pain in the area of the kidneys as well as any signs of sepsis (such as chills, fever, and hypotension). If irrigation is ordered, never use more than 10 ml of sterile saline solution.*

## PRECAUTIONS

● Be aware that retrograde ureteropyelography must be done carefully in the patient with urinary stasis caused by ureteral obstruction to prevent further injury to the ureter.

● Know that this test is contraindicated in the pregnant patient unless the benefits of the procedure outweigh the risks to the fetus.

## NORMAL FINDINGS

Following a normal cystoscopic examination, ureteral catheterization, and injection of contrast medium through the catheters, opacification of the pelves and calyces should occur immediately. Normal structures should be outlined clearly and should appear symmetrical in bilateral testing. Ureters should fill uniformly and appear normal in size and course. Inspiratory and expiratory exposures, when superimposed, normally create two outlines of the renal pelvis ¾" (2 cm) apart.

## ABNORMAL FINDINGS

Incomplete or delayed drainage reflects an obstruction, most commonly at the ureteropelvic junction. Enlargement of the components of the collecting system or delayed emptying of contrast medium may indicate obstruction due to a tumor, a blood clot, a stricture, or calculi.

Perinephric inflammation or suppuration commonly causes fixation of the kidney on the same side, resulting in a single sharp radiographic outline of the collecting system when inspiratory and expiratory exposures are superimposed. Upward, downward, or lateral renal displacement can result from a renal abscess or tumor or from a perinephric abscess. Neoplasms can cause displacement of either pole or of the entire kidney.

## INTERFERING FACTORS

● Previous contrast studies or presence of stool or gas in the bowel (possible poor imaging)

# *Retrograde urethrography*

Used almost exclusively in men, retrograde urethrography requires instillation or injection of a contrast medium into the urethra and permits visualization of its membranous, bulbar, and penile portions.

Although visualization of the anterior portion of the urethra is excellent with this test alone, the posterior portion is more effectively outlined by retrograde urethrography in tandem with voiding cystourethrography.

## PURPOSE

● To diagnose urethral strictures, diverticula, and congenital anomalies

● To assess urethral lacerations or other trauma

● To assist with follow-up examination after surgical repair of the urethra

## PATIENT PREPARATION

● Explain to the patient that retrograde urethrography diagnoses urethral structural problems. Inform him that he need not restrict food and fluids.

● Describe the test, including who will perform it and where it will take place.

● Inform the patient that he may experience some discomfort when the catheter is inserted and when the contrast medium is instilled through the catheter.

- Tell the patient that he may hear loud, clacking sounds as the X-ray films are made.
- Make sure that the patient or a responsible family member has signed an informed consent form.
- Check the patient's history for hypersensitivity to iodine-containing foods, such as shellfish, or contrast media.
- Administer any prescribed sedatives just before the procedure and instruct the patient to void before leaving the unit.

## PROCEDURE AND POSTTEST CARE

### For men

- The patient is placed in a recumbent position on the examining table. Anteroposterior exposures of the bladder and urethra are made, and the resulting films studied for radiopaque densities, foreign bodies, or calculi.
- The glans and meatus are cleaned with an antiseptic solution. The catheter is filled with the contrast medium before insertion to eliminate air bubbles.
- Although no lubricant should be used, the tip of the catheter may be dipped in sterile water to facilitate insertion.
- The catheter is inserted until the balloon portion is inside the meatus; the balloon is then inflated with 1 to 2 ml of water, which prevents the catheter from slipping during the procedure.
- The patient then assumes the right posterior oblique position, with his right thigh drawn up to a 90-degree angle and the penis placed along its axis. The left thigh is extended.
- The contrast medium is injected through the catheter. After three-fourths of the contrast medium has been injected, the first X-ray film is exposed while the remainder of the contrast medium is being injected. Left lateral oblique views may also be taken.
- Fluoroscopic control may be helpful, especially for evaluating urethral injury.

### For women and children

- In women, this test may be used when urethral diverticula are suspected. A double-balloon catheter is used, which occludes the bladder neck from above and the external meatus from below.
- In children, the procedure is the same as for adults except that a smaller catheter is used, depending on the size of the child.

**Alert** *Watch all patients for chills and fever related to extravasation of contrast medium into the general circulation for 12 to 24 hours after retrograde urethrography. Also observe for signs of sepsis and allergic manifestations.*

## PRECAUTIONS

- Be aware that retrograde urethrography should be performed cautiously in the patient with a urinary tract infection (UTI).
- Monitor the patient for a UTI. If urethral trauma is present, monitor for stricture, infection, and urinary extravasation. Prepare him for surgery, if indicated.

## NORMAL FINDINGS

The membranous, bulbar, and penile portions of the urethra—and occasionally the prostatic portion—appear normal in size, shape, and course.

## ABNORMAL FINDINGS

Radiographs obtained during retrograde urethrography may show the following abnormalities: urethral diverticula, fistulas, strictures, false passages, calculi, and lacerations; congenital anomalies, such as urethral valves and perineal hypospadias; and, rarely, tumors (in less than 1% of cases).

## INTERFERING FACTORS

- None significant

## *Rheumatoid factor*

The rheumatoid factor (RF) test is the most useful immunologic test for confirming rheumatoid arthritis (RA). In this disease, "renegade" immunoglobulin (Ig) G and IgA antibodies, produced by lymphocytes in the synovial joints, react with IgM antibody to produce immune complexes, complement activation, and tissue destruction. How IgG molecules become antigenic is still unknown, but they may be altered by aggregating with viruses or other antigens. Techniques for detecting RF include the sheep cell agglutination test and the latex fixation test. Although the presence of this autoantibody is diagnostically useful, it may not be etiologically related to RA.

## PURPOSE
● To confirm RA, especially when clinical diagnosis is doubtful

## PATIENT PREPARATION
● Explain to the patient that the RA test helps confirm RA.
● Inform the patient that he need not restrict food and fluids.
● Tell the patient that the test requires a blood sample. Explain who will perform the venipuncture and when and where the test will take place.
● Explain to the patient that he may experience slight discomfort from the tourniquet and needle puncture.

## PROCEDURE AND POSTTEST CARE
● Perform a venipuncture and collect the sample in a 7-ml clot-activator tube.
● Because a patient with RA may be immunologically compromised, keep the venipuncture site clean and dry for 24 hours.
● Check regularly for signs of infection.
● Apply direct pressure to the venipuncture site until bleeding stops.
● If a hematoma develops at the venipuncture site, apply pressure.

## PRECAUTIONS
● Label the sample with the patient's name, the hospital or blood bank number, the date, and the phlebotomist's initials.
● Handle the sample gently and send it to the laboratory immediately.

## REFERENCE VALUES
The normal RF titer is less than 1:20; a normal rheumatoid screening test is nonreactive.

## ABNORMAL FINDINGS
Non-RA and RA populations aren't clearly separated with regard to the presence of RF: 25% of patients with RA have a nonreactive titer; 8% of non-RA patients are reactive at greater than 39 IU/ml, and only 3% of non-RA patients are reactive at greater than 80 IU/ml.

Patients with various non-RA diseases characterized by chronic inflammation may test positive for RF. These diseases include systemic lupus erythematosus, polymyositis, tuberculosis, infectious mononucleosis, syphilis, viral hepatic disease, and influenza.

## INTERFERING FACTORS
● Inadequately activated complement (possible false-positive)
● Serum with high lipid or cryoglobulin levels (possible false-positive, requiring a repeat test after restricting fat intake)
● Serum with high IgG levels (possible false-negative due to competition with IgG on the surface of latex particles or sheep red blood cells used as substrate)

# Rh typing

The Rhesus (Rh) system classifies blood by the presence or absence of Rh antigen, called *Rho(D) factor,* on the surface of red blood cells (RBCs). In Rh typing, a patient's RBCs are mixed with serum containing anti-Rho(D) antibodies and are observed for agglutination. If agglutination occurs, the Rho(D) antigen is present, and the patient's blood is typed Rh-positive; if agglutination doesn't occur, the antigen is absent, and the patient's blood is typed Rh-negative.

Prospective blood donors are fully tested to exclude the Du variant, a weak variant of the D antigen, before being classified as having Rh-negative blood. People who have this antigen are considered Rh-positive donors, but are generally transfused as Rh-negative recipients.

## PURPOSE
● To establish blood type according to the Rh system
● To help determine the donor's compatibility before transfusion
● To determine if the patient will require an Rho(D) immune globulin injection

## PATIENT PREPARATION
● Explain to the patient that Rh typing determines or verifies blood group to ensure safe blood transfusion.
● Inform the patient that he need not restrict food and fluids.
● Tell the patient that the test requires a blood sample. Explain who will perform the venipuncture and when and where the test will take place.
● Explain to the patient that he may experience slight discomfort from the tourniquet and needle puncture.

- Check the patient's history for recent administration of dextran, I.V. contrast media, or drugs that may alter results.

## PROCEDURE AND POSTTEST CARE
- Perform a venipuncture and collect the sample in a 7-ml EDTA tube.
- Apply direct pressure to the venipuncture site until bleeding stops.
- If a hematoma develops at the venipuncture site, apply pressure.
- If necessary, give the pregnant patient a card identifying that she may need to receive Rho(D) injection.

## PRECAUTIONS
- Label the sample with the patient's name, the hospital or blood bank number, the date, and the phlebotomist's initials.
- Handle the sample gently and send it to the laboratory immediately.
- If a transfusion is ordered, be sure a transfusion request form accompanies the sample to the laboratory.

## FINDINGS
Classified as Rh-positive or Rh-negative, donor blood may be transfused only if it's compatible with the recipient's blood.

If an Rh-negative woman delivers an Rh-positive neonate or aborts a fetus whose Rh type is unknown, she should receive an Rho(D) injection within 72 hours to prevent hemolytic disease of the neonate in future births.

## INTERFERING FACTORS
- Recent administration of dextran or I.V. contrast media (cellular aggregation resembling antibody-mediated agglutination)
- Cephalosporins, levodopa (Dopar), and methyldopa (Aldomet) (possible false-positive for the Du antigen due to positive direct antiglobulin [Coombs'] test)

## *Routine urinalysis*

A routine urinalysis tests for urinary and systemic disorders. This test evaluates physical characteristics (color, odor, turbidity, and opacity) of urine; determines specific gravity and pH; detects and measures protein, glucose, and ketone bodies; and examines sediment for blood cells, casts, and crystals.

Diagnostic laboratory methods include visual examination, reagent strip screening, refractometry for specific gravity, and microscopic inspection of centrifuged sediment.

## PURPOSE
- To screen the patient's urine for renal or urinary tract disease (see *Urine cytology*)
- To help detect metabolic or systemic disease unrelated to renal disorders
- To detect substances (drugs)

## PATIENT PREPARATION
- Explain to the patient that the routine urinalysis aids in the diagnosis of renal or urinary tract disease and helps evaluate overall body function.
- Inform the patient that he need not restrict food and fluids.
- Notify the laboratory and physician of medications the patient is taking that may affect laboratory results; they may need to be restricted.

## PROCEDURE AND POSTTEST CARE
- Collect a random urine specimen of at least 15 ml.
- Obtain a first-voided morning specimen if possible.
- Inform the patient that he may resume his usual diet and medications, as ordered.

## PRECAUTIONS
- Strain the specimen to catch stones or stone fragments if the patient is being evaluated for renal colic.
- Carefully pour the urine through an unfolded 4″ × 4″ gauze pad or a fine-mesh sieve placed over the specimen container.
- Send the specimen to the laboratory immediately.
- Refrigerate the specimen if analysis will be delayed longer than 1 hour.

## NORMAL FINDINGS
See *Normal findings in routine urinalysis,* page 400.

## ABNORMAL FINDINGS
Nonpathologic variations in normal values may result from diet, nonpathologic conditions, specimen collection time, and other factors. (See *Drugs that influence routine urinaly-*

# URINE CYTOLOGY

Epithelial cells line the urinary tract and exfoliate easily into the urine, so a simple cytologic examination of these cells can aid diagnosis of urinary tract disease. Although urine cytology isn't performed routinely, it's useful for detecting cancer and inflammatory diseases of the renal pelvis, ureters, bladder, and urethra. It's especially useful for detecting bladder cancer in high-risk groups, such as smokers, people who work with aniline dyes (such as leather workers), and patients who have already received treatment for bladder cancer. Urine cytology can also determine whether bladder lesions that appear on X-rays are benign or malignant. This test can also detect cytomegalovirus infection and other viral disease.

To perform the test, the patient must collect a 100- to 300-ml clean-catch urine specimen 3 hours after his last voiding. (He should not use the first-voided specimen of the morning.) The urine specimen is sent to the cytology laboratory immediately so that it can be examined before the cells begin to degenerate.

## PREPARING THE SPECIMEN
The specimen is prepared in one of the following ways and stained with Papanicolaou stain:
♦ *Centrifuge* — After the urine is spun down, the sediment is smeared on a glass slide and stained for examination.

♦ *Filter* — Urine is poured through a filter, which traps the cells so that they can be stained and examined directly.
♦ *Cytocentrifuge* — After the urine is centrifuged, the sediment is resuspended and placed on slides, which are spun in a cytocentrifuge and stained for examination.

## IMPLICATIONS OF RESULTS
Normal urine is relatively free from cellular debris, but should have some epithelial and squamous cells that appear normal under a microscope. Identification of malignant cells or other signs of malignancy may indicate cancer of the kidney, renal pelvis, ureters, bladder, or urethra. It could also indicate a metastatic tumor.

An overgrowth of epithelial cells, an excess of red blood cells, or the presence of leukocytes or atypical cells may indicate a lower urinary tract inflammation, which can result from prostatic hyperplasia, urinary calculi, bladder diverticula, strictures, or malformation.

Large intranuclear inclusions may indicate a cytomegalovirus infection, which usually affects the renal tubular epithelium. This type of viral infection commonly occurs in cancer patients undergoing chemotherapy and transplant patients receiving immunosuppressant drugs. Cytoplasmic inclusion bodies may also indicate measles and may precede the characteristic Koplik's spots.

---

*sis results,* pages 401 and 402.) For example, specific gravity influences urine color and odor. As specific gravity increases, urine becomes darker and its odor becomes stronger.

Urine pH, which is greatly affected by diet and medications, influences the appearance of urine and the composition of crystals. An alkaline pH (above 7.0) — characteristic of a vegetarian diet — causes turbidity and the formation of phosphate, carbonate, and amorphous crystals. An acid pH (below 7.0) — typical of a high-protein diet — produces turbidity and the formation of oxalate, cystine, leucine, tyrosine, amorphous urate, and uric acid crystals.

Protein, normally absent from the urine, may be present in a benign condition known as orthostatic (postural) proteinuria. Most

common in patients ages 10 to 20, this condition is intermittent, appears after prolonged standing, and disappears after recumbency. Transient benign proteinuria can also occur with fever, exposure to cold, emotional stress, or strenuous exercise. Systemic diseases that may cause proteinuria include lymphoma, hepatitis, diabetes mellitus, toxemia, hypertension, lupus erythematosus, and febrile illnesses.

Sugars, usually absent from the urine, may appear under normal conditions. The most common sugar in urine is glucose. Transient nonpathologic glycosuria may result from emotional stress or pregnancy and may follow ingestion of a high-carbohydrate meal.

# NORMAL FINDINGS IN ROUTINE URINALYSIS

| ELEMENT | FINDINGS |
| --- | --- |
| **MACROSCOPIC** | |
| Color | ◆ Straw to dark yellow |
| Odor | ◆ Slightly aromatic |
| Appearance | ◆ Clear |
| Specific gravity | ◆ 1.005 to 1.035 |
| pH | ◆ 4.5 to 8 |
| Protein | ◆ None |
| Glucose | ◆ None |
| Ketone bodies | ◆ None |
| Bilirubin | ◆ None |
| Urobilinogen | ◆ Normal |
| Hemoglobin | ◆ None |
| Erythrocytes (red blood cells [RBCs]) | ◆ None |
| Nitrites (bacteria) | ◆ None |
| Leukocytes (white blood cells [WBCs]) | ◆ None |
| **MICROSCOPIC** | |
| RBCs | ◆ 0 to 2/highpower field |
| WBCs | ◆ 0 to 5/highpower field |
| Epithelial cells | ◆ 0 to 5/highpower field |
| Casts | ◆ None, except 1 to 2 hyaline casts/low-power field |
| Crystals | ◆ Present |
| Bacteria | ◆ None |
| Yeast cells | ◆ None |
| Parasites | ◆ None |

Centrifuged urine sediment contains cells, casts, crystals, bacteria, yeast, and parasites. Red blood cells (RBCs) commonly don't appear in urine without pathologic significance; however, strenuous exercise can cause hematuria.

The following abnormal findings generally suggest pathologic conditions:
● Color — Color change can result from diet, drugs, and many diseases.
● Odor — In diabetes mellitus, starvation, and dehydration, a fruity odor accompanies formation of ketone bodies. In urinary tract infections (UTIs), a fetid odor commonly is associated with *Escherichia coli.* Maple syrup urine disease and phenylketonuria also cause distinctive odors.

Other abnormal odors include those similar to a brewery, sweaty feet, cabbage, fish, and sulfur.
● Turbidity — Turbid urine may contain red or white cells, bacteria, fat, or chyle and may reflect renal infection.

● Specific gravity — Low specific gravity (less than 1.005) is characteristic of diabetes insipidus, nephrogenic diabetes insipidus, acute tubular necrosis, increased fluid intake, diuretics, and pyelonephritis. Fixed specific gravity, in which values remain 1.010 regardless of fluid intake, occurs in chronic glomerulonephritis with severe renal damage. High specific gravity (greater than 1.035) occurs in nephrotic syndrome, dehydration, acute glomerulonephritis, heart failure, liver failure, and shock.
● pH — Alkaline urine pH may result from vegetarian diet, Fanconi's syndrome, UTI caused by urea-splitting bacteria (*Proteus* and *Pseudomonas*), and metabolic or respiratory alkalosis. Acid urine pH is associated with intake of large amounts of meat, renal tuberculosis, pyrexia, phenylketonuria, alkaptonuria, and acidosis.
● Protein — Proteinuria suggests renal failure or disease (including nephrosis, glomerulosclerosis, glomerulonephritis, nephrolithia-

# DRUGS THAT INFLUENCE ROUTINE URINALYSIS RESULTS

## DRUGS THAT CHANGE URINE COLOR
Chlorzoxazone (orange to purple-red)
Deferoxamine mesylate (red)
Fluorescein sodium I.V. (yellow-orange)
Furazolidone (brown)
Iron salts (black)
Levodopa (dark)
Methylene blue (blue-green)
Metronidazole (dark)
Nitrofurantoin (brown)
Oral anticoagulants, indandione derivatives (orange)
Phenazopyridine (orange, red, or orange-brown)
Phenolphthalein (red to purple-red)
Phenolsulfonphthalein (pink or red)
Phenothiazines (dark)
Quinacrine (deep yellow)
Riboflavin (yellow)
Rifabutin (red-orange)
Rifampin (red-orange)
Sulfasalazine (orange-yellow)
Sulfobromophthalein (red)

## DRUGS THAT CAUSE URINE ODOR
Antibiotics
Paraldehyde
Vitamins

## DRUGS THAT INCREASE SPECIFIC GRAVITY
Albumin
Dextran
Glucose
Radiopaque contrast media

## DRUGS THAT DECREASE pH
Ammonium chloride
Ascorbic acid
Diazoxide
Methenamine
Metolazone

## DRUGS THAT INCREASE pH
Amphotericin B
Carbonic anhydrase inhibitors
Mafenide
Potassium citrate
Sodium bicarbonate

## DRUGS THAT CAUSE FALSE-POSITIVE RESULTS FOR PROTEINURIA
Acetazolamide (Combistix)
Aminosalicylic acid (sulfosalicylic acid or Extons method)
Cephalothin in large doses (sulfosalicylic acid method)
Dichlorphenamide
Methazolamide
Nafcillin (sulfosalicylic acid method)
Sodium bicarbonate
Tolbutamide (sulfosalicylic acid method)
Tolmetin (sulfosalicylic acid method)

## DRUGS THAT CAUSE TRUE PROTEINURIA
Aminoglycosides
Amphotericin B
Bacitracin
Cephalosporins
Cisplatin
Etretinate
Gold preparations
Isotretinoin
Nonsteroidal anti-inflammatory drugs
Phenylbutazone
Polymyxin B
Sulfonamides
Trimethadione

## DRUGS THAT CAN CAUSE EITHER TRUE PROTEINURIA OR FALSE-POSITIVE RESULTS
Penicillin in large doses (except with Ames reagent strips)
Sulfonamides (sulfosalicylic acid method)

## DRUGS THAT CAUSE FALSE-POSITIVE RESULTS FOR GLYCOSURIA
Aminosalicylic acid (Benedict's test)
Ascorbic acid (Clinistix, Diastix, Tes-Tape)
Ascorbic acid in large doses (Clinitest tablets)
Cephalosporins (Clinitest tablets)
Chloral hydrate (Benedict's test)
Chloramphenicol (Clinitest tablets)
Isoniazid (Benedict's test)
Levodopa (Clinistix, Diastix, Tes-Tape)
Levodopa in large doses (Clinitest tablets)
Methyldopa (Tes-Tape)

(continued)

# DRUGS THAT INFLUENCE ROUTINE URINALYSIS RESULTS
## (continued)

### DRUGS THAT CAUSE FALSE-POSITIVE RESULTS FOR GLYCOSURIA (continued)
Nalidixic acid (Benedict's test or Clinitest tablets)
Nitrofurantoin (Benedict's test)
Penicillin G in large doses (Benedict's test)
Phenazopyridine (Clinistix, Diastix, Tes-Tape)
Probenecid (Benedict's test, Clinitest tablets)
Salicylates in large doses (Clinitest tablets, Clinistix, Diastix, Tes-Tape)
Streptomycin (Benedict's test)
Tetracycline (Clinistix, Diastix, Tes-Tape)
Tetracyclines, due to ascorbic acid buffer (Benedict's test, Clinitest tablets)

### DRUGS THAT CAUSE TRUE GLYCOSURIA
Ammonium chloride
Asparaginase
Carbamazepine
Corticosteroids
Dextrothyroxine
Lithium carbonate
Nicotinic acid (large doses)
Phenothiazines (long-term)
Thiazide diuretics

### DRUGS THAT CAUSE FALSE-POSITIVE RESULTS FOR KETONURIA
Levodopa (Ketostix, Labstix)
Phenazopyridine (Ketostix or Gerhardt's reagent strip shows atypical color)
Phenolsulfonphthalein (Rothera's test)
Phenothiazines (Gerhardt's reagent strip shows atypical color)
Salicylates (Gerhardt's reagent strip shows reddish color)
Sulfobromophthalein (Bili-Labstix)

### DRUGS THAT CAUSE TRUE KETONURIA
Ether (anesthesia)
Insulin (excessive doses)

Isoniazid (intoxication)
Isopropyl alcohol (intoxication)

### DRUGS THAT INCREASE WHITE BLOOD CELL COUNT
Allopurinol
Ampicillin
Aspirin (toxicity)
Kanamycin
Methicillin

### DRUGS THAT CAUSE HEMATURIA
Amphotericin B
Coumarin derivatives
Methenamine in large doses
Methicillin
Para-aminosalicylic acid
Phenylbutazone
Sulfonamides

### DRUGS THAT CAUSE CASTS
Amphotericin B
Aspirin (toxicity)
Bacitracin
Ethacrynic acid
Furosemide
Gentamicin
Isoniazid
Kanamycin
Neomycin
Penicillin
Radiographic agents
Streptomycin
Sulfonamides

### DRUGS THAT CAUSE CRYSTALS (IF URINE IS ACIDIC)
Acetazolamide
Aminosalicylic acid
Ascorbic acid
Nitrofurantoin
Theophylline
Thiazide diuretics

sis, nephrotic syndrome, and polycystic kidney disease) or, possibly, multiple myeloma.
● Sugars — Glycosuria usually indicates diabetes mellitus, but may result from pheochromocytoma, Cushing's syndrome, im-paired tubular reabsorption, advanced renal disease, and increased intracranial pressure. I.V. solutions containing glucose and total parenteral nutrition containing from 10% to 50% glucose can cause glucose to spill over

the renal threshold, leading to glycosuria. Fructosuria, galactosuria, and pentosuria generally suggest rare hereditary metabolic disorders (except for lactosuria during pregnancy and breast-feeding). However, an alimentary form of pentosuria and fructosuria may follow excessive ingestion of pentose or fructose. When the liver fails to metabolize these sugars, they spill into the urine because the renal tubules don't reabsorb them.

● Ketone bodies — Ketonuria occurs in diabetes mellitus when cellular energy needs exceed available cellular glucose. In the absence of glucose, cells metabolize fat for energy. Ketone bodies — the end products of incomplete fat metabolism — accumulate in plasma and are excreted in the urine. Ketonuria may also occur in pregnancy, salicylate overdose, starvation states, low- or no-carbohydrate diets, and following diarrhea or vomiting.

● Bilirubin — Bilirubin in urine may occur in liver disease resulting from obstructive jaundice or hepatotoxic drugs or toxins or from fibrosis of the biliary canaliculi (which may occur in cirrhosis).

● Urobilinogen — Intestinal bacteria in the duodenum change bilirubin into urobilinogen. The liver reprocesses the remainder into bile. Increased urobilinogen in the urine may indicate liver damage, hemolytic disease, or severe infection. Decreased levels may occur with biliary obstruction, inflammatory disease, antimicrobial therapy, severe diarrhea, or renal insufficiency.

● Cells — Hematuria indicates bleeding within the genitourinary tract and may result from infection, obstruction, inflammation, trauma, tumors, glomerulonephritis, renal hypertension, lupus nephritis, renal tuberculosis, renal vein thrombosis, renal calculi, hydronephrosis, pyelonephritis, scurvy, malaria, parasitic infection of the bladder, subacute bacterial endocarditis, polyarteritis nodosa, and hemorrhagic disorders. Strenuous exercise or exposure to toxic chemicals may also cause hematuria. An excess of white blood cells (WBCs) in urine usually implies urinary tract inflammation, especially cystitis or pyelonephritis. WBC and WBC casts in urine suggest renal infection or noninfective inflammatory disease. Numerous epithelial cells suggest renal tubular degeneration, such as heavy metal poisoning, eclampsia, and kidney transplant rejection.

● Casts (plugs of gelled proteinaceous material [high-molecular-weight mucoprotein]) — Casts form in the renal tubules and collecting ducts by agglutination of protein cells or cellular debris and are flushed loose by urine flow. Excessive numbers of casts indicate renal disease. Hyaline casts are associated with renal parenchymal disease, inflammation, trauma to the glomerular capillary membrane, and some physiologic states (such as after exercise); epithelial casts, with renal tubular damage, nephrosis, eclampsia, amyloidosis, and heavy metal poisoning; coarse and fine granular casts, with acute or chronic renal failure, pyelonephritis, and chronic lead intoxication; fatty and waxy casts, with nephrotic syndrome, chronic renal disease, and diabetes mellitus; RBC casts, with renal parenchymal disease (especially glomerulonephritis), renal infarction, subacute bacterial endocarditis, vascular disorders, sickle cell anemia, scurvy, blood dyscrasias, malignant hypertension, collagen disease, and acute inflammation; and WBC casts, with acute pyelonephritis and glomerulonephritis, nephrotic syndrome, pyogenic infection, and lupus nephritis.

● Crystals — Some crystals normally appear in urine, but numerous calcium oxalate crystals suggest hypercalcemia or ethylene glycol ingestion. Cystine crystals (cystinuria) reflect an inborn error of metabolism.

● Other components — Bacteria, yeast cells, and parasites in urine sediment reflect genitourinary tract infection or contamination of external genitalia. Yeast cells, which may be mistaken for RBCs, are identifiable by their ovoid shape, lack of color, variable size and, frequently, signs of budding. The most common parasite in sediment is *Trichomonas vaginalis,* which causes vaginitis, urethritis, and prostatovesiculitis.

## INTERFERING FACTORS

● Strenuous exercise before routine urinalysis (may cause transient myoglobulinuria)

● Insufficient urinary volume, less than 2 ml (possible limitation of the range of procedures)

● Foods, such as beets, berries, and rhubarb (false change in color)

● Certain drugs (see *Drugs that influence routine urinalysis results,* pages 401 and 402)

● Highly dilute urine such as in diabetes insipidus

# Rubella antibodies

Although rubella (German measles) is generally a mild viral infection in children and young adults, it can produce severe infection in the fetus, resulting in spontaneous abortion, stillbirth, or congenital rubella syndrome. Because rubella infection normally induces immunoglobulin (Ig) G and IgM antibody production, measuring rubella antibodies can determine present infection as well as immunity resulting from past infection. The hemagglutination inhibition test is the most commonly used serologic test for rubella antibodies.

Suspected cases of congenital rubella may be confirmed if rubella-specific IgM antibodies are present in the infant's serum. Immune status in adults can be confirmed by an existing IgG-specific titer.

Exposure risk (when the immunity status is unknown) may be evaluated using two serum samples. The first sample should be drawn in the acute phase of clinical symptoms. If clinical symptoms aren't apparent, the sample should be drawn as soon as possible after the suspected exposure. The second sample should be drawn 3 to 4 weeks later during the convalescent phase.

## PURPOSE
- To diagnose rubella infection, especially congenital infection
- To determine susceptibility to rubella in children and in women of childbearing age

## PATIENT PREPARATION
- Explain to the patient that the rubella antibodies test diagnoses or evaluates susceptibility to rubella.
- Inform the patient that she need not restrict food and fluids.
- Tell the patient that this test requires a blood sample and that if a current infection is suspected, a second blood sample will be needed in 2 to 3 weeks to identify a rise in the titer.
- Explain who will perform the venipuncture and when and where the test will take place.
- Explain to the patient that she may experience slight discomfort from the tourniquet and needle puncture.

## PROCEDURE AND POSTTEST CARE
- Perform a venipuncture and collect the sample in a 7-ml clot-activator tube.
- Apply direct pressure to the venipuncture site until bleeding stops.
- If a hematoma develops at the venipuncture site, apply pressure.
- Instruct the patient to return for an additional blood test, when appropriate.
- If a woman of childbearing age is found to be susceptible to rubella, explain that vaccination can prevent rubella and that she must wait at least 3 months after the vaccination to become pregnant or risk permanent damage or death to the fetus.
- If the pregnant patient is found to be susceptible to rubella, instruct her to return for follow-up rubella antibody tests to detect possible subsequent infection.
- If the test confirms rubella in a pregnant patient, provide emotional support. As needed, refer her for appropriate counseling.

## PRECAUTIONS
- Handle the specimen gently to prevent hemolysis.

## REFERENCE VALUES
A titer of 1:8 or less indicates little or no immunity against rubella; titer more than 1:10 indicates adequate protection against rubella.

IgM results are reported as positive or negative.

## ABNORMAL FINDINGS
Hemagglutination inhibition antibodies normally appear 2 to 4 days after the onset of the rash, peak in 3 to 4 weeks, and then slowly decline but remain detectable for life. A fourfold or greater rise from the acute to the convalescent titer indicates a recent rubella infection.

**Alert** *The presence of rubella-specific IgM antibodies indicates recent infection in an adult and congenital rubella in an infant.*

## INTERFERING FACTORS
- None significant

S

## SARS viral testing

Severe acute respiratory syndrome (SARS) viral testing involves the use of one of three different tests to identify infection with the SARS virus. The SARS virus is a coronavirus (CoV) that causes a pneumonia-like infection. The incubation period is approximately 8 to 10 days. Typically the person has traveled to an area or lives in an area in which the infection has been identified. Usually SARS testing isn't performed unless there's a high index of suspicion, that is, groups of cases have developed for which the cause of other infections has been ruled out.

The three tests used for SARS testing include:
● Enzyme-linked immunosorbent assay (ELISA) — identifies antibodies to the SARS virus, usually about 20 days after the onset of symptoms
● Immunofluorescence assay — identifies antibodies to the SARS virus, possibly as early as 10 days after infection; however, this test can be time consuming because it involves growing the virus in the laboratory
● Reverse transcriptase-polymerase chain reaction (RT-PCR) — identifies the genetic information of ribonucleic acid in the virus; it's helpful in identifying the infection early on, with results available as early as within 2 days.

Specimens for SARS testing may be obtained from the nasopharyngeal, oropharyngeal, or bronchoalveolar area; trachea; pleural fluid; sputum; or postmortem tissue. Testing with RT-PCR usually involves serum and blood specimens.

### PURPOSE
● To identify the SARS CoV as the cause of the infection

### PATIENT PREPARATION
● Explain to the patient that the SARS viral test is used to identify the organism causing respiratory tract infection.
● Tell the patient about the types of specimens that will be collected. Explain when the specimens will be collected and how.
● If the specimen will be collected by expectoration, encourage fluid intake the night before collection to help sputum production, unless contraindicated by a fluid restriction. Teach the patient how to expectorate by taking three deep breaths and forcing a deep cough; emphasize that sputum isn't the same as saliva, which is unacceptable for culturing. Tell him to brush his teeth and gargle with water before the specimen collection to reduce contaminating oropharyngeal bacteria.
● If the specimen will be collected by swabbing the area, warn the patient that he may feel a slight itching sensation.
● If the specimen will be collected by tracheal suctioning, tell the patient that he'll experience discomfort as the catheter passes into the trachea.
● If the specimen will be collected by bronchoscopy, instruct the patient to fast for 6 hours before the procedure.
● Make sure the patient or a responsible family member has signed an informed consent form.

## PROCEDURE AND POSTTEST CARE
● Put on gloves.

### Washing or aspirating of nasopharyngeal area
● Have the patient sit with his head tilted slightly back.
● Insert a syringe filled with 1 to 1.5 ml of saline (non-bacteriostatic) into one nostril and instill the saline.
● Attach a small plastic catheter or tubing to the syringe and flush it with 2 to 3 ml of saline.
● Insert the tubing into the nostril and aspirate the secretions; then repeat in the other nostril.

### Swabbing of the nasopharyngeal or oropharyngeal area
● Obtain sterile swabs that have plastic sticks and Dacron or rayon tips.

**Alert** *Never use cotton-tipped applicators or swabs with wooden sticks. Some viruses can become inactivated by the substances contained in these swabs, thereby interfering with RT-PCR testing.*
● Insert the swab into the nostril and let it remain there for several seconds to absorb the secretions; if swabbing the oropharyngeal area, run the swab along the posterior pharynx and tonsils. Avoid touching the tongue.

### Expectorating of sputum
● Have the patient rinse his mouth with water.
● Instruct the patient to cough deeply and expectorate into the sterile dry container.

### Collecting of blood and plasma specimens
● Perform a venipuncture and collect 5 to 10 ml of whole blood in a serum separator tube (for serum RT-PCR or ELISA antibody testing) or an EDTA tube (for plasma testing).

### Collecting of other specimens
● Assist with tracheal suctioning, bronchoscopy, or thoracentesis as appropriate.

### All tests
● Make sure that all specimens are placed in the appropriate sterile container for transport.

● Dispose of equipment properly; seal the container in a biohazard bag before sending it to the laboratory.
● Label the container with the patient's name. Include on the test request form the nature and origin of the specimen, the date and time of collection, the initial diagnosis, and any current antimicrobial therapy.
● Provide mouth care as indicated.

## PRECAUTIONS
● Be sure to wear gloves when performing the procedure and handling specimens; adhere to your facility's infection control policies at all times.
● Because the patient may cough violently during suctioning, wear gloves, a mask and, if necessary, a gown to avoid exposure to pathogens.
● Send the specimen to the laboratory immediately after collection.

## NORMAL FINDINGS
Normally, the specimens would test negative for antibodies to the SARS virus.

## ABNORMAL FINDINGS
The specimens test positive for the SARS virus, indicating infection with SARS. SARS is diagnosed when positive test results occur:
● in a single specimen, which is tested at two distinct times
● in two specimens from two different areas
● in two specimens from the same area but tested on different days.

## INTERFERING FACTORS
● None significant

## Semen analysis

Semen analysis is a simple, inexpensive, and reasonably definitive test that's used in many applications, including evaluating a man's fertility. Fertility analysis usually includes measuring seminal fluid volume, performing sperm counts, and microscopic examination of spermatozoa. Sperm are counted in much the same way that white blood cells, red blood cells, and platelets are counted in a blood sample. Motility and morphology are studied microscopically after staining a drop of semen.

If analysis detects an abnormality, additional tests (for example, liver, thyroid, pituitary, or adrenal function tests) may be performed to identify the underlying cause and to screen for metabolic abnormalities (such as diabetes mellitus). Significant abnormalities — such as greatly decreased sperm count or motility or a marked increase in morphologically abnormal forms — may require testicular biopsy.

Semen analysis can also be used to detect semen on a rape victim, to identify the blood group of an alleged rapist, or to prove sterility in a paternity suit. (See *Identifying semen for medicolegal purposes*, **page 408**.) Some laboratories offer specialized semen tests such as screening for antibodies to spermatozoa.

## Purpose
- To evaluate male fertility in an infertile couple
- To substantiate the effectiveness of a vasectomy
- To detect semen on the body or clothing of a suspected rape victim or elsewhere at the crime scene
- To identify blood group substances to exonerate or incriminate a criminal suspect
- To rule out paternity on grounds of complete sterility

## Patient preparation
### For fertility evaluation
- Provide written instructions, and inform the patient that obtaining the most desirable specimen requires masturbation, ideally in a physician's office or laboratory.
- Tell the patient to follow the instructions given to him regarding the period of sexual continence before the test because doing so may increase his sperm count. Some physicians specify a fixed number of days, usually between 2 and 5; others advise a period of continence equal to the usual interval between episodes of sexual intercourse.
- If the patient prefers to collect the specimen at home, emphasize the importance of delivering the specimen to the laboratory within 1 hour after collection. Warn him not to expose the specimen to extreme temperatures or to direct sunlight (which can also increase its temperature). Ideally, the specimen should remain at body temperature until liquefaction is complete (about 20 minutes). To

deliver a semen specimen during cold weather, suggest that the patient keep the specimen container in a coat pocket on the way to the laboratory to protect the specimen from exposure to cold.
- Alternative collection methods include coitus interruptus or the use of a condom. For collection by coitus interruptus, instruct the patient to withdraw immediately before ejaculation and to deposit the ejaculate in a suitable specimen container. For collection by condom, tell the patient to first wash the condom with soap and water, rinse it thoroughly, and allow it to dry completely. (Powders or lubricants applied to the condom may be spermicidal.) Special sheaths that don't contain spermicide are also available for semen collection. After collection, instruct him to tie the condom, place it in a glass jar, and promptly deliver it to the laboratory.
- Fertility may also be determined by collecting semen from the woman after coitus to assess the ability of the spermatozoa to penetrate the cervical mucus and remain active. For the postcoital cervical mucus test, instruct the patient to report for examination 1 to 2 days before ovulation as determined by basal temperature records. A urine luteinizing hormone-releasing hormone test may help predict ovulation in the patient with an irregular cycle. Instruct the couple to abstain from intercourse for 2 days and then to have sexual intercourse 2 to 8 hours before the examination. Remind them to avoid using lubricants. Explain to the patient scheduled for this test that the procedure takes only a few minutes. Tell her that she'll be placed in the lithotomy position and that a speculum will be inserted into the vagina to collect the specimen. She may feel some pressure, but usually no pain.

### For semen collection from a rape victim
- Explain to the patient that the examiner will try to obtain a semen specimen from her vagina. For more information, see the appendix Sexual assault testing.
- Prepare the victim for insertion of the speculum as you would the patient scheduled for postcoital examination.
- Handle the victim's clothes as little as possible. If her clothes are moist, put them in a paper bag — not a plastic bag (which causes seminal stains and secretions to mold). La-

# Identifying semen for medicolegal purposes

Spermatozoa (or their fragments) persist in the vagina for more than 72 hours after sexual intercourse. This duration allows detection and positive identification of semen from vaginal aspirates or smears or from stains on clothing, other fabrics, skin, or hair, which is commonly necessary for medicolegal purposes, usually in connection with rape or homicide investigations. Spermatozoa taken from the vagina of an exhumed body that has been properly embalmed and remains reasonably intact can also be identified.

To determine which stains or fluids require further investigation, clothing or other fabrics can be scanned with ultraviolet light to detect the typical green-white fluorescence of semen. Soaking appropriate samples of clothing, fabric, or hair in physiologic saline solution elutes the semen and spermatozoa. Deposits of dried semen can be gently sponged from the victim's skin.

The two most common tests to identify semen are the determination of *acid phosphatase concentration* (the more sensitive test) and *microscopic examination* for the presence of spermatozoa. Acid phosphatase appears in semen in significantly greater concentrations than in other body fluids. In microscopic examination, spermatozoa or head fragments can be identified on stained smears prepared directly from vaginal scrapings or aspirates or from the concentrated sediment of eluates or lavages.

Like other body fluids, semen contains the soluble A, B, and H blood group substances in approximately 80% of males who are genetically determined secretors (males who have the dominant secretor gene in a homozygous or heterozygous state). Thus, the male who has group A blood and is a secretor has soluble blood group A substance in his seminal fluid and group A substance on the surface of his red blood cells. This fact can be of considerable medicolegal importance. Semen analysis can demonstrate that the semen of a suspect in a rape or homicide investigation is different from or consistent with semen found in or on the victim's body.

---

bel the bag properly, and send it to the laboratory immediately.
● Provide emotional support by speaking to the patient calmly and reassuringly. Encourage her to express her fears and anxieties. Listen sympathetically.
● If the patient is scheduled for vaginal lavage, tell the rape victim to expect a cold sensation when saline solution is instilled to wash out the specimen.
● Help the patient relax by instructing her to breathe deeply and slowly through her mouth.
● Instruct the victim to urinate just before the test, but warn her not to wipe the vulva afterward because doing so may remove semen.

## PROCEDURE AND POSTTEST CARE
● Obtain a semen specimen for a fertility study by asking the patient to collect semen in a clean plastic specimen container.
● A specimen is obtained from the vagina of a rape victim by direct aspiration, saline lavage, or a direct smear of vaginal contents using a Papanicolaou stick or, less desirably, a cotton applicator stick. Dried smears are usually collected from the suspected rape victim's skin by gently washing the skin with a small piece of gauze moistened with physiologic saline solution.
● Prepare direct smears on glass microscopic slides after labeling the frosted end. Immediately place smeared slides in Coplin jars containing 95% ethanol.
● Before postcoital examination, the examiner wipes excess mucus from the external cervix and collects the specimen by direct aspiration of the cervical canal using a 1-ml tuberculin syringe without a cannula or needle.
● Inform a patient who's undergoing infertility studies that test results should be available in 24 hours.
● Refer the suspected rape victim to an appropriate specialist for counseling — a gynecologist, psychiatrist, clinical psychologist, nursing specialist, member of the clergy, or representative of a community support group such as Women Organized Against Rape.

## PRECAUTIONS

● If the patient prefers to collect the specimen during coitus interruptus, tell him he must prevent any loss of semen during ejaculation.

● Deliver all specimens, regardless of the source or method of collection, to the laboratory within 1 hour.

● Protect semen specimens for fertility studies from extremes of temperature and direct sunlight during delivery to the laboratory.

● Never lubricate the vaginal speculum. Oil or lubrication hinders examination of spermatozoa by interfering with smear preparation and staining and by inhibiting sperm motility through toxic ingredients. Instead, moisten the speculum with water or physiologic saline solution.

● Use extreme caution in securing, labeling, and delivering all specimens to be used for medicolegal purposes. You may be asked to testify when, where, and from whom the specimen was obtained; the specimen's general appearance and identifying features; steps taken to ensure the specimen's integrity; and when, where, and to whom the specimen was delivered for analysis. If your facility or clinic uses routing requests for such specimens, fill them out carefully and place them in the permanent medicolegal file.

## NORMAL FINDINGS

Normal semen volume ranges from 0.7 to 6.5 ml. Paradoxically, the semen volume of many men in infertile couples is increased. Abstinence for 1 week or more results in progressively increased semen volume. (With abstinence of up to 10 days, sperm counts increase, sperm motility progressively decreases, and sperm morphology stays the same.) Liquefied semen is generally highly viscid, translucent, and gray-white, with a musty or acrid odor. After liquefaction, specimens of normal viscosity can be poured in drops. Normally, semen is slightly alkaline with a pH of 7.3 to 7.9.

Other normal characteristics of semen are immediate coagulation and liquefaction within 20 minutes; a normal sperm count of 20 to 150 million/ml or greater; normal morphology in 40% of spermatozoa; and 20% or more of spermatozoa showing progressive motility within 4 hours of collection.

The normal postcoital cervical mucus test shows 10 to 20 motile spermatozoa per microscopic high-power field and spinnbarkeit (a measurement of the tenacity of the mucus) of at least 4" (10 cm). These findings indicate adequate spermatozoa and receptivity of the cervical mucus. Shaking or dead sperm may indicate antisperm antibodies.

## ABNORMAL FINDINGS

Abnormal semen isn't synonymous with infertility. Only one viable spermatozoon is needed to fertilize an ovum. Although a normal sperm count is 20 million/ml or more, many men with sperm counts below 1 million/ml have fathered normal children. Only men who can't deliver any viable spermatozoa in their ejaculate during sexual intercourse are absolutely sterile. Nevertheless, subnormal sperm counts, decreased sperm motility, and abnormal morphology are usually associated with decreased fertility.

Other tests may be necessary to evaluate the patient's general health, metabolic status, or the function of specific endocrine glands (pituitary, thyroid, adrenal, or gonadal).

## INTERFERING FACTORS

● Poor timing of test within the menstrual cycle (abnormal postcoital test results)

● Previous cervical conization or cryotherapy and some medications such as clomiphene citrate (possible abnormal postcoital test results due to changes in cervical mucus)

● Delayed transport of the specimen, exposure to extreme temperatures or direct sunlight, or the presence of toxic chemicals in the container or the condom (possible decrease in number of viable sperm)

● An incomplete specimen — for example, from improper collection technique (decrease in specimen volume)

## *Sentinel node location before biopsy*

Sentinel node location before biopsy is a procedure that involves identifying and then localizing the nodes before a biopsy is performed. A sentinel lymph node is the first node in the lymphatic basin into which a primary tumor site drains. Apparently, the histology of the sentinel node will reflect the histology of the rest of the nodes in that basin. So, if that sentinel node is identified and found to be negative for tumor invasion, it's assumed that the rest of the nodes are also negative for tumor. For example, in breast cancer, if the hypothesis is proven true, axillary lymph node dissections and their resulting morbidity could be avoided.

Sentinel node location is performed using one of three techniques; the techniques are usually combined to increase the likelihood of identifying the sentinel node. The first technique is lymphoscintigraphy, performed with nuclear medicine using injected technetium-99m ($^{99m}$Tc), a radioactive isotope. The second technique uses a nuclear radiation probe that produces sound to detect the node. The third technique uses the injection of blue dye.

## PURPOSE

- To aid in diagnosing breast cancer or malignant melanoma
- To identify the sentinel lymph node and evaluate it for the presence or absence of tumor cells, indicating nodal metastasis
- To detect metastasis, map all sentinel nodes, and stage and monitor cancers of the breast, head, neck, and skin and malignant melanoma (lymphoscintigraphy)
- To provide auditory confirmation of nodal involvement (nuclear radiation probe)
- To provide visual confirmation of nodal involvement and map tumor route (blue dye injection)

## PATIENT PREPARATION

- Explain to the patient the three techniques for sentinel node location before biopsy that may be used to evaluate a particular lymph node will determine if cancer has spread into the lymph system. Tell the patient that if the results are positive, surgery usually occurs shortly afterward.
- Inform the patient that she may be moved to the operating room for the nuclear radiation probe and blue dye injection techniques.
- Provide routine preoperative care as ordered, including maintaining the patient on nothing-by-mouth status.
- For the lymphoscintigraphy for breast cancer, tell the patient that a radioactive substance will be injected subcutaneously into the breast and nearby the area of the suspected tumor. For malignant melanoma, tell the patient that four to six injections will be made under the skin around the tumor site or where previous surgery had been done.

- For the nuclear radiation probe, tell the patient that a radioactive substance will be administered and the probe will be applied to area to identify the radioactive area.
- For the blue dye injection, tell the patient that the dye will be injected between the toes and hands, between the second and third fingers.
- Explain that the site of the lymph nodes will be marked with an indelible pen.
- Warn the patient that if blue dye is used, the skin may develop a slight blue coloration that will fade in about 6 to 12 hours and that urine may turn blue temporarily.
- Offer emotional support as necessary.

## PROCEDURE AND POSTTEST CARE

- The patient is positioned on the table in the nuclear medicine suite.
- A standard dose of $^{99m}$Tc is injected circumferentially around the margins of a palpable mass using a 25G needle. For a nonpalpable mass, injections are guided with ultrasound or mammographic techniques. If the tumor has already been excised, the injections are made around the tumor bed.

### Lymphoscintigraphy

- Images of the axilla are taken with a gamma camera. The location of the sentinel node is marked on the skin in indelible ink and noted on a data sheet. If nuclear radiation probe is to follow, the patient is moved to the operating room.

### Nuclear radiation probe

- A sound-radiation gamma probe is applied to locate the area of radioactivity detector as sound.

### Blue dye injection

- Blue dye is injected into the feet in the web between the toes, and in the hands between the second and third fingers.
- Within 10 to 15 minutes of the dye injection, a small incision is made in the axilla over the suspected location of the sentinel lymph node. The surgeon follows the trail of stained lymphatics to the sentinel lymph node.

## All tests

● The axilla is then checked for remaining radioactivity; if none is noted, the procedure concludes.

● Because of the radioactivity, the sentinel lymph node is maintained in formalin for 24 to 48 hours before it can be processed.

● Monitor the site of injection for the radioactive substance, noting any signs of bleeding or inflammation.

● Prepare the patient for additional surgery if necessary.

● Provide emotional support and guidance, helping to explain the results and their implications.

## PRECAUTIONS

● Be aware that because $^{99m}$Tc is a radioactive substance, all radiation precautions must be implemented. Staff members need to be monitored for radiation exposure. Radiation levels need to be determined in the nuclear medicine suite and the operating room postsurgically.

● Know that rare cases of allergy to the $^{99m}$Tc or blue dye have been noted; the patient should be observed for signs and symptoms of allergic reaction (skin changes and respiratory difficulties).

## NORMAL FINDINGS

Normal findings include absence of any evidence of tumor activity in the lymph node and no blockage of lymphatic drainage.

## ABNORMAL FINDINGS

Sentinel node location before biopsy identifies metastasis to the lymph nodes and its mode of spread. Obstruction to lymph circulation may be seen as asymmetry.

## INTERFERING FACTORS

● Allergy to a radioactive substance

● Inability to raise arm to allow access to axilla

● Administration of radioactive substance into an inaccurate location or improper administration of substance

# 17-hydroxycortico-steroids, urine

The 17-hydroxycorticosteroid (17-OHCS) test measures urine levels of 17-OHCS — metabolites of the hormones that regulate glyconeogenesis. More than 80% of all urinary 17-OHCS are metabolites of cortisol, the primary adrenocortical steroid. Test findings thus reflect cortisol secretion and, indirectly, adrenocortical function.

Urine 17-OHCS levels are most accurately determined from a 24-hour specimen because cortisol secretion varies diurnally and in response to stress and many other factors. Column chromatography and spectrophotofluorimetry with the Porter-Silber reagent are used to measure 17-OHCS levels.

Levels of plasma cortisol, urine-free cortisol, and urine 17-ketosteroids may be measured and corticotropin stimulation and suppression testing performed to confirm test results. Of these, urine-free cortisol is a more sensitive and specific test for hypercortisolism.

## PURPOSE

● To assess adrenocortical function

## PATIENT PREPARATION

● Explain to the patient that the urine 17-OHCS test evaluates how his adrenal glands are functioning.

● Inform the patient that he should restrict food and fluids that will alter test results (coffee, tea) and avoid excessive physical exercise and stressful situations during the collection period.

● Tell the patient that the test requires collection of urine over a 24-hour period, and instruct him in the proper collection technique.

● Notify the laboratory and physician of medications the patient is taking that may affect test results; they may need to be restricted.

## PROCEDURE AND POSTTEST CARE

● Collect the patient's urine over a 24-hour period, discarding the first specimen and retaining the last. Use a bottle containing a preservative to prevent deterioration of the specimen. Label the specimen appropriately, including the patient's gender on the request forms.

● Instruct the patient that he may resume his usual activities, diet, and medications, as ordered.

## PRECAUTIONS

● Refrigerate the specimen or place it on ice during the collection period.

## REFERENCE VALUES

Normally, urine 17-OHCS values range from 4.5 to 12 mg/24 hours in males (SI, 12.4 to 33.1 µmol/d) and from 2.5 to 10 mg/24 hours in females (SI, 6.9 to 27.6 µmol/d). In children ages 8 to 12, levels are less than 4.5 mg/24 hours (SI, < 12.4 µmol/d); in children younger than age 8, levels are normally less than 1.5 mg/24 hours (SI, < 4.14 µmol/d).

## ABNORMAL FINDINGS

Elevated urine 17-OHCS levels may indicate Cushing's syndrome, an adrenal carcinoma or adenoma, or a pituitary tumor. Increased levels may also occur in the patient with virilism, hyperthyroidism, or severe hypertension. Extreme stress induced by such conditions as acute pancreatitis and eclampsia also causes urine 17-OHCS levels to rise above normal.

Low urine 17-OHCS levels may indicate Addison's disease, hypopituitarism, or myxedema.

## INTERFERING FACTORS

● Ascorbic acid, chloral hydrate, chlordiazepoxide, glutethimide, hydroxyzine, iodides, meprobamate, methenamine, penicillin G, phenothiazines, quinidine, quinine, and spironolactone (possible increase)
● Estrogens, hormonal contraceptives, hydralazine (Apresoline), nalidixic acid (NegGram), phenothiazines, phenytoin (Dilantin), and thiazide diuretics (possible decrease)

## *17-ketogenic steroids, urine*

Using spectrophotofluorimetry, the 17-ketogenic steroids (17-KGS) test determines urine levels of 17-KGS, which consist of the 17-hydroxycorticosteroids — cortisol and its

metabolites, for example — and other adrenocortical steroids, such as pregnanetriol, that can be oxidized in the laboratory to 17-ketosteroids. Because 17-KGS represent such a large group of steroids, this test provides an excellent overall assessment of adrenocortical function. For accurate diagnosis of a specific disease, 17-KGS levels must be compared with results of other tests, including plasma corticotropin, plasma cortisol, corticotropin stimulation, single-dose metyrapone, and dexamethasone suppression.

## PURPOSE

● To evaluate adrenocortical and testicular function
● To aid in the diagnosis of Cushing's syndrome and Addison's disease

## PATIENT PREPARATION

● Explain to the patient that the urine 17-KGS test evaluates adrenal function.
● Inform the patient that he need not restrict food and fluids, but should avoid excessive physical exercise and stressful situations during the collection period.
● Tell the patient that the test requires urine collection over a 24-hour period, and teach him how to collect the specimen correctly.
● Notify the laboratory and physician of medications the patient is taking that may affect test results; they may need to be restricted.

## PROCEDURE AND POSTTEST CARE

● Collect the patient's urine over a 24-hour period, discarding the first specimen and retaining the last. Use a bottle containing a preservative to keep the specimen at a pH of 4.0 to 4.5. Appropriately label the specimen and laboratory requisition requests with the patient's gender.
● Instruct the patient that he may resume his usual activities and medications, as ordered.

## PRECAUTIONS

● Refrigerate the specimen or keep it on ice during the collection period.
● Send the specimen to the laboratory as soon as collection is complete.

## REFERENCE VALUES

Normally, urine 17-KGS levels range from 4 to 14 mg/24 hours (SI, 13 to 49 µmol/d) in males and from 2 to 12 mg/24 hours (SI, 7 to 42 µmol/d) in females. Children ages 11 to 14 excrete 2 to 9 mg/24 hours (SI, 7 to 31 µmol/d); younger children and infants excrete 0.1 to 4 mg/24 hours (SI, 0.3 to 14 µmol/d).

## ABNORMAL FINDINGS

Elevated urine 17-KGS levels indicate hyperadrenalism, which may occur in Cushing's syndrome, adrenogenital syndrome (congenital adrenal hyperplasia), and adrenal carcinoma or adenoma. Levels also rise with severe physical stress (burns, infections, or surgery, for example) or emotional stress.

Low levels may reflect hypoadrenalism, which may occur in Addison's disease and may also be associated with panhypopituitarism, cretinism, and general wasting.

## INTERFERING FACTORS

● Corticotropin, hydralazine, meprobamate, oleandomycin, penicillin, phenothiazines, and spironolactone (possible increase)
● Long-term corticosteroid therapy, estrogens, quinine, reserpine, and thiazide diuretics (possible decrease)
● Carbamazepine, cephalothin, dexamethasone, nalidixic acid, and tiaprofenic acid (possible increase or decrease)

# 17-ketosteroids, urine

The 17-ketosteroids (17-KS) is a fractionation test that uses the spectrophotofluorimetric technique to measure urine levels of 17-KS. Steroids and steroid metabolites characterized by a ketone group on carbon 17 in the steroid nucleus, 17-KS originate primarily in the adrenal glands, but also in the testes and ovaries.

Although not all 17-KS are androgens, they cause androgenic effects. For example, excessive secretion of 17-KS may result in hirsutism and may increase clitoral or phallic size; in utero, elevated 17-KS levels may cause a female fetus to develop a male urogenital tract. Because 17-KS don't include all the androgens (testosterone, for example, the most potent androgen), these levels provide only a rough estimate of androgenic activity. To provide additional information about an-

drogen secretion, plasma testosterone levels may be measured concurrently.

## PURPOSE

● To aid in the diagnosis of adrenal and gonadal dysfunction
● To aid in the diagnosis of adrenogenital syndrome (congenital adrenal hyperplasia)
● To monitor cortisol therapy in the treatment of adrenogenital syndrome

## PATIENT PREPARATION

● Explain to the patient that the urine 17-KS test evaluates hormonal balance.
● Inform the patient that he need not restrict food and fluids, but should avoid excessive physical exercise and stressful situations during the collection period.
● Tell the patient that the test requires urine collection over a 24-hour period, and instruct him in the proper collection technique.
● Notify the laboratory and physician of medications the patient is taking that may affect test results; they may need to be restricted.

## PROCEDURE AND POSTTEST CARE

● Collect the patient's urine over a 24-hour period, discarding the first sample and retaining the last. Use a bottle containing a preservative to keep the specimen at a pH of 4.0 to 4.5. Appropriately label the specimen and laboratory requisition requests with the patient's gender.
● Instruct the patient that he may resume his usual activities and medications, as ordered.

## PRECAUTIONS

● Refrigerate the specimen or place it on ice during the collection period.
● Send the specimen to the laboratory as soon as collection is complete.

## REFERENCE VALUES

Normally, urine 17-KS values range from 10 to 25 mg/24 hours (SI, 35 to 87 µmol/d) in males and from 4 to 6 mg/24 hours (SI, 4 to 21 µmol/d) in females. Children between ages 10 and 14 excrete 1 to 6 mg/24 hours (SI, 2 to 21 µmol/d); children younger than age 10 excrete less than 3 mg/24 hours (SI, < 10 µmol/d).

For more information about specific steroids in the 17-KS group, the 17-KS frac-

# NORMAL VALUES FOR THE 17-KETOSTEROID FRACTIONATION TEST

Through gas-liquid chromatography, the 17-ketosteroid (17-KS) fractionation test shows which specific steroids in the 17-KS group are elevated or suppressed and thus aids differential diagnosis of conditions suggested by abnormal 17-KS levels. Note that 17-KS levels are measured in milligrams per 24 hours

| STEROID | ADULT MALE | ADULT FEMALE | MALE AGES 10 TO 15 | FEMALE AGES 10 TO 15 |
|---------|-----------|--------------|--------------------|-----------------------|
| Androsterone | 0.9 to 6.1 | 0 to 3.1 | 0.2 to 2 | 0.5 to 2.5 |
| Dehydroepiandrosterone | 0 to 3.1 | 0 to 1.5 | < 0.4 | < 0.4 |
| Etiocholanolone | 0.9 to 5.2 | 0.1 to 3.5 | 0.1 to 1.6 | 0.7 to 3.1 |
| 11-hydroxyandrosterone | 0.2 to 1.6 | 0 to 1.1 | 0.1 to 1.1 | 0.2 to 1 |
| 11-hydroxyetiocholanolone | 0.1 to 0.9 | 0.1 to 0.8 | < 0.3 | 0.1 to 0.5 |
| 11-ketoandrosterone | 0 to 0.5 | 0 to 0.3 | < 0.1 | < 0.1 |
| 11-ketoetiocholanolone | 0 to 1.6 | 0 to 1 | < 0.3 | 0.1 to 0.5 |
| Pregnanetriol | 0.2 to 2 | 0 to 1.4 | 0.2 to 0.6 | 0.1 to 0.6 |

tionation test may be performed. (See *Normal values for the 17-ketosteroid fractionation test.*)

## ABNORMAL FINDINGS

Elevated urine 17-KS levels may result from adrenal hyperplasia, carcinoma or adenoma, or adrenogenital syndrome. In females, elevated levels may also indicate ovarian dysfunction, such as polycystic ovary (Stein-Leventhal) syndrome, lutein cell tumor of the ovary, or androgenic arrhenoblastoma. In males, elevated 17-KS levels may indicate interstitial cell tumor of the testis. Characteristically, 17-KS levels also rise during pregnancy, severe stress, chronic illness, or debilitating disease.

Depressed urine 17-KS levels may result from Addison's disease, panhypopituitarism, eunuchoidism, or castration and may occur in cretinism, myxedema, and nephrosis. When this test is used to monitor cortisol therapy for adrenogenital syndrome, 17-KS levels typically return to normal with adequate cortisol administration.

## INTERFERING FACTORS

- Presence of menstrual blood in the specimen
- Antibiotics, corticotropin, dexamethasone, meprobamate, oleandomycin, phenothiazines, and spironolactone (possible increase)
- Estrogens, ethacrynic acid, penicillin, and phenytoin (possible decrease)
- Nalidixic acid and quinine (possible increase or decrease)

# Sex chromosome tests

Although sex chromosome tests can screen for abnormalities in the number of sex chromosomes, the faster, simpler, and more accurate full karyotype (chromosome analysis) has all but replaced them. Sex chromosome tests are usually indicated for abnormal sexual development, ambiguous genitalia, amen-

| BOTH SEXES AGES 6 TO 9 | BOTH SEXES AGES 3 TO 5 | BOTH SEXES AGES 1 TO 2 | BOTH SEXES BIRTH TO AGE 1 |
| --- | --- | --- | --- |
| 0.1 to 1 | < 0.3 | < 0.3 | < 0.1 |
| < 0.2 | < 0.1 | < 0.1 | < 0.1 |
| 0.3 to 1 | < 0.7 | < 0.4 | < 0.1 |
| 0.4 to 1 | < 0.4 | < 0.3 | < 0.3 |
| 0.1 to 0.5 | < 0.4 | < 0.1 | < 0.1 |
| < 0.1 | < 0.1 | < 0.1 | < 0.1 |
| 0.1 to 0.5 | < 0.4 | < 0.1 | < 0.1 |
| < 0.3 | < 0.1 | < 0.1 | < 0.1 |

orrhea, and suspected chromosomal abnormalities.

## PURPOSE
- To quickly screen for abnormal sexual development (X and Y chromatin tests)
- To aid in the assessment of an infant with ambiguous genitalia (X chromatin test)
- To determine the number of Y chromosomes in an individual (Y chromatin test)

## PATIENT PREPARATION
- Explain to the patient or his parents, if appropriate, why the sex chromosome test is being performed.
- Tell the patient that the test requires that the inside of his cheek be scraped to obtain a specimen and who will perform the test.
- Assure the patient that the test takes only a few minutes, but may require a follow-up chromosome analysis.
- Inform the patient that the laboratory generally requires as long as 4 weeks to complete the analysis.

## PROCEDURE AND POSTTEST CARE
- Scrape the buccal mucosa firmly with a wooden or metal spatula at least twice to obtain a specimen of healthy cells (vaginal mucosa is used, rarely, in young women).
- Rub the spatula over the glass slide, making sure the cells are evenly distributed.
- Spray the slide with a cell fixative and send it to the laboratory with a brief patient history and indications for the test.

## PRECAUTIONS
- Make sure the buccal mucosa is scraped firmly to ensure a sufficient number of cells.
- Check that the specimen isn't saliva, which contains no cells.

## NORMAL FINDINGS
A normal female (XX) has only one X chromatin mass (the number of X- chromatin masses discernible is one less than the number of X chromosomes in the cells examined). For various reasons, an X-chromatin mass is ordinarily discernible in only 20% to

# Sex chromosome anomalies

| DISORDER AND CHROMOSOMAL ANEUPLOIDY | CAUSE AND INCIDENCE | PHENOTYPIC FEATURES |
|---|---|---|
| **KLINEFELTER'S SYNDROME** | | |
| ◆ 47,XXY<br>◆ 48,XXXY<br>◆ 49,XXXXY<br>◆ 48,XXYY<br>◆ 49,XXXYY | ◆ Nondisjunction or improper chromatid separation during anaphase I or II of oogenesis or spermatogenesis results in abnormal gamete<br>◆ 1 per 1,000 male births | ◆ Syndrome usually inapparent until puberty<br>◆ Small penis and testes<br>◆ Sparse facial and abdominal hair; feminine distribution of pubic hair<br>◆ Somewhat enlarged breasts (gynecomastia)<br>◆ Sexual dysfunction<br>◆ Truncal obesity<br>◆ Sterility<br>◆ Possible mental retardation (greater incidence with increased X chromosomes) |
| **POLYSOMY Y** | | |
| ◆ 47,XYY | ◆ Nondisjunction during anaphase II of spermatogenesis causes both Y chromosomes to pass to the same pole and results in a YY sperm<br>◆ 1 per 1,000 male births | ◆ Above-average stature (commonly over 72″ [182.9 cm])<br>◆ Increased incidence of severe acne<br>◆ May display aggressive, psychopathic, or criminal behavior<br>◆ Normal fertility<br>◆ Learning disabilities |
| **TURNER'S SYNDROME** | | |
| ◆ 45,XO<br>◆ Mosaics: XO/XX or XO/XXX<br>◆ Aberrations of X chromosomes, including deletion of short arm of one X chromosome, presence of a ring chromosome, or presence of an isochromosome on the long arm of an X chromosome | ◆ Nondisjunction during anaphase I or II of spermatogenesis results in sperm without any sex chromosomes<br>◆ 1 per 3,500 female births (most common chromosome complement in first-trimester abortions) | ◆ Short stature (usually under 57″ [144.8 cm])<br>◆ Webbed neck<br>◆ Low posterior hairline<br>◆ Broad chest with widely spaced nipples<br>◆ Underdeveloped breasts<br>◆ Juvenile external genitalia<br>◆ Primary amenorrhea common<br>◆ Congenital heart disease (30% with coarctation of the aorta)<br>◆ Renal abnormalities<br>◆ Sterility from underdeveloped internal reproductive organs (ovaries are only strands of connective tissue)<br>◆ No mental retardation, but possible problems with space perception and orientation |

| DISORDER AND CHROMOSOMAL ANEUPLOIDY | CAUSE AND INCIDENCE | PHENOTYPIC FEATURES |
|---|---|---|
| **OTHER X POLYSOMES** | | |
| ◆ 47,XXX | ◆ Nondisjunction at anaphase I or II of oogenesis | |
| | ◆ 1 per 1,400 female births | ◆ Commonly, no obvious anatomic abnormalities<br>◆ Normal fertility |
| ◆ 48,XXXX | ◆ Rare<br>◆ Rare | ◆ Mental retardation<br>◆ Ocular hypertelorism<br>◆ Reduced fertility |
| ◆ 49,XXXXX | | ◆ Severe mental retardation<br>◆ Ocular hypertelorism with uncoordinated eye movement<br>◆ Abnormal sexual organ development<br>◆ Various skeletal anomalies |

50% of the buccal mucosal cells of a normal woman.

A normal male (XY) has only one Y-chromatin mass (the number of Y-chromatin masses equals the number of Y chromosomes in the cells examined).

## ABNORMAL FINDINGS

In most laboratories, if less than 20% of the cells in a buccal smear contain an X-chromatin mass, some cells are presumed to contain only one X chromosome, necessitating full karyotyping. A person with a female phenotype and a positive Y-chromatin mass runs a high risk of developing a malignancy in the intra-abdominal gonads. In such cases, removal of these gonads is indicated and should generally be performed before age 5.

The patient and his parents require genetic counseling after the cause of chromosomal abnormal sexual development has been identified. A medical team comprising physicians, psychologists, psychiatrists, and educators must decide the child's sex if a child is phenotypically of one sex and genotypically of the other. This careful evaluation should be made early to prevent developmental problems related to incorrect gender identification. (See *Sex chromosome anomalies*.)

## INTERFERING FACTORS

● Obtaining saliva instead of buccal cells (false specimen)
● Cell deterioration due to failure to apply cell fixative to the slide
● Presence of bacteria or wrinkles in the cell membrane, analysis of degenerative cells, or use of an outdated stain

# Sickle cell test

The sickle cell test, also known as the *hemoglobin (Hb) S test,* is used to detect sickle cells, which are severely deformed, rigid erythrocytes that may slow blood flow. Sickle cell trait (characterized by heterozygous Hb S) is found almost exclusively in blacks — 0.2% of blacks born in the United States have sickle cell disease.

Although the sickle cell test is useful as a rapid screening procedure, it may produce erroneous results. Hb electrophoresis should be performed to confirm the diagnosis if sickle cell disease is strongly suspected.

## PURPOSE
- To identify sickle cell disease and sickle cell trait (see *Identifying sickle cell trait*)

## PATIENT PREPARATION
- Explain to the patient that the Hb S test is used to detect sickle cell disease.
- Tell the patient that a blood sample will be taken. Explain who will perform the venipuncture and when.
- Explain to the patient that he may feel slight discomfort from the tourniquet and the needle puncture.

*Age alert*  If the patient is an infant or child, explain to his parents that a small amount of blood will be taken from his finger or earlobe.

- Check the patient's history for a blood transfusion within the past 3 months.
- Inform the patient that he need not restrict food and fluids.

## PROCEDURE AND POSTTEST CARE
- Perform a venipuncture and collect the sample in a 3- or 4.5-ml EDTA tube.

*Age alert*  For young children, collect capillary blood in a microcollection device.

- If a hematoma develops at the venipuncture site, apply pressure. If the hematoma is large, monitor pulses distal to the phlebotomy site.
- Make sure subdermal bleeding has stopped before removing pressure.

## PRECAUTIONS
- Be sure to completely fill the collection tube and invert it gently several times to thoroughly mix the sample and the anticoagulant.
- Don't shake the tube vigorously.

## NORMAL FINDINGS
Results of the Hb S test are reported as positive or negative. A negative result suggests the absence of Hb S.

## ABNORMAL FINDINGS
A positive result may indicate the presence of sickle cells, but Hb electrophoresis is needed to further diagnose the sickling tendency of cells. Rarely, in the absence of Hb S, other abnormal Hb may cause sickling.

## INTERFERING FACTORS
- Hb concentration less than 10%, elevated Hb S levels in infants under age 6 months, or transfusion within 3 months of the test (possible false-negative)

# Signal-averaged electrocardiography

Signal averaging is the amplification, averaging, and filtering of an electrocardiogram (ECG) signal that's recorded on the body surface by orthogonal leads. The recording detects high-frequency, low-amplitude cardiac electrical signals in the last part of the QRS complex and in the ST segment. In patients who have survived an acute myocardial infarction (MI), these distinctive signals, called *late potentials,* may represent delayed disorganized activity in abnormal areas of the myocardium at the interface of fibrous scar tissue and normal tissue. This activity can lead to life-threatening ventricular arrhythmias.

In this computerized procedure, each electrode lead input is amplified, its voltage is measured or sampled at intervals of 1 msec or less, and each sample is converted into a digital number. The ECG is thereby converted from an analogue voltage waveform into a series of digital numbers that are, in essence, a computer-readable ECG of 100 or more QRS complexes.

## PURPOSE

- To detect late potentials and evaluate the risk of life-threatening arrhythmias

## PATIENT PREPARATION

- Explain to the patient that signal-averaged ECG is used to evaluate his heart's electrical activity and the potential for developing a life-threatening arrhythmia.
- Inform the patient that the test will be performed by a technician who has been specially trained to monitor recording and computerized equipment used to analyze the signal-averaged ECG.
- Describe the test, including who will perform it, where it will take place, and how long it will last.
- Tell the patient that electrodes will be attached to his arms, legs, and chest and that the procedure is painless.
- Explain to the patient that during the test, he'll be asked to lie still and breathe normally and that doing so is important because limb movement or the sound of his voice will distort the recording.
- Inform the patient that he need not restrict food and fluids.
- Record on the patient's chart any use of antiarrhythmics.

## PROCEDURE AND POSTTEST CARE

- Place the patient in the supine position. If he can't tolerate lying flat, help him into semi-Fowler's position.
- Have the patient expose his chest, both ankles, and both wrists for electrode placement. If the patient is a woman, provide a chest drape until the chest leads are applied.
- The test is performed by a technician who's specially trained to operate the recording and computer equipment used in analyzing the signal-averaged ECG.

- The technician gathers the multiple inputs necessary for signal averaging from standard orthogonal bipolar X, Y, and Z leads over a series of ECG cycles. The average is taken over a large number of beats, typically 100 or more.
- After the test is completed, disconnect the equipment. If suction cups were used, be sure to wash the conductive gel from the patient's skin.

## PRECAUTIONS

- Be aware that the recording equipment and other nearby electrical equipment should be properly grounded to prevent electrical interference.
- Know that tissue-electrode artifacts can be minimized by lightly sanding the skin with fine sandpaper (no. 220), wiping with alcohol, and using silver-silver chloride electrodes.
- Urge the patient to lie as quietly and motionlessly as possible to avoid signal distortion.

## NORMAL FINDINGS

A QRS complex without low potentials is considered normal.

The areas of interest in the signal-averaged ECG are the:
- duration of the filtered QRS complex (QRST), which indicates how long the completion of the QRS complex is delayed by late potentials
- amount of energy in the late potentials, as indicated by the root mean square (RMS) voltage in the terminal 40 msec of the QRS complex (RMS40)
- duration of the late potentials, as indicated by the duration of the low-amplitude signals of less than 40 µV in the terminal QRS region.

The preceding values can be read either from the signal-averaged ECG itself or from the computer system.

Defining a late potential and scoring a signal-averaged ECG as normal or abnormal are highly dependent on technique. Representative criteria include when late potentials exist when the filtered QRS complex is longer than 114 msec, when there's less than 20 µV RMS of signal in the terminal 40 msec of the filtered QRS, or when the terminal portion of the filtered QRS remains below 40 µV for longer than 38 msec.

## ABNORMAL FINDINGS

Identifying late potentials after the QRS complex indicates a risk of ventricular arrhythmias. Late potentials are most common and of greater prognostic value in the patient who has sustained an MI. The patient who doesn't have late potentials is at low risk for serious ventricular arrhythmias and sudden death. Although the predictive accuracy of a positive signal-averaged ECG is relatively low, it has been advocated as a screening test for the patient who should undergo electrophysiologic testing.

## INTERFERING FACTORS

- Artifact from skeletal muscle movement (possible need to administer a muscle relaxant)
- Electromagnetic interference (possible need to shield and twist input cables to reduce noise)
- Poor tissue-electrode contact (production of artifact)
- Antiarrhythmic drugs

# Skeletal computed tomography

Skeletal computed tomography (CT) provides a series of tomograms, translated by a computer and displayed on a monitor, representing cross-sectional images of various layers (or slices) of bone. This technique can reconstruct cross-sectional, horizontal, sagittal, and coronal plane images.

Taking collimated (parallel) radiographs increases the number of radiation density calculations the computer makes, thereby improving the degree of resolution and thus specificity and accuracy. Hundreds of thousands of readings of radiation levels absorbed by tissues may be combined to depict anatomic slices of varying thickness.

## PURPOSE

- To determine the existence and extent of primary bone tumors, skeletal metastases, soft-tissue tumors, injuries to ligaments or tendons, and fractures
- To diagnose joint abnormalities difficult to detect by other methods

## PATIENT PREPARATION

- Explain to the patient that skeletal CT allows visualization of bones and joints. If contrast medium isn't ordered, tell him that he need not restrict food and fluids. If contrast medium is ordered, instruct him to fast for 4 hours before the test.
- Explain to the patient who will perform the procedure and where it will take place. Reassure him that the procedure is painless.
- Explain to the patient that he'll be positioned on an X-ray table inside a CT scanner and asked to lie still; the computer-controlled scanner will revolve around him taking multiple scans. Stress that he should lie as still as possible because movement may cause distorted images.
- If a contrast medium is used, tell the patient that he may feel flushed and warm and may experience a transient headache, a salty or metallic taste, and nausea or vomiting after its injection. Reassure him that these reactions are normal.
- Instruct the patient to wear a radiologic examining gown and remove all metal objects and jewelry in the X-ray field.

⚠ **Alert** *Check the patient's history for hypersensitivity reactions to iodine, shellfish, or contrast media. Mark such reactions in the chart and notify the physician, who may order prophylactic medications or choose not to use a contrast medium.*

- If the patient appears restless or apprehensive about the procedure, a mild sedative may be prescribed.
- Make sure that the patient or a responsible family member has signed an informed consent form, if required.

## PROCEDURE AND POSTTEST CARE

- Place the patient in a supine position on an X-ray table and tell him to lie as still as possible.
- The table is slid into the circular opening of the CT scanner. The scanner revolves around the patient, taking radiographs at preselected intervals.
- After the first set of scans is taken, the patient is removed from the scanner and a contrast medium is administered, if necessary.
- Observe the patient for signs and symptoms of a hypersensitivity reaction, including pruritus, rash, and respiratory difficulty, for 30 minutes after the contrast medium has been injected.

- After contrast medium I.V. injection, the patient is moved back into the scanner and another series of scans is taken. The images obtained from the scan are displayed on a monitor during the procedure and stored on magnetic tape to create a permanent record for subsequent study.
- If contrast media is used, observe for a delayed allergic reaction and treat as necessary. (Diphenhydramine [Benadryl] is the drug of choice.)
- Encourage fluids to assist in eliminating the contrast medium.
- Tell the patient that he may resume his usual diet and activities, if appropriate.
- Provide comfort measures and pain medication, as ordered, because of prolonged positioning on the table.

## PRECAUTIONS
- Know that this procedure is contraindicated during pregnancy.
- Be aware that this test is contraindicated in a patient who's hypersensitive to iodine, shellfish, or contrast media, or in a patient with renal insufficiency (if he isn't on dialysis).
- Be aware that the patient may experience strong feelings of claustrophobia or anxiety when inside the CT body scanner. In this case, a mild sedative may be ordered to help reduce anxiety.
- For the patient with significant bone or joint pain, administer analgesics so that he can lie still comfortably during the scan.

## NORMAL FINDINGS
The scan should reveal no disease in the bones or joints. It produces crisp images of the structure while blurring or eliminating details of surrounding structures.

## ABNORMAL FINDINGS
Because of its ability to display cross-sectional anatomy, CT scanning is useful for imaging the shoulder, spine, hip, and pelvis. The cross-sectional view eliminates the confusing shadows of superimposed structures that occur with conventional radiographs. The scan can reveal primary bone tumors and soft-tissue tumors as well as skeletal metastasis. It can also reveal joint abnormalities difficult to detect by other methods.

## INTERFERING FACTORS
- Claustrophobia (possible interference with the patient's ability to lie in the scanner for long periods)
- Excessive patient movement
- Failure to remove metallic objects from the examination field (possible poor imaging)

# Skeletal magnetic resonance imaging

A noninvasive technique, skeletal magnetic resonance imaging (MRI) produces clear and sensitive images of bone and soft tissue. The scan provides superior contrast of body tissues and allows imaging of multiple planes, including direct sagittal and coronal views in regions that can't be easily visualized with X-rays or computed tomography scans. MRI eliminates any risks associated with exposure to X-ray beams and causes no known harm to cells.

MRI is most easily generated from the proton of the hydrogen atom. Each water molecule has two hydrogen atoms, but the distribution of water molecules varies according to specific body tissue. For example, bone is considered "dry" because it doesn't contain much hydrogen. Consequently, bone produces a weak signal and can't be visualized. However, normal bone marrow has the brightest signal and can be seen well.

## PURPOSE
- To evaluate bony and soft-tissue tumors
- To identify changes in bone marrow composition
- To identify spinal disorders

## PATIENT PREPARATION
- Make sure the scanner can accommodate the patient's weight and abdominal girth.
- Explain to the patient that skeletal MRI assesses bone and soft tissue. Tell him who will perform the test and where it will take place.
- Explain to the patient that although MRI is painless and involves no exposure to radiation from the scanner, a contrast medium may be used, depending on the type of tissue being studied.
- If the patient is claustrophobic or if extensive time is required for scanning, explain

to him that a mild sedative may be administered to reduce anxiety. Open scanners have been developed for use on the patient with extreme claustrophobia or morbid obesity, but tests using such machines take longer.

- Tell the patient that he must lie flat, and describe the test procedure.
- Explain to the patient that he'll hear the scanner clicking, whirring, and thumping as it moves inside its housing.
- Reassure the patient that he'll be able to communicate with the technician at all times.
- Instruct the patient to remove all metallic objects, including jewelry, hairpins, or watches.
- Ask whether the patient has any surgically implanted joints, pins, clips, valves, pumps, or pacemakers containing metal that could be attracted to the strong MRI magnet. If he does, he won't be able to have the test.
- Make sure that the patient or a responsible family member has signed an informed consent form, if required.

## PROCEDURE AND POSTTEST CARE

- At the scanner room door, check the patient one last time for metal objects.
- The patient is placed on a narrow, padded, nonmetallic table that moves into the scanner tunnel. Fans continuously circulate air in the tunnel, and a call bell or intercom is used to maintain verbal contact.
- Remind the patient to remain still throughout the procedure.
- While the patient lies within the strong magnetic field, the area to be studied is stimulated with radio-frequency waves.
- If the test is prolonged with the patient lying flat, monitor him for orthostatic hypotension.
- Provide comfort measures and pain medication as needed and ordered because of prolonged positioning in the scanner.
- After the test, tell the patient that he may resume his usual activity.
- Provide emotional support to the patient with claustrophobia or anxiety over his diagnosis.

## PRECAUTIONS

- Be aware that MRI can't be performed on a patient with a pacemaker, intracranial aneurysm clip, or other ferrous metal implants. Ventilators, I.V. infusion pumps, oxygen tanks, and other metallic or computer-based equipment must be kept out of the MRI area.
- If the patient is unstable, make sure an I.V. line without metal components is in place and that all equipment is compatible with MRI imaging. If necessary, monitor the patient's oxygen saturation, cardiac rhythm, and respiratory status during the test. An anesthesiologist may be needed to monitor a heavily sedated patient.
- Make sure that the technician maintains verbal contact with the conscious patient.

## NORMAL FINDINGS

MRI should reveal no disease in bone, muscles, and joints.

## ABNORMAL FINDINGS

MRI is excellent for visualizing diseases of the spinal canal and cord and for identifying primary and metastatic bone tumors. It's beneficial in anatomic delineation of muscles, ligaments, and bones. The images show superior contrast of body tissues and sharply define healthy, benign, and malignant tissues.

## INTERFERING FACTORS

- Excessive patient movement
- Patient inability to fit into scanner

# Skin biopsy

Skin biopsy is the removal of a small piece of tissue under local anesthesia from a lesion suspected of being malignant or from other dermatoses. One of three techniques may be used: shave biopsy, punch biopsy, or excisional biopsy. Shave biopsy uses a scalpel to slice a superficial specimen from the site. Punch biopsy removes an oval core from the center of a lesion down to the dermis or subcutaneous tissue. Excisional biopsy removes the entire lesion with a small border of normal skin.

Lesions suspected of being malignant usually have changed color, size, or appearance or have failed to heal properly after injury. Fully developed lesions should be selected for biopsy whenever possible because they provide more diagnostic information than lesions that are resolving or in early developing stages.

## PURPOSE
- To provide differential diagnosis among basal cell carcinoma, squamous cell carcinoma, malignant melanoma, and benign growths
- To diagnose chronic bacterial or fungal skin infections

## PATIENT PREPARATION
- Explain to the patient that the biopsy provides a specimen for microscopic study.
- Describe the procedure to the patient, and answer his questions.
- Inform the patient that he need not restrict food and fluids.
- Tell the patient who will perform the procedure and when and where it will be done.
- Tell the patient that he'll receive a local anesthetic to minimize pain during the procedure.
- Make sure the patient or a responsible family member has signed an informed consent form.
- Check the patient's history for hypersensitivity to the local anesthetic.

## PROCEDURE AND POSTTEST CARE
- Position the patient comfortably, and clean the biopsy site before the local anesthetic is administered.

### Shave biopsy
- The protruding growth is cut off at the skin line with a #15 scalpel, and the tissue is placed immediately in a properly labeled specimen bottle containing 10% formalin solution.
- Apply pressure to the area to stop the bleeding.

### Punch biopsy
- The skin surrounding the lesion is pulled taut, and the punch is firmly introduced into the lesion and rotated to obtain a tissue specimen. The plug is lifted with forceps or a needle and severed as deeply into the fat layer as possible.
- The specimen is placed in a properly labeled specimen bottle containing 10% formalin solution or in a sterile container, if indicated.

- Closing the wound depends on the size of the punch: A 3-mm punch requires only an adhesive bandage, a 4-mm punch requires one suture, and a 6-mm punch requires two sutures.

### Excisional biopsy
- A #15 scalpel is used to excise the entire lesion; the elliptical incision is made as wide and as deep as necessary.
- The tissue specimen is removed and placed immediately in a properly labeled specimen bottle containing 10% formalin solution.
- Apply pressure to the site to stop bleeding.
- The wound is closed using 4-0 suture. If the incision is large, skin grafting may be required.

### All procedures
- Check the biopsy site for bleeding.
- If the patient experiences pain, administer an analgesic as ordered.
- Advise the patient with sutures to keep the area as clean and dry as possible. Facial sutures are removed in 3 to 5 days; trunk sutures, in 7 to 14 days. Tell the patient with adhesive strips to leave them in place for 14 to 21 days or until they fall off.

## PRECAUTIONS
- Send the specimen to the laboratory immediately.

## NORMAL FINDINGS
Normal skin consists of squamous epithelium (epidermis) and fibrous connective tissue (dermis).

## ABNORMAL FINDINGS
Histologic examination of the tissue specimen may reveal a benign or malignant lesion. Benign growths include cysts, seborrheic keratoses, warts, pigmented nevi (moles), keloids, dermatofibromas, and multiple neurofibromas.

Malignant tumors include basal cell carcinoma, squamous cell carcinoma, and malignant melanoma. Basal cell carcinoma occurs on hair-bearing skin; the most common location is the face, including the nose and its folds. Squamous cell carcinoma most commonly appears on the lips, mouth, and genitalia. Malignant melanoma, the deadliest skin cancer, can spread through the body by way of the lymphatic system and blood vessels.

Cultures can be used to detect chronic bacterial and fungal infections in which flora are relatively sparse.

## INTERFERING FACTORS
- Improper selection of the biopsy site
- Inability to obtain appropriate specimen

# Skull radiography

Although skull radiography is of limited value in assessing patients with head injuries, skull X-rays are extremely valuable for studying abnormalities of the skull base and cranial vault, congenital and perinatal anomalies, and systemic diseases that produce bone defects of the skull. For more accurate assessment of head injuries as well as of skull and head abnormalities, nonenhanced computed tomography studies of the head are done.

Skull radiography evaluates the three groups of bones that comprise the skull: the calvaria (vault), the mandible (jaw bone), and the facial bones. The calvaria and the facial bones are closely connected by immovable joints with irregular serrated edges called *sutures*. The skull bones form an anatomic structure so complex that a complete skull examination requires several radiologic views of each area.

## PURPOSE
- To detect fractures in the patient with head trauma
- To aid in the diagnosis of pituitary tumors
- To detect congenital anomalies
- To detect metabolic and endocrinologic disorders

## PATIENT PREPARATION
- Explain to the patient that his head will be immobilized and that several X-rays of his skull will be taken from various angles.
- Tell the patient that skull radiography helps to determine the presence of anomalies and helps establish a diagnosis.
- Tell the patient who will perform the test and when and where it will take place.

- Explain to the patient that he need not restrict food and fluids and that the test will cause no discomfort.
- Tell the patient to remove glasses, dentures, jewelry, or any metallic objects that would be in the X-ray field.

## PROCEDURE AND POSTTEST CARE
- Have the patient recline on the X-ray table or sit in a chair.
- Tell the patient to remain still during the procedure.
- Use foam pads, sandbags, or a headband to immobilize the patient's head and increase comfort.
- Five views of the skull are taken: left and right lateral, anteroposterior Towne's, posteroanterior Caldwell, and axial (or base).
- Films are developed and checked for quality before the patient leaves the area.

## PRECAUTIONS
- None

## NORMAL FINDINGS
A radiologist interprets the X-rays, evaluating the size, shape, thickness, and position of the cranial bones as well as the vascular markings, sinuses, and sutures.

## ABNORMAL FINDINGS
Skull radiography is commonly used to diagnose fractures of the vault or base, although basilar fractures may not show on the film if the bone is dense. This test may confirm congenital anomalies and may show erosion, enlargement, or decalcification of the sella turcica that result from increased intracranial pressure (ICP). A marked rise in ICP may cause the brain to expand and press against the inner bony table of the skull, yielding visible marks or impressions.

In such conditions as osteomyelitis (with possible skull calcification) and chronic subdural hematomas, X-rays may show abnormal areas of calcification. The X-rays can detect neoplasms within brain substances that contain calcium (such as oligodendrogliomas or meningiomas) or the midline shifting of a calcified pineal gland caused by a space-occupying lesion.

Radiography may also detect other changes in bone structure — for example, those that arise from metabolic disorders, such as acromegaly or Paget's disease.

## INTERFERING FACTORS

● Improper positioning of the patient and excessive head movement (possible poor imaging)
● Failure to remove radiopaque objects from the X-ray field (possible poor imaging)

# Small-bowel biopsy

Small-bowel biopsy is used to evaluate diseases of the intestinal mucosa, which may cause malabsorption or diarrhea. It produces larger specimens than those produced by endoscopic biopsy and allows removal of tissue from areas beyond an endoscope's reach. (See *Endoscopic biopsy of the GI tract,* page 426.)

Several similar types of capsules are available for tissue collection. In each, a mercury-weighted bag is attached to one end of the capsule; a thin polyethylene tube about 5′ (1.5 m) long is attached to the other end. When the bag, capsule, and tube are in place in the small bowel, suction on the tube draws the mucosa into the capsule and closes it, cutting off the piece of tissue within. Although this is an invasive procedure, it causes little pain and rarely causes complications.

Small-bowel biopsy verifies the diagnosis of some diseases, such as Whipple's disease, and may help confirm others such as tropical sprue. Capsule biopsy is also an invasive procedure, but it causes little pain and complications are rare.

## PURPOSE

● To help diagnose diseases of the intestinal mucosa

## PATIENT PREPARATION

● Explain to the patient that the small-bowel biopsy is used to identify intestinal disorders.
● Describe the procedure to the patient, and answer his questions.
● Instruct the patient to restrict food and fluids for at least 8 hours before the test.
● Tell the patient who will perform the biopsy and when and where it will be done.
● Make sure the patient or a responsible family member has signed an informed consent form.

● Make sure that coagulation tests have been performed and that the results are recorded on the patient's chart.
● Withhold aspirin and anticoagulants, as ordered. If these drugs must be continued, note this on the laboratory request.

## PROCEDURE AND POSTTEST CARE

● Check the tubing and the mercury bag for leaks.
● Lightly lubricate the tube and capsule with a water-soluble lubricant, and moisten the mercury bag with water.
● Spray the back of the patient's throat with a local anesthetic to decrease gagging.
● Ask the patient to sit upright.
● The capsule is placed in the patient's pharynx, and he's asked to flex his neck and swallow as the tube is advanced.
● If a local anesthetic is used to control the gag reflex, the patient must not receive any fluids to help him swallow the capsule.
● Place the patient on his right side; the tube is then advanced another 20″ (50.8 cm). The tube's position is checked by fluoroscopy or by instilling air through the tube and listening with a stethoscope for air to enter the stomach.
● Next, the tube is advanced 2″ to 4″ (5 to 10 cm) at a time to pass the capsule through the pylorus. (Talk to the patient about food to stimulate the pylorus and help the capsule pass.)
● When fluoroscopy confirms that the capsule has passed the pylorus, keep the patient on his right side to allow the capsule to move into the second and third portions of the small bowel.
● Tell the patient that he may hold the tube loosely to one side of his mouth if it makes him more comfortable.
● Capsule position is checked again by fluoroscopy. When the capsule is at or beyond the ligament of Treitz, the biopsy sample can be taken. (The physician will determine the biopsy site.)
● Place the patient in a supine position so that the capsule's position can be verified fluoroscopically. A 100-ml glass syringe is placed on the end of the tube, and steady suction is applied to close the capsule and cut off a tissue specimen. Suction is maintained on the syringe as the tube and capsule are removed; then the suction is released.

# ENDOSCOPIC BIOPSY OF THE GI TRACT

Endoscopy allows direct visualization of the GI tract and any site that requires biopsy of tissue specimens for histologic analysis. This relatively painless procedure helps detect, support diagnosis of, or monitor GI tract disorders. Its complications, notably hemorrhage, perforation, and aspiration, are rare.

Endoscopic biopsy of the GI tract can be used to diagnose cancer, lymphoma, amyloidosis, candidiasis, and gastric ulcers; to support a diagnosis of Crohn's disease, chronic ulcerative colitis, gastritis, esophagitis, and melanosis coli in laxative abuse; and to monitor progression of Barrett's esophagus, multiple gastric polyps, colon cancer and polyps, and chronic ulcerative colitis.

## PREPARING THE PATIENT

Careful patient preparation is vital for this procedure. Describe the procedure to the patient, and reassure him that he'll be able to breathe with the endoscope in place. Tell him to fast for at least 8 hours before the procedure. For lower GI biopsy, clean the bowel. Make sure the patient or a responsible family member has signed an informed consent form.

Just before the procedure, administer the prescribed sedative to the patient. He should be relaxed but not asleep because his cooperation is necessary to promote smooth passage of the endoscope. Spray the back of his throat with a local anesthetic to suppress his gag reflex. Have suction equipment and bipolar cauterization electrodes available to prevent aspiration and excessive bleeding.

## OBTAINING THE SAMPLE

After the endoscope is passed into the upper or lower GI tract and a lesion, node, or other abnormal area is visualized, a biopsy forceps is pushed through a channel in the endoscope until this, too, can be seen. The forceps are then opened, positioned at the biopsy site, and closed on the tissue. The closed forceps and tissue specimen are removed from the endoscope, and the tissue is taken from the forceps. Then the forceps may be used to cauterize any remaining abnormal tissue to stop bleeding.

The specimen is placed mucosal side up on fine-mesh gauze or filter paper and then placed in a labeled biopsy bottle containing fixative. When all specimens have been collected, the endoscope is removed. Specimens are sent to the laboratory immediately.

---

This release opens the capsule and exposes the specimen, mucosal side down.

- The specimen is gently removed with forceps, placed mucosal side up on a piece of mesh, and then placed in a biopsy bottle with required fixative.
- As ordered, resume the patient's diet after confirming return of the gag reflex.
- Although complications are rare, watch for signs of hemorrhage, bacteremia with transient fever and pain, and bowel perforation. Tell the patient to report abdominal pain or bleeding.

## PRECAUTIONS

**Alert** *Keep suction equipment nearby to prevent aspiration if the patient vomits.*

- Don't allow the patient to bite the tubing.
- Handle the tissue carefully, and place it correctly on the slide.

- Send the specimen to the laboratory immediately.
- Be aware that small-bowel biopsy is contraindicated in an uncooperative patient, one taking aspirin or anticoagulants, and the patient with uncontrolled coagulation disorders.

## NORMAL FINDINGS

A normal small-bowel biopsy specimen consists of fingerlike villi, crypts, columnar epithelial cells, and round cells.

## ABNORMAL FINDINGS

Small-bowel tissue that reveals histologic changes in cell structure may indicate Whipple's disease, abetalipoproteinemia, lymphoma, lymphangiectasia, eosinophilic enteritis, and such parasitic infections as giardiasis and coccidiosis. Abnormal specimens may also suggest celiac sprue, tropical sprue, infectious gastroenteritis, intraluminal bacterial overgrowth, folate and vitamin $B_{12}$ deficiency, radiation enteritis, and malnutrition, but such disorders require further studies.

## INTERFERING FACTORS
● Failure to fast before biopsy (possible poor specimen or vomiting and aspiration)
● Mechanical failure of the biopsy capsule or hole in the tubing (possible difficulty in removing tissue specimen)
● Inability of patient to remain still or keep from coughing during the procedure

# Sodium, serum

The sodium test is used to measure serum levels of sodium in relation to the amount of water in the body. Sodium, the major extracellular cation, affects body water distribution, maintains osmotic pressure of extracellular fluid, and helps promote neuromuscular function. It also helps maintain acid-base balance and influences chloride and potassium levels.

Because extracellular sodium concentration helps the kidneys to regulate body water (decreased sodium levels promote water excretion and increased levels promote retention), serum levels of sodium are evaluated in relation to the amount of water in the body. For example, a sodium deficit (hyponatremia) refers to a decreased level of sodium in relation to the body's water level. (See *Fluid imbalances,* page 428.) The body normally regulates this sodium-water balance through aldosterone, which inhibits sodium excretion and promotes its resorption (with water) by the renal tubules to maintain balance. Low sodium levels stimulate aldosterone secretion; elevated sodium levels depress it.

## PURPOSE
● To evaluate fluid-electrolyte and acid-base balance and related neuromuscular, renal, and adrenal functions

## PATIENT PREPARATION
● Explain to the patient that the serum sodium test is used to determine the sodium content of the blood.

● Tell the patient that the test requires a blood sample. Explain who will perform the venipuncture and when.
● Explain to the patient that he may experience slight discomfort from the tourniquet and the needle puncture.
● Inform the patient that he need not restrict food and fluids.
● Notify the laboratory and physician of medications the patient is taking that may affect test results; they may need to be restricted.

## PROCEDURE AND POSTTEST CARE
● Perform a venipuncture and collect the sample in a 3- or 4-ml clot-activator tube.
● Apply direct pressure to the venipuncture site until bleeding stops.
● If a hematoma develops at the venipuncture site, apply pressure.
● Instruct the patient to resume any medications discontinued before the test, as ordered.

## PRECAUTIONS
● Handle the sample gently to prevent hemolysis.

## REFERENCE VALUES
Normally, serum sodium levels range from 135 to 145 mEq/L (SI, 135 to 145 mmol/L).

## ABNORMAL FINDINGS
Sodium imbalance can result from a loss or gain of sodium or from a change in the patient's state of hydration. Increased serum sodium levels (hypernatremia) may be due to inadequate water intake, water loss in excess of sodium (such as diabetes insipidus, impaired renal function, prolonged hyperventilation and, rarely, severe vomiting or diarrhea), and sodium retention (such as aldosteronism). Hypernatremia can also result from excessive sodium intake.

⊛ **Alert** *In the patient with hypernatremia and associated loss of water, observe for signs of thirst, restlessness, dry and sticky mucous membranes, flushed skin, oliguria, and diminished reflexes. If increased total body sodium causes water retention, observe for hypertension, dyspnea, edema, and heart failure.*

Abnormally low serum sodium levels (hyponatremia) may result from inadequate sodium intake or excessive sodium loss due to profuse sweating, GI suctioning, diuretic

## FLUID IMBALANCES

This chart lists the causes, signs and symptoms, and diagnostic test findings associated with hypervolemia (increased fluid volume) and hypovolemia (decreased fluid volume).

| CAUSES | SIGNS AND SYMPTOMS | LABORATORY FINDINGS |
|---|---|---|
| **HYPERVOLEMIA** | | |
| ◆ Increased water intake<br>◆ Decreased water output due to renal disease<br>◆ Heart failure<br>◆ Excessive ingestion or infusion of sodium chloride<br>◆ Long-term administration of adrenocortical hormones<br>◆ Excessive infusion of isotonic solutions | ◆ Increased blood pressure, pulse rate, body weight, and respiratory rate<br>◆ Bounding peripheral pulses<br>◆ Moist pulmonary crackles<br>◆ Moist mucous membranes<br>◆ Moist respiratory secretions<br>◆ Edema<br>◆ Weakness<br>◆ Seizures and coma due to swelling of brain cells | ◆ Decreased red blood cell (RBC) count, hemoglobin concentration, packed cell volume, serum sodium concentration (dilutional decrease), and urine specific gravity |
| **HYPOVOLEMIA** | | |
| ◆ Decreased water intake<br>◆ Fluid loss due to fever, diarrhea, or vomiting<br>◆ Systemic infection<br>◆ Impaired renal concentrating ability<br>◆ Fistulous drainage<br>◆ Severe burns<br>◆ Hidden fluid in body cavities | ◆ Increased pulse and respiratory rates<br>◆ Decreased blood pressure and body weight<br>◆ Weak and thready peripheral pulses<br>◆ Thick, slurred speech<br>◆ Thirst<br>◆ Oliguria<br>◆ Anuria<br>◆ Dry skin | ◆ Increased RBC count, hemoglobin concentration, packed cell volume, serum sodium concentration, and urine specific gravity |

therapy, diarrhea, vomiting, adrenal insufficiency, burns, and chronic renal insufficiency with acidosis. Urine sodium determinations are usually more sensitive to early changes in sodium balance and should be evaluated simultaneously with serum sodium findings.

**Alert** *In the patient with hyponatremia, watch for apprehension, lassitude, headache, decreased skin turgor, abdominal cramps, and tremors that may progress to seizures.*

### INTERFERING FACTORS

● Most diuretics (decrease by promoting sodium excretion)
● Chlorpropamide, lithium, and vasopressin (decrease by inhibiting water excretion)
● Corticosteroids (increase by promoting sodium retention)
● Antihypertensives, such as hydralazine, methyldopa, and reserpine (possible increase due to sodium and water retention)

## Sputum culture

Bacteriologic examination of sputum (material raised from the lungs and bronchi) is an important aid to the management of lung disease. During passage through the throat and oropharynx, sputum specimens are commonly contaminated with indigenous bacterial flora, such as alpha-hemolytic streptococci, *Neisseria* species, diphtheroids, some *Haemophilus* species, pneumococci, staphylococci, and yeasts such as *Candida*.

Pathogenic organisms typically found in sputum include *Streptococcus pneumoniae, Mycobacterium tuberculosis, Klebsiella pneumoniae* (and other Enterobacteriaceae), *Haemophilus influenzae, Staphylococcus aureus,* and *Pseudomonas aeruginosa.* Other pathogens, such as *Pneumocystis carinii, Legionella* species, *Mycoplasma pneumoniae,* and respiratory viruses, may exist in the sputum and can cause lung disease, but they usually require serologic or histologic diagnosis rather than diagnosis by sputum culture.

The usual method of specimen collection is expectoration (which may require ultrasonic nebulization, hydration, physiotherapy, or postural drainage); other methods include tracheal suctioning and bronchoscopy. (See *Using an in-line trap,* page 430.)

A Gram stain of expectorated sputum must be examined to ensure that it's a representative specimen of secretions from the lower respiratory tract (many white blood cells [WBCs], few epithelial cells) rather than one contaminated by oral flora (few WBCs, many epithelial cells). Careful examination of an acid-fast smear of sputum may provide presumptive evidence of a mycobacterial infection such as tuberculosis.

## PURPOSE

● To isolate and identify the cause of pulmonary infection, thus aiding in the diagnosis of respiratory diseases (most commonly bronchitis, tuberculosis, lung abscess, and pneumonia)

## PATIENT PREPARATION

● Explain to the patient that the sputum culture is used to identify the organism causing respiratory tract infection.
● Tell the patient that the test requires a sputum specimen and who will collect the specimen and when.
● If the suspected organism is *M. tuberculosis,* tell the patient that as many as three consecutive morning specimens may be required.
● If testing is for tuberculosis, explain that cultures for tuberculosis may take some time to develop and that specimens may need to be collected on at least three consecutive mornings; therefore, diagnosis of this disor-

der generally depends on clinical symptoms, a smear for acid-fast bacilli, a chest X-ray, and response to a purified protein derivative skin test.
● If the specimen will be collected by expectoration, encourage fluid intake the night before collection to help sputum production, unless contraindicated by a fluid restriction. Teach the patient how to expectorate by taking three deep breaths and forcing a deep cough; emphasize that sputum isn't the same as saliva, which is unacceptable for culturing. Tell him to brush his teeth and gargle with water before the specimen collection to reduce contaminating oropharyngeal bacteria.
● If the specimen will be collected by tracheal suctioning, tell the patient that he'll experience discomfort as the catheter passes into the trachea.
● If the specimen will be collected by bronchoscopy, instruct the patient to fast for 6 hours before the procedure.
● Make sure that the patient or a responsible family member has signed an informed consent form.
● Tell the patient that he'll receive a local anesthetic just before the test to minimize discomfort during passage of the tube.

## PROCEDURE AND POSTTEST CARE
### Expectoration

● Put on gloves.
● Instruct the patient to cough deeply and expectorate into the container. If the cough is nonproductive, use chest physiotherapy or a heated aerosol spray (nebulization) to induce sputum. Using sterile technique, close the container securely.
● Dispose of equipment properly; seal the container in a leakproof bag before sending it to the laboratory.

### Tracheal suctioning

● Administer oxygen to the patient before and after the procedure if necessary.
● Attach the sputum trap to the suction catheter. Using sterile gloves, lubricate the catheter with normal saline solution, and pass it through the patient's nostril without suction. (He'll cough when the catheter passes through the larynx.) Advance the catheter into the trachea. Apply suction for no longer than 15 seconds to obtain the specimen.

# USING AN IN-LINE TRAP

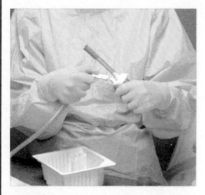

Push the suction tubing onto the male adapter of the in-line trap.

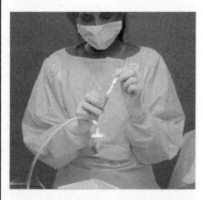

With one hand, insert the suction catheter into the rubber tubing of the trap. Then suction the patient.

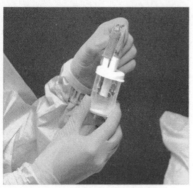

After suctioning, disconnect the in-line trap from the suction tubing and catheter. To seal the container, connect the rubber tubing to the female adapter of the trap.

- Stop suction and gently remove the catheter. Discard the catheter and gloves in the proper receptacle. Then detach the in-line sputum trap from the suction apparatus, and cap the opening.

## Bronchoscopy
- After a local anesthetic is sprayed into the patient's throat or after he gargles with a local anesthetic, the bronchoscope is inserted through the pharynx and trachea into the bronchus.
- Secretions are then collected with a bronchial brush or aspirated through the inner channel of the scope using an irrigating solution, such as normal saline solution, if necessary.
- After the specimen is obtained, the bronchoscope is removed.

*Alert During and after bronchoscopy, observe the patient carefully for signs of hypoxemia (change in mental status), laryngospasm (laryngeal stridor), bronchospasm (paroxysms of coughing or wheezing), pneumothorax (dyspnea, cyanosis, pleural pain, tachycardia), perforation of the trachea or bronchus (subcutaneous crepitus), and trauma to respiratory structures (blood-tinged sputum, coughing up blood). Also check for difficulty in breathing or swallowing. Don't give liquids until the gag reflex returns.*

## All collection methods
- Provide good mouth care.
- Label the container with the patient's name. Include on the test request form the nature and origin of the specimen, the date and time of collection, the initial diagnosis, and any current antimicrobial therapy.

## PRECAUTIONS
- Know that tracheal suctioning is contraindicated in the patient with esophageal varices.

*Alert In a patient with asthma or chronic bronchitis, watch for aggravated bronchospasms when using normal saline solution or acetylcysteine in an aerosol.*

- During tracheal suctioning, suction for only 5 to 10 seconds at a time. Never suction longer than 15 seconds. If the patient becomes hypoxic or cyanotic, remove the catheter immediately and administer oxygen.
- Wear gloves when performing the procedure and handling specimens.
- Because the patient may cough violently during suctioning, be sure to wear gloves, a mask and, if necessary, a gown to avoid exposure to pathogens.
- Don't use more than 20% propylene glycol with water as an inducer for a specimen scheduled for tuberculosis culturing because higher concentrations inhibit the growth of *M. tuberculosis*. (If propylene glycol isn't available, use 10% to 20% acetylcysteine with water or saline solution.)
- Send the specimen to the laboratory immediately after collection.

## NORMAL FINDINGS
Flora commonly found in the respiratory tract include alpha-hemolytic streptococci, *Neisseria* species, and diphtheroids. The presence of normal flora doesn't rule out infection.

## ABNORMAL FINDINGS
Because sputum is invariably contaminated with normal oropharyngeal flora, a culture isolate must be interpreted in light of the patient's overall clinical condition. Isolation of *M. tuberculosis* is always a significant finding.

## INTERFERING FACTORS
- Failure to report current or recent antimicrobial therapy on the laboratory request (possible false-negative)
- Collection over an extended period, which may cause pathogens to deteriorate or become overgrown by commensals (not accepted as a valid specimen by laboratories)

# Stool culture

Normal bacterial flora in stool include several potentially pathogenic organisms. Bacteriologic examination is valuable for identifying pathogens that cause overt GI disease — such as typhoid and dysentery — and carrier states. A sensitivity test may follow isolation of the pathogen. The most common pathogenic organisms of the GI tract are *Shigella,* *Salmonella,* and *Campylobacter jejuni*. Less common pathogenic organisms include *Vibrio cholerae, Clostridium botulinum, Clostridium difficile, Clostridium perfringens, Staphylococcus aureus,* enterotoxigenic *Escherichia coli, Bacillus cereus, Yersinia enterocolitica, Aeromonas hydrophila,* and *V. parahaemolyticus*. (See *Pathogens of the GI tract,* page 432.) Identifying these organ-

# Pathogens of the GI tract

The presence of the following pathogens in a stool culture may indicate certain disorders.

**Aeromonas hydrophila:** gastroenteritis, which causes diarrhea, especially in children

**Bacillus cereus:** food poisoning, acute gastroenteritis (rare)

**Campylobacter jejuni:** gastroenteritis

**Clostridium botulinum:** Food poisoning and infant botulism (a possible cause of sudden infant death syndrome)

**Toxin-producing Clostridium difficile:** pseudomembranous enterocolitis

**Clostridium perfringens:** food poisoning

**Enterotoxigenic Escherichia coli:** gastroenteritis (resembles cholera or shigellosis)

**Salmonella:** gastroenteritis, typhoid fever, nontyphoidal salmonellosis, paratyphoid fever

**Shigella:** shigellosis, bacillary dysentery

**Staphylococcus aureus:** food poisoning, suppression of normal bowel flora from antimicrobial therapy

**Vibrio cholerae:** cholera

**Vibrio parahaemolyticus:** food poisoning, especially seafood

**Yersinia enterocolitica:** gastroenteritis, enterocolitis (resembles appendicitis), mesenteric lymphadenitis, ileitis

---

isms is vital to treat the patient, to prevent possibly fatal complications (especially in a debilitated patient), and to confine these severe infectious diseases. A sensitivity test may follow isolation of the pathogen.

Some viruses, such as rotavirus and parvovirus, may also cause GI symptoms. However, these viruses can be detected only by immunoassay or electron microscopy. Stool culture may detect other viruses, such as enterovirus, which can cause aseptic meningitis.

## PURPOSE
* To identify pathogenic organisms caused by GI disease
* To identify carrier states

## PATIENT PREPARATION
* Explain to the patient that the stool culture is used to determine the cause of GI distress or to determine if he's a carrier of infectious organisms.
* Advise the patient that he need not restrict food and fluids.
* Tell the patient that the test requires the collection of a stool specimen on 3 consecutive days.
* Check the patient's history for dietary patterns, recent antimicrobial therapy, and recent travel that might suggest endemic infections or infestations.

## PROCEDURE AND POSTTEST CARE
* Collect a stool specimen directly into the container. If the patient isn't ambulatory, collect the specimen in a clean, dry bedpan and, using a tongue blade, transfer the specimen to the container.
* If you must collect the specimen by rectal swab, insert the swab past the anal sphincter, rotate it gently, and withdraw it. Then place the swab in the appropriate container.
* Check with the laboratory for the proper collection procedure before obtaining a specimen for a virus test.
* Label the specimen with the patient's name, physician's name, facility number, and date and time of collection.
* Indicate the suspected cause of enteritis and current antimicrobial therapy on the laboratory request.

## PRECAUTIONS
* Wear gloves when performing the procedure and handling the specimen.
* If the patient uses a bedpan or a diaper, avoid contaminating the stool specimen with urine.
* The specimen must represent the first, middle, and last portion of the stool passed. Be sure to include mucoid and bloody portions.

- Put the specimen container in a leakproof bag.
- Send the specimen to the laboratory immediately. Trophozoites and cysts may be destroyed if exposed to heat, cold, or a delay in delivery to the laboratory.
- Specimens should be collected before antimicrobial therapy is started.

## NORMAL FINDINGS
A large percentage of normal fecal flora consists of anaerobes, including non-spore-forming bacilli, clostridia, and anaerobic streptococci. The remaining percentage consists of aerobes, including gram-negative bacilli (predominantly *E. coli* and other *Enterobacteriaceae,* plus small amounts of *Pseudomonas*), gram-positive cocci (mostly enterococci), and a few yeasts.

## ABNORMAL FINDINGS
The most common pathogenic organisms of the GI tract are *Shigella, Salmonella,* and *Campylobacter jejuni.* Less common pathogenic organisms include *V. cholerae, V. parahaemolyticus, C. botulinum, C. difficile, C. perfringens, S. aureus, enterotoxigenic E. coli,* and *Y. enterocolitica.* Isolation of some pathogens indicates bacterial infection in the patient with acute diarrhea and may require antimicrobial sensitivity tests. Normal fecal flora may include *C. difficile, E. coli,* and other organisms. Therefore, isolation of these organisms may require further tests to demonstrate invasiveness or toxin production.

Isolation of pathogens such as *C. botulinum* indicates food poisoning; the pathogens must also be isolated from the contaminated food. In a patient undergoing long-term antimicrobial therapy, isolation of large numbers of *S. aureus* or yeast may indicate infection. (Asymptomatic carrier states are also indicated by these enteric pathogens.) Isolation of enteroviruses may indicate aseptic meningitis.

If a stool culture shows no unusual growth, detection of viruses by immunoassay or electron microscopy may be used to diagnose nonbacterial gastroenteritis. Highly increased polymorphonuclear leukocytes in fecal material may indicate an invasive pathogen.

## INTERFERING FACTORS
- Contamination of the specimen by urine (possible injury to or destruction of enteric pathogens)
- Antimicrobial therapy (possible decrease in bacterial growth)
- Recent barium studies (possible interference in detecting parasites)

# *Stool examination*
---

Examination of a stool specimen can detect several types of intestinal parasites. Some of these parasites live in nonpathogenic symbiosis; others cause intestinal disease. In the United States, the most common parasites include the roundworms *Ascaris lumbricoides* and *Necator americanus* (commonly called *hookworm*); the tapeworms *Diphyllobothrium latum, Taenia saginata* and, rarely, *T. solium;* the amoeba *Entamoeba histolytica;* and the flagellate *Giardia lamblia. Cyclospora* can also be detected in stool examination for ova and parasites.

Detection of pinworm requires a different collection method. (See *Collection procedure for pinworm,* page 434.)

## PURPOSE
- To confirm or rule out intestinal parasitic infection and disease

## PATIENT PREPARATION
- Explain to the patient that the stool examination detects intestinal parasitic infection.
- Instruct the patient to avoid treatments with castor or mineral oil, bismuth, magnesium or antidiarrheal compounds, barium enemas, and antibiotics for 7 to 10 days before the test.
- Tell the patient that the test requires three stool specimens — one every other day or every third day. Up to six specimens may be required to confirm the presence of *E. histolytica.*
- If the patient has diarrhea, assess recent dietary and travel history.
- Check the patient's history for use of antiparasitic drugs, such as tetracycline, paromomycin (Humatin), metronidazole (Flagyl), and iodoquinol (Yodoxin), within 2 weeks of the test.

## PROCEDURE AND POSTTEST CARE

● Put on gloves and collect a stool specimen directly in the container. If the patient is bedridden, collect the specimen in a clean, dry bedpan, and then, using a tongue blade, transfer it into a properly labeled container.

● Note on the laboratory request the date and time of collection and the specimen consistency. Also record recent or current antimicrobial therapy and any pertinent history.

● Tell the patient that he may resume his usual medications, as ordered.

## PRECAUTIONS

● Don't contaminate the stool specimen with urine, which can destroy trophozoites.

● Don't collect stool from a toilet bowl because water is toxic to trophozoites and may contain organisms that interfere with test results.

● Send the specimen to the laboratory immediately. If a liquid or soft stool specimen can't be examined within 30 minutes of passage, place some of it in a preservative; if a formed stool specimen can't be examined immediately, refrigerate it or place it in preservative.

● If the entire stool can't be sent to the laboratory, include macroscopic worms or worm segments as well as bloody and mucoid portions of the specimen.

● Use gloves when performing the procedure and handling the specimen, disposing of equipment, sealing the container, and transporting the specimen. Dispose of gloves after specimen collection and transport.

## NORMAL FINDINGS

No parasites or ova should appear in stool.

## ABNORMAL FINDINGS

The presence of *E. histolytica* confirms amebiasis; *G. lamblia,* giardiasis. However, the extent of infection depends on the degree of tissue invasion. If amebiasis is suspected, but stool examinations are negative, specimen collection after saline catharsis using buffered sodium biphosphate or during sigmoidoscopy may be necessary. If giardiasis is suspected, but stool examinations are negative, examination of duodenal contents may be necessary.

Because injury to the host is difficult to detect — even when helminth ova or larvae appear — the number of worms is usually correlated with the patient's clinical symptoms to distinguish between helminth infestation and helminth diseases. Eosinophilia may also indicate parasitic infection. Helminths may migrate from the intestinal tract, producing pathologic changes in other parts of the body. For example, the roundworm *Ascaris* may perforate the bowel wall, causing peritonitis, or may migrate to the lungs, causing pneumonitis. Hookworms can cause hypochromic microcytic anemia secondary to bloodsucking and hemorrhage, especially in the patient with an iron-deficient diet. The tapeworm *D. latum* may cause megaloblastic anemia by removing vitamin $B_{12}$.

## INTERFERING FACTORS

● Presence of urine (false-negative results)
● Excessive heat or cold
● Recent barium studies (possible interference with detection of organism)

# *Stool examination for rotavirus antigen*

Rotaviruses are the most common cause of infectious diarrhea in infants and young children. They're most prevalent in children ages

3 months to 2 years during the winter months. Clinical features include diarrhea, vomiting, fever, and abdominal pain. Symptoms of infection may range from mild in adults to severe in young children, especially hospitalized infants.

Detection of human rotaviruses typically requires sensitive, specific enzyme immunoassays that provide results within minutes or hours (depending on the assay) because human rotaviruses don't replicate efficiently in laboratory cell cultures.

## PURPOSE

● To obtain a laboratory diagnosis of rotavirus gastroenteritis

## PATIENT PREPARATION

● Explain the purpose of the stool examination for rotavirus antigen to the patient or his parents if the patient is a child.
● Inform the patient that the test requires a stool specimen.
● Collect the specimens during the prodromal and acute stages of clinical infection to ensure detection of the viral antigens by enzyme immunoassay.

## PROCEDURE AND POSTTEST CARE

● Usually, a stool specimen (1 g in a screwcapped tube or vial) is used to detect rotaviruses. If a microbiological transport swab is used, it must be heavily stained with stool to be diagnostically productive for rotavirus.
● Monitor the patient's intake and output and provide him with fluids to avoid dehydration caused by vomiting and diarrhea.

## PRECAUTIONS

● Avoid using collection containers with preservatives, metal ions, detergents, and serum, which may interfere with the assay.
● Store stool specimens for up to 24 hours at 35° to 46° F (2° to 8° C). If a longer period of storage or shipment is necessary, freeze specimens at –4° F (–20° C) or colder. Repeated freezing and thawing will cause the specimen to deteriorate and yield misleading results.
● Don't store the specimen in a self-defrosting freezer.
● Use gloves when obtaining or handling all specimens.

## NORMAL FINDINGS

Rotavirus shouldn't appear in the specimen. Detection by enzyme immunoassay is laboratory evidence of current infection with the organism.

## ABNORMAL FINDINGS

Rotavirus isn't normally detectable in the stool. It can infect all age-groups but is generally more severe in young children than in adults. Rotavirus infections are easily transmitted in group settings, such as nursing homes, preschools, and day-care centers. Transmission is presumed to occur from person to person by the fecal-oral route. In a health care facility setting, nosocomial spread of this viral infection can cause significant harm.

## INTERFERING FACTORS

● Collection of a specimen in containers with preservatives, such as detergents, metal ions, or serum (decreased number of pathogens)

## *Sweat test*

The sweat test is a quantitative measurement of electrolyte concentrations (primarily sodium and chloride) in sweat, usually performed using pilocarpine iontophoresis (pilocarpine is a sweat inducer). Although this test is primarily used to confirm cystic fibrosis (CF) in children, it's also performed in adults to determine if they're homozygous or heterozygous for CF. Genetic testing for CF also has become available. (See *Tag-It Cystic Fibrosis Kit,* page 436.)

## PURPOSE

● To confirm or exclude the diagnosis of CF

## PATIENT PREPARATION

● Explain the sweat test to the child (if he's old enough to understand), using clear, simple terms.
● Inform the child and his parents that there are no restrictions on diet, medication, or activity before the test.
● Tell the child who will perform the test and where.

# TAG-IT CYSTIC FIBROSIS KIT

The U.S. Food and Drug Administration approved the use of a deoxyribonucleic acid (DNA) test for diagnosing cystic fibrosis (CF). The test, called the *Tag-It Cystic Fibrosis Kit*, is a blood test that screens for genetic mutations and variations in the cystic fibrosis transmembrane conductance regulator (CFTR) gene. This test identifies 23 genetic mutations and 4 variations in the CFTR gene. It also screens for 16 additional mutations in the gene that are involved in many cases of CF.

The test is recommended for use in detecting and identifying these mutations and variations in the gene as a means for determining carrier status in adults, screening neonates, and for confirming diagnostic testing in neonates and children. There are over 1,300 genetic variations in the CFTR gene responsible for causing CF. Therefore, the test isn't recommended as the only means for diagnosing CF. Test results need to be viewed along with the patient's condition, ethnic background, and family history. Additionally, genetic counseling is suggested to help patients understand the results and their implications.

● Tell the child that he may feel a slight tickling sensation during the procedure, but won't feel any pain.

● Encourage the parents to assist with preparations and to stay with their child during the test. Their presence will minimize the child's anxiety.

## PROCEDURE AND POSTTEST CARE

● Wash the area that will undergo iontophoresis with distilled water and dry it. (The flexor surface of the right forearm is commonly used or, when the patient's arm is too small to secure electrodes [as with an infant], the right thigh.)

● Place a gauze pad saturated with premeasured pilocarpine solution on the positive electrode; place the pad saturated with normal saline solution on the negative electrode.

● Apply both electrodes to the area to undergo iontophoresis and secure them with straps. Lead wires to the analyzer are given a current of 4 mA in 15 to 20 seconds. Iontophoresis will continue at 15- to 20-second intervals for 5 minutes.

● Try to distract the child with a book, television, toy, or another diversion if he becomes nervous or frightened during the test.

● Remove both electrodes after iontophoresis.

● Discard the pads, clean the skin with distilled water, and then dry it.

● Using forceps, place a dry gauze pad or filter paper (previously weighed on a gram scale) on the area that underwent iontophoresis.

● Cover the pad or filter paper with a slightly larger piece of plastic and seal the edges of the plastic with waterproof adhesive tape.

● Leave the gauze pad or filter paper in place for about 30 to 40 minutes. (The appearance of droplets on the plastic usually indicates induction of an adequate amount of sweat.)

● Remove the pad or filter paper with the forceps, place it immediately in the weighing bottle, and insert the stopper in the bottle. (The difference between the first and second weights indicates the weight of the sweat specimen collected.)

● Wash the area that underwent iontophoresis with soap and water and dry it thoroughly. If the area looks red, reassure the patient that this is normal and will disappear within a few hours.

● Tell the patient or his parents that he may resume his usual activities.

## PRECAUTIONS

● Always perform iontophoresis on the right arm (or right thigh) rather than on the left.

● Never perform iontophoresis on the chest, especially in a child, because the current can induce cardiac arrest.

● Use battery-powered equipment to prevent electric shock, if possible.

- Stop the test immediately if the patient complains of a burning sensation, which usually indicates that the positive electrode is exposed or positioned improperly. Adjust the electrode and continue the test.
- Make sure at least 100 mg of sweat is collected for analysis.
- Carefully seal the gauze pad or filter paper in the weighing bottle and immediately send the bottle to the laboratory.

## REFERENCE VALUES

Normal sodium values in sweat range from 10 to 30 mEq/L (SI, 10 to 30 mmol/L). Normal chloride values range from 10 to 35 mEq/L (SI, 10 to 35 mmol/L).

## ABNORMAL FINDINGS

Sodium concentrations of 50 to 60 mEq/L (SI, 50 to 60 mmol/L) strongly suggests CF. Concentrations above 60 mEq/L (SI, > 60 mmol/L) with typical clinical features confirm the diagnosis.

Only a few conditions other than CF result in elevated sweat electrolyte levels — most notably, untreated adrenal insufficiency as well as type I glycogen storage disease, vasopressin-resistant diabetes insipidus, meconium ileus, and renal failure.

In women, sweat electrolyte levels fluctuate cyclically; chloride concentrations usually peak 5 to 10 days before onset of menses, and most women retain fluid before menses. Men also show fluctuations up to 70 mEq/L (SI, 70 mmol/L). However, CF is the only condition that raises sweat electrolyte levels above 80 mEq/L (SI, 80 mmol/L).

## INTERFERING FACTORS

- Dehydration or edema, especially in the collection area
- Failure to obtain an adequate amount of sweat, a common problem in neonates
- Presence of pure salt depletion, common during hot weather (possible false normal)
- Failure to clean the skin thoroughly or to use sterile gauze pads (possible false high)
- Failure to seal the gauze pad or filter paper carefully (possible false-high electrolyte levels due to evaporation)

# Synovial fluid analysis

In synovial fluid aspiration, or arthrocentesis, a sterile needle is inserted into a joint space — most commonly the knee — to obtain a fluid specimen for analysis. This procedure is indicated for the patient with undiagnosed articular disease and symptomatic joint effusion, a condition marked by the excessive accumulation of synovial fluid. Although rare, complications associated with synovial fluid aspiration include joint infection and hemorrhage leading to hemarthrosis (accumulation of blood within the joint).

## PURPOSE

- To aid differential diagnosis of arthritis, particularly septic or crystal-induced arthritis
- To identify the cause and nature of joint effusion
- To relieve the pain and distention resulting from the accumulation of fluid within the joint
- To administer a drug locally (usually corticosteroids)

## PATIENT PREPARATION

- Describe synovial fluid analysis to the patient and answer his questions.
- Explain that this test helps determine the cause of joint inflammation and swelling and also helps relieve the associated pain.
- Instruct the patient to fast for 6 to 12 hours before the test if glucose testing of synovial fluid is ordered; otherwise, inform him that he need not restrict food and fluids.
- Tell the patient who will perform the test and when and where it will be done.
- Warn the patient that although he'll receive a local anesthetic, he may still feel slight pain when the needle penetrates the joint capsule.
- Make sure that the patient or a responsible family member has signed an informed consent form.
- Check the patient's history for hypersensitivity to iodine compounds (such as povidone-iodine), procaine, lidocaine, or other local anesthetics.
- Administer a sedative as ordered.

## PROCEDURE AND POSTTEST CARE

● Position the patient and explain that he'll need to maintain this position throughout the procedure.

● Clean the skin over the puncture site with surgical detergent and alcohol.

● Paint the site with tincture of povidone-iodine and allow it to air-dry for 2 minutes.

● Know that after the local anesthetic is administered, the aspirating needle is quickly inserted through the skin, subcutaneous tissue, and synovial membrane into the joint space.

● Be aware that as much fluid as possible is aspirated into the syringe; at least 15 ml should be obtained, although a smaller amount is usually adequate for analysis.

● Assist as appropriate to maintain the joint (except for the area around the puncture site) wrapped with an elastic bandage to compress the free fluid into this portion of the sac, ensuring maximal fluid collection.

● If a corticosteroid is being injected, prepare the dose as necessary. For instillation, the syringe is detached, leaving the needle in the joint, and the syringe containing the steroid is attached to the needle instead.

● After the steroid is injected and the needle withdrawn, wipe the puncture site with an alcohol pad.

● Apply pressure to the puncture site for about 2 minutes to prevent bleeding, and then apply a sterile dressing.

● If synovial fluid glucose levels are being measured, perform a venipuncture to obtain a specimen for blood glucose analysis.

● Apply ice or cold packs to the affected joint for 24 to 36 hours after aspiration to decrease pain and swelling. Use pillows for support. If a large quantity of fluid was aspirated, apply an elastic bandage to stabilize the joint.

● If the patient's condition permits, tell him that he may resume his usual activity immediately after the procedure. However, warn him to avoid excessive use of the affected joint for a few days even if pain and swelling subside.

● Watch for increased pain or fever; these signs and symptoms may indicate joint infection.

● Be careful when handling the dressings and linens of the patient with drainage from the joint space, especially if septic arthritis is confirmed or suspected.

● Tell the patient that he may resume his usual diet, as ordered.

## PRECAUTIONS

● Wear gloves when handling all specimens.

● Don't perform the test in areas of skin or wound infections.

● Use strict sterile technique throughout aspiration to prevent contamination of the joint space or the synovial fluid specimen.

● Add an anticoagulant to the specimen, according to the laboratory tests requested. Gently invert the tube several times to mix the specimen and anticoagulant adequately.

### For cultures

● Obtain 2 to 5 ml of synovial fluid and, if possible, inoculate the medium immediately. Otherwise, add one or two drops of heparin to the specimen.

### For cytologic analysis

● Add 5 mg of EDTA or one or two drops of heparin to 2 to 5 ml of synovial fluid.

### For glucose analysis

● Add potassium oxalate, as specified by the laboratory, to 3 to 5 ml of fluid.

### For crystal examination

● Add heparin if specified by the laboratory.

### For other studies

● For general appearance and clot evaluation, obtain 2 to 5 ml of synovial fluid, but don't add an anticoagulant.

● Send the properly labeled specimens to the laboratory immediately after collection — gonococci are particularly labile. If a white blood cell (WBC) count is being obtained as well, clearly label the specimen SYNOVIAL FLUID and CAUTION: DON'T USE ACID DILUENTS.

## NORMAL FINDINGS

Routine examination includes gross analysis for color, clarity, quantity, viscosity, pH, and the presence of a mucin clot as well as microscopic analysis for WBC count and differential. Special examination includes microbiological analysis for formed elements (including crystals) and bacteria, serologic analysis, and chemical analysis for such components as glucose, protein, and enzymes.

## ABNORMAL FINDINGS

Synovial fluid examination may reveal various joint diseases, including noninflammatory disease (traumatic arthritis and osteoarthritis), inflammatory disease (systemic lupus erythematosus, rheumatic fever, pseudogout, gout, and rheumatoid arthritis), and septic disease (tuberculous and septic arthritis).

## INTERFERING FACTORS

- Failure to adhere to dietary restrictions
- Specimen contamination
- Acid diluents added to the specimen for WBC count (alteration in cell count)

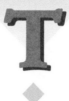

# T- and B-lymphocyte assays

Lymphocytes — key cells in the immune syste — have the capacity to recognize antigens through special receptors found on their surfaces. The two primary kinds of lymphocytes, T and B cells, originate in the bone marrow. T cells mature under the influence of the thymus gland; B cells evolve without thymic influence.

Cell separation is used to isolate lymphocytes from other cellular blood elements. In this method, a whole blood sample is layered on Ficoll-Hypaque in a narrow tube, which is then centrifuged. Granulocytes and erythrocytes form a sediment at the bottom of the tube, and lymphocytes, monocytes, and platelets form a distinct band at the Ficoll-Hypaque-plasma interface.

This procedure recovers approximately 80% of the lymphocytes, but doesn't differentiate between T and B cells. The percentage of T and B cells is determined by attaching a label or marker and by using different identification techniques. The E-rosette assay identifies T cells, which tend to form unstable clusterlike shapes (or rosettes) after exposure to sheep red blood cells at 39.2° F (4° C). Direct immunofluorescence detects B cells, which have monoclonal immunoglobulin on their surfaces; unlike T cells, B cells present receptors for complement as well as for Fc portions of immunoglobulin.

Null cells, which make up the remainder of the lymphocytes, possess Fc receptors but no other detectable surface markers, and presently have no diagnostic significance. Null cells are usually determined by subtracting the sum of T and B cells from total lymphocytes.

## PURPOSE
- To aid in the diagnosis of primary and secondary immunodeficiency diseases
- To distinguish between benign and malignant lymphocytic proliferative diseases
- To monitor the patient's response to therapy

## PATIENT PREPARATION
- Explain to the patient that the T- and B-lymphocyte assays measure certain white blood cells.
- Tell the patient that this test requires a blood sample. Explain who will perform the venipuncture and when.
- Explain to the patient that he may experience slight discomfort from the tourniquet and the needle puncture.

## PROCEDURE AND POSTTEST CARE
- Perform a venipuncture and collect the sample in a 7 ml tube.
- Apply direct pressure to the venipuncture site until bleeding stops.
- Because the patient with T- and B-cell changes may have a compromised immune system, keep the venipuncture site clean and dry. If a hematoma develops at the venipuncture site, apply pressure.

## PRECAUTIONS
- Fill the collection tube completely and invert it gently several times to mix the sample and the anticoagulant adequately.

- Send the sample to the laboratory immediately to ensure viable lymphocytes.
- If antilymphocyte antibodies are suspected, as in autoimmune disease, notify the laboratory.

## REFERENCE VALUES

T-cell and B-cell values may differ from one laboratory to another, depending on test technique and different age groups. Generally, for patients older than age 18, T cells constitute 68% to 75% of total lymphocytes; B cells, 10% to 20%; and null cells, 5% to 20%. The total lymphocyte count ranges from 1,500 to 3,000/µl, the T-cell count varies from 1,400 to 2,700/µl, and the B-cell count ranges from 270 to 640/µl. These counts are higher in children.

## ABNORMAL FINDINGS

An abnormal T-cell or B-cell count suggests but doesn't confirm specific diseases. The B-cell count is elevated in chronic lymphocytic leukemia (thought to be a B-cell malignancy), multiple myeloma, Waldenström's macroglobulinemia, and DiGeorge syndrome (a congenital T-cell deficiency). The B-cell count decreases in acute lymphocytic leukemia and in certain congenital or acquired immunoglobulin deficiency diseases. In other immunoglobulin deficiency diseases, especially if only one immunoglobulin class is deficient, the B-cell count remains normal.

Though the T-cell count rises rarely in infectious mononucleosis, it does so more commonly in multiple myeloma and acute lymphocytic leukemia. T cells decrease in congenital T-cell deficiency diseases, such as DiGeorge, Nezelof, and Wiskott-Aldrich syndromes, and in certain B-cell proliferative disorders, such as chronic lymphocytic leukemia, Waldenström's macroglobulinemia, and acquired immunodeficiency syndrome.

Normal T-cell and B-cell counts don't necessarily ensure a competent immune system. In autoimmune diseases, such as systemic lupus erythematosus and rheumatoid arthritis, T and B cells may be present in normal numbers but may not be functionally competent.

## INTERFERING FACTORS

- Exposing the sample to temperature extremes

- Changes in health status from the effects of chemotherapy, radiography, steroid or immunosuppressive therapy, stress, or surgery (possible rapid change in T- and B-cell counts)
- Immunoglobulins, such as autologous antilymphocyte antibodies, that sometimes occur in autoimmune disease (possible change in results)

# Technetium pyrophosphate scanning

Technetium pyrophosphate scanning (also called *hot spot myocardial imaging* or *infarct avid imaging*) is used to detect a recent myocardial infarction (MI) and to determine its extent. This test uses an I.V. tracer isotope (technetium 99m [$^{99m}$Tc] pyrophosphate). $^{99m}$Tc accumulates in damaged myocardial tissue (possibly by combining with calcium in the damaged myocardial cells), where it forms a "hot spot" on a scan made with a scintillation camera. Such hot spots first appear within 12 hours of infarction, are most apparent after 48 to 72 hours, and usually disappear after 1 week. Hot spots that persist longer than 1 week usually suggest ongoing myocardial damage.

## PURPOSE

- To confirm a recent MI
- To help define the size and location of an MI
- To assess the prognosis after an acute MI

## PATIENT PREPARATION

- Explain to the patient that technetium pyrophosphate scanning helps assess if the heart muscle is injured.
- Inform the patient that he need not restrict food and fluids. Tell him who will perform the test and where it will take place.
- Inform the patient that he'll receive an I.V. tracer isotope 2 or 3 hours before the procedure and that multiple images of his heart will be made.
- Reassure the patient that the injection causes only slight discomfort, that the scan itself is painless, and that the test involves

less exposure to radiation than does a chest X-ray.

- Instruct the patient to remain quiet and motionless while he's being scanned.
- Make sure that the patient or a responsible family member has signed an informed consent form.

## PROCEDURE AND POSTTEST CARE

- Usually, 20 millicuries of $^{99m}Tc$ pyrophosphate are injected I.V. into the antecubital vein.
- After 2 or 3 hours, the patient is placed in a supine position and electrocardiography electrodes are attached for continuous monitoring during the test.
- Generally, scans are taken with the patient in several positions, including anterior, left anterior oblique, right anterior oblique, and left lateral. Each scan takes 10 minutes.

## PRECAUTIONS

- Although there have been no documented adverse effects to this radioisotope, be alert for adverse reactions to the injected contrast medium.

## NORMAL FINDINGS

A normal technetium pyrophosphate scan shows no isotope in the myocardium.

## ABNORMAL FINDINGS

The isotope is taken up by the sternum and ribs, and their activity is compared with the heart's; 2+, 3+, and 4+ activity (equal to or greater than bone) indicates a positive myocardial scan. The technetium pyrophosphate scan can reveal areas of $^{99m}Tc$ accumulation, or hot spots, in damaged myocardium, particularly 48 to 72 hours after onset of an acute MI; however, hot spots are apparent as early as 12 hours after an acute MI. In most cases, hot spots disappear after 1 week; in some, they persist for several months if necrosis continues in the area of infarction.

Knowing where the infarct is makes it possible to anticipate complications and to plan care. About 25% of patients with unstable angina pectoris show hot spots due to subclinical myocardial necrosis and may require coronary arteriography and bypass grafting.

## INTERFERING FACTORS

- Isotope accumulation (in about 10% of patients, may result from ventricular aneurysm associated with dystrophic calcification, pulmonary neoplasm, recent cardioversion, or valvular heart disease due to severe calcification)

# Tensilon test

The Tensilon test involves careful observation of the patient after I.V. administration of Tensilon (edrophonium chloride), a rapid, short-acting anticholinesterase that improves muscle strength by increasing muscle response to nerve impulses.

It's especially useful in diagnosing myasthenia gravis, an abnormality of the myoneural junction in which nerve impulses fail to induce normal muscular responses. Patients with myasthenia gravis experience extreme fatigue at the end of the day and after repetitive activity or stress. Results of other procedures, including electromyography, may supplement Tensilon test findings in diagnosing this disease.

## PURPOSE

- To aid in the diagnosis of myasthenia gravis
- To aid in differentiating between myasthenic and cholinergic crises
- To monitor oral anticholinesterase therapy

## PATIENT PREPARATION

- Explain to the patient that the Tensilon test helps determine the cause of muscle weakness.
- Describe the test, including who will perform it, where it will take place, and how long it will last.
- Don't describe the exact response that will be evaluated; the patient's foreknowledge can affect the test's objectivity.
- Explain to the patient that a small tube will be inserted into a vein in his arm and that a drug will be administered periodically. He'll be asked to make repetitive muscle movements and his reactions will be observed. To ensure accuracy, the test may be repeated several times.

- Advise the patient that the Tensilon may produce some unpleasant adverse effects, but reassure him that someone will be with him at all times and that any reactions will quickly disappear.
- Check the patient's history for medications that affect muscle function, anticholinesterase therapy, drug hypersensitivities, and respiratory disease. Withhold medications, as ordered. If the patient is receiving anticholinesterase therapy, note this on the requisition request; include the time of the most recent dose.
- Make sure that the patient or a responsible family member has signed an informed consent form.

## PROCEDURE AND POSTTEST CARE

- Begin an I.V. infusion of dextrose 5% in water ($D_5W$) or normal saline solution.
- When performing the test on an adult patient suspected of having myasthenia gravis, 2 mg of Tensilon are administered initially. Before the rest of the dose is administered, the physician may want to fatigue the muscles by asking the patient to perform various exercises, such as looking up until ptosis develops, counting to 100 until his voice diminishes, or holding his arms above his shoulders until they drop. When the muscles are fatigued, the remaining 8 mg of Tensilon are administered over 30 seconds.
- Some physicians may prefer to begin the test with a placebo injection to evaluate the patient's muscle response more accurately. The placebo isn't necessary if cranial muscles are being tested because cranial strength can't be simulated voluntarily.
- After Tensilon is administered, the patient is asked to perform repetitive muscle movements, such as opening and closing his eyes and crossing and uncrossing his legs. Closely observe the patient for improved muscle strength. If muscle strength doesn't improve within 3 to 5 minutes, the test may be repeated.
- To differentiate between a myasthenic and cholinergic crisis, 1 to 2 mg of Tensilon is infused. After the infusion, continually monitor the patient's vital signs. Watch closely for respiratory distress and be prepared to provide respiratory assistance.
- If muscle strength doesn't improve, more Tensilon is infused cautiously — 1 mg at a time up to a maximum of 5 mg — and the patient is observed for distress.
- Neostigmine is administered immediately if the test demonstrates myasthenic crisis; atropine is administered for cholinergic crisis.
- To evaluate oral anticholinesterase therapy, 2 mg of Tensilon is infused 1 hour after the patient's last dose of the anticholinesterase. The patient is observed carefully for adverse effects and muscle response.
- After Tensilon administration, the I.V. line is kept open at a rate of 20 ml/hour until all of the patient's responses have been evaluated.
- When the test is complete, discontinue the I.V. and check the patient's vital signs.
- Check the puncture site for hematoma, excessive bleeding, and swelling.
- Tell the patient that he may resume his usual medications, as ordered.

## PRECAUTIONS

- Because of the systemic adverse reactions Tensilon may produce, be aware that this test may be contraindicated in the patient with hypotension, bradycardia, apnea, or mechanical obstruction of the intestine or urinary tract.
- Know that the patient with a respiratory ailment, such as asthma, should receive atropine during the test to minimize adverse reactions to Tensilon.
- Stay with the patient during the test and observe him closely for adverse reactions.

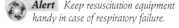 **Alert** *Keep resuscitation equipment handy in case of respiratory failure.*

## NORMAL FINDINGS

Someone who doesn't have myasthenia gravis usually develops fasciculation in response to Tensilon. The physician must interpret the responses carefully to distinguish normal ones from those signalling myasthenia gravis.

## ABNORMAL FINDINGS

If the patient has myasthenia gravis, muscle strength should improve promptly after administration of Tensilon. The degree of improvement depends on the muscle group being tested; improvement is usually obvious within 30 seconds. Although the maximum benefit lasts only several minutes, lingering effects may persist — for example, up to 2 hours in a patient receiving prednisone. The patient with myasthenia gravis shows improved muscle strength in this test; in some cases, the patient responds slightly, and the test may need to be repeated to confirm the diagnosis.

The test may yield inconsistent results if myasthenia gravis affects only the ocular muscles, as in mild or early forms of the disorder. It may produce a positive response in motor neuron disease and in some neuropathies and myopathies. The response is usually less dramatic and less consistent than in myasthenia gravis.

The patient in myasthenic crisis shows brief improvement in muscle strength after Tensilon administration. The patient in cholinergic crisis (anticholinesterase overdose) may experience exaggerated muscle weakness. If Tensilon increases the patient's muscle strength without increasing adverse effects, oral anticholinesterase therapy can be increased. If Tensilon decreases muscle strength in a person with severe adverse reactions, therapy should be reduced. If the test shows no change in muscle strength and only mild adverse effects occur, therapy should remain the same.

## INTERFERING FACTORS
- Prednisone (possible delay of Tensilon's effect on muscle strength)
- Anticholinergics and quinidine (inhibit the action of Tensilon)
- Muscle relaxants and procainamide (inhibit normal muscle response)

## Testosterone

The principal androgen secreted by the interstitial cells of the testes (Leydig cells), testosterone induces puberty in the male and maintains male secondary sex characteristics.

Prepubertal levels of testosterone are low. Increased testosterone secretion during puberty stimulates growth of the seminiferous tubules and sperm production; it also contributes to the enlargement of external genitalia, accessory sex organs (such as prostate glands), and voluntary muscles and to the growth of facial, pubic, and axillary hair.

Testosterone production begins to increase at the onset of puberty and continues to rise during adulthood. Production begins to taper off at about age 40 and eventually

drops to about one-fifth the peak level by age 80. In women, the adrenal glands and ovaries secrete small amounts of testosterone.

This competitive protein-binding test measures plasma or serum testosterone levels. When combined with measurement of plasma gonadotropin levels (follicle-stimulating hormone and luteinizing hormone), it's a reliable aid in the evaluation of gonadal dysfunction in men and women.

## PURPOSE
- To facilitate differential diagnosis of male sexual precocity in boys younger than age 10 (True precocious puberty must be distinguished from pseudoprecocious puberty.)
- To aid differential diagnosis of hypogonadism (Primary hypogonadism must be distinguished from secondary hypogonadism.)
- To evaluate male infertility or other sexual dysfunction
- To evaluate hirsutism and virilization in women

## PATIENT PREPARATION
- Explain to the patient that the testosterone test helps determine if male sex hormone secretion is adequate.
- Inform the patient that he need not restrict food and fluids.
- Tell the patient that the test requires a blood sample. Explain who will perform the venipuncture and when.
- Explain to the patient that he may experience slight discomfort from the tourniquet and needle puncture.

## PROCEDURE AND POSTTEST CARE
- Perform a venipuncture and collect a serum sample in a 7-ml clot-activator tube.
- If plasma is to be collected, use a heparinized tube.
- Indicate the patient's age, sex, and history of hormone therapy on the laboratory request.
- Apply direct pressure to the venipuncture site until bleeding stops.
- If a hematoma develops at the venipuncture site, apply pressure.

## PRECAUTIONS
- Handle the sample gently to prevent hemolysis and send it to the laboratory promptly.

Be aware that the sample is stable and requires no refrigeration or preservative for up to 1 week. Frozen samples are stable for at least 6 months.

## REFERENCE VALUES

Normal testosterone levels are (laboratory values may vary slightly):
- males — 300 to 1,200 ng/dl (SI, 10.4 to 41.6 nmol/L)
- females — 20 to 80 ng/dl (SI, 0.7 to 2.8 nmol/L).

*Age alert* *Prepubertal children have lower testosterone values when compared with prepubescent adolescents and adults.*

## ABNORMAL FINDINGS

Increased testosterone levels can occur with a benign adrenal tumor or cancer, hyperthyroidism, and incipient puberty. In women with ovarian tumors or polycystic ovary syndrome, testosterone levels may rise, leading to hirsutism.

Low testosterone levels can indicate primary hypogonadism (as in Klinefelter's syndrome) or secondary hypogonadism (hypogonadotropic eunuchoidism) from hypothalamic-pituitary dysfunction. Low levels can also follow orchiectomy, testicular or prostate cancer, delayed male puberty, estrogen therapy, and cirrhosis of the liver.

*Age alert* *Elevated testosterone levels in prepubertal boys may indicate true sexual precocity due to excessive gonadotropin secretion or pseudoprecocious puberty due to male hormone production by a testicular tumor. They can also indicate congenital adrenal hyperplasia, which results in precocious puberty in boys (from ages 2 to 3) and pseudohermaphroditism and milder virilization in girls.*

## INTERFERING FACTORS

- Exogenous sources of estrogens and androgens, thyroid and growth hormones, and other pituitary-based hormones
- Estrogens (decrease in free testosterone levels, increasing sex hormone-binding globulin, which binds testosterone)
- Androgens (possible increase)

# Thallium imaging

Also called *cold spot myocardial imaging* or *thallium scintigraphy,* thallium imaging evaluates myocardial blood flow after I.V. injection of the radioisotope thallium-201 or Cardiolite. The main difference between these tracers is that Cardiolite has a better energy spectrum for imaging. Cardiolite requires living myocardial cells for uptake and allows for imaging the myocardial blood flow before and after reperfusion. This sequence allows for better estimation of myocardial salvage. Because thallium, the physiologic analogue of potassium, concentrates in healthy myocardial tissue but not in necrotic or ischemic tissue, areas of the heart with a normal blood supply and intact cells rapidly take it up. Areas with poor blood flow and ischemic cells fail to take up the isotope and appear as "cold spots" on a scan.

This test is performed in a resting state or after stress. Resting imaging can detect acute myocardial infarction (MI) within the first few hours of symptoms, but doesn't distinguish an old from a new infarct. Stress imaging, performed after the patient exercises on a treadmill until he experiences angina or rate-limiting fatigue, can assess known or suspected coronary artery disease (CAD) and can evaluate the effectiveness of antianginal therapy or balloon angioplasty and the patency of grafts after coronary artery bypass grafting (CABG). Possible complications of stress testing include arrhythmias, angina pectoris, and MI.

## PURPOSE

- To assess myocardial scarring and perfusion
- To demonstrate the location and extent of acute or chronic MI, including transmural and postoperative infarction (resting imaging)
- To diagnose CAD (stress imaging)
- To evaluate the patency of grafts after CABG
- To evaluate the effectiveness of antianginal therapy or balloon angioplasty (stress imaging)

## PATIENT PREPARATION

- Explain to the patient that thallium imaging helps determine if any areas of the heart muscle aren't receiving an adequate blood supply.

- If the patient is undergoing stress imaging, instruct him to restrict alcohol, tobacco, and nonprescribed medications for 24 hours before the test and to have nothing by mouth for 3 hours before the test.
- Describe the test, including who will perform it and where it will take place. Explain that additional scans may be required.
- Tell the patient that he'll receive an I.V. radioactive tracer and that multiple images of his heart will be scanned.
- Explain to the patient that it's important to lie still when images are taken.
- Warn the patient that he may experience discomfort from skin abrasion during preparation for electrode placement. Assure him that the test involves minimal radiation exposure.
- Make sure that the patient or a responsible family member has signed an informed consent form.
- Tell the patient undergoing stress imaging to wear walking shoes during the treadmill exercise and to report fatigue, pain, or shortness of breath immediately.

## PROCEDURE AND POSTTEST CARE
### Resting imaging
- Optimally, within the first few hours of symptoms of a MI, the patient receives an injection of I.V. thallium or Cardiolite and scanning begins after 10 minutes.
- If further scanning is required, have the patient rest and restrict food and beverages other than water.

### Stress imaging
- The patient, wired with electrodes, walks on a treadmill at a regulated pace that's gradually increased, while the electrocardiogram (ECG), blood pressure, and heart rate are monitored.
- When the patient reaches peak stress, the examiner injects 1.5 to 3 millicuries of thallium into the antecubital vein and then flushes it with 10 to 15 ml of normal saline solution or an infusion of Cardiolite.
- The patient exercises an additional 45 to 60 seconds to permit circulation and uptake of the isotope, and then lies on his back under the scintillation camera.
- If the patient is asymptomatic, the precordial leads are removed. Scanning begins

after 10 minutes with the patient in the anterior, left anterior oblique, and left lateral positions.
- Additional scans may be taken after the patient rests and, rarely, after 24 hours. Taking a scan after the patient rests is helpful in differentiating between an ischemic area and an infarcted or scarred area of the myocardium.

## PRECAUTIONS
- Be aware that contraindications include impaired neuromuscular function, pregnancy, locomotor disturbances, acute MI or myocarditis, aortic stenosis, acute infection, unstable metabolic conditions (such as diabetes), digoxin toxicity, and recent pulmonary infarction.
- Have emergency medical equipment readily available, if needed.
- **Alert** *Stop stress imaging at once if the patient develops chest pain, dyspnea, fatigue, syncope, hypotension, ischemic ECG changes, significant arrhythmias, or critical signs and symptoms (pale, clammy skin, confusion, or staggering).*

## NORMAL FINDINGS
Imaging should show normal distribution of the isotope throughout the left ventricle and no defects (cold spots). The results may be normal if the patient has narrowed coronary arteries but adequate collateral circulation.

## ABNORMAL FINDINGS
Persistent defects indicate an MI; transient defects (those that disappear after 3 to 6 hours of rest) indicate ischemia from CAD. After coronary artery bypass surgery, improved regional perfusion suggests patency of the graft. Increased perfusion after taking antianginal drugs can show that those drugs relieve ischemia. Improved perfusion after balloon angioplasty suggests increased coronary flow.

## INTERFERING FACTORS
- Cold spots (possible result of sarcoidosis, myocardial fibrosis, cardiac contusion, attenuation due to soft tissue, apical cleft, coronary spasm, and artifacts, such as implants and electrodes)
- Absence of cold spots in the presence of CAD (possibly due to insignificant obstruction, inadequate stress, delayed imaging, collateral circulation, or single-vessel disease,

particularly of the right or left circumflex coronary arteries)

# Thoracic computed tomography

Thoracic computed tomography (CT) provides cross-sectional views of the chest by passing an X-ray beam from a computerized scanner through the body at different angles. CT scanning may be done with or without an injected contrast medium, which is primarily used to highlight blood vessels and to allow greater visual discrimination.

This test provides a three-dimensional image and is especially useful in detecting small differences in tissue density. The thoracic CT scan may replace mediastinoscopy in the diagnosis of mediastinal masses and Hodgkin's disease; its value in the evaluation of pulmonary disease is proven.

## PURPOSE

● To locate suspected neoplasms (such as in Hodgkin's disease), especially with mediastinal involvement
● To identify an abnormal morphology noted on chest X-ray
● To differentiate coin-sized calcified lesions (indicating tuberculosis) from tumors
● To differentiate emphysema or bronchopleural fistula from lung abscess
● To distinguish tumors adjacent to the aorta from aortic aneurysms
● To detect the invasion of a neck mass in the thorax
● To evaluate primary malignancy that may metastasize to the lungs, especially in the patient with a primary bone tumor, soft-tissue sarcoma, or melanoma
● To evaluate the mediastinal lymph nodes
● To evaluate the severity of lung disease such as emphysema
● To detect a dissection or leak of an aortic aneurysm or aortic arch aneurysm
● To plan radiation treatment

## PATIENT PREPARATION

● Explain to the patient that the thoracic CT provides cross-sectional views of the chest and distinguishes small differences in tissue density.

● If a contrast medium won't be used, inform the patient that he need not restrict food and fluids. If the test is to be performed with contrast enhancement, instruct him to fast for 4 hours before the test.
● Tell the patient who will perform the test and when and where it will take place.
● Inform the patient that he'll be positioned on an X-ray table that moves into the center of a large ring-shaped piece of X-ray equipment and that the equipment may be noisy.
● Inform the patient that a contrast medium may be injected into a vein in his arm. If so, he may experience nausea, warmth, flushing of the face, and a salty or metallic taste. Reassure him that these symptoms are normal and that radiation exposure is minimal.
● Tell the patient not to move during the test, but to breathe normally until told to follow specific breathing instructions. Instruct him to remove all jewelry and metallic objects from the X-ray field.
● Check the patient's history for hypersensitivity to iodine, shellfish, or contrast media.
● Make sure that the patient or a responsible family member has signed an informed consent form, if required.

## PROCEDURE AND POSTTEST CARE

● After the patient is placed in a supine position on the X-ray table and the contrast medium has been injected, the machine scans the patient at different angles while the computer calculates small differences in the densities of various tissues, water, fat, bone, and air.
● This information is displayed as a printout of numerical values and as a projection on a monitor. Images may be recorded for further study.
● Watch the patient for signs of delayed hypersensitivity to the contrast medium (itching, hypotension or hypertension, or respiratory distress).
● After the test, encourage the patient to drink lots of fluids.

## PRECAUTIONS

● Know that thoracic CT scanning is contraindicated during pregnancy.
● Keep in mind that the test is also contraindicated — if a contrast medium is used — in a person who has a history of hy-

# COMPARING ABNORMAL AND NORMAL THORACIC CT SCANS

In abnormal thoracic computed tomography (CT) scan (top), note atelectasis in the right middle lobe and cancer in the right hilum. The normal scan (bottom) shows no such deviations.

**Abnormal scan**

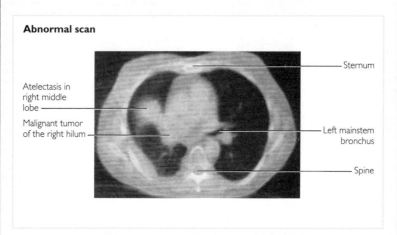

- Sternum
- Atelectasis in right middle lobe
- Malignant tumor of the right hilum
- Left mainstem bronchus
- Spine

**Normal scan**

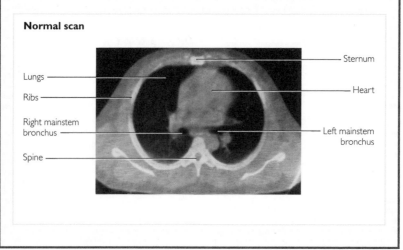

- Sternum
- Lungs
- Ribs
- Heart
- Right mainstem bronchus
- Left mainstem bronchus
- Spine

persensitivity reactions to iodine, shellfish, or contrast media.

## NORMAL FINDINGS
Black-and-white areas on a thoracic CT scan refer, respectively, to air and bone densities. Shades of gray correspond to water, fat, and soft-tissue densities. (See *Comparing abnormal and normal thoracic CT scans.*)

## ABNORMAL FINDINGS
Abnormal thoracic CT findings include tumors, nodules, cysts, aortic aneurysms, enlarged lymph nodes, pleural effusion, and accumulations of blood, fluid, or fat.

## INTERFERING FACTORS

- Failure to remove metallic objects from the scanning field (possible poor imaging)
- Inability of patient to remain still during the procedure
- An obese patient (may be too heavy for scanning table)

# Thoracoscopy

In thoracoscopy, an endoscope is inserted directly into the chest wall to view the pleural space, thoracic walls, mediastinum, and pericardium. It's used for diagnostic and therapeutic purposes and can sometimes replace traditional thoracotomy. Thoracoscopy reduces morbidity (by reducing the use of open chest surgery) and postoperative pain, decreases surgical and anesthesia time, and allows faster recovery.

## PURPOSE

- To diagnose pleural disease
- To obtain biopsy specimens
- To treat pleural conditions, such as cysts, blebs, and effusions
- To perform wedge resections

## PATIENT PREPARATION

- Explain to the patient that thoracoscopy permits visual examination of the chest wall to view the pleural space, thoracic wall, mediastinum, and pericardium.
- Describe the procedure. Caution the patient that an open thoracotomy may still be needed for diagnosis or treatment and that general anesthesia may be required.
- Instruct the patient not to eat or drink for 10 to 12 hours before the procedure.
- Make sure that the appropriate preoperative tests (such as pulmonary function and coagulation tests, electrocardiography, and chest X-ray) have been performed and that an informed consent form has been signed.
- Tell the patient that he'll have a chest tube and drainage system in place after surgery. Reassure him that analgesics will be available.

## PROCEDURE AND POSTTEST CARE

- The patient is anesthetized, and a double-lumen endobronchial tube is inserted.
- The lung on the operative side is collapsed, and a small intercostal incision (approximately 1' long) is made through which a trocar is inserted.
- A lens is then inserted to view the area and assess thoracoscopy access.
- Two or three more small incisions (approximately 1' long) are made, and trocars are placed to insert suction and dissection instruments.
- The camera lens and instruments are moved from site to site as needed.
- After thoracoscopy, the lung is reexpanded, a chest tube is placed through one incision site, and a water-sealed drainage system is attached. The other incisions are closed with adhesive strips and dressed.
- Monitor the patient's postoperative vital signs as per facility policy or every 15 minutes for 1 hour, every 30 minutes for 2 hours, every hour for 2 hours, and then every 4 hours.
- Assess the patient's respiratory status and the patency of the chest drainage system.
- Give analgesics as needed for pain and monitor the patient for adverse effects.

## PRECAUTIONS

- Send specimens to the laboratory immediately.
- Know that thoracoscopy is contraindicated in the patient who has coagulopathies or lesions near major blood vessels, who has extensive pleural disease or pleural adhesions, or who can't be adequately oxygenated with one lung.

⚠ *Alert  Be alert for complications, although rare, including hemorrhage, nerve injury, perforation of the diaphragm, air emboli, and tension pneumothorax.*

## NORMAL FINDINGS

A normal pleural cavity contains a small amount of lubricating fluid that facilitates movement of the lung and chest wall. The parietal and visceral layers are lesion-free and can separate from each other.

## ABNORMAL FINDINGS

Lesions — such as tumors, ulcers, and bleeding sites — adjacent to or involving the pleura or mediastinum can be seen and biopsies can be taken. Diagnosis may include carcinoma, empyema, pleural effusion, tuberculosis, or an inflammatory process. Areas of blebs can be removed by wedge resection to reduce the risk of repeat episodes of spontaneous pneumothorax.

## INTERFERING FACTORS
● Extensive disease or inaccessibility (may prevent thoracoscopy)
● Excessive bleeding during the procedure (may require open thoracotomy)
● Use of antiseptic mouthwash

# Throat culture

A throat culture is used primarily to isolate and identify pathogens, thus allowing early treatment of pharyngitis and prevention of sequelae, such as rheumatic heart disease and glomerulonephritis. It's also used to screen for carriers of *Neisseria meningitidis*. In rare instances, a throat culture may be used to identify *Corynebacterium diphtheriae* or *Bordetella pertussis*. Although a throat culture may also be used to identify *Candida albicans*, direct potassium hydroxide preparation usually provides the same information faster.

A throat culture requires swabbing the throat, streaking a culture plate, and allowing the organisms to grow for isolation and identification of pathogens. A Gram-stained smear may provide preliminary identification, which may guide clinical management and determine the need for further tests. Culture results are considered in relation to the patient's clinical status, recent antimicrobial therapy, and amount of normal flora.

## PURPOSE
● To isolate and identify group A beta-hemolytic streptococci
● To screen asymptomatic carriers of pathogens, especially *N. meningitidis*

## PATIENT PREPARATION
● Explain to the patient that the throat culture is used to identify microorganisms that may be causing his symptoms or to screen for asymptomatic carriers.

● Inform the patient that he need not restrict food and fluids.
● Tell the patient that a specimen will be collected from his throat and who will collect the specimen and when.
● Describe the procedure, and warn the patient that he may gag during the swabbing.
● Check the patient's history for recent antimicrobial therapy. Determine immunization history if it's pertinent to the preliminary diagnosis.

## PROCEDURE AND POSTTEST CARE
● Tell the patient to tilt his head back and close his eyes.
● With the throat well illuminated, check for inflamed areas using a tongue blade.
● Swab the tonsillar areas from side to side; include inflamed or purulent sites.
● Don't touch the tongue, cheeks, or teeth with the swab.
● Immediately place the swab in the culture tube.
● If a commercial sterile collection and transport system is used, crush the ampule and force the swab into the medium to keep the swab moist.
● Note recent antimicrobial therapy on the laboratory request; label the specimen with the patient's name, the physician's name, the date and time of collection, and the origin of the specimen; indicate the suspected organism, especially *C. diphtheriae* (requires two swabs and a special growth medium), *B. pertussis* (requires a nasopharyngeal culture and a special growth medium), and *N. meningitidis* (requires enriched selective media).
● Nonculture antigen testing methods can be used to detect group A streptococcal antigen in as few as 5 minutes. Cultures are then performed on negative specimens.

## PRECAUTIONS
● Procure the throat specimen before beginning antimicrobial therapy.
● Wear gloves when performing the procedure and handling specimens.
● Send the specimen to the laboratory immediately. Unless a commercial sterile collection and transport system is used, keep the container upright during transport.
  **Alert** *Be aware that laryngospasm may occur after the throat culture is obtained if the*

*patient has epiglottiditis or diphtheria. Keep resuscitation equipment nearby.*

## NORMAL FINDINGS
Normal throat flora include nonhemolytic and alpha-hemolytic streptococci, *Neisseria* species, staphylococci, diphtheroids, some *Haemophilus* species, pneumococci, yeasts, enteric gram-negative rods, spirochetes, *Veillonella* species, and *Micrococcus* species.

## ABNORMAL FINDINGS
Pathogens that may be cultured include group A beta-hemolytic streptococci (*Streptococcus pyogenes*), which can cause scarlet fever and pharyngitis; *C. albicans,* which can cause thrush; *C. diphtheriae,* which can cause diphtheria; and *B. pertussis,* which can cause whooping cough. The laboratory report should indicate the prevalent organisms and the quantity of pathogens cultured.

## INTERFERING FACTORS
● Failure to report recent or current antimicrobial therapy on the laboratory request (possible false-negative)
● More than a 15-minute delay in sending the specimen to the laboratory
● Use of antiseptic mouthwash

## Thyroid biopsy

Thyroid biopsy is the excision of a thyroid tissue specimen for histologic examination. This procedure is indicated in patients with thyroid enlargement or nodules (even if serum triiodothyronine [$T_3$] and thyroxine [$T_4$] levels are normal), breathing and swallowing difficulties, vocal cord paralysis, weight loss, hemoptysis, and a sensation of fullness in the neck. It's commonly performed when noninvasive tests, such as thyroid ultrasonography and scans, are abnormal or inconclusive. Coagulation studies should always precede thyroid biopsy.

Thyroid tissue may be obtained with a hollow needle under local anesthesia or during open (surgical) biopsy under general anesthesia. Fine-needle aspiration with a cytologic smear examination can aid in diagnosis and replace an open biopsy. Open biopsy, performed in the operating room, provides more information than needle biopsy; it also permits direct examination and immediate excision of suspicious tissue.

## PURPOSE
● To differentiate between benign and malignant thyroid disease
● To help diagnose Hashimoto's disease, hyperthyroidism, and nontoxic nodular goiter

## PATIENT PREPARATION
● Describe the thyroid biopsy to the patient, and answer his questions.
● Explain that this test permits microscopic examination of a thyroid tissue specimen.
● Inform the patient that he need not restrict food and fluids (unless he receives a general anesthetic).
● Tell the patient who will perform the biopsy and when and where it will be done.
● Make sure the patient or a responsible family member has signed an informed consent form.
● Check the patient's history for hypersensitivity to anesthetics or analgesics.
● Tell the patient that he'll receive a local anesthetic to minimize pain during the procedure but may experience some pressure when the tissue specimen is procured.
● Check the results of the patient's coagulation studies, and make sure they're in his chart.
● Advise the patient that he may have a sore throat the day after the test.
● Administer a sedative to the patient 15 minutes before biopsy.

## PROCEDURE AND POSTTEST CARE
● For needle biopsy, place the patient in the supine position with a pillow under his shoulder blades. (This position pushes the trachea and thyroid forward and allows the neck veins to fall backward.)
● Prepare the skin over the biopsy site.
● As the examiner prepares to inject the local anesthetic, warn the patient not to swallow.
● After the anesthetic is injected, the carotid artery is palpated and the biopsy needle is inserted parallel to the thyroid cartilage to prevent damage to the deep structures and the larynx.
● When the specimen is obtained, the needle is removed and the specimen is placed in formalin immediately.

- Apply pressure to the biopsy site to stop bleeding. If bleeding continues for more than a few minutes, press on the site for up to an additional 15 minutes. Apply an adhesive bandage. (Bleeding may persist in a patient with a prolonged prothrombin time [PT] or partial thromboplastin time [PTT] or in a patient with a large, vascular thyroid with distended veins.)
- To make the patient more comfortable, place him in the semi-Fowler's position; tell him to avoid straining the biopsy site by putting both hands behind his neck when he sits up.

🔷 *Alert   Watch for tenderness or redness, and report signs of bleeding at the biopsy site immediately. Check the back of the patient's neck and his pillow for bleeding every hour for 8 hours. Observe for difficult breathing due to edema or hematoma, with resultant tracheal collapse.*

- Keep the biopsy site clean and dry.

## PRECAUTIONS
- Know that thyroid biopsy should be used cautiously in the patient with coagulation defects, as indicated by a prolonged PT or PTT.
- Immediately place the specimen in formalin solution because cell breakdown in the tissue specimen begins immediately after excision.

## NORMAL FINDINGS
Histologic examination of normal tissue shows fibrous networks dividing the gland into pseudolobules that are made up of follicles and capillaries. Cuboidal epithelium lines the follicle walls and contains the protein thyroglobulin, which stores $T_4$ and $T_3$.

## ABNORMAL FINDINGS
Malignant tumors appear as well-encapsulated, solitary nodules of uniform but abnormal structure. Papillary carcinoma is the most common thyroid cancer. Follicular carcinoma, a less common form, strongly resembles normal cells.

Benign tumors, such as nontoxic nodular goiter, demonstrate hypertrophy, hyperplasia, and hypervascularity. Distinct histologic patterns characterize subacute granulomatous thyroiditis, Hashimoto's thyroiditis, and hyperthyroidism.

Because thyroid tumors are usually multicentric and small, a negative histologic report doesn't rule out cancer.

## INTERFERING FACTORS
- Inability to obtain a representative tissue specimen

# Thyroid ultrasonography

In thyroid ultrasonography, high-frequency sound waves emitted from a transducer are directed at the thyroid gland and reflected back to produce structural images on a monitor.

When a mass is located by palpation or by thyroid imaging, thyroid ultrasonography can differentiate between a cyst and a tumor larger than ¼" (1 cm) with a high degree of accuracy. This test is also used to evaluate thyroid nodules during pregnancy because it doesn't require use of radioactive iodine.

## PURPOSE
- To evaluate thyroid structure
- To differentiate between a cyst and a solid tumor
- To monitor the size of the thyroid gland during suppressive therapy

## PATIENT PREPARATION
- Describe thyroid ultrasonography to the patient, and explain that this test defines the size and shape of the thyroid gland.
- Inform the patient that he need not restrict food and fluids.
- Tell the patient who will perform the procedure, when and where it will take place, and that it's painless and safe.

## PROCEDURE AND POSTTEST CARE
- The patient is placed in a supine position with a pillow under his shoulder blades to hyperextend his neck.
- His neck is coated with water-soluble conductive gel.
- The transducer then scans the thyroid, projecting its echographic image on the oscilloscope screen.
- The image on the monitor is photographed for subsequent examination.
- Accurate visualization of the anterior portion of the thyroid requires use of a short-focused transducer.

- Thoroughly clean the patient's neck to remove the conductive gel.

## PRECAUTIONS
- None

## NORMAL FINDINGS
Thyroid ultrasonography exhibits a uniform echo pattern throughout the gland.

## ABNORMAL FINDINGS
Cysts appear as smooth-bordered, echo-free areas with enhanced sound transmission; adenomas and carcinomas appear either solid and well demarcated with identical echo patterns or, less commonly, solid with cystic areas. Carcinoma infiltrating the gland may not be well demarcated.

Identification of a tumor is generally followed up by fine needle aspiration or an excisional biopsy to determine malignancy.

## INTERFERING FACTORS
- None significant

# Thyroid-stimulating hormone, serum

Thyroid-stimulating hormone (TSH), or thyrotropin, promotes increases in the size, number, and activity of thyroid cells and stimulates the release of triiodothyronine and thyroxine. These hormones affect total body metabolism and are essential for normal growth and development.

This test measures serum TSH levels by radioimmunoassay. It can detect primary hypothyroidism and determine whether the hypothyroidism results from thyroid gland failure or from pituitary or hypothalamic dysfunction. Normal serum TSH levels rule out primary hypothyroidism. This test may not distinguish between low-normal and subnormal levels, especially in secondary hypothyroidism.

## PURPOSE
- To confirm or rule out primary hypothyroidism and distinguish it from secondary hypothyroidism
- To monitor drug therapy in the patient with primary hypothyroidism

## PATIENT PREPARATION
- Explain to the patient that the serum thyroid-stimulating hormone test helps assess thyroid gland function.
- Tell the patient that the test requires a blood sample. Explain who will perform the venipuncture and when.
- Explain to the patient that he may experience slight discomfort from the tourniquet and the needle puncture.
- Withhold steroids, thyroid hormones, aspirin, and other medications that may influence test results, as ordered. If they must be continued, note this on the laboratory request.
- Keep the patient relaxed and recumbent for 30 minutes before the test.

## PROCEDURE AND POSTTEST CARE
- Between 6 a.m. and 8 a.m., perform a venipuncture and collect the sample in a 5-ml clot-activator tube.
- Apply direct pressure to the venipuncture site until bleeding stops.
- If a hematoma develops at the venipuncture site, apply pressure.
- Instruct the patient that he may resume medications discontinued before the test, as ordered.

## PRECAUTIONS
- Handle the sample gently to prevent hemolysis.

## REFERENCE VALUES
Normal TSH values range from undetectable to 15 µIU/ml (SI, undetectable to 15 mU/L).

## ABNORMAL FINDINGS
TSH levels may be slightly elevated in euthyroid patients with thyroid cancer. Levels that exceed 20 µIU/ml (SI, > 20 mU/L) suggest primary hypothyroidism or, possibly, endemic goiter.

Low or undetectable TSH levels may be normal, but occasionally indicate secondary hypothyroidism (with inadequate secretion of TSH or thyrotropin-releasing hormone [TRH]). Low TSH levels may also result from hyperthyroidism (Graves' disease) and thyroiditis; both are marked by hypersecretion of thyroid hormones, which suppresses TSH release. Provocative testing with TRH is necessary to confirm the diagnosis. (See *TRH challenge test.*)

## INTERFERING FACTORS
● Use of aspirin, steroids, thyroid hormones (alteration in test results)

# Thyroid-stimulating immunoglobulin

Thyroid-stimulating immunoglobulin (TSI), formerly called *long-acting thyroid stimulator,* appears in the blood of most patients with Graves' disease. This autoantibody reacts with the cell-surface receptors that usually combine with thyroid-stimulating hormone (TSH). TSI reacts with these receptors, activates intracellular enzymes, and promotes epithelial cell activity that functions outside the normal feedback regulation mechanism for TSH. It stimulates the thyroid gland to produce and excrete excessive amounts of thyroid hormone.

Reportedly, 90% of people with Graves' disease have elevated TSI levels. Positive results of this test strongly suggest Graves' disease, despite normal routine thyroid tests in patients still suspected of having Graves' disease or progressive exophthalmos.

## PURPOSE
● To aid in the evaluation of suspected thyroid disease

● To aid in the diagnosis of suspected thyrotoxicosis, especially in patients with exophthalmos
● To monitor treatment of thyrotoxicosis

## PATIENT PREPARATION
● Explain to the patient that the TSI test evaluates thyroid function, as appropriate.
● Tell the patient that the test requires a blood sample. Explain who will perform the venipuncture and when.
● Explain to the patient that he may experience slight discomfort from the tourniquet and the needle puncture.

## PROCEDURE AND POSTTEST CARE
● Perform a venipuncture and collect the sample in a 5-ml clot-activator tube.
● Apply direct pressure to the venipuncture site until bleeding stops.
● If a hematoma develops at the venipuncture site, apply pressure.
● If the patient had a radioactive iodine scan within 48 hours of the test, note this on the laboratory request.

## PRECAUTIONS
● Handle the sample gently to prevent hemolysis and send it to the laboratory immediately.

## REFERENCE VALUES
TSI doesn't normally appear in serum. However, it's considered normal at levels equal to or greater than 1.3 index.

## ABNORMAL FINDINGS

Increased TSI levels are associated with exophthalmos, Graves' disease (thyrotoxicosis), and recurrence of hyperthyroidism.

## INTERFERING FACTORS

● Administration of radioactive iodine within 48 hours of the test

## Thyroxine-binding globulin, serum

The thyroxine-binding globulin (TBG) test measures the serum level of TBG, the predominant protein carrier for circulating thyroxine ($T_4$) and triiodothyronine ($T_3$). TBG values may be identified by saturating the sample for TBG determination with radioactive $T_4$, then subjecting this to electrophoresis and measuring the amount of TBG by the amount of radioactive $T_4$ by radioimmunoassay.

Any condition that affects TBG levels and subsequent binding capacity also affects the amount of free $T_4$ ($FT_4$) in circulation. An underlying TBG abnormality renders tests for total $T_3$ and $T_4$ inaccurate, but doesn't affect the accuracy of tests for free $T_3$ ($FT_3$) and $FT_4$.

## PURPOSE

● To evaluate abnormal thyrometabolic states that don't correlate with thyroid hormone ($T_3$ or $T_4$) values (for example, a patient with overt signs of hypothyroidism and a low $FT_4$ level with a high total $T_4$ level due to a marked increase of TBG secondary to hormonal contraceptives)
● To identify TBG abnormalities

## PATIENT PREPARATION

● Explain to the patient that the serum TBG test helps evaluate thyroid function.
● Tell the patient that the test requires a blood sample. Explain who will perform the venipuncture and when.
● Explain to the patient that he may experience slight discomfort from the tourniquet and the needle puncture.
● Withhold medications that may affect the accuracy of test results, such as estrogens, anabolic steroids, phenytoin, salicylates, or thyroid preparations, as ordered. If they must be continued, note this on the laboratory request. (They may be continued to determine if prescribed drugs are affecting TBG levels.)

## PROCEDURE AND POSTTEST CARE

● Perform a venipuncture, and collect the sample in a 7-ml clot activator tube.
● Apply direct pressure to the venipuncture site until bleeding stops.
● If a hematoma develops at the venipuncture site, apply pressure.
● Instruct the patient that he may resume medications discontinued before the test, as ordered.

## PRECAUTIONS

● Handle the sample gently to prevent hemolysis.

## REFERENCE VALUES

Normal values for TBG by immunoassay range from 16 to 32 µg/dl (SI, 120 to 180 mg/ml).

## ABNORMAL FINDINGS

Elevated TBG levels may indicate hypothyroidism or congenital (genetic) excess, some forms of hepatic disease, or acute intermittent porphyria. TBG levels normally rise during pregnancy and are high in neonates. Suppressed levels may indicate hyperthyroidism or congenital deficiency and can occur in active acromegaly, nephrotic syndrome, and malnutrition associated with hypoproteinemia, acute illness, or surgical stress.

Patients with TBG abnormalities require additional testing, such as the serum $FT_3$ and $T_4$ tests, to evaluate thyroid function more precisely.

## INTERFERING FACTORS

● Estrogens, including hormonal contraceptives, and phenothiazines such as perphenazine (increase)
● Androgens, prednisone, phenytoin, and high doses of salicylates (decrease)

## Thyroxine, serum

Thyroxine ($T_4$) is an amine secreted by the thyroid gland in response to thyroid-stimulating hormone (TSH) and, indirectly, thyrotropin-releasing hormone. The rate of secretion is normally regulated by a complex system of negative and positive feedback involving the thyroid, anterior pituitary, and hypothalamus. The suspected precursor, or prohormone, of triiodothyronine ($T_3$), $T_4$ is believed to convert to $T_3$ by monodeiodination, which occurs mainly in the liver and kidneys.

Only a fraction of $T_4$ (about 0.05%) circulates freely in the blood; the rest binds strongly to plasma proteins, primarily thyroxine-binding globulin (TBG). This minute fraction is responsible for the clinical effects of thyroid hormone. TBG binds so tenaciously that $T_4$ survives in the plasma for a relatively long time, with a half-life of about 6 days. This immunoassay, one of the most common thyroid diagnostic tools, measures the total circulating $T_4$ level when TBG is normal. An alternative test is the Murphy-Pattee or $T_4$ (D), based on competitive protein binding.

## PURPOSE
- To evaluate thyroid function
- To aid diagnosis of hyperthyroidism and hypothyroidism
- To monitor the patient's response to antithyroid medication in hyperthyroidism or to thyroid replacement therapy in hypothyroidism (TSH estimates are needed to confirm hypothyroidism.)

## PATIENT PREPARATION
- Explain to the patient that the serum $T_4$ test helps evaluate thyroid gland function.
- Inform the patient that he need not fast or restrict activity.
- Tell the patient that the test requires a blood sample. Explain who will perform the venipuncture and when.
- Withhold medications that may interfere with test results, as ordered. If they must be continued, note this on the laboratory request. If this test is being performed to monitor thyroid therapy, the patient should continue to receive daily thyroid supplements.

## PROCEDURE AND POSTTEST CARE
- Perform a venipuncture and collect the sample in a 7-ml clot-activator tube.
- Send the sample to the laboratory immediately so that the serum can be separated.
- Apply direct pressure to the venipuncture site until bleeding stops.
- If a hematoma develops at the venipuncture site, apply pressure.
- Instruct the patient that he may resume medications discontinued before the test, as ordered.

## PRECAUTIONS
- Handle the sample gently to prevent hemolysis.

## REFERENCE VALUES
Normally, total $T_4$ levels range from 5 to 13.5 µg/dl (SI, 60 to 165 mmol/L).

## ABNORMAL FINDINGS
Abnormally elevated $T_4$ levels are consistent with primary and secondary hyperthyroidism, including excessive $T_4$ (levothyroxine) replacement therapy (factitious or iatrogenic hyperthyroidism). Subnormal levels suggest primary or secondary hypothyroidism or may be due to $T_4$ suppression by normal, elevated, or replacement $T_3$ levels. In doubtful cases of hypothyroidism, TSH levels may be indicated.

Normal $T_4$ levels don't guarantee euthyroidism; for example, normal readings occur in $T_3$ toxicosis. Overt signs of hyperthyroidism require further testing.

## INTERFERING FACTORS
- Hereditary factors and hepatic disease (possible increase or decrease in TBG)
- Protein-wasting disease (such as nephrotic syndrome) and androgens (possible decrease in TBG)
- Estrogens, levothyroxine, methadone, and progestins (increase)
- Free fatty acids, heparin, iodides, liothyronine sodium, lithium, methylthiouracil, phenylbutazone, phenytoin, propylthiouracil, salicylates (high doses), steroids, sulfonamides, and sulfonylureas (decrease)
- Clofibrate (possible increase or decrease)

# TORCH test

The TORCH test helps detect exposure to pathogens involved in congenital and neonatal infections. TORCH is an acronym for

Toxoplasmosis, Rubella, Cytomegalovirus, and Herpes simplex antibodies. These pathogens are commonly associated with congenital and neonatal infections that aren't clinically apparent and may cause severe central nervous system impairment. This test detects specific immunoglobulin M-associated antibodies in infant blood.

## PURPOSE
- To aid in the diagnosis of acute, congenital, and intrapartum infections

## PATIENT PREPARATION
- Explain to the infant's parents the purpose of the TORCH test and mention that the test requires a blood sample.
- Tell the parents who will perform the venipuncture and when.
- Explain that the infant may experience slight discomfort from the tourniquet and the needle puncture.

## PROCEDURE AND POSTTEST CARE
- Obtain a 3-ml sample of venous or cord blood.
- Apply direct pressure to the venipuncture site until bleeding stops.
- If a hematoma develops at the venipuncture site, apply pressure.

## PRECAUTIONS
- Handle the sample gently to prevent hemolysis.
- Send the sample to the laboratory immediately.
- Don't freeze the sample.

## NORMAL FINDINGS
Normal test results are negative for TORCH agents.

## ABNORMAL FINDINGS
Toxoplasmosis is diagnosed by sequential examination that shows rising antibody titers, changing titers, and serologic conversion from negative to positive; a titer of 1:256 suggests recent Toxoplasma infection.

In infants less than 6 months old, rubella infection is associated with a marked and persistent rise in complement-fixing antibody titer over time. Persistence of rubella antibody in an infant after age 6 months strongly suggests congenital infection. Congenital rubella is associated with cardiac anomalies, neurosensory deafness, growth retardation, and encephalitic symptoms.

Detection of herpes antibodies in cerebrospinal fluid with signs of herpetic encephalitis and persistent herpes simplex virus type 2 antibody levels confirms herpes simplex infection in a neonate without obvious herpetic lesions.

## INTERFERING FACTORS
- None significant

# *Total carbon dioxide content*

When carbon dioxide ($CO_2$) pressure in red blood cells exceeds 40 mm Hg, $CO_2$ spills out of the cells and dissolves in plasma. There it may combine with water to form carbonic acid, which in turn may dissociate into hydrogen and bicarbonate ions.

The total $CO_2$ content test is used to measure the total concentration of all forms of $CO_2$ in serum, plasma, or whole blood samples. It's commonly ordered for patients with respiratory insufficiency and is usually included in an assessment of electrolyte balance. Test results are most significant when considered with pH and arterial blood gas values.

Because about 90% of $CO_2$ in serum is in the form of bicarbonate, this test closely assesses bicarbonate levels. Total $CO_2$ content reflects the adequacy of gas exchange in the lungs and the efficiency of the carbonic acid–bicarbonate buffer system, which maintains acid-base balance and normal pH.

## PURPOSE
- To help evaluate acid-base balance

## PATIENT PREPARATION
- Explain to the patient that the total $CO_2$ content test is performed to measure the amount of $CO_2$ in the blood.
- Tell the patient that the test requires a blood sample. Explain who will perform the venipuncture and when.
- Explain to the patient that he may experience discomfort from the tourniquet and the needle puncture.

- Inform the patient that he need not restrict food and fluids.
- Notify the laboratory and physician of medications the patient is taking that may affect test results; they may need to be restricted.

## PROCEDURE AND POSTTEST CARE
- Perform a venipuncture.
- When $CO_2$ content is measured along with electrolytes, a 3- or 4-ml clot activator tube may be used.
- When this test is performed alone, a heparinized tube is appropriate.
- Apply direct pressure to the venipuncture site until the bleeding has stopped.
- If a hematoma develops at the venipuncture site, apply pressure.
- Instruct the patient that he may resume any medications discontinued before the test, as ordered.

## PRECAUTIONS
- Fill the tube completely to prevent diffusion of $CO_2$ into the vacuum.

## REFERENCE VALUES
Normally, total $CO_2$ levels range from 22 to 26 mEq/L (SI, 22 to 26 mmol/L). Levels may vary, depending on the patient's sex and age.

## ABNORMAL FINDINGS
High $CO_2$ levels may occur in metabolic alkalosis, respiratory acidosis, primary aldosteronism, and Cushing's syndrome. $CO_2$ levels may also increase after excessive loss of acids, such as severe vomiting and continuous gastric drainage.

Decreased $CO_2$ levels are common in metabolic acidosis. Decreased total $CO_2$ levels in metabolic acidosis also result from loss of bicarbonate. Levels may decrease in respiratory alkalosis.

## INTERFERING FACTORS
- Excessive use of corticotropin, cortisone, or thiazide diuretics; excessive ingestion of alkali or licorice (increase)
- Acetazolamide, ammonium chloride, dimercaprol, methicillin, paraldehyde, and salicylates; ingestion of ethylene glycol or methyl alcohol (decrease)

# Total cholesterol

The total cholesterol test, the quantitative analysis of serum cholesterol, is used to measure the circulating levels of free cholesterol and cholesterol esters; it reflects the level of the two forms in which this biochemical compound appears in the body. High serum cholesterol levels may be associated with an increased risk of coronary artery disease (CAD). A 3-minute skin test is now available for use in physician offices. (See *Skin test for cholesterol.*)

## PURPOSE
- To assess the risk of CAD
- To evaluate fat metabolism
- To aid in the diagnosis of nephrotic syndrome, pancreatitis, hepatic disease, hypothyroidism, and hyperthyroidism
- To assess the efficacy of lipid-lowering drug therapy

## PATIENT PREPARATION
- Explain to the patient that the total cholesterol test is used to assess the body's fat metabolism.
- Tell the patient that the test requires a blood sample. Explain who will perform the venipuncture and when.
- Explain to the patient that he may experience slight discomfort from the tourniquet and the needle puncture.
- Instruct the patient not to eat or drink for 12 hours before the test, but that he may have water.
- Notify the laboratory and physician of medications the patient is taking that may affect test results; they may need to be restricted.

## PROCEDURE AND POSTTEST CARE
- Perform a venipuncture and collect the sample in a 4-ml EDTA tube. The patient should be in a sitting position for 5 minutes before the blood is drawn. Fingersticks can also be used for initial screening when using an automated analyzer.
- Apply direct pressure to the venipuncture site until bleeding stops.

● Instruct the patient that he may resume his usual diet and medications discontinued before the test, as ordered.

## PRECAUTIONS
● Send the sample to the laboratory immediately.

## REFERENCE VALUES
Total cholesterol concentrations vary with age and gender. Total cholesterol values are:
● adult males — (desirable) less than 205 mg/dl (SI, < 5.3 mmol/L)
● adults females — (desirable) less than 190 mg/dl (SI, < 4.9 mmol/L).

*Age alert* *Desirable total cholesterol levels in children ages 12 to 18 are less than 170 mg/dl (SI, < 4.4 mmol/L).*

## ABNORMAL FINDINGS
Elevated serum cholesterol levels (hypercholesterolemia) may indicate a risk of CAD as well as incipient hepatitis, lipid disorders, bile duct blockage, nephrotic syndrome, obstructive jaundice, pancreatitis, and hypothyroidism.

Low serum cholesterol levels (hypocholesterolemia) are commonly associated with malnutrition, cellular necrosis of the liver, and hyperthyroidism. Abnormal cholesterol levels commonly necessitate further testing to pinpoint the cause.

## INTERFERING FACTORS
● Chlortetracycline, cholestyramine, clofibrate, colestipol, dextrothyroxine, haloperidol, neomycin, and niacin (decrease)
● Chlorpromazine, epinephrine, hormonal contraceptives, trifluoperazine, and trimethadione (increase)
● Androgens (possible variable effect)

## *Total hemoglobin*

Total hemoglobin (Hb) is used to measure the amount of Hb found in a deciliter (dl, or 100 ml) of whole blood. It's usually part of a complete blood count. Hb concentration correlates closely with the red blood cell (RBC) count and affects the Hb-RBC ratio (mean corpuscular hemoglobin [MCH] and mean corpuscular hemoglobin concentration [MCHC]).

## PURPOSE
● To measure the severity of anemia or polycythemia and to monitor response to therapy
● To obtain data for calculating the MCH and MCHC

## PATIENT PREPARATION
● Explain to the patient that the total Hb test is used to detect anemia or polycythemia or to assess his response to treatment.

- Tell the patient that a blood sample will be taken. Explain who will perform the venipuncture and when.
- Explain to the patient that he may feel slight discomfort from the tourniquet and the needle puncture.

*Age alert* *If the patient is an infant or child, explain to the parents that a small amount of blood will be taken from his finger or earlobe.*

- Inform the patient that he need not restrict food and fluids.

## PROCEDURE AND POSTTEST CARE

- For adults and older children, perform a venipuncture and collect the sample in a 3- or 4.5-ml EDTA tube.

*Age alert* *For younger children and infants, collect the sample by fingerstick or heelstick in a microcollection device with EDTA.*

- If a hematoma develops at the venipuncture site, apply pressure. If the hematoma is large, monitor pulses distal to the venipuncture site.
- Make sure subdermal bleeding has stopped before removing pressure.

## PRECAUTIONS

- Completely fill the collection tube and invert it gently several times to thoroughly mix the sample and the anticoagulant.
- Handle the sample gently to prevent hemolysis.

## REFERENCE VALUES

Hb concentration varies depending on the type of sample drawn and the patient's sex:
- adult males — 14 to 17.4 g/dl (SI, 140 to 174 g/L)
- adult females — 12 to 16 g/dl (SI, 120 to 160 g/L).

*Age alert* *Reference values for infants and children also vary depending on age:*
- *neonates — 17 to 22 g/dl (SI, 170 to 220 g/L)*
- *1 week — 15 to 20 g/dl (SI, 150 to 200 g/L)*
- *1 month — 11 to 15 g/dl (SI, 110 to 150 g/L)*
- *2 months to 6 months — 10.7 to 17.3 g/dL (SI, 107 to 173 g/L)*
- *6 months to 1 year — 9.9 to 14.5 g/dL (SI, 99 to 145 g/L)*
- *1 year to 6 years — 9.5 to 14.1 g/dL (SI, 95 to 141 g/L)*
- *6 years to 16 years — 10.3 to 14.9 g/dL (SI, 103 to 149 g/L)*
- *16 years to 18 years — 11.1 to 15.7 g/dL (SI, 111 to 157 g/L)*

Those who are more active or who live in high altitudes may have higher values.

## ABNORMAL FINDINGS

Low Hb concentration may indicate anemia, recent hemorrhage, or fluid retention, causing hemodilution.

Elevated Hb suggests hemoconcentration from polycythemia or dehydration.

## INTERFERING FACTORS

- Hemoconcentration due to prolonged tourniquet constriction
- Extremely high white blood cell counts, lipemia, or RBCs that are resistant to lysis (false-high)

# Total urine estrogens

The total urine estrogens test is a quantitative analysis of total urine levels of estradiol, estrone, and estriol — the major estrogens present in significant amounts in urine. A common method for measuring total urine estrogen levels involves purification by gel filtration, followed by spectrophotofluorimetry. Supplementary tests that may provide further information about ovarian function include cytologic examination of vaginal smears, measurement of urine levels of pregnanediol and follicle-stimulating hormone, and evaluation of response to a progesterone injection. Supplementary tests that may provide further information about testicular function may include testicular examination and testosterone and androgen studies.

## PURPOSE

- To evaluate ovarian/testicular activity
- To help determine the cause of amenorrhea and female hyperestrogenism
- To aid in the diagnosis of tumors of ovarian, adrenocortical, or testicular origin
- To assess fetoplacental status

## PATIENT PREPARATION

- Explain to the female patient that the total urine estrogens test helps evaluate ovarian function; to the pregnant patient that this test helps evaluate fetal development and placental function; and to the male patient that this test helps evaluate testicular function.

- Inform the patient that the test requires collection of urine over a 24-hour period.
- Advise the patient that he need not restrict food and fluids.
- If the 24-hour specimen is to be collected at home, teach the patient the proper collection technique.
- Notify the laboratory and physician of medications the patient is taking that may affect test results; they may need to be restricted.

## PROCEDURE AND POSTTEST CARE

- Collect the patient's urine over a 24-hour period, discarding the first specimen and retaining the last. Use a bottle containing a preservative to keep the specimen at a pH of 3.0 to 5.0.
- If the patient is pregnant, note the approximate week of gestation on the laboratory request.
- If the patient isn't pregnant, note the stage of her menstrual cycle.
- Instruct the patient that she may resume her usual medications, as ordered.

## PRECAUTIONS

- Refrigerate the specimen or keep it on ice during the collection period.

## NORMAL FINDINGS

In nonpregnant females, total urine estrogen levels rise and fall during the menstrual cycle, peaking shortly before midcycle, decreasing immediately after ovulation, increasing through the life of the corpus luteum, and decreasing greatly as the corpus luteum degenerates and menstruation begins.

Total estrogen levels range as follows:
- Nonpregnant females — 4 to 60 mcg/24 hours.

Pregnant females:
- First trimester — 0 to 800 mcg/24 hours
- Second trimester — 800 to 5,000 mcg/24 hours
- Third trimester — 5,000 to 50,000 mcg/24 hours.

In postmenopausal females, values are less than 10 mcg/24 hours. In males, total estrogen levels range from 4 to 25 mcg/24 hours.

## ABNORMAL FINDINGS

Decreased total urine estrogen levels may reflect ovarian agenesis, primary ovarian insufficiency (due to Stein-Leventhal syndrome, for example), or secondary ovarian insufficiency (due to pituitary or adrenal hypofunction or metabolic disturbances).

Elevated total estrogen levels in the nonpregnant female may indicate tumors of ovarian or adrenocortical origin, adrenocortical hyperplasia, or a metabolic or hepatic disorder. In a male, elevated total estrogen levels are associated with testicular tumors.

Elevated total urine estrogen levels are normal during pregnancy; serial determinations should show a rising titer.

## INTERFERING FACTORS

- Ampicillin, cascara sagrada, hydrochlorothiazide, meprobamate, methenamine mandelate, phenazopyridine hydrochloride, phenolphthalein, phenothiazines, senna, steroid hormones, and tetracyclines (possible increase or decrease)

# *Transcranial Doppler studies*

Transcranial Doppler studies provide information about the presence, quality, and changing nature of circulation to an area of the brain by measuring the velocity of blood flow through cerebral arteries. Narrowed blood vessels produce high velocities, indicating possible stenosis or vasospasm. High velocities may also indicate an arteriovenous malformation.

## PURPOSE

- To measure the velocity of blood flow through certain cerebral vessels
- To detect and monitor the progression of cerebral vasospasm
- To determine whether collateral blood flow exists before surgical ligation or radiologic occlusion of diseased vessels

## PATIENT PREPARATION

- Explain the purpose of the transcranial Doppler study to the patient (or to his family).

# COMPARING VELOCITY WAVEFORMS

A normal transcranial Doppler signal is usually characterized by mean velocities that fall within the normal reported values. Additional information can be gathered by evaluating the shape of the velocity waveform.

## EFFECT OF SIGNIFICANT PROXIMAL VESSEL OBSTRUCTION

A delayed systolic upstroke can be seen in a waveform when significant proximal vessel obstruction is present.

**Normal**

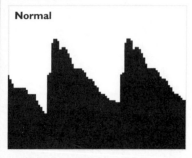

**Proximal vessel obstruction**

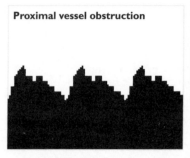

## EFFECT OF INCREASED CEREBROVASCULAR RESISTANCE

Changes in cerebrovascular resistance, as occur with increased intracranial pressure, cause a decrease in diastolic flow.

**Normal**

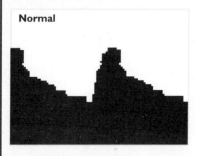

**Increased resistance**

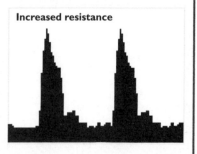

● Tell the patient that the test will be done while he lies on a bed or stretcher or sits in a reclining chair (or it can be performed at the bedside if he's too ill to be moved to the laboratory).

● Describe the procedure. Explain that a small amount of gel will be applied to his skin and that a probe will be used to transmit a signal to the artery being studied. Tell the patient that it usually takes less than 1 hour, depending on the number of vessels to be examined and any interfering factors.

● Tell the patient that he need not restrict food and fluids.

## PROCEDURE AND POSTTEST CARE

● Have the patient recline in a chair or on a stretcher or bed.

● A small amount of conductive gel is applied to the transcranial window (an area where bone is thin enough to allow the Doppler signal to enter and be detected); the most common approaches are temporal, transorbital, and through the foramen magnum.

● The technician directs the signal toward the artery being studied and records the velocities detected. In a complete study, the middle cerebral arteries, anterior cerebral arteries, posterior cerebral arteries, ophthalmic arteries, carotid siphon, vertebral arteries, and basilar artery are studied.

● The Doppler signal waveforms may be printed for later analysis and can be transmitted to varying depths (measured in millimeters).

● When the study is completed, wipe away the conductive gel.

## PRECAUTIONS

● Make sure to remove turban head dressings or thick dressings over the test site.

## NORMAL FINDINGS

The type of waveforms and velocities obtained indicate whether a disorder exists.

## ABNORMAL FINDINGS

Although this test commonly isn't definitive, high velocities are typically abnormal and suggest that blood flow is too turbulent or the vessel is too narrow. (See *Comparing velocity waveforms*.)

After the transcranial Doppler study and before surgery, the patient may undergo cerebral angiography to further define cerebral blood flow patterns and locate the exact vascular abnormality.

## INTERFERING FACTORS

● Failure to remove dressings over the test site (possible poor imaging)

## *Transesophageal echocardiography*

Transesophageal echocardiography combines ultrasound with endoscopy to give a better view of the heart's structures. In this procedure, a small transducer is attached to the end of a gastroscope and inserted into the esophagus, allowing images to be taken from the posterior aspect of the heart. This method causes less tissue penetration and interference from chest wall structures and produces high-quality images of the thoracic aorta, except for the superior ascending aorta, which is shadowed by the trachea.

This test is appropriate for inpatients and outpatients, for patients under general anesthesia, and for critically ill, intubated patients.

## PURPOSE

● To visualize and evaluate:
  – thoracic and aortic disorders, such as dissection and aneurysm
  – valvular disease, especially in the mitral valve and in prosthetic devices
  – endocarditis
  – congenital heart disease
  – intracardiac thrombi
  – cardiac tumors
  – valvular repairs

## PATIENT PREPARATION

● Explain to the patient that transesophageal echocardiography allows visual examination of heart function and structures.

● Tell the patient who will perform the test, when it's scheduled, and that he'll need to fast for 6 hours before the test.

● Review the patient's medical history for possible contraindications to the test, such as esophageal obstruction or varices, GI bleeding, previous mediastinal radiation therapy, or severe cervical arthritis.

● Ask the patient about any allergies and note them on the chart.

● Before the test, have the patient remove any dentures or oral prostheses and note any loose teeth.

● Explain to the patient that his throat will be sprayed with a topical anesthetic and that he may gag when the tube is inserted.

● Tell the patient that an I.V. line will be inserted to administer sedation before the procedure and that he may feel slight discomfort from the tourniquet and the needle puncture. Reassure him that he'll be made as comfortable as possible and that his blood pressure and heart rate will be monitored continuously.

● Make sure that the patient or a responsible family member has signed an informed consent form.

## PROCEDURE AND POSTTEST CARE

● Connect the patient to a cardiac monitor, the automated blood pressure cuff, and pulse oximetry probe so that all parameters can be assessed during the procedure.

● Help the patient lie down on his left side and administer the prescribed sedative.

● The back of the patient's throat is sprayed with a topical anesthetic.

● A bite block is placed in his mouth and he's instructed to close his lips around it.

A gastroscope is introduced and advanced 12″ to 14″ (30 to 35 cm) to the level of the right atrium. To visualize the left ventricle, the scope is advanced 16″ to 18″ (40 to 45 cm).

Ultrasound images are recorded and then reviewed after the procedure.

Monitor the patient's vital signs and oxygen levels for any changes.

Keep the patient in a supine position until the sedative wears off.

Encourage the patient to cough after the procedure while lying on his side or sitting upright.

**Alert** *Don't give the patient food or water until the gag response returns.*

If the procedure is done on an outpatient basis, make sure someone is available to drive the patient home.

Treat sore throat symptomatically.

## PRECAUTIONS

Keep resuscitation equipment readily available.

Have suction equipment nearby to avoid aspiration if vomiting occurs.

Be aware that vasovagal responses may occur with gagging, so observe the cardiac monitor closely.

Use pulse oximetry to detect hypoxia.

If bleeding occurs, stop the procedure immediately.

Know that laryngospasm, arrhythmias, or bleeding increase the risk of complications. If any of these occurs, postpone the test.

## NORMAL FINDINGS

Transesophageal echocardiography should reveal no cardiac problems.

## ABNORMAL FINDINGS

Transesophageal echocardiography can reveal thoracic and aortic disorders, endocarditis, congenital heart disease, intracardiac thrombi, or tumors and it can evaluate valvular disease or repairs. Findings may include aortic dissection or aneurysm, mitral valve disease, or congenital defects such as patent ductus arteriosus.

## INTERFERING FACTORS

Inability of the patient to cooperate

Using a transesophageal approach (restricts visualization of the left atrial appendage and ascending or descending aorta)

Hyperinflation of lungs due to such causes as chronic obstructive pulmonary disease or mechanical ventilation (possible poor imaging)

# *Transferrin*

A quantitative analysis of serum transferrin (siderophilin) levels is used to evaluate iron metabolism. Transferrin is a glycoprotein formed in the liver. It transports circulating iron obtained from dietary sources or the breakdown of red blood cells by reticuloendothelial cells to bone marrow for use in hemoglobin synthesis or to the liver, spleen, and bone marrow for storage. A serum iron level is usually obtained simultaneously.

## PURPOSE

To determine the iron-transporting capacity of the blood

To evaluate iron metabolism in iron deficiency anemia

## PATIENT PREPARATION

Explain to the patient that the transferrin test is used to determine the cause of anemia.

Tell the patient that the test requires a blood sample. Explain who will perform the venipuncture and when.

Explain to the patient that he may experience slight discomfort from the tourniquet and the needle puncture.

Inform the patient that he need not restrict food and fluids.

Notify the laboratory and physician of medications the patient is taking that may affect test results; they may need to be restricted.

## PROCEDURE AND POSTTEST CARE

Perform a venipuncture and collect the sample in a 4-ml clot-activator tube.

Apply direct pressure to the venipuncture site until bleeding stops.

If a hematoma develops at the venipuncture site, apply pressure.

Inform the patient that he may resume his usual medications discontinued before the test, as ordered.

## PRECAUTIONS
- Handle the sample gently to prevent hemolysis.
- Send the sample to the laboratory immediately.

## REFERENCE VALUES
Normal serum transferrin values range from 200 to 400 mg/dl (SI, 2 to 4 g/L).

## ABNORMAL FINDINGS
Inadequate transferrin levels may lead to impaired hemoglobin synthesis and, possibly, anemia. Low serum levels may indicate inadequate transferrin production due to hepatic damage or excessive protein loss from renal disease. Decreased transferrin levels may also result from acute or chronic infection and cancer. Increased serum transferrin levels may indicate severe iron deficiency.

## INTERFERING FACTORS
- Hormonal contraceptives and late pregnancy (possible increase)

## Triglycerides

Serum triglyceride analysis provides quantitative analysis of triglycerides — the main storage form of lipids — which constitute about 95% of fatty tissue. Although not in itself diagnostic, the triglyceride test permits early identification of hyperlipidemia and the risk of coronary artery disease (CAD).

## PURPOSE
- To screen for hyperlipidemia or pancreatitis
- To help identify nephrotic syndrome and the individual with poorly controlled diabetes mellitus
- To assess the risk of CAD
- To calculate the low-density lipoprotein cholesterol level using the Friedewald equation

## PATIENT PREPARATION
- Explain to the patient that the triglyceride test is used to detect fat metabolism disorders.

- Tell the patient that the test requires a blood sample. Explain who will perform the venipuncture and when.
- Explain to the patient that he may experience slight discomfort from the tourniquet and the needle puncture.
- Instruct the patient to fast for at least 12 hours before the test and to abstain from alcohol for 24 hours. Tell him that he may drink water.
- Notify the laboratory and physician of medications the patient is taking that may affect test results; they may need to be restricted.

## PROCEDURE AND POSTTEST CARE
- Perform a venipuncture and collect a sample in a 4-ml EDTA tube.
- Apply direct pressure to the venipuncture site until bleeding stops.
- If a hematoma develops at the venipuncture site, apply pressure.
- Instruct the patient that he may resume his usual diet and medications discontinued before the test, as ordered.

## PRECAUTIONS
- Send the sample to the laboratory immediately.
- Avoid prolonged venous occlusion; remove the tourniquet within 1 minute of application.

## REFERENCE VALUES
Triglyceride values vary with age and sex. There's some controversy about the most appropriate normal ranges, but values of 44 to 180 mg/dl (SI, 0.44 to 2.01 mmol/L) for adult men and 10 to 190 mg/dl (SI, 0.11 to 2.21 mmol/L) for adult women are widely accepted.

## ABNORMAL FINDINGS
Increased or decreased serum triglyceride levels suggest a clinical abnormality; additional tests are required for a definitive diagnosis.

A mild to moderate increase in serum triglyceride levels indicates biliary obstruction, diabetes mellitus, nephrotic syndrome, endocrinopathies, or overconsumption of alcohol. Markedly increased levels without an identifiable cause reflect congenital hyperlipoproteinemia and necessitate lipoprotein phenotyping to confirm the diagnosis.

Decreased serum triglyceride levels are rare and occur mainly in malnutrition and abetalipoproteinemia.

## INTERFERING FACTORS
- Use of a glycol-lubricated collection tube
- Antilipemics (decreased serum lipid levels)
- Cholestyramine and colestipol (decreased cholesterol levels, but increased or having no effect on triglyceride levels)
- Alcohol, corticosteroids (long-term use), estrogen, ethyl furosemide, hormonal contraceptives, and miconazole (increase)
- Clofibrate, dextrothyroxine, gemfibrozil, and niacin (decreased cholesterol and triglyceride levels)
- Probucol (decreased cholesterol levels, but variable effect on triglyceride levels)

# *Triiodothyronine uptake*

Triiodothyronine ($T_3$) uptake, also called the *$T_3$ uptake test,* indirectly measures free thyroxine ($FT_4$) levels by demonstrating the availability of serum protein-binding sites for thyroxine ($T_4$). The results of $T_3$ uptake are frequently combined with a $T_4$ radioimmunoassay or $T_4$ (D) (competitive protein-binding test) to determine the $FT_4$ index, a mathematical calculation thought to reflect $FT_4$ by correcting for thyroxine-binding globulin (TBG) abnormalities.

The $T_3$ uptake test has become less popular recently because rapid tests for $T_3$, $T_4$, and thyroid-stimulating hormone are readily available.

## PURPOSE
- To aid diagnosis of hypothyroidism and hyperthyroidism when TBG is normal
- To aid diagnosis of primary disorders of TBG levels

## PATIENT PREPARATION
- Explain to the patient that the $T_3$ uptake test helps evaluate thyroid function.
- Tell the patient that the test requires a blood sample. Explain who will perform the venipuncture and when.

- Explain to the patient that he may experience slight discomfort from the tourniquet and the needle puncture.
- Tell the patient that the laboratory requires several days to complete the analysis.
- Withhold medications that may interfere with test results, such as estrogens, androgens, phenytoin, salicylates, and thyroid preparations, as ordered. If they must be continued, note this on the laboratory request.

## PROCEDURE AND POSTTEST CARE
- Perform a venipuncture and collect the sample in a 7-ml clot-activator tube.
- Apply direct pressure to the venipuncture site until bleeding stops.
- If a hematoma develops at the venipuncture site, apply pressure.
- Instruct the patient that he may resume medications discontinued before the test, as ordered.

## PRECAUTIONS
- Handle the sample gently to prevent hemolysis.

## REFERENCE VALUES
Normal $T_3$ uptake values are 25% to 35%.

## ABNORMAL FINDINGS
A high $T_3$ uptake percentage in the presence of elevated $T_4$ levels indicates hyperthyroidism (implying few TBG free binding sites and high $FT_4$ levels). A low uptake percentage, together with low $T_4$ levels, indicates hypothyroidism (implying more TBG free binding sites and low $FT_4$ levels). Thus, in primary thyroid disease, $T_4$ and $T_3$ uptake vary in the same direction; availability of binding sites varies inversely.

Discordant variance in $T_4$ and $T_3$ uptake suggests a TBG abnormality. For example, a high $T_3$ uptake percentage and a low or normal $FT_4$ level suggest decreased TBG levels. Such decreased levels may result from protein loss (as in nephrotic syndrome), decreased production (due to androgen excess or genetic or idiopathic causes), or competition for $T_4$ binding sites by certain drugs (phenylbutazone, phenytoin, and salicylates). Conversely, a low $T_3$ uptake percentage and a high or normal $FT_4$ level suggest increased TBG levels. Such increased levels may be due to exogenous or endogenous estrogen (pregnancy) or result from idiopathic causes. Thus, in primary disorders of TBG levels, measured $T_4$ and free sites change in the same direction.

## INTERFERING FACTORS
● Radioisotope scans performed before sample collection
● Anabolic steroids, heparin, phenytoin, salicylates (high dose), thyroid preparations, and warfarin (possible increase in TBG and thyroxine-binding protein electrophoresis)
● Antithyroid agents, clofibrate, estrogen, hormonal contraceptives, and thiazide diuretics (decreased uptake)

# Troponin

Cardiac troponin I (cTnI) and cardiac troponin T (cTnT) are proteins in the striated cells that are extremely specific markers of cardiac damage. When injury occurs to the myocardial tissue, these proteins are released into the bloodstream. Elevations in troponin levels can be seen within 1 hour of myocardial infarction (MI) and will persist for a week or longer.

## PURPOSE
● To detect and diagnose acute MI and reinfarction
● To evaluate possible causes of chest pain

## PATIENT PREPARATION
● Explain to the patient that the troponin test helps assess myocardial injury and that multiple samples may be drawn to detect fluctuations in serum levels.
● Inform the patient he need not restrict foods and fluids.
● Tell the patient that the test requires a blood sample. Explain who will perform the venipuncture and when.
● Explain to the patient that he may feel slight discomfort from the tourniquet and the needle puncture.

## PROCEDURE AND POSTTEST CARE
● Perform a venipuncture and collect the specimen in a 7-ml clot-activator tube.
● If a hematoma develops at the venipuncture site, apply pressure.

## PRECAUTIONS
● Obtain each specimen on schedule and note the date and collection time on each.

## REFERENCE VALUES
Laboratory results may vary. Some laboratories may call a test positive if it shows any detectable levels, and others may give a range for abnormal results. Normally, cTnI levels are less than 0.35 mcg/L (SI, < 0.35 µg/L). cTnT levels are less than 0.1 mcg/L (SI, < 0.1 µ/L). cTnI levels greater than 2.0 mcg/L (SI, > 2.0 µ/L) suggest cardiac injury. Results of a qualitative cTnT rapid immunoassay that are greater than 0.1 mcg/L (SI, > 0.1 µ/L) are considered positive for cardiac injury. As long as tissue injury continues, the troponin levels will remain high.

## ABNORMAL FINDINGS
Troponin levels rise rapidly and are detectable within 1 hour of myocardial cell injury. cTnI levels aren't detectable in a person without cardiac injury.

## INTERFERING FACTORS
● Sustained vigorous exercise (increase in absence of significant cardiac damage)
● Cardiotoxic drugs such as doxorubicin (increase)
● Renal disease and certain surgical procedures (possible increase)

# Tuberculin skin tests

Tuberculin skin tests are used to screen for previous infection by the tubercle bacillus. They're routinely performed in children, young adults, and patients with radiographic findings that suggest this infection. In the old tuberculin (OT) and purified protein derivative (PPD) tests, intradermal injection of the tuberculin antigen causes a delayed hypersensitivity reaction in patients with active or dormant tuberculosis (TB).

The Mantoux test uses a single-needle intradermal injection of PPD, permitting precise measurement of the dose. Multipuncture tests, such as the tine test, MonoVacc tests, and Aplitest, use intradermal injections with tines impregnated with OT or PPD. Because they require less skill and are more rapidly administered, multipuncture tests are generally used for screening. A positive multipuncture test usually requires a Mantoux test for confirmation.

## PURPOSE
- To distinguish TB from blastomycosis, coccidioidomycosis, and histoplasmosis
- To identify people who need diagnostic investigation for TB because of possible exposure

## PATIENT PREPARATION
- Explain to the patient that the tuberculin skin test helps detect TB.
- Tell the patient that the test requires an intradermal injection, which may cause him discomfort.
- Check the patient's history for active TB, the results of previous skin tests, and hypersensitivities.
- If the patient has had TB, don't perform a skin test.
- If the patient has had a positive reaction to previous skin tests, consult the physician or follow your facility's policy.
- If the patient has had an allergic reaction to acacia, don't perform an OT test because this product contains acacia.
- If you're performing a tuberculin test on an outpatient, instruct him to return at the specified time so that test results can be read.
- Inform the patient that a positive reaction to a skin test appears as a red, hard, raised area at the injection site. Although the area may itch, instruct him not to scratch it.
- Stress that a positive reaction doesn't always indicate active TB.

## PROCEDURE AND POSTTEST CARE
- Ask the patient to sit and support his extended arm on a flat surface.
- Clean the volar surface of the upper forearm with alcohol and allow the area to dry completely.

### Mantoux test
- Perform an intradermal injection.

### Multipuncture test
- Remove the protective cap on the injection device to expose the four tines.
- Hold the patient's forearm in one hand, stretching the skin of the forearm tightly. Then, with your other hand, firmly depress

the device into the patient's skin without twisting it.
- Hold the device in place for at least 1 second before removing it.
- If you've applied sufficient pressure, you'll see four puncture sites and a circular depression made by the device on the patient's skin.

### Both tests
- Record where the test was given, the date and time, and when the results are to be read. Tuberculin skin tests are generally read 48 to 72 hours after injection; the MonoVacc test can be read 48 to 96 hours after the test.
- If ulceration or necrosis develops at the injection site, apply cold soaks or a topical steroid.

## PRECAUTIONS
- Know that tuberculin skin tests are contraindicated in the patient with current reactions to smallpox vaccinations, a rash, a skin disorder, or active TB.
- Don't perform a skin test in areas with excessive hair, acne, or insufficient subcutaneous tissue, such as over a tendon or bone.
- Know that if the patient is known to be hypersensitive to skin tests, you should use a first-strength dose in the Mantoux test to avoid necrosis at the puncture site.
- Have epinephrine available to treat a possible anaphylactic or acute hypersensitivity reaction.

## NORMAL FINDINGS
In tuberculin skin tests, normal findings show negative or minimal reactions. In the Mantoux test, no induration may appear or the patient may develop induration less than 5 mm in diameter.

In the tine and Aplitest tests, no vesiculation or induration may appear or the patient may develop induration less than 2 mm in diameter. In the MonoVacc tests, no induration appears.

## ABNORMAL FINDINGS
A positive tuberculin reaction indicates previous infection by tubercle bacilli. It doesn't distinguish between an active and a dormant infection or provide a definitive diagnosis. If a positive reaction occurs, sputum smear and culture and chest radiography are necessary for further information.

In the Mantoux test, induration 5 to 9 mm in diameter indicates a borderline reaction; larger induration, a positive reaction. Because patients infected with atypical mycobacteria other than tubercle bacilli may have borderline reactions, repeat testing is necessary.

In the tine or Aplitest tests, vesiculation indicates a positive reaction; induration 2 mm in diameter without vesiculation requires confirmation by the Mantoux test. Any induration in the MonoVacc test indicates a positive reaction; however, it requires confirmation by the Mantoux test.

## INTERFERING FACTORS

● Subcutaneous injection, usually indicated by erythema greater than 10 mm in diameter without induration
● Corticosteroids, other immunosuppressants, and live vaccine viruses, such as measles, mumps, rubella, and polio, within 4 to 6 weeks before the test (possible suppression of skin reaction)

*Age alert* *In elderly people and patients with viral infection, malnutrition, febrile illness, uremia, immunosuppressive disorders, or miliary TB (possible suppression of skin reaction) can interfere with test results.*

● Less than 10-week period since infection (possible suppression of skin reaction)
● Improper dilution, dosage, or storage of the tuberculin

# Tumor markers (CA 15-3 [27, 29]; CA 19-9; CA-125; and CA-50)

Tumor markers are substances produced and secreted by tumor cells to help determine tumor activity. They can be found in the serum of the cancer patient. Specific tests are ordered depending on the type of cancer the patient has. The CA 15-3 antigen (breast-cystic fluid protein or BCFP) may be used in conjunction with carcinoembryonic antigen and is helpful particularly in the breast cancer patient (CA 27, metastatic breast cancer, breast-cystic fluid protein 29, BCFP). CA 19-9 carbohydrate antigen may be ordered in the patient with pancreas, hepatobiliary, or lung cancer. The CA-125 glycoprotein antigen and serum carbohydrate antigen is commonly associated with types of ovarian cancers. The CA-50 may be ordered in the patient with GI or pancreatic cancer.

A combination of markers may be used due to low sensitivity and specificity of the markers. Few tumor markers meet U.S. Food and Drug Administration approval due to their controversy of their role in cancer diagnosis and treatment.

## PURPOSE

● To assist tumor staging and identify possible metastasis
● To monitor and detect disease recurrence
● To assess the patient's response to therapy

## PATIENT PREPARATION

● Explain the purpose of the particular tumor marker test ordered and that it may be helpful in the patient's disorder, as appropriate.
● Specific directions from the laboratory or cancer center should be followed for the particular test ordered. Fasting may be involved and factors may be identified that may interfere with test results. Note interfering factors on the appropriate laboratory requests.
● Tell the patient that the test requires a blood sample. Explain who will perform the venipuncture and when.
● Explain to the patient that he may experience slight discomfort from the tourniquet and the needle puncture.

## PROCEDURE AND POSTTEST CARE

● Obtain a 10-ml venous sample as ordered, in the tube specified by the laboratory or cancer center and transport the sample as directed.
● Apply direct pressure to the venipuncture site until bleeding stops.
● If a hematoma develops at the venipuncture site, apply pressure.

## PRECAUTIONS

● Consult the laboratory or cancer center as to specific patient preparation required (fasting, identifying interfering factors).
● Transport the specimen as directed.
● Handle the sample gently to prevent hemolysis.

## REFERENCE VALUES

Normal values for these tumor markers are:

- CA 15-3 (27, 29) — less than 30 U/ml
- CA 19-9 — less than 70 U/ml
- CA-125 — less than 34 U/ml
- CA-50 — less than 17 U/ml.

## ABNORMAL FINDINGS

CA 15-3 (27, 29) is greatly increased in metastatic breast cancer; it's also increased in pancreas, lung, colorectal, ovarian, and liver cancers. It decreases with therapy; an increase after therapy suggests progressive disease.

CA 19-9 is increased in pancreas, hepatobiliary, and lung cancers. It may be mildly increased in gastric and colorectal cancers.

CA-125 is increased in epithelial ovary, fallopian tube, endometrial, endocervix, pancreas, and liver cancers. It's less increased in colon, breast, lung, and GI cancers.

CA-50 is increased in GI and pancreatic cancers.

## INTERFERING FACTORS

- Benign breast or ovarian disease (increased CA 15-3 [27, 29])
- Cholecystitis, cirrhosis, cystic fibrosis, gallstones, and pancreatitis (minimal elevations in CA 19-9)
- Acute and chronic hepatitis, ascites, endometriosis, GI disease, Meig's syndrome, menstruation, pancreatitis, pelvic inflammatory disease, peritonitis, pleural effusion, pregnancy, and pulmonary disease (increased CA 125)

---

## 2-hour postprandial plasma glucose

---

Also called the *2-hour postprandial blood sugar test,* the 2-hour postprandial plasma glucose procedure is a valuable screening tool for detecting diabetes mellitus. The test is performed when the patient demonstrates symptoms of diabetes (polydipsia and polyuria) or when results of the fasting plasma glucose test suggest diabetes.

## PURPOSE

- To aid in the diagnosis of diabetes mellitus

- To monitor drug or diet therapy in the patient with diabetes mellitus

## PATIENT PREPARATION

- Explain to the patient that the 2-hour postprandial plasma glucose test is used to evaluate glucose metabolism and to detect diabetes.
- Tell the patient that the test requires a blood sample. Explain who will perform the venipuncture and when.
- Explain to the patient that he may experience slight discomfort from the tourniquet and the needle puncture.
- Tell the patient to eat a balanced meal or one containing 75 to 100 g of carbohydrates before the test and then fast for 2 hours. Instruct him to avoid smoking and strenuous exercise after the meal.
- Notify the laboratory and physician of medications the patient is taking that may affect test results; they may need to be restricted.

## PROCEDURE AND POSTTEST CARE

- Perform a venipuncture and collect the sample in a 5-ml clot-activator tube.
- Apply direct pressure to the venipuncture site until bleeding stops.
- If a hematoma develops at the venipuncture site, apply pressure.
- Instruct the patient that he may resume his usual diet, medications, and activity discontinued before the test, as ordered.

## PRECAUTIONS

- Send the sample to the laboratory immediately or refrigerate it.
- Specify on the laboratory request when the patient last ate, the sample collection time, and when the last pretest dose of insulin or oral antidiabetic drug was given.
- If the sample is to be drawn by a technician, tell the patient the exact time the venipuncture must be performed.

## REFERENCE VALUES

*Age alert* In the patient who doesn't have diabetes, postprandial glucose values are less than 140 mg/dl (SI, < 7.8 mmol/L) by the glucose oxidase or hexokinase method; levels are slightly elevated in people over age 50.

## ABNORMAL FINDINGS

Two-hour postprandial blood glucose values of 100 to 125 mg/dL (SI, 5.6 to 6.9 mmol/L) indicate impaired glucose tolerance. Values of 140 mg/dL (SI, 7.8 mmol/L) to 199 mg/dL (SI, 11.0 mmol/L) indicate diabetes mellitus. High levels may also occur with pancreatitis, Cushing's syndrome, acromegaly, and pheochromocytoma. Hyperglycemia may also be caused by hyperlipoproteinemia (especially type III, IV, or V), chronic hepatic disease, nephrotic syndrome, brain tumor, sepsis, gastrectomy with dumping syndrome, eclampsia, anoxia, and seizure disorders.

Low glucose levels occur in hyperinsulinism, insulinoma, von Gierke's disease, functional and reactive hypoglycemia, myxedema, adrenal insufficiency, congenital adrenal hyperplasia, hypopituitarism, malabsorption syndrome, and some cases of hepatic insufficiency.

## INTERFERING FACTORS

- Recent illness, infection, or pregnancy (possible increase)
- Acetaminophen, if using the glucose oxidase or hexokinase method (possible false-positive)
- Arginine, benzodiazepines, chlorthalidone, corticosteroids, dextrothyroxine, diazoxide, epinephrine, furosemide, hormonal contraceptives, recent I.V. glucose infusions, lithium, large doses of nicotinic acid, phenolphthalein, phenothiazines, phenytoin, thiazide diuretics, and triamterene (increase)
- Ethacrynic acid (possible increase); large doses in patients with uremia (possible decrease)
- Amphetamines, beta-adrenergic blockers, clofibrate, ethanol, insulin, monoamine oxidase inhibitors, and oral antidiabetic drugs (possible decrease)
- Strenuous exercise or stress (possible decrease)
- Glycolysis caused by failure to refrigerate the sample or to send it to the laboratory immediately (possible decrease)

# Ultrasonography of the abdominal aorta

In ultrasonography of the abdominal aorta, a transducer directs high-frequency sound waves into the abdomen over a wide area from the xiphoid process to the umbilical region. The echoing sound waves are displayed on a monitor to indicate internal organs, the vertebral column, and the size and course of the abdominal aorta and other major vessels.

## PURPOSE
- To detect and measure a suspected abdominal aortic aneurysm (findings may be supported and refined by angiography or computed tomography angiography)
- To detect and measure the expansion of a known abdominal aortic aneurysm

## PATIENT PREPARATION
- Explain to the patient that ultrasonography allows examination of the abdominal aorta.
- Instruct the patient to fast for 12 hours before the test to minimize bowel gas and motility.
- Tell the patient who will perform the test, where it will take place, that the lights may be lowered, and that he'll feel only slight pressure.
- Describe the procedure. Tell the patient that mineral oil or a gel, which may feel cool, will be applied to his abdomen.
- Explain that a transducer will pass over his skin, from the costal margins to the um-

bilicus or slightly below, directing safe, painless, and inaudible sound waves into the abdominal vessels and organs.
- Reassure the patient with a known aneurysm that the sound waves won't cause rupture.
- Instruct the patient to remain still during scanning and to hold his breath when requested.
- If ordered, give simethicone to reduce bowel gas.

## PROCEDURE AND POSTTEST CARE
- The patient is placed in a supine position, and conductive gel or mineral oil is applied to his abdomen.
- Longitudinal scans are made at ⅛" to ¾" (0.5- to 2-cm) intervals left and right of the midline until the entire abdominal aorta is outlined; transverse scans are made at ⅜" to ¾" (1- to 2-cm) intervals from the xiphoid to the bifurcation at the common iliac arteries.
- The patient may be placed in the right and left lateral positions.
- Appropriate views are photographed or videotaped.
- Remove the conductive gel from the patient's skin.
- Instruct the patient that he may resume his usual diet and medications, as ordered.

   *Alert* *Aneurysms may expand and dissect rapidly, so check the patient's vital signs frequently. Remember that the sudden onset of constant abdominal or back pain accompanies rapid expansion of the aneurysm; sudden, excruciating pain with weakness, sweating, tachycardia, and hypotension signals rupture.*

## PRECAUTIONS
● None

## NORMAL FINDINGS
In adults, the normal abdominal aorta tapers from about 1" to ⅝" (2.5 to 1.5 cm) in diameter along its length from the diaphragm to the bifurcation. It descends through the retroperitoneal space, anterior to the vertebral column and slightly left of the midline. Four of its major branches are usually well visualized: the celiac trunk, the renal arteries, the superior mesenteric artery, and the common iliac arteries.

## ABNORMAL FINDINGS
The luminal diameter of the abdominal aorta greater than 1⅛" (3.8 cm) suggests aneurysm; greater than 2¾" (7 cm), aneurysm with high risk of rupture.

## INTERFERING FACTORS
● Bowel gas and motility, excessive body movement, severe dyspnea, and surgical wounds
● Residual barium from GI contrast studies within the past 24 hours
● Air introduced during endoscopy within the past 12 to 24 hours
● Mesenteric fat in the obese patient

## *Ultrasonography of the gallbladder and biliary system*

In ultrasonography of the gallbladder and biliary system, a focused beam of high-frequency sound waves passes into the right upper quadrant of the abdomen, creating echoes that vary with changes in tissue density. These echoes are converted to images on a screen, indicating the size, shape, and position of the gallbladder and biliary system.

## PURPOSE
● To confirm a diagnosis of cholelithiasis
● To diagnose acute cholecystitis
● To distinguish between obstructive and nonobstructive jaundice

## PATIENT PREPARATION
● Explain to the patient that ultrasonography allows examination of the gallbladder and biliary system.
● Instruct the patient to eat a fat-free meal in the evening and then to fast for 8 to 12 hours before the procedure, if possible; this promotes accumulation of bile in the gallbladder and enhances ultrasonic visualization.
● Tell the patient who will perform the procedure and when and where it will take place.
● Tell the patient that the room may be darkened slightly to aid visualization on the screen.
● Describe the procedure. Tell the patient that a transducer will pass smoothly over his abdomen in direct contact with his skin, but assure him that he'll feel only mild pressure.
● Instruct the patient to remain as still as possible during the procedure and to hold his breath when requested to ensure that the gallbladder is in the same position for each scan.

## PROCEDURE AND POSTTEST CARE
● The patient is placed in a supine position.
● A water-soluble conductive gel is applied to the face of the transducer.
● Transverse and longitudinal oblique scans of the gallbladder are taken at ⅜" (1-cm) intervals, starting at the level of the xiphoid and moving laterally to the right subcostal area. Longitudinal oblique scans are taken at 5-mm intervals parallel to the long axis of the gallbladder marked on the patient's skin, beginning medial to the gallbladder and continuing through to its lateral border.
● During each scan, the patient is asked to inhale deeply and to hold his breath. (If the gallbladder is positioned deeply under the right costal margin, a scan may be taken through the intercostal spaces while the patient holds his breath.)
● The patient is then placed in a left lateral decubitus position and is scanned beneath the right costal margin. (This position and scanning angle may displace and allow detection of stones lodged in the gallbladder neck and cystic duct region.)
● Scanning with the patient erect helps demonstrate mobility or fixity of suspicious

echogenic areas. Views may be photographed for later study.

- Remove the conductive gel from the patient's skin.
- Inform the patient that he may resume his usual diet.

## PRECAUTIONS

- Keep the patient in a fasting state to prevent the excretion of bile in the gallbladder. Even smelling greasy foods, such as popcorn, can cause the gallbladder to empty.

## NORMAL FINDINGS

The normal gallbladder is sonolucent; it appears circular on transverse scans and pear-shaped on longitudinal scans. Although the size of the gallbladder varies, its outer walls normally appear sharp and smooth. Intrahepatic radicles seldom appear because the flow of sonolucent bile is extremely fine. The cystic duct may also be indistinct — the result of folds known as *Heister's valves* that line the cystic duct lumen. When visualized, the cystic duct has a serpentine appearance. The common bile duct, in contrast, has a linear appearance, but is sometimes obscured by overlying bowel gas.

## ABNORMAL FINDINGS

Gallstones within the gallbladder lumen or the biliary system typically appear as mobile, echogenic areas, usually associated with an acoustic shadow. The size of gallstones generally parallels the size of their shadows; gallstones 5 mm or larger usually produce shadows. However, if the gallbladder is distended with bile, gallstones as small as 1 mm can be detected because of the acoustic contrast between liquid bile and solid gallstones. Detecting stones in the biliary ducts, which contain little bile, may be difficult. When the gallbladder is shrunken or fully impacted with gallstones, inadequate bile may likewise make gallstone detection difficult, and the gallbladder itself might not be detectable. In this case, an acoustic shadow in the gallbladder fossa indicates cholelithiasis; the presence of such a shadow in the cystic and common bile ducts can also indicate cholelithiasis.

Polyps and carcinoma within the gallbladder lumen are distinguished from gallstones by their fixity. Polyps usually appear as sharply defined, echogenic areas; carcinoma appears as a poorly defined mass, commonly associated with a thickened gallbladder wall.

Biliary sludge within the gallbladder lumen appears as a fine layer of echoes that slowly gravitates to the dependent portion of the gallbladder as the patient changes position. Although biliary sludge may arise without accompanying disease, it may also result from obstruction and can predispose the patient to gallstone formation.

Acute cholecystitis is indicated by an enlarged gallbladder with thickened, double-rimmed walls, usually with gallstones within the lumen. There may also be precholecystic fluid. In chronic cholecystitis, the walls of the gallbladder appear thickened; the organ itself, however, is generally contracted. In obstructive jaundice, ultrasonography readily demonstrates a dilated biliary system and, usually, a dilated gallbladder. Dilated intrahepatic radicles appear tortuous and irregular; a dilated gallbladder usually loses its characteristic pear shape, becoming spherical.

Biliary obstruction may result from intrinsic factors, such as a gallstone or small carcinoma within the biliary system. (Ultrasonography can't distinguish between these two echogenic masses.) Alternatively, it may result from extrinsic factors, such as a mass in the hepatic portal vein that compresses the cystic duct and interferes with bile drainage from the intrahepatic radicles, or from disease in the head of the pancreas that obstructs the common bile duct. Such disease includes carcinoma and pancreatitis, although ultrasonography can't distinguish between the two.

When ultrasonography fails to clearly define the site of biliary obstruction, percutaneous transhepatic cholangiography or endoscopic retrograde cholangiopancreatography should be performed.

## INTERFERING FACTORS

- Failure to observe pretest dietary restrictions
- Overlying bowel gas or retained barium from a previous test (possible poor imaging)
- Deficiency of body fluids in a dehydrated patient, obscuring boundaries between organs and tissue structures (possible poor imaging)

# Ultrasonography of the liver

Ultrasonography of the liver produces images by channeling high-frequency sound waves into the right upper quadrant of the abdomen. Resultant echoes are converted to cross-sectional images on a monitor; different shades of gray depict various tissue densities. Ultrasonography can show intrahepatic structures and organ size, shape, and position.

This procedure is indicated in patients with jaundice with no known cause, unexplained hepatomegaly and abnormal biochemical test results, suspected metastatic tumors and elevated serum alkaline phosphatase levels, and recent abdominal trauma.

When used with liver-spleen scanning, ultrasonography can define cold spots (focal defects that fail to pick up the radionuclide) as tumors, abscesses, or cysts; it also provides better views of the periportal and perihepatic spaces than liver-spleen scanning. If ultrasonography fails to provide definitive diagnosis, computed tomography (CT), gallium scanning, or liver biopsy may yield more information.

## PURPOSE
- To distinguish between obstructive and nonobstructive jaundice
- To screen for hepatocellular disease
- To detect hepatic metastases and hematomas
- To define cold spots as tumors, abscesses, or cysts

## PATIENT PREPARATION
- Explain to the patient that ultrasonography allows examination of the liver. Tell him who will perform the test and where it will take place.
- Instruct the patient to fast for 8 to 12 hours before the test to reduce bowel gas, which hinders ultrasound transmission.
- Describe the procedure. Tell the patient a transducer will pass smoothly over his abdomen, channeling sound waves into the liver, but assure him that he'll feel only mild pressure.

- Instruct the patient to remain as still as possible during the procedure and to hold his breath when requested.

## PROCEDURE AND POSTTEST CARE
- The patient is placed in a supine position.
- A water-soluble conductive gel is applied to the face of the transducer.
- Transverse scans are taken at $3/8''$ (1-cm) intervals, using a single-sweep technique between the costal margins. Although this technique demonstrates the left lobe of the liver and part of the right lobe, sector scans through the intercostal spaces are used to view the remainder of the right lobe.
- Scans are taken longitudinally from the right border of the liver to the left.
- For better demonstration of the right lateral dome, oblique cephalad-angled scans may be taken beneath the right costal margin.
- Scans are then taken parallel to the hepatic portal, at a 45-degree angle toward the superior right lateral dome, to examine the peripheral anatomy, portal venous system, common bile duct, and biliary tree. Clear images are photographed for later study.
- During each scan, ask the patient to hold his breath briefly in deep inspiration to displace the liver caudally from the costal margin and the ribs to aid visualization.
- Remove the conductive gel from the patient's skin.
- Inform the patient that he may resume his usual diet.

## PRECAUTIONS
- None

## NORMAL FINDINGS
The liver normally demonstrates a homogeneous, low-level echo pattern, interrupted only by the different echo patterns of its portal and hepatic veins, the aorta, and the inferior vena cava. Hepatic veins appear completely sonolucent; portal veins have margins that are highly echogenic.

## ABNORMAL FINDINGS
In obstructive jaundice, ultrasonography shows dilated intrahepatic biliary radicles and extrahepatic ducts. Conversely, in nonobstructive jaundice, ultrasonography shows a biliary tree of normal diameter.

Ultrasonographic characteristics of hepatocellular disease are generally nonspecific, and disorders in early stages can escape detection; liver-spleen scanning is a more sensitive diagnostic tool. In cirrhosis, ultrasonography may demonstrate variable liver size; dilated, tortuous portal branches associated with portal hypertension; and an irregular echo pattern with increased echo amplitude, causing overall increased attenuation. Demonstration of splenomegaly by spleen ultrasonography or liver-spleen scanning aids diagnosis. In fatty infiltration of the liver, ultrasonography may show hepatomegaly and a regular echo pattern that, although greater in echo amplitude than that of a normal parenchyma, doesn't alter attenuation.

Ultrasonographic characteristics of metastases in the liver vary widely; metastases may appear either hypoechoic or echogenic, poorly defined or well defined. For example, metastatic lymphomas and sarcomas are generally hypoechoic; mucin-secreting adenocarcinoma of the colon is highly echogenic. Liver biopsy is necessary to confirm the tumor type. Serial ultrasonography may be used to monitor the effectiveness of therapy.

Primary hepatic tumors also present a varied appearance and may mimic metastases, requiring angiography and liver biopsy for definitive diagnosis. Hepatomas are the most common malignant tumors in adults; hepatoblastomas are most common in children. Benign tumors are far less common than malignant ones.

Abscesses usually appear as sonolucent masses with ill-defined, slightly thickened borders and accentuated posterior wall transmission; scattered internal echoes, caused by necrotic debris, may also be present. Because they produce similar echo patterns, intrahepatic abscesses are occasionally mistaken for hematomas, necrotic metastases, or hemorrhagic cysts. Gas-containing intrahepatic abscesses, which may be echogenic, are sometimes confused with solid intrahepatic lesions. Subphrenic abscesses occur between the diaphragm and the liver; subhepatic abscesses appear inferior to the liver and anterior to the upper pole of the right kidney. Ascitic fluid resembles a subhepatic abscess, but lacks internal echoes and has a more regular border.

Cysts usually appear as spherical, sonolucent areas with well-defined borders and accentuated posterior wall transmission. When a cyst can't be distinguished from an abscess or necrotic metastases, gallium scanning, CT, and angiography should be performed.

Hematomas — either intrahepatic or subcapsular — usually result from trauma. Intrahepatic hematomas appear as poorly defined, relatively sonolucent masses and may have scattered internal echoes due to clotting; serial ultrasonography can differentiate between a hematoma and a cyst or tumor as the hematoma becomes smaller. Subcapsular hematoma may appear as a focal, sonolucent mass on the periphery of the liver or as a diffuse, sonolucent area surrounding part of the liver.

## INTERFERING FACTORS

● Overlying ribs and gas or residual barium in the stomach or colon (possible misleading results)
● Deficiency of body fluids in a dehydrated patient, obscuring boundaries between organs and tissue structures (possible misleading results)

# Ultrasonography of the pancreas

In ultrasonography of the pancreas, cross-sectional images are produced by channeling high-frequency sound waves into the epigastric region and converting the resultant echoes to real-time images, which are displayed on a monitor. The pattern varies with tissue density and indicates the size, shape, and position of the pancreas and surrounding viscera.

## PURPOSE

● To aid in the diagnosis of pancreatitis, pseudocysts, and pancreatic carcinoma

## PATIENT PREPARATION

● Explain to the patient that ultrasonography permits examination of the pancreas.
● Instruct the patient to fast for 8 to 12 hours before the procedure to reduce bowel gas.
● Tell the patient who will perform the procedure, when and where it will take place, and that the room may be darkened slightly to aid visualization on the monitor.

# COMPARING NORMAL AND ABNORMAL IMAGES OF THE PANCREAS

The ultrasound view on the left shows a normal pancreas (outlined in color). The ultrasound view on the right shows a diffusely enlarged pancreas due to pancreatitis. The color outline indicates the extent of enlargement.

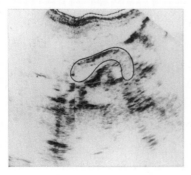 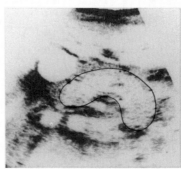

● If the patient is a smoker, ask him to abstain before the test to eliminate the risk of swallowing air while inhaling, which interferes with test results.
● Describe the procedure. Tell the patient a transducer will pass smoothly over his epigastric region, channeling sound waves into the pancreas, but assure him that he'll only feel mild pressure.
● Tell the patient he'll be asked to inhale deeply during scanning, and instruct him to remain still during the procedure.

## PROCEDURE AND POSTTEST CARE
● The patient is placed in a supine position.
● A water-soluble conductive gel or mineral oil is applied to the abdomen and, with the patient at full inspiration, transverse scans are taken at ³⁄₈″ (1-cm) intervals, starting from the xiphoid and moving caudally; longitudinal scans are taken to view the head, body, and tail of the pancreas in sequence; scanning the right anterior oblique view allows imaging of the head and body of the pancreas; oblique sagittal scans are used to view the portal vein; and scanning from the sagittal view images the vena cava.

● When good ultrasonography views are obtained, they're photographed for later study.
● Remove the conductive gel from the patient's skin.
● Inform the patient that he may resume his usual diet.

## PRECAUTIONS
● None

## NORMAL FINDINGS
The pancreas normally demonstrates a coarse, uniform echo pattern and usually appears more echogenic than does the adjacent liver. (See *Comparing normal and abnormal images of the pancreas.*)

## ABNORMAL FINDINGS
Alterations in the size, contour, and parenchymal texture of the pancreas characterize pancreatic disease. An enlarged pancreas with decreased echogenicity and distinct borders suggests pancreatitis. A well-defined mass with an essentially echo-free interior indicates pseudocyst; an ill-defined mass with scattered internal echoes or a mass in the head of the pancreas (obstructing the common bile duct) and a large noncontracting gallbladder suggest pancreatic carcinoma.

Subsequent computed tomography scan and biopsy of the pancreas may be necessary to confirm a diagnosis.

## INTERFERING FACTORS

- Gas or residual barium in the stomach and intestine (possible poor imaging)
- Deficiency of body fluids in a dehydrated patient, obscuring boundaries between organs and tissue structures (possible poor imaging)
- Obesity (possible poor imaging)
- Fatty infiltration of the pancreas (possible poor imaging)

# Ultrasonography of the spleen

In ultrasonography of the spleen, a focused beam of high-frequency sound waves passes into the left upper quadrant of the abdomen, creating echoes that vary with changes in tissue density. These echoes are displayed on a monitor as real-time images that indicate the size, shape, and position of the spleen and surrounding viscera.

Ultrasonography is indicated in patients with an upper left quadrant mass of unknown origin; with known splenomegaly, to evaluate changes in splenic size; with left-upper-quadrant pain and local tenderness; and with recent abdominal trauma.

## PURPOSE

- To demonstrate splenomegaly
- To monitor the progression of primary and secondary splenic disease and to evaluate the effectiveness of therapy
- To evaluate the spleen after abdominal trauma
- To help detect splenic cysts and subphrenic abscesses

## PATIENT PREPARATION

- Explain to the patient that ultrasonography allows examination of the spleen.
- Tell the patient who will perform the test, when and where it will take place, and that the room may be darkened slightly to aid visualization on the monitor.
- Instruct the patient to fast for 8 to 12 hours before the procedure, if possible; do-

ing so reduces the amount of gas in the bowel, improving sound wave transmission.
- Describe the procedure. Tell the patient that a transducer will pass smoothly over his abdomen in direct contact with his skin, but assure him that he'll feel only mild pressure.
- Instruct the patient to remain as still as possible during the procedure and to hold his breath when requested to aid visualization.

## PROCEDURE AND POSTTEST CARE

- Because the procedure for ultrasonography varies depending on the size of the spleen and the patient's physique, the patient is usually repositioned several times; the transducer scanning angle or path is also changed.
- Generally, the patient is first placed in a supine position, with his chest uncovered.
- A water-soluble conductive gel is applied to the face of the transducer, and transverse scans of the spleen are taken at $3/8"$ to $3/4"$ (1- to 2-cm) intervals, beginning at the level of the diaphragm and moving posteriorly, while the transducer is angled anteromedially.
- The patient is then placed in a right lateral decubitus position, and transverse scans are taken through the intercostal spaces using a sectoring motion.
- A pillow may be placed under the patient's right side to help separate the intercostal spaces, making it easier to position the transducer face between them.
- Longitudinal scans are taken from the axilla toward the iliac crest.
- To prevent rib artifacts and to obtain the best view of the splenic parenchyma, oblique scans are taken by passing the transducer face along the intercostal spaces.
- During each scan, the patient may be asked to hold his breath briefly at various stages of inspiration.
- Good views are photographed for later study.
- Remove the conductive gel from the patient's skin.
- Inform the patient that he may resume his usual diet.

## PRECAUTIONS

- None

## NORMAL FINDINGS

The splenic parenchyma normally demonstrates a homogeneous, low-level echo pattern; its individual vascular channels aren't usually apparent. The superior and lateral splenic borders are clearly defined, each having a convex margin. The undersurface and medial borders, in contrast, show indentations from surrounding organs (stomach, left kidney, and pancreas). The hilar region, where the vascular pedicle enters the spleen, commonly produces an area of highly reflective echoes. The medial surface is generally concave, which helps differentiate between left-upper-quadrant masses and an enlarged spleen. Even when splenomegaly is present, the spleen generally remains concave medially unless a space-occupying lesion distorts this contour.

## ABNORMAL FINDINGS

Ultrasonography can show splenomegaly, but it usually doesn't indicate the cause; a computed tomography (CT) scan can provide more specific information. Splenomegaly is generally accompanied by increased echogenicity. Enlarged vascular channels are commonly visible, especially in the hilar region. If space-occupying lesions distort the splenic contour, liver-spleen scanning should be performed to confirm splenomegaly.

Abdominal trauma may result in splenic rupture or subcapsular hematoma. In splenic rupture, ultrasonography demonstrates splenomegaly and an irregular, sonolucent area (the presence of free intraperitoneal fluid); however, these findings must be confirmed by arteriography. In subcapsular hematoma, ultrasonography shows splenomegaly as well as a double contour, altered splenic position, and a relatively sonolucent area on the spleen's periphery. The double contour results from blood accumulation between the splenic parenchyma and the intact splenic capsule. As the spleen enlarges, a transverse section shows its anterior margin extending more anteriorly than the aorta. Ultrasonography may be difficult and painful after abdominal trauma because the transducer may have to pass across fractured ribs and contusions; CT scanning, which differentiates blood and fluid in the peritoneal space, should be used instead.

In subphrenic abscess, ultrasonography shows a sonolucent area beneath the diaphragm. Clinical findings may differentiate between abscess and blood or fluid accumulation.

Used with liver-spleen scanning, ultrasonography differentiates cold spots as cystic or solid lesions. It shows cysts as spherical, sonolucent areas with well defined, regular margins with acoustic enhancement behind them. When ultrasonography fails to identify a cyst as splenic or extrasplenic — especially if the cyst is located in the upper pole of the left kidney and the adrenal gland or in the tail of the pancreas — a CT scan and arteriography are used. Ultrasonography can readily clarify cystic cold spots, but using a CT scan with a contrast medium is superior for evaluating primary and metastatic tumors. Ultrasonography usually fails to identify tumors associated with lymphoma and chronic leukemias because these resemble tumors of the splenic parenchyma.

## INTERFERING FACTORS

● Overlying ribs, an aerated left lung, or gas or residual barium in the colon or stomach (possible poor imaging)
● Deficiency of body fluids in a dehydrated patient, obscuring boundaries between organs and tissue structures (possible poor imaging)
● Body physique affecting the spleen's shape or adjacent masses displacing the spleen (possible poor imaging, may be mistaken for splenomegaly)
● Splenic trauma (possible difficulty in tolerating the procedure)

# Upper GI and small-bowel series

The upper GI and small-bowel series is the fluoroscopic examination of the esophagus, stomach, and small intestine after ingestion of barium sulfate, a contrast agent. As the barium passes through the digestive tract, fluoroscopy outlines peristalsis and the mucosal contours of the respective organs, and spot films record significant findings. This test is indicated in patients who have upper GI symptoms (difficulty swallowing, regurgitation, burning or gnawing epigastric pain), signs of small-bowel disease (diarrhea, weight loss), and signs of GI bleeding (hematemesis, melena).

Although this test can detect various mucosal abnormalities, subsequent biopsy is typically necessary to rule out malignancy or distinguish specific inflammatory diseases. Oral cholecystography, barium enema, and routine X-rays should always precede this test because retained barium clouds anatomic detail on X-ray films.

## PURPOSE

- To detect hiatal hernia, diverticula, and varices
- To aid in the diagnosis of strictures, blockages, ulcers, tumors, regional enteritis, and malabsorption syndrome
- To help detect motility disorders

## PATIENT PREPARATION

- Explain to the patient that the upper GI and small-bowel series uses ingested barium and X-ray films to examine the esophagus, stomach, and small intestine.
- Tell the patient to consume a low-residue diet for 2 to 3 days before the test and then to fast and avoid smoking after midnight the night before the test.
- Describe the test, including who will perform it and when and where it will take place.
- Encourage the patient to bring reading material.
- Inform the patient that he'll be placed on an X-ray table that rotates into vertical, semivertical, and horizontal positions.
- Explain to the patient that he'll be adequately secured and assisted to the supine, prone, and side-lying positions.
- Describe the milkshake consistency and chalky taste of the barium mixture. Although it's flavored, the patient may find its taste unpleasant, but tell him he must drink 16 to 20 oz (475 to 590 ml) for a complete examination.
- Inform the patient that his abdomen may be compressed to ensure proper coating of the stomach or intestinal walls with barium or to separate overlapping bowel loops.
- As ordered, withhold most oral medications after midnight and anticholinergics and opioids for 24 hours because these drugs affect small intestinal motility. Antacids, histamine-2 receptor antagonists, and proton pump inhibitors are also sometimes withheld for several hours if gastric reflux is suspected.

- Just before the procedure, instruct the patient to put on a gown without snap closures and to remove jewelry, dentures, hair clips, or other objects that might obscure anatomic detail on the X-ray films.

## PROCEDURE AND POSTTEST CARE

- After the patient is secured in a supine position on the X-ray table, the table is tilted until the patient is erect, and the heart, lungs, and abdomen are examined fluoroscopically.
- The patient is instructed to take several swallows of the barium suspension, and its passage through the esophagus is observed. (Occasionally, the patient is given a thick barium suspension, especially when esophageal disease is strongly suspected.)
- During fluoroscopic examination, spot films of the esophagus are taken from lateral angles and from right and left posteroanterior angles.
- When barium enters the stomach, the patient's abdomen is palpated or compressed to ensure adequate coating of the gastric mucosa.
- To perform a double-contrast examination, the patient is instructed to sip the barium through a perforated straw. As he does so, a small amount of air is also introduced into the stomach, permitting detailed examination of the gastric rugae, and spot films of significant findings are taken. The patient is then instructed to ingest the remaining barium suspension and the filling of the stomach and emptying into the duodenum are observed fluoroscopically.
- Two series of spot films of the stomach and duodenum are taken from posteroanterior, anteroposterior, lateral, and oblique angles, with the patient erect and then in a supine position.
- The passage of barium into the remainder of the small intestine is then observed fluoroscopically, and spot films are taken at 30- to 60-minute intervals until the barium reaches the region of the ileocecal valve. If abnormalities in the small intestine are detected, the area is palpated and compressed to help clarify the defect, and a spot film is taken. The examination ends when the barium enters the cecum.
- Make sure additional X-rays haven't been ordered before allowing the patient food, fluids, and oral medications (if applicable).

- Tell the patient to drink plenty of fluid (unless contraindicated) to help eliminate the barium.
- Administer a cathartic or enema to the patient. Tell the patient that his stool will be light colored for 24 to 72 hours. Record and describe any stool passed by the patient in the health care facility. Barium retention in the intestine may cause obstruction or fecal impaction, so notify the physician if the patient doesn't pass the barium within 2 to 3 days. Also, barium retention may affect scheduling of other GI tests.
- Instruct the patient to tell the physician of abdominal fullness or pain or a delay in return to brown stools.

## PRECAUTIONS

- Be aware that the upper GI and small-bowel series may be contraindicated in the patient with obstruction or perforation of the digestive tract. Barium may intensify the obstruction or seep into the abdominal cavity. Sometimes a small-bowel series is performed to find a "transition zone." If a perforation is suspected, Gastrografin (a water-soluble contrast medium) rather than barium may be used.
- Know that the test is contraindicated in the pregnant patient because of radiation's possible teratogenic effects.

## NORMAL FINDINGS

After the barium suspension is swallowed, it pours over the base of the tongue into the pharynx and is propelled by a peristaltic wave through the entire length of the esophagus in about 2 seconds. The bolus evenly fills and distends the lumen of the pharynx and esophagus, and the mucosa appears smooth and regular. When the peristaltic wave reaches the base of the esophagus, the cardiac sphincter opens, allowing the bolus to enter the stomach. After passage of the bolus, the cardiac sphincter closes.

As barium enters the stomach, it outlines the characteristic longitudinal folds called *rugae,* which are best observed using the double-contrast technique. When the stomach is completely filled with barium, its outer contour appears smooth and regular without evidence of flattened, rigid areas suggestive of intrinsic or extrinsic lesions.

After barium enters the stomach, it quickly empties into the duodenal bulb through relaxation of the pyloric sphincter. Although the mucosa of the duodenal bulb is relatively smooth, circular folds become apparent as barium enters the duodenal loop. These folds deepen and become more numerous in the jejunum. The barium temporarily lodges between these folds, producing a speckled pattern on the X-ray film. As barium enters the ileum, the circular folds become less prominent and, except for their broadness, resemble those in the duodenum. The film also shows that the diameter of the small intestine tapers gradually from the duodenum to the ileum.

## ABNORMAL FINDINGS

X-ray studies of the esophagus may reveal strictures, tumors, hiatal hernia, diverticula, varices, and ulcers (particularly in the distal esophagus). Benign strictures usually dilate the esophagus, whereas malignant ones cause erosive changes in the mucosa. Tumors produce filling defects in the column of barium, but only malignant ones change the mucosal contour. Nevertheless, biopsy is necessary for definitive diagnosis of esophageal strictures and tumors.

Motility disorders, such as esophageal spasm, are usually difficult to detect because spasms are erratic and transient; manometry, which measures the length and pressure of peristaltic contractions and evaluates cardiac sphincter function, is generally performed to detect such disorders. However, achalasia (cardiospasm) is strongly suggested when the distal esophagus has a beaklike appearance. Gastric reflux appears as a backflow of barium from the stomach into the esophagus.

X-ray studies of the stomach may reveal tumors and ulcers. Malignant tumors, usually adenocarcinomas, appear as filling defects on the X-ray film and usually disrupt peristalsis. Benign tumors, such as adenomatous polyps and leiomyomas, appear as outpouchings of the gastric mucosa and generally don't affect peristalsis. Ulcers occur most commonly in the stomach and duodenum (particularly in the duodenal bulb), and these two areas are thus examined together. Benign ulcers usually demonstrate evidence of partial or complete healing and are characterized by radiating folds extending to the edge of the ulcer crater. Malignant ulcers, usually associated with a suspicious mass, generally have radiating folds that extend beyond the ulcer crater to the edge of the mass. However, biopsy is necessary for definitive diagnosis of tumors and ulcers.

Occasionally, this test detects signs that suggest pancreatitis or pancreatic carcinoma. Such signs include edematous changes in the mucosa of the antrum or duodenal loop or dilation of the duodenal loop. These findings mandate further studies for pancreatic disease, such as endoscopic retrograde cholangiopancreatography, abdominal ultrasonography, or computed tomography scanning.

X-ray studies of the small intestine may reveal regional enteritis, malabsorption syndrome, and tumors. Although regional enteritis may not be detected in its early stages, small ulcerations and edematous changes develop in the mucosa as the disease progresses. Edematous changes, segmentation of the barium column, and flocculation characterize malabsorption syndrome. Filling defects occur with Hodgkin's disease and lymphosarcoma.

## INTERFERING FACTORS
- Excess air in the small bowel (possible poor imaging)
- Failure to remove metallic objects in the X-ray field (possible poor imaging)

# *Urea clearance*

The urea clearance test is a quantitative analysis of urine levels of urea, the main nitrogenous component in urine and the end product of protein metabolism. (See *How urea is formed.*)

After filtration by the glomeruli, roughly 40% of the urea is reabsorbed by the renal tubules. Because of this reabsorption, urea clearance was once considered a precise fraction (60%) of the glomerular filtration rate (GFR). However, because the reabsorption rate of urea varies with the amount of water reabsorbed, this test actually assesses overall renal function; the creatinine clearance test provides a more accurate evaluation of the GFR.

In urea clearance, blood urea content and the total amount of urea excreted in the urine are proportional only when the rate of urine flow is 2 ml/minute or higher (maximal clearance). At lower flow rates, the test's accuracy decreases. The equation for determining urea clearance is $C = (U \times V) \div$ by P; it's similar to the equation used for creatinine clearance.

## PURPOSE
- To assess overall renal function

## PATIENT PREPARATION
- Explain to the patient that the urea clearance test evaluates kidney function.
- Instruct the patient to fast from midnight before the test and to abstain from exercise before and during the test.
- Tell the patient that the test requires two timed urine specimens and one blood sample.
- Tell him how the urine specimens will be collected, who will perform the venipuncture and when, and that he may experience slight discomfort from the tourniquet and the needle puncture.
- Check the patient's medication history for drugs that may affect urea clearance.
- Review your findings with the laboratory and then notify the physician; he may want to restrict these medications.

## PROCEDURE AND POSTTEST CARE
- Instruct the patient to empty his bladder and discard the urine. Then give him water to drink to ensure adequate urine output.
- Collect two specimens 1 hour apart, and mark the collection time on the laboratory request.
- Perform a venipuncture anytime during the collection period and collect the sample in a 7-ml red-top tube.
- If a hematoma develops at the venipuncture site, apply pressure.
- Tell the patient that he may resume his usual diet, activities, and medications, as ordered.

## PRECAUTIONS
- Because this is a clearance test, make sure the patient empties his bladder completely and that the total amount of urine is collected from each hour's specimen.
- Send each specimen to the laboratory as soon as it's collected.
- If the patient is catheterized, empty the drainage bag before beginning the specimen collection.
- Handle the blood sample gently to prevent hemolysis, and send it to the laboratory immediately.

## How urea is formed

Urea, the main nitrogenous component in urine, is the final product of protein metabolism. Amino acids absorbed by the intestinal villi pass from the portal vein into the liver. Because the liver stores only small amounts of amino acids — which are later returned to the blood for use in the synthesis of enzymes, hormones, or new protoplasm — the excess is converted into other substances, such as glucose, glycogen, and fat.

Before this conversion, the amino acids are deaminated — they lose their nitrogenous amino groups. These amino groups are then converted to ammonia. Because ammonia is extremely toxic, especially to the brain, it must be removed as quickly as it's formed. (Serious liver disease causes elevated blood ammonia levels and eventually leads to hepatic coma.)

In the liver, ammonia combines with carbon dioxide to form urea, which is released into the blood and ultimately secreted in urine.

## REFERENCE VALUES

Normally, urea clearance ranges from 64 to 99 ml/minute with maximal clearance. If the flow rate is less than 2 ml/minute, normal clearance is 41 to 68 ml/minute. (If the urine flow rate is less than 1 ml/minute, this test shouldn't be performed.)

## ABNORMAL FINDINGS

Low urea clearance values may indicate decreased renal blood flow (due to shock or renal artery obstruction), acute or chronic glomerulonephritis, advanced bilateral chronic pyelonephritis, acute tubular necrosis, or nephrosclerosis. Low clearance rates may also result from advanced bilateral renal lesions (as in polycystic kidney disease, renal tuberculosis, or cancer), bilateral ureteral obstruction, heart failure, or dehydration.

High urea clearance rates usually aren't diagnostically significant.

## INTERFERING FACTORS

● Failure of patient to empty his bladder completely (the most common error in this test)
● Caffeine, milk, or small doses of epinephrine (increase)
● Antidiuretic hormone or large doses of epinephrine (decrease)
● Amphotericin B, corticosteroids, streptomycin, and thiazide diuretics

# Uric acid, serum and urine

The uric acid test is used to measure serum levels of uric acid, the major end metabolite of purine. Disorders of purine metabolism, rapid destruction of nucleic acids, and conditions marked by impaired renal excretion characteristically raise serum uric acid levels.

A quantitative analysis of urine uric acid levels may supplement serum uric acid testing when seeking to identify disorders that alter production or excretion of uric acid (such as gout, leukemia, and renal dysfunction).

The most specific laboratory method for detecting uric acid is spectrophotometric absorption after treatment of the specimen with the enzyme uricase.

## PURPOSE

● To confirm the diagnosis of gout
● To help detect renal dysfunction
● To detect enzyme deficiencies and metabolic disturbances that affect uric acid production such as gout (urine uric acid)

## PATIENT PREPARATION

● Explain to the patient that the uric acid test is used to detect gout and kidney dysfunction.
● Tell the patient that the test requires a blood sample or urine sample as appropriate. Explain who will perform the venipuncture or how and when the urine will be collected.

- Notify the laboratory and physician of medications the patient is taking that may affect test results; they may need to be restricted.

### Serum uric acid
- Explain to the patient that he may experience slight discomfort from the tourniquet and the needle puncture.
- Instruct the patient to fast for 8 hours before the test.

### Urine uric acid
- Anticipate the need for a diet low or high in purines before or during urine collection.
- Tell the patient that the test requires urine collection over a 24-hour period, and teach him the proper collection technique.

## PROCEDURE AND POSTTEST CARE
### Serum uric acid
- Perform a venipuncture and collect the sample in a 3- or 4-ml clot-activator tube.
- Apply direct pressure to the venipuncture site until bleeding stops.
- If a hematoma develops at the venipuncture site, apply pressure.

### Urine uric acid
- Collect the patient's urine over a 24-hour period, discarding the first specimen and retaining the last.

### Both tests
- Inform the patient that he may resume his usual diet and medications discontinued before the test, as ordered.

## PRECAUTIONS
- Handle the blood sample gently to prevent hemolysis.
- Send the urine specimen to the laboratory immediately after the collection is completed.

## REFERENCE VALUES
Uric acid concentrations in men normally range from 3.4 to 7 mg/dl (SI, 202 to 416 µmol/L); in women, normal levels range from 2.3 to 6 mg/dl (SI, 143 to 357 µmol/L).

Normal urine uric acid values vary with diet, but generally are 250 to 750 mg/24 hours (SI, 1.48 to 4.43 mmol/d).

## ABNORMAL FINDINGS
Increased serum uric acid levels may indicate gout or impaired kidney function. Levels may also rise in heart failure, glycogen storage disease (type I, von Gierke's disease), infections, hemolytic and sickle cell anemia, polycythemia, neoplasms, and psoriasis. Low serum uric acid levels may indicate defective tubular absorption (such as Fanconi's syndrome) or acute hepatic atrophy.

Elevated urine uric acid levels may result from chronic myeloid leukemia, polycythemia vera, multiple myeloma, early remission in pernicious anemia, lymphosarcoma and lymphatic leukemia during radiotherapy, or tubular reabsorption defects, such as Fanconi's syndrome and hepatolenticular degeneration (Wilson's disease).

Low urine uric acid levels occur in gout (when associated with normal uric acid production but inadequate excretion) and in severe renal damage such as that resulting from chronic glomerulonephritis, diabetic glomerulosclerosis, and collagen disorders.

## INTERFERING FACTORS
### Serum uric acid
- Low doses of aspirin, ethambutol, loop diuretics, pyrazinamide, thiazides, and vincristine (possible increase)
- Acetaminophen, ascorbic acid, and levodopa (possible false-high if using colorimetric method)
- Aspirin in high doses (possible decrease)
- Alcohol abuse, high-purine diet, starvation, and stress (possible increase)

### Urine uric acid
- Diuretics, such as benzthiazide, ethacrynic acid, and furosemide (decrease); alcohol, allopurinol, phenylbutazone, probenecid, pyrazinamide, salicylates, vitamin C and warfarin (Coumadin) (increase)
- High-purine diet (increase)
- Low-purine diet (decrease)

## *Urinary calculi*

Urinary calculi (urolithiasis or, more commonly, urinary stones) are insoluble substances most commonly formed of the mineral salts — calcium oxalate, calcium phosphate, magnesium ammonium phosphate,

## TYPES AND CAUSES OF CALCULI

**A**

*Calcium oxalate calculi* usually result from idiopathic hypercalciuria, a condition that reflects absorption of calcium from the bowel.

**B**

*Calcium phosphate calculi* usually result from primary hyperparathyroidism, which causes excessive reabsorption of calcium from bone.

**C**

*Cystine calculi* result from primary cystinuria, an inborn error of metabolism that prevents renal tubular reabsorption of cystine.

**D**

*Urate calculi* result from gout, dehydration (causing elevated uric acid levels), acidic urine, or hepatic dysfunction.

**E**

*Magnesium ammonium phosphate calculi* result from the presence of urea-splitting organisms, such as *Proteus*, which raises ammonia concentration and makes urine alkaline.

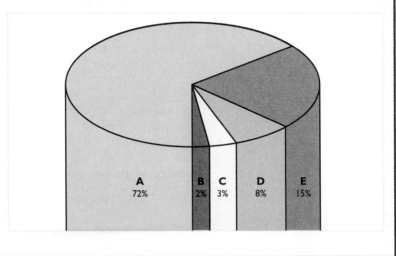

| A | B | C | D | E |
|---|---|---|---|---|
| 72% | 2% | 3% | 8% | 15% |

urate, or cystine. (See *Types and causes of calculi.*) They may appear anywhere in the urinary tract and range in size from microscopic to several centimeters. Calculi usually possess well-defined nuclei composed of bacteria, fibrin, blood clots, or epithelial cells that are enclosed in a protein matrix. Mineral salts accumulate around this matrix in layers, causing progressive enlargement.

Formation of calculi can result from reduced urinary volume, increased excretion of mineral salts, urinary stasis, pH changes, and decreased protective substances. Calculi commonly form in the kidney, pass into the ureter, and are excreted in the urine. Because not all calculi pass spontaneously, they may require surgical extraction or pulverization

using extracorporeal shock-wave lithotripsy. Calculi don't always cause symptoms, but when they do, hematuria is most common. If calculi obstruct the ureter, they may cause severe flank pain, dysuria, and urinary retention, frequency, and urgency.

To test for urinary calculi, the patient must have all his urine carefully strained to remove any calculi. Qualitative chemical analysis then reveals the calculi's composition, which helps to identify their causes.

### PURPOSE

- To detect and analyze calculi in the urine

## PATIENT PREPARATION

• Explain to the patient that the urinary calculi test detects urinary calculi and that laboratory analysis will reveal their composition.
• Tell the patient that his urine will be collected and strained.
• Advise the patient that he need not restrict food and fluids.
• Inform the patient that medication to control pain will be administered.

## PROCEDURE AND POSTTEST CARE

• Have the patient void into the strainer.
• Inspect the strainer carefully because calculi may be minute, looking like gravel or sand.
• Document the appearance of the calculi and the number, if possible.
• Place the calculi in a properly labeled container.
• Send the container to the laboratory immediately for prompt analysis.
• Observe the patient for severe flank pain, dysuria, and urinary retention, frequency, or urgency. Hematuria should subside.

## PRECAUTIONS

• Keep the strainer and urinal or bedpan within the patient's reach if he has received analgesics because he may be drowsy and unable to get out of bed to void.

## NORMAL FINDINGS

Normally, calculi aren't present in urine.

## ABNORMAL FINDINGS

More than one-half of all calculi in urine are of mixed composition, containing two or more mineral salts; calcium oxalate is the most common component. Determining the calculi's composition helps identify various metabolic disorders, guiding proper treatment and prevention measures.

## INTERFERING FACTORS

• None significant

---

# Urine culture

---

Laboratory examination and culture of urine are used to evaluate urinary tract infections (UTIs), especially bladder infections. Urine in the kidneys and bladder is normally sterile, but a urine specimen may contain various organisms due to bacteria in the urethra and on external genitalia.

Bacteriuria generally results from one prevalent bacteria type; the presence of more than two bacterial species in a specimen strongly suggests contamination during collection. A single negative culture doesn't always rule out infection; a quantitative examination of urine culture is needed.

Significant results of urine culture are possibly only after quantitative examination. To distinguish between true bacteriuria and contamination, it's necessary to know the number or organisms in a milliliter of urine, estimated by a culture technique known as *colony count*. In addition, a quick centrifugation test can determine where a UTI originates. (See *Quick centrifugation test*.)

Clean-voided midstream collection, rather than suprapubic aspiration of catheterization, is now the method of choice for obtaining a urine specimen.

## PURPOSE

• To diagnose UTI
• To monitor microorganism colonization after urinary catheter insertion

## PATIENT PREPARATION

• Explain to the patient that the urine culture is used to detect UTIs.
• Inform the patient that the test requires a urine specimen and that no restriction of food and fluids is necessary.
• Instruct him how to collect a clean-voided midstream specimen; emphasize that external genitalia must be cleaned thoroughly.
• If appropriate, explain catheterization or suprapubic aspiration to the patient, and inform him that he may experience some discomfort during specimen collection.
• For the patient with suspected tuberculosis, specimen collection may be required on three consecutive mornings.
• Check the patient's history for current antimicrobial therapy.

## PROCEDURE AND POSTTEST CARE

• Collect a urine specimen, as ordered.
• When obtaining a specimen from an indwelling urinary catheter, clamp the tubing below the collection port to collect a specimen in the tubing. Then use an alcohol pad

to clean the port. Next, using a sterile needle and syringe, aspirate a 4-ml specimen from the port, and transfer it into a sterile specimen cup.

● Seal the cup with a sterile lid, and send it to the laboratory immediately. If transport is delayed longer than 30 minutes, store the specimen at 39.2° F (4° C) or place it on ice, unless a urine transport tube containing preservative is used.

● Instruct the patient to wash his hands, then clean the urethral area with antiseptic towelettes. Tell the patient to begin urinating in the toilet, then stop and continue to urinate into the sterile cup, without touching the inside of the cup.

● Record on the laboratory request the suspected diagnosis, the collection time and method, current antimicrobial therapy, and fluid- or drug-induced diuresis.

## PRECAUTIONS

● Wear gloves when performing the procedure and handling specimens.

● Collect at least 3 ml of urine, but don't fill the specimen cup more than halfway.

## NORMAL FINDINGS

Culture results of sterile urine are usually reported as "no growth," which typically indicates the absence of a UTI.

## ABNORMAL FINDINGS

Bacterial counts of 100,000/ml or more of a single microbe species indicate a probable UTI. Counts under 100,000/ml may be significant, depending on the patient's age, sex, history, and other individual factors. Counts under 10,000/ml usually suggest that the organisms are contaminants, except in symptomatic patients, those with urologic disorders, and those whose urine specimens were collected by suprapubic aspiration. A special test for acid-fast bacteria isolates *Mycobacterium tuberculosis,* thus indicating tuberculosis of the urinary tract.

Isolation of more than two species of organisms or of vaginal or skin organisms usually suggests contamination and requires a repeat culture. Prolonged catheterization or urinary diversion may cause polymicrobial infection.

## INTERFERING FACTORS

● Improper collection technique

---

### QUICK CENTRIFUGATION TEST

The quick centrifugation test can determine whether the source of a urinary tract infection is in the lower tract (bladder) or the upper tract (kidneys). The test involves centrifugation of urine in a test tube, followed by staining of the sediment with fluorescein. If one-quarter of the bacteria fluoresce when viewed under a fluorescent microscope, an upper tract infection is present; if bacteria don't fluoresce, a lower tract infection is present.

---

● Antimicrobial therapy and fluid- or drug-induced diuresis (possible decrease)

# Urobilinogen, urine

The urobilinogen test detects impaired liver function by measuring urine levels of urobilinogen, the colorless, water-soluble product that results from the reduction of bilirubin by intestinal bacteria. Absent or altered urobilinogen levels can indicate hepatic damage or dysfunction. Increased urine urobilinogen levels may indicate hemolysis of red blood cells.

Quantitative analysis of urine urobilinogen involves the addition of a reagent to a 2-hour urine specimen. The resulting color reaction is read promptly by spectrophotometry.

## PURPOSE

● To aid in the diagnosis of extrahepatic obstruction such as blockage of the common bile duct

● To aid in the differential diagnosis of hepatic and hematologic disorders

## PATIENT PREPARATION

● Explain to the patient that the urine urobilinogen test helps assess liver and biliary tract function.

● Inform the patient that he need not restrict food and fluids, except for bananas, which he should avoid for 48 hours before the test.

● Tell the patient that the test requires a 2-hour urine specimen, and teach him how to collect it.

● Notify the laboratory and physician of medications the patient is taking that may affect test results; they may need to be restricted.

## PROCEDURE AND POSTTEST CARE

● Most laboratories request a random urine specimen; others prefer a 2-hour specimen, usually during the afternoon (ideally, between 1 p.m. and 3 p.m.), when urobilinogen levels peak.

● Instruct the patient that he may resume his usual diet and medications, as ordered.

## PRECAUTIONS

**Alert** *Send the specimen to the laboratory immediately after collection. This test must be performed within 30 minutes of collection because urobilinogen quickly oxidizes into an orange compound called urobilin.*

## REFERENCE VALUES

Normally, urine urobilinogen values are 0.1 to 0.8 EU/2 hours (SI, 0.1 to 0.8 EU/ 2 hours) or 0.5 to 4.0 EU/24 hours (SI, 0.5 to 4.0 EU/d).

## ABNORMAL FINDINGS

Absence of urine urobilinogen may result from complete obstructive jaundice, cholestasis, or treatment with broad-spectrum antibiotics, which destroy the intestinal bacterial flora. Low urine urobilinogen levels may result from congenital enzymatic jaundice (hyperbilirubinemia syndromes) or from treatment with drugs that acidify urine, such as ammonium chloride or ascorbic acid.

Elevated levels may indicate hemolytic jaundice, hemolytic or pernicious anemia, hepatitis, or cirrhosis.

## INTERFERING FACTORS

● Para-aminosalicylic acid, phenazopyridine, phenothiazines, procaine, and sulfonamides (possible decrease)

● Acetazolamide and sodium bicarbonate (increase)

● Bananas eaten up to 48 hours before the test (increase)

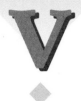

# Vaginal ultrasonography

In vaginal ultrasonography, a probe inserted into the vagina reflects high-frequency sound waves to a transducer, forming an image of the pelvic structures. This study allows better evaluation of pelvic anatomy and earlier diagnosis of pregnancy. It also circumvents the poor visualization encountered with obese patients.

## PURPOSE
● To establish pregnancy with fetal heart motion as early as 5 to 6 weeks' gestation
● To determine ectopic pregnancy
● To evaluate abnormal pregnancy
● To diagnose fetal abnormalities and placental location
● To visualize retained products of conception
● To evaluate adnexal diseases, such as tubo-ovarian abscess, hydrosalpinx, and ovarian masses
● To evaluate the uterine lining (in cases of dysfunctional uterine bleeding and post-menopausal bleeding)
● To monitor follicular growth during infertility treatment

## PATIENT PREPARATION
● Describe the vaginal ultrasonography to the patient and explain the reason for the test.
● Assure the patient that the procedure is safe.

## PROCEDURE AND POSTTEST CARE
● The patient is placed in the lithotomy position. If the sonographer is a male, a female assistant should be present during the examination.
● Water-soluble conductive gel is placed on the transducer tip to allow better sound transmission and a protective sheath is placed over the transducer.
● Place more lubricant on the sheathed transducer tip to allow for its gentle insertion into the vagina by the patient or the sonographer. Allowing the patient to introduce the probe may decrease her anxiety.
● To observe the pelvic structures, rotate the probe 90 degrees to one side and then the other.

## PRECAUTIONS
● None

## NORMAL FINDINGS
If the patient isn't pregnant, the uterus and ovaries are normal in size and shape. The body of the uterus lies on the superior surface of the bladder; the uterine tubes are attached laterally. The ovaries are located on the lateral pelvic walls, with the external iliac vessels above the ureter posteroinferiorly and covered by the fimbria of the uterine tubes medially. If the patient is pregnant, the gestational sac and fetus are of normal size for the gestational date.

## ABNORMAL FINDINGS
Vaginal ultrasonography may reveal an empty uterus if the patient was pregnant. Free peritoneal fluid may be visible in the pelvic

cavity, indicating possible peritonitis. Ectopic pregnancies may also be visible in the pelvic cavity.

## INTERFERING FACTORS
- Mistaking the bowel for the ovaries
- Small tubal mass (possible difficulty in detecting ectopic pregnancies)

# Vanillylmandelic acid, urine

Using spectrophotofluorimetry, the vanillylmandelic acid (VMA) test determines urine levels of VMA, a phenolic acid. VMA is the catecholamine metabolite that's normally most prevalent in the urine and is the product of hepatic conversion of epinephrine and norepinephrine; urine VMA levels reflect endogenous production of these major catecholamines. Like the test for urine total catecholamines, this test helps to detect catecholamine-secreting tumors — especially pheochromocytoma — and helps evaluate adrenal medulla function, the primary site of catecholamine production.

The VMA test ideally should be performed on a 24-hour urine specimen (not a random specimen) to overcome the effects of diurnal variations in catecholamine secretion. Other catecholamine metabolites — metanephrine, normetanephrine, and homovanillic acid (HVA) — may be measured at the same time. If evaluating hypertension, specimen collection may be of greatest value during the hypertensive episode.

## PURPOSE
- To help detect pheochromocytoma, neuroblastoma, and ganglioneuroma
- To evaluate the function of the adrenal medulla

## PATIENT PREPARATION
- Explain to the patient that the urine VMA test evaluates hormonal secretion.
- Instruct the patient to restrict foods and beverages containing phenolic acid, such as coffee, tea, bananas, citrus fruits, chocolate, and vanilla, and carbonated beverages for 3 days before the test.

- Advise the patient to avoid stressful situations and excessive physical activity during the urine collection period.
- Tell the patient that the test requires collection of urine over a 24-hour period, and teach him the proper collection technique.
- Notify the laboratory and physician of medications the patient is taking that may affect test results; they may need to be restricted.

## PROCEDURE AND POSTTEST CARE
- Collect the patient's urine over a 24-hour period, discarding the first specimen and retaining the last. Use a bottle containing a preservative to keep the specimen at a pH of 3.0.
- Instruct the patient that he may resume his usual activities, diet, and medications, as ordered.

## PRECAUTIONS
- Refrigerate the specimen or keep it on ice during the collection period.
- Send the specimen to the laboratory immediately after the collection is completed.

## REFERENCE VALUES
Normally, VMA levels in adults are 2 to 7 mg/24 hours (SI, 1 to 35 μmol/d).

## ABNORMAL FINDINGS
Elevated urine VMA levels may result from a catecholamine-secreting tumor. Further testing, such as measurement of urine HVA levels to rule out pheochromocytoma, is necessary for precise diagnosis. If pheochromocytoma is confirmed, the patient may be tested for multiple endocrine neoplasia, an inherited condition commonly associated with pheochromocytoma. (Family members of a patient with confirmed pheochromocytoma should also be carefully evaluated for multiple endocrine neoplasia.)

## INTERFERING FACTORS
- Excessive exercise or emotional stress (increase)
- Epinephrine, lithium carbonate, methocarbamol, and norepinephrine, (increase); chlorpromazine, clonidine, guanethidine, monoamine oxidase inhibitors, and reserpine (decrease); levodopa and salicylates (increase or decrease)

# Venereal Disease Research Laboratory test

The Venereal Disease Research Laboratory (VDRL) test, a flocculation test, is widely used to screen for primary and secondary syphilis. Although the test has diagnostic significance during the first two stages of syphilis, transient or permanent biologic false-positive reactions can make accurate interpretation difficult. A biologic false-positive reaction can result from viral or bacterial infection, chronic systemic illness, or non-syphilitic treponemal disease. Usually, a serum sample is used in the VDRL test, but this test may also be performed on a cerebrospinal fluid (CSF) specimen obtained by lumbar puncture to test for tertiary syphilis. The VDRL test of CSF is less sensitive than the fluorescent treponemal antibody absorption test.

The rapid plasma reagin test can also be used to diagnose syphilis. (See *Rapid plasma reagin test.*)

## PURPOSE
● To screen for primary and secondary syphilis
● To confirm primary or secondary syphilis in the presence of syphilitic lesions
● To monitor the patient's response to treatment

## PATIENT PREPARATION
● Explain to the patient that the VDRL test detects syphilis.
● Inform the patient that the disease usually goes undetected in the general population because the majority of infected people don't know they're infected, thus remain untreated.
● Tell the patient that he need not restrict food, fluids, or medications, but should abstain from alcohol for 24 hours before the test.
● Tell the patient that the test requires a blood sample. Explain who will perform the venipuncture and when.
● Explain to the patient that he may experience slight discomfort from the tourniquet and the needle puncture.

## RAPID PLASMA REAGIN TEST

The rapid plasma reagin (RPR) test is a rapid, macroscopic serologic test that's an acceptable substitute for the Venereal Disease Research Laboratory (VDRL) test in diagnosing syphilis. The RPR test, available as a kit, uses a cardiolipin antigen to detect reagin, the antibody relatively specific for *Treponema pallidum,* the causative agent of syphilis.

In the RPR test, the patient's serum is mixed with cardiolipin on a plastic-coated card, rotated mechanically, and then examined with the unaided eye. If flocculation occurs, the test sample is diluted until no visible reaction occurs. The last dilution to show visible flocculation is the titer of the reagin antibody.

In the RPR test, as in the VDRL test, normal serum shows no flocculation.

## PROCEDURE AND POSTTEST CARE
● Perform a venipuncture and collect the sample in a 7-ml clot-activator tube.
● Apply direct pressure to the venipuncture site until bleeding stops.
● If a hematoma develops at the venipuncture site, apply pressure.
● If the test is nonreactive or borderline, but syphilis hasn't been ruled out, instruct the patient to return for follow-up testing. Explain that borderline test results don't necessarily mean that he's free from the disease.
● If the test is reactive, explain the importance of proper treatment. Provide the patient with further information about sexually transmitted diseases and how they're spread and stress the need for antibiotic therapy. Report the results to state public health authorities and prepare the patient for mandatory inquiries.
● If the test is reactive, but the patient shows no clinical signs of syphilis, explain that many uninfected people show false-positive reactions. Stress the need for further specific tests to rule out syphilis.

## PRECAUTIONS
● Handle the specimen carefully to prevent hemolysis.

## NORMAL FINDINGS

Normal serum shows no flocculation and is reported as a nonreactive test.

## ABNORMAL FINDINGS

Definite flocculation is reported as a reactive test; slight flocculation is reported as a weakly reactive test. A reactive VDRL test occurs in about 50% of patients with primary syphilis and in nearly all patients with secondary syphilis. If syphilitic lesions exist, a reactive VDRL test is diagnostic. If no lesions are evident, a reactive VDRL test necessitates repeated testing. Biologic false-positive reactions can be caused by conditions unrelated to syphilis; for example, infectious mononucleosis, malaria, leprosy, hepatitis, systemic lupus erythematosus, rheumatoid arthritis, and nonsyphilitic treponemal diseases, such as pinta and yaws.

A nonreactive test doesn't rule out syphilis because *Treponema pallidum* causes no detectable immunologic changes in the serum for 14 to 21 days after infection. Darkfield microscopy of exudate from suspicious lesions can provide early diagnosis by identifying the causative spirochetes.

A reactive VDRL test using a CSF specimen indicates neurosyphilis, which can follow the primary and secondary stages in patients who remain untreated.

## INTERFERING FACTORS

- Ingestion of alcohol within 24 hours of the test (possible transient nonreactive results)
- Immunosuppression (possible nonreactive results)

# *Vertebral radiography*

Vertebral radiography visualizes all or part of the vertebral column. A commonly performed test, it's used to evaluate the vertebrae for deformities, fractures, dislocations, tumors, and other abnormalities. Bone films determine bone density, texture, erosion, and changes in bone relationships. X-rays of the cortex of the bone reveal the presence of any widening, narrowing, and signs of irregularity. Joint X-rays can reveal the presence of fluid, spur formation, narrowing, and changes in the joint structure.

The type and extent of vertebral radiography depends on the patient's clinical condition. For example, a patient with lower back pain requires only study of the lumbar and sacral segments.

## PURPOSE

- To detect vertebral fractures, dislocations, subluxations, and deformities
- To detect vertebral degeneration, infection, and congenital disorders
- To detect disorders of the intervertebral disks
- To determine the vertebral effects of arthritic and metabolic disorders

## PATIENT PREPARATION

- Explain to the patient that vertebral radiography permits examination of the spine.
- Inform the patient that he need not restrict food and fluids.
- Tell the patient the test requires X-rays. Also tell him who will perform the test and when where it will take place.
- Advise the patient that he'll be placed in various positions for the X-rays.
- Tell the patient that although some positions may cause slight discomfort, his cooperation is needed to ensure accurate results.
- Stress to the patient that he must keep still and hold his breath during the procedure.

## PROCEDURE AND POSTTEST CARE

- The procedure varies considerably, depending on the vertebral segment being examined.
- Initially, the patient is placed in a supine position on the X-ray table for an anteroposterior view.
- The patient may be repositioned for lateral or right and left oblique views; specific positioning depends on the vertebral segment or adjacent structure of interest.
- Analgesics or local heat applications may relieve pain.

## PRECAUTIONS

- Know that vertebral radiography is contraindicated during the first trimester of pregnancy, unless the benefits outweigh the risk of fetal radiation exposure.

⊛ *Alert Be sure to exercise extreme caution when handling a trauma patient with suspected spinal injuries, particularly of the cervical* area. He should be filmed while on the stretcher to avoid further injury during transfer to the radiographic table.

## NORMAL FINDINGS

Normal vertebrae show no fractures, subluxations, dislocations, curvatures, or other abnormalities. Specific positions and spacing of the vertebrae vary with the patient's age.

*Age alert* *In the lateral view, adult vertebrae are aligned to form four alternately concave and convex curves. The cervical and lumbar curves are convex anteriorly; the thoracic and sacral curves are concave anteriorly. Although the structure of the coccyx varies, it usually points forward and downward. Neonatal vertebrae form only one curve, which is concave anteriorly.*

## ABNORMAL FINDINGS

The vertebral radiograph readily shows spondylolisthesis, fractures, subluxations, dislocations, wedging, and such deformities as kyphosis, scoliosis, and lordosis.

To confirm other disorders, spinal structures and their spatial relationships on the radiograph must be examined, and the patient's history and clinical status must be considered. These disorders include congenital abnormalities, such as torticollis (wryneck), absence of sacral or lumbar vertebrae, hemivertebrae, and Klippel-Feil syndrome; degenerative processes, such as hypertrophic spurs, osteoarthritis, and narrowed disk spaces; tuberculosis (Pott's disease); benign or malignant intraspinal tumors; ruptured disk and cervical disk syndrome; and systemic disorders, such as rheumatoid arthritis, Charcot's disease, ankylosing spondylitis, osteoporosis, and Paget's disease.

Depending on X-ray results, definitive diagnosis may also require additional tests, such as myelography or computed tomography scanning.

## INTERFERING FACTORS

● Improper positioning of the patient or patient movement (possible poor imaging)

---

# Voiding cystourethrography

In voiding cystourethrography, a contrast medium is instilled by gentle syringe pressure or gravity into the bladder through a urethral catheter. Fluoroscopic films or overhead radiographs demonstrate bladder filling and then show excretion of the contrast medium as the patient voids.

## PURPOSE

● To detect abnormalities of the bladder and urethra, such as vesicoureteral reflux, neurogenic bladder, prostatic hyperplasia, urethral strictures, or diverticula

## PATIENT PREPARATION

● Explain to the patient that voiding cystourethrography permits assessment of the bladder and urethra.
● Inform the patient that he need not restrict food and fluids.
● Tell the patient who will perform the test and when and where it will take place.
● Inform the patient that a catheter will be inserted into his bladder and that a contrast medium will be instilled through the catheter.
● Tell the patient that he may experience a feeling of fullness and an urge to void when the contrast medium is instilled. Explain that X-rays will be taken of his bladder and urethra and that he'll be asked to assume various positions.
● Make sure that the patient or a responsible family member has signed an informed consent form.

*Alert* *Check the patient's history for hypersensitivity to contrast media or iodine-containing foods such as shellfish; note sensitivities on the chart and notify the physician.*
● Administer a sedative, if prescribed, just before the procedure.

## PROCEDURE AND POSTTEST CARE

● The patient is placed in a supine position, and an indwelling urinary catheter is inserted into the bladder.
● The contrast medium is instilled through the catheter until the bladder is full.
● The catheter is clamped, and X-rays are exposed with the patient in supine, oblique, and lateral positions.
● The catheter is removed, and the patient assumes the right oblique position (right leg flexed to 90 degrees, left leg extended, penis parallel to right leg) and begins to void.
● Four high-speed exposures of the bladder and urethra, coned down to reduce radiation

exposure, are usually made on one film during voiding.

- If the right oblique view doesn't delineate both ureters, the patient is asked to stop urinating and to begin again in the left oblique position.
- The most reliable voiding cystourethrograms are obtained with the patient recumbent. The patient who can't void recumbent may do so standing (not sitting).
- Expression cystourethrography may have to be performed, under a general anesthetic, for a young child who can't void on command.

**Alert** *Observe and record the time, color, and volume of the patient's voidings. Report hematuria if present after the third voiding.*

- Encourage the patient to drink large quantities of fluids to reduce burning on urination and to flush out residual contrast medium.

**Alert** *Monitor the patient for chills and fever related to extravasation of contrast material or urinary sepsis.*

- If stricture is present, prepare for surgery, as indicated.
- Monitor the patient for symptoms of urinary tract infection.

## PRECAUTIONS

- Know that voiding cystourethrography is contraindicated in the patient with an acute or exacerbated urethral or bladder infection or an acute urethral injury.
- Be aware that hypersensitivity to the contrast medium may also contraindicate this test.

## NORMAL FINDINGS

Delineation of the bladder and urethra shows normal structure and function, with no regurgitation of contrast medium into the ureters.

## ABNORMAL FINDINGS

Voiding cystourethrography may show urethral stricture, vesical or urethral diverticula, ureterocele, cystocele, prostate enlargement, vesicoureteral reflux, or neurogenic bladder. The severity and location of such abnormalities are then evaluated to determine whether surgical intervention is necessary.

## INTERFERING FACTORS

- Embarrassment (inhibits the patient from voiding on command)
- Interrupted or less vigorous voiding, muscle spasm, or incomplete sphincter relaxation (due to urethral trauma during catheterization)
- Presence of contrast media from recent tests, stool, or gas in the bowel (possible poor imaging)

# W-Z

## White blood cell count and differential

A white blood cell (WBC) count, also called a *leukocyte count,* is part of a complete blood count. It indicates the number of white cells in a microliter (µl, or cubic millimeter) of whole blood.

WBC counts may vary by as much as 2,000 cells/µl (SI, $2 \times 10^9$/L) on any given day due to strenuous exercise, stress, or digestion. The WBC count may increase or decrease significantly in certain diseases, but is diagnostically useful only when the patient's white cell differential and clinical status are considered.

The WBC differential is used to evaluate the distribution and morphology of WBCs, providing more specific information about a patient's immune system than does the WBC count alone.

WBCs are classified as one of five major types of leukocytes — neutrophils, eosinophils, basophils, lymphocytes, and monocytes — and the percentage of each type is determined. The differential count is the percentage of each type of WBC in the blood. The total number of each type of WBC is obtained by multiplying the percentage of each type by the total WBC count.

High levels of these leukocytes are associated with various allergic diseases and reactions to parasites. An eosinophil count is sometimes ordered as a follow-up test when an elevated or depressed eosinophil level is reported.

## PURPOSE
### WBC count
- To determine infection or inflammation
- To determine the need for further tests, such as bone marrow biopsy
- To monitor response to chemotherapy or radiation therapy

### WBC differential
- To evaluate the body's capacity to resist and overcome infection
- To detect and identify various types of leukemia (see *Performing a LAP stain,* page 496)
- To determine the stage and severity of an infection
- To detect allergic reactions and parasitic infections and assess their severity (eosinophil count)
- To distinguish viral from bacterial infections

## PATIENT PREPARATION
- Explain to the patient that the WBC count and differential test is used to detect an infection or inflammation (WBC count) or evaluate the immune system (WBC differential).
- Tell the patient that a blood sample will be taken. Explain who will perform the venipuncture and when.
- Explain to the patient that he may feel slight discomfort from the tourniquet and needle puncture.

# PERFORMING A LAP STAIN

Levels of leukocyte alkaline phosphatase (LAP), an enzyme found in neutrophils, may be altered by infection, stress, chronic inflammatory diseases, Hodgkin's disease, and hematologic disorders. Most of these conditions elevate LAP levels; only a few—notably chronic myelogenous leukemia (CML)—depress them. Thus, this test is usually used to differentiate CML from other disorders that produce an elevated white blood cell count.

## PROCEDURE

To perform the LAP stain, a blood sample is obtained by venipuncture or fingerstick. The venous blood sample is collected in a 7-ml *green-top* tube and transported immediately to the laboratory, where a blood smear is prepared; the peripheral blood sample is smeared on a 3" glass slide and fixed in cold formalin-methanol. The blood smear is then stained to show the amount of LAP present in the cytoplasm of the neutrophils. One hundred neutrophils are counted and assessed; each is assigned a score of 0 to 4, according to the degree of LAP staining. Normally, values for LAP range from 40 to 100, depending on the laboratory's standards.

## IMPLICATIONS OF RESULTS

Depressed LAP values typically indicate CML; however, values may also be low in paroxysmal nocturnal hemoglobinuria, aplastic anemia, and infectious mononucleosis. Elevated levels may indicate Hodgkin's disease, polycythemia vera, or a neutrophilic leukemoid reaction—a response to such conditions as infection, chronic inflammation, or pregnancy.

After a diagnosis of CML, the LAP stain may also be used to help detect onset of the blastic phase of the disease, when LAP levels typically rise. However, LAP levels also increase toward normal in response to therapy; because of this, test results must be correlated with the patient's condition.

---

- Inform the patient that he need not restrict food and fluids but that he should avoid strenuous exercise for 24 hours before the test. Also tell him that he should avoid eating a heavy meal before the test.
- If the patient is being treated for an infection, advise him that this test will be repeated to monitor his progress.
- Notify the laboratory and physician of medications the patient is taking that may affect test results; they may need to be restricted.

## PROCEDURE AND POSTTEST CARE

- Perform a venipuncture and collect the sample in a 3- or 4.5-ml EDTA tube.
- If a hematoma develops at the venipuncture site, apply pressure. If the hematoma is large, monitor pulses distal to the venipuncture site.
- Make sure subdermal bleeding has stopped before removing pressure.

- Instruct the patient that he may resume his usual diet, activity, and medications discontinued before the test, as ordered.
- A patient with severe leukopenia may have little or no resistance to infection and requires infection control precautions.

## PRECAUTIONS

- Completely fill the sample collection tube.
- Invert the sample gently several times to mix the sample and the anticoagulant.

## REFERENCE VALUES

The WBC count ranges from 4,000 to 10,000/µl (SI, 4 to 10 × 10$^9$/L).

For normal values for the five types of WBCs classified in the differential for adults and children, see *Interpreting WBC differential values*. For an accurate diagnosis, differential test results must always be interpreted in relation to the total WBC count.

# Interpreting WBC differential values

The differential count measures the types of white blood cells (WBCs) as a percentage of the total WBC count (the relative value). The absolute value is obtained by multiplying the relative value of each cell type by the total WBC count. The relative and absolute values must be considered to obtain an accurate diagnosis.

For example, consider a patient whose WBC count is 6,000/μl (SI, 6 × 10⁹/L) and whose differential shows 30% (SI, 0.3) neutrophils and 70% (SI, 0.7) lymphocytes. His relative lymphocyte count seems to be quite high (lymphocytosis), but when this figure is multiplied by his WBC count (6,000 × 70% = 4,200 lymphocytes/μl), (SI, [6 × 10⁹/L] × 0.7 = 4.2 × 10⁹/L lymphocytes), it's well within the normal range.

However, this patient's neutrophil count (30%; SI, 0.3) is low; when this figure is multiplied by the WBC count (6,000 × 30% = 1,800 neutrophils/ml) (SI, [6 × 10⁹/L] × 0.30 = 1.8 × 10⁹/L neutrophils), the result is a low absolute number, which may mean depressed bone marrow.

The normal percentages of WBC type in adults are:
Neutrophils — 54% to 75% (SI, 0.54 to 0.75)
Eosinophils — 1% to 4% (SI, 0.01 to 0.04)
Basophils — 0% to 1% (SI, 0 to 0.01)
Monocytes — 2% to 8% (SI, 0.02 to 0.08)
Lymphocytes — 25% to 40% (SI, 0.25 to 0.4).

## ABNORMAL FINDINGS

An elevated WBC count (leukocytosis) commonly signals infection, such as an abscess, meningitis, appendicitis, or tonsillitis. A high count may also result from leukemia and tissue necrosis due to burns, myocardial infarction, or gangrene.

A low WBC count (leukopenia) indicates bone marrow depression that may result from viral infections or from toxic reactions, such as those following treatment with antineoplastics, ingestion of mercury or other heavy metals, or exposure to benzene or arsenicals. Leukopenia characteristically accompanies influenza, typhoid fever, measles, infectious hepatitis, mononucleosis, and rubella.

Abnormal differential patterns provide evidence for many disease states and other conditions. (See *Influence of disease on blood cell count,* pages 498 and 499.)

## INTERFERING FACTORS
### WBC count

- Digestion, exercise, or stress
- Anticonvulsants, such as phenytoin derivatives; anti-infectives, such as flucytosine (Ancobon) and metronidazole (Flagyl); most antineoplastics; nonsteroidal anti-inflammatory drugs such as indomethacin (Indocin); and thyroid hormone antagonists (decrease)

### WBC differential

- Anticonvulsants, capreomycin (Capastat sulfate), cephalosporins, D-penicillamine, desipramine (Norpramin), gold compounds, indomethacin (Indocin), isoniazid, methysergide (increase or decrease eosinophil count), nalidixic acid (NegGram), novobiocin, para-aminosalicylic acid, paromomycin (Humatin), penicillins, phenothiazines, procainamide (Procanbid) (decrease eosinophil count), rifampin, streptomycin, sulfonamides, and tetracyclines (increase count by provoking an allergic reaction)

# INFLUENCE OF DISEASE ON BLOOD CELL COUNT

| CELL TYPE | HOW AFFECTED |
|-----------|--------------|

## NEUTROPHILS

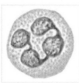

*Increased by:*
- ◆ Infections: osteomyelitis, otitis media, salpingitis, septicemia, gonorrhea, endocarditis, smallpox, chickenpox, herpes, Rocky Mountain spotted fever
- ◆ Ischemic necrosis due to myocardial infarction, burns, carcinoma
- ◆ Metabolic disorders: diabetic acidosis, eclampsia, uremia, thyrotoxicosis
- ◆ Stress response due to acute hemorrhage, surgery, excessive exercise, emotional distress, third trimester of pregnancy, childbirth
- ◆ Inflammatory diseases: rheumatic fever, rheumatoid arthritis, acute gout, vasculitis, myositis

*Decreased by:*
- ◆ Bone marrow depression due to radiation or cytotoxic drugs
- ◆ Infections: typhoid, tularemia, brucellosis, hepatitis, influenza, measles, mumps, rubella, infectious mononucleosis
- ◆ Hypersplenism: hepatic disease and storage diseases
- ◆ Collagen vascular disease such as systemic lupus erythematosus (SLE)
- ◆ Folic acid or vitamin $B_{12}$ deficiency

## EOSINOPHILS

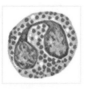

*Increased by:*
- ◆ Allergic disorders: asthma, hay fever, food or drug sensitivity, serum sickness, angioneurotic edema
- ◆ Parasitic infections: trichinosis, hookworm, roundworm, amebiasis
- ◆ Skin diseases: eczema, pemphigus, psoriasis, dermatitis, herpes
- ◆ Neoplastic diseases: chronic myelocytic leukemia (CML), Hodgkin's disease, metastases and necrosis of solid tumors

*Decreased by:*
- ◆ Stress response
- ◆ Cushing's syndrome

## BASOPHILS

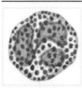

*Increased by:*
- ◆ CML, Hodgkin's disease, ulcerative colitis, chronic hypersensitivity states

*Decreased by:*
- ◆ Hyperthyroidism
- ◆ Ovulation, pregnancy
- ◆ Stress

## LYMPHOCYTES

*Increased by:*
- ◆ Infections: tuberculosis (TB), hepatitis, infectious mononucleosis, mumps, rubella, cytomegalovirus
- ◆ Thyrotoxicosis, hypoadrenalism, ulcerative colitis, immune diseases, lymphocytic leukemia

*Decreased by:*
- ◆ Severe debilitating illnesses: heart failure, renal failure, advanced TB
- ◆ Defective lymphatic circulation, high levels of adrenal corticosteroids, immunodeficiency due to immunosuppressives

| CELL TYPE | HOW AFFECTED |
| --- | --- |

### MONOCYTES

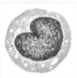

*Increased by:*
- ◆ Infections: subacute bacterial endocarditis, TB, hepatitis, malaria
- ◆ Collagen vascular disease: SLE, rheumatoid arthritis
- ◆ Carcinomas
- ◆ Monocytic leukemia
- ◆ Lymphomas

---

# *Wound culture*

Performed to confirm infection, a wound culture is a microscopic analysis of a specimen from a lesion. Wound cultures may be aerobic, for detection of organisms that usually appear in a superficial wound, or anaerobic, for organisms that need little or no oxygen and appear in areas of poor tissue perfusion, such as postoperative wounds, ulcers, and compound fractures. Indications for wound culture include fever as well as inflammation and drainage in damaged tissue.

## PURPOSE
- To identify an infectious microbe in a wound

## PATIENT PREPARATION
- Explain to the patient that the wound culture is used to identify infectious microbes.
- Describe the procedure, informing the patient that a drainage specimen from the wound is withdrawn by a syringe or removed on sterile cotton swabs.
- Tell the patient who will collect the specimen.

## PROCEDURE AND POSTTEST CARE
- Put on gloves, prepare a sterile field, and clean the area around the wound with antiseptic solution.
- For an aerobic culture, express the wound and swab as much exudate as possible, or insert the swab deeply into the wound and gently rotate. Immediately place the swab in the aerobic culture tube.
- For an anaerobic culture, insert the swab deeply into the wound, gently rotate, and immediately place the swab in the anaerobic culture tube. (See *Anaerobic specimen collector,* page 500.) Or, insert the needle into the wound, aspirate 1 to 5 ml of exudate into the syringe, and immediately inject the exudate into the anaerobic culture tube. If the needle is covered with a rubber stopper, the aspirate may be sent to the laboratory in the syringe.
- Record on the laboratory request recent antimicrobial therapy, the source of the specimen, and the suspected organism. Label the specimen container with the patient's name, the physician's name, the facility number, the wound site, and the time of collection.
- Dress the wound.

## PRECAUTIONS
- Clean the area around the wound thoroughly to limit contamination of the culture by normal skin flora, such as diphtheroids, *Staphylococcus epidermidis,* and alpha-hemolytic streptococci. Don't clean the area around a perineal wound.
- Make sure no antiseptic enters the wound.
- Obtain exudate from the entire wound, using more than one swab if necessary.
- Because some anaerobes die in the presence of even a small amount of oxygen, place the specimen in the culture tube quickly; take care that no air enters the tube; and check that double stoppers are secure.

# ANAEROBIC SPECIMEN COLLECTOR

Some anaerobes die when exposed to oxygen. To facilitate anaerobic collection and culturing, tubes filled with carbon dioxide ($CO_2$) or nitrogen are used for oxygen-free transport.

The anaerobic specimen collector shown here consists of a rubber-stopper tube filled with $CO_2$, a small inner tube, and a swab attached to a plastic plunger. The drawing below left shows the tube before specimen collection. The small inner tube containing the swab is held in place by the rubber stopper.

After specimen collection (below right), the swab is quickly replaced in the inner tube, and the plunger is depressed. This procedure separates the inner tube from the stopper, forcing it into the larger tube and exposing the specimen to the $CO_2$-rich environment.

The tube should be kept upright.

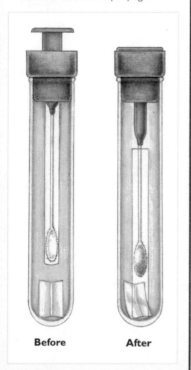

**Before**        **After**

● Keep the specimen container upright, and send it to the laboratory within 15 minutes to prevent growth or deterioration of microbes.

● Wear gloves during the procedure and when handling the specimen, and take necessary isolation precautions when sending the specimen to the laboratory.

## NORMAL FINDINGS
Normally, no pathogenic organisms are present in a clean wound.

## ABNORMAL FINDINGS
The most common aerobic pathogens for wound infection include *S. aureus,* group A beta-hemolytic streptococci, *Proteus, Escherichia coli* and other *Enterobacteriaceae,* and some *Pseudomonas* species; the most common anaerobic pathogens include some *Clostridium, Peptococcus, Bacteroides,* and *Streptococcus* species.

## INTERFERING FACTORS
● Failure to report recent or current antimicrobial therapy (possible false-negative)
● Use of inappropriate transport medium, allowing the specimen to dry and the bacteria to deteriorate

# SEXUAL ASSAULT TESTING

# QUICK-REFERENCE GUIDE
# TO LABORATORY TEST RESULTS

# SELECTED REFERENCES

# INDEX
—◆—

# SEXUAL ASSAULT TESTING

◆

Each facility or agency has a specific protocol for specimen collection in cases involving sexual assault. Specimens can be collected from various sources, including blood, hair, nails, tissues, and body fluids such as urine, semen, saliva, and vaginal secretions. In addition, evidence can be obtained from the results of diagnostic tests, such as computed tomography and radiography. Regardless of the protocol or specimen source, accurate and precise specimen collection is essential in conjunction with thorough, objective documentation because in many cases, this information will be used as evidence in legal proceedings.

Many institutions have a Sexual Assault Nurse Examiner (SANE) available to care for patients who are victims of sexual assault. SANEs are skilled rape crisis professionals who can evaluate the victim and collect specimens. They may also be called upon at a later date to testify in legal proceedings.

## GENERAL GUIDELINES FOR COLLECTING SPECIMENS

If you're responsible for collecting specimens in a sexual assault, follow these important guidelines:
- Be knowledgeable about your facility's policy and procedures for specimen collection in sexual assault cases.
- When obtaining specimens, be sure to collect them from the victim and, if possible, from the suspect.
- Check with local law enforcement agencies about additional specimens that may be needed; for example, trace evidence, such as soot, grass, gravel, glass, or other debris.
- Wear gloves and change them frequently; use disposable equipment and instruments if possible.
- Avoid coughing, sneezing, or talking over specimens or touching your face, nose, or mouth when collecting specimens.
- Include the victim's clothing as part of the collection procedure.
- Place all items collected in a paper bag.

⚠ **Alert**  *Never allow a specimen or item considered as evidence to be left unattended.*

- Document each item or specimen collected; have another person witness each collection and document it.
- Obtain photographs of all injuries for documentation.
- Include written documentation of the victim's physical and psychological condition on first encounter, throughout specimen collection, and afterward.

## PATIENT PREPARATION
- Assess the patient's ability to undergo the specimen collection procedure.
- Explain the procedures that the patient will undergo, what specimens will be collected and from where, and provide emotional support throughout.
- Obtain consent from the patient or family for specimens to be obtained.
- Ask patient if she would like someone, such as a family member, friend, or other person to stay with her during the specimen collection.
- Ensure patient privacy throughout the collection procedure.

## Specimen collection

When possible, obtain a special Sexual Assault Evidence Collection Kit, which contains the necessary items for specimen collection based on the evidence required by the local crime laboratory. In addition, the kit contains a form that's to be completed, signed, and dated by the examiner. Keep in mind that when collecting specimens for moist secretions, typically a one-swab technique is used; if secretions are dry, then a two-swab technique is used.

Before obtaining any specimens, inspect the genital area using a Wood's lamp. This device uses long wave ultraviolet light to scan the area for secretions and aids in identifying areas of trauma.

### Clothing for specimen collection
* Ask the patient to stand on a clean piece of examination paper if he or she is able to stand; if the patient can't stand, then have the patient remain on the examination table or bed.
* Have the patient remove each article of clothing, one at a time, and place each article in a separate, clean paper bag.
* If the clothing is wet, allow it to dry first before placing the item into the paper bag.

**Alert** *Never use plastic bags to collect clothing. Plastic promotes bacterial growth and can destroy DNA.*

* Fold the examination paper onto itself and place it into a clean paper bag.
* Fold over, seal, label, and initial each bag.

### Vaginal or cervical secretion collection
* Swab the vaginal area thoroughly with four swabs; swab the cervical area with two swabs, making sure to keep the vaginal swabs separate from the cervical swabs.
* Run the vaginal swabs over a slide (supplied in the kit) and allow the slide and swabs to air dry; do the same for the cervical swabs.
* Place the vaginal swabs in the swab container and close it; place the slide in the cardboard sleeve, close it and tape it shut; repeat this procedure for the cervical swabs.
* Place the swab container and cardboard sleeve into the envelope, and seal it securely.
* Complete the information as provided on the front of the envelope; if both vaginal and cervical swabs are obtained, use a separate envelope for each.

### Anal secretion collection
* Moisten a single swab with sterile water.
* Insert the swab gently into the patient's rectum approximately $1\frac{1}{4}''$ (3 cm).
* Rotate the swab gently and then remove it.
* Allow the swab to air dry and then place it in an envelope.
* Seal and label the envelope appropriately.

### Penile secretion collection
* Moisten a single swab with sterile water.
* Swab the entire external surface of the penis.
* Repeat this at least one more time (so that at least two swabs are obtained).
* Allow the swab to air dry and then place it in an envelope.
* Seal and label the envelope appropriately.

### Pubic hair collection
* Use the comb provided in the kit and comb through the pubic hair.
* Collect approximately 20 to 30 pubic hairs and place them in the envelope.
* Alternatively, obtain 20 to 30 plucked hairs from the patient; allow the patient the option of plucking own pubic hair.
* Place the hair in the envelope, seal and label it appropriately.

### Blood samples
* After performing a venipuncture, obtain at least 5 ml of blood in an EDTA tube.
* Write the patient's name and date on the label of the tube.
* Remove the DNA stain card from the kit and label it with the patient's name.
* Using the blood collected in this tube, withdraw 1 ml of blood and apply blood to each of the four circles on the card, completely filling each circle if possible.
* Let the card air dry and then place the card in the envelope.
* Seal and label the envelope appropriately.
* Place the blood tube into the tube holder supplied in the kit and seal the holder with tape supplied in the kit (may be referred to as evidence tape).

- Place the tube and holder in the zippered bag provided.
- Collect additional blood samples to test for pregnancy; sexually transmitted diseases, such as gonorrhea, chlamydia, and syphilis; or toxicology as appropriate and send to the laboratory immediately.

## Urine specimens
- Obtain a random urine specimen from the patient; if necessary, obtain the urine specimen via catheterization.

## SPECIMEN STORAGE AND TRANSPORT
- Refrigerate blood samples obtained.
- Place all other specimens in the specimen kit and keep the kit at room temperature.
- Give all the specimens to the police when they arrive.

## SPECIMEN CARE AFTER COLLECTION
- Be sure to follow the directions in the kit precisely to ensure that the chain of evidence is followed.
- Document all specimens collected, including type, location, time and patient's name, identification number and any other relevant information. Include photographs as appropriate, making sure to also include relevant information on the photo.
- Provide follow-up counseling and support to the patient.
- If necessary, administer ordered medications, such as tetanus or antibiotics.
- Make sure that the patient has a support person to accompany home.
- Arrange for referral to local support group or follow up with a trained counselor.

# QUICK-REFERENCE GUIDE TO LABORATORY TEST RESULTS

---

## A

**Acetylcholine receptor antibodies, serum**
Negative

**Acid mucopolysaccharides, urine**
Adults: <13.3 µg glucuronic acid/mg/creatinine/24 hours

**Acid phosphatase, serum**
0 to 3.7 U/L (SI, 0 to 3.7 U/L)

**Adrenocorticotropic hormone, plasma**
<120 pg/ml (SI, <26.4 pmol/L)

**Alanine aminotransferase**
8 to 50 IU/L (SI, 0.14 to 0.85 µkat/L)

**Aldosterone, serum**
● Supine individuals: 3 to 16 ng/dl (SI, 80 to 440 pmol/L)
● Upright individuals: 7 to 30 ng/dl (SI, 190 to 832 pmol/L)

**Aldosterone, urine**
3 to 19 µg/24 hours (SI, 8 to 51 nmol/d)

**Alkaline phosphatase, peritoneal fluid**
● Males >18 years: 90 to 239 U/L (SI, 90 to 239 U/L)
● Females <45 years: 76 to 196 U/L (SI, 76 to 196 U/L); >45 years: 87 to 250 U/L (87 to 250 U/L)

**Alkaline phosphatase, serum**
45 to 115 U/L (SI, 45 to 115 U/L)

**Alpha-fetoprotein serum**
Males and nonpregnant, females: <15 ng/ml (SI, <15 mg/L)

**Ammonia, peritoneal fluid**
<50 ng/dl (SI, <29 µmol/L)

**Amniotic fluid analysis**
● Lecithin-sphingomyelin ratio: >2
● Meconium: absent (except in breech presentation)
● Phosphatidylglycerol: present

**Amylase, peritoneal fluid**
138 to 404 U/L (SI, 138 to 404 U/L)

**Amylase, serum**
Adults ≥18 years: 26 to 102 U/L (SI, 0.4 to 1.74 µkat/L)

**Amylase, urine**
1 to 17 U/hour (SI, 0.017 to 0.29 µkat/h)

**Androstenedione (radioimmunoassay)**
● Males: 75 to 205 ng/dl (SI, 2.6 to 7.2 nmol/L)
● Females: 85 to 275 ng/dl (SI, 3.0 to 9.6 nmol/L)

**Angiotensin-converting enzyme**
Adults ≥ 20 years: 8 to 52 U/L (SI, 0.14 to 0.88 µkat/L)

**Anion gap**
8 to 14 mEq/L (SI, 8 to 14 mmol/L)

**Antibody screening, serum**
Negative

**Antidiuretic hormone, serum**
1 to 5 pg/ml (SI, 1 to 5 ng/L)

**Antiglobulin test, direct**
Negative

**Antimitochondrial antibodies, serum**
Negative

**Anti-smooth-muscle antibodies, serum**
Negative

**Antistreptolysin-O, serum**
- Preschoolers and adults: 85 Todd units/ml
- School-age children: 170 Todd units/ml

**Antithrombin III**
80% to 120% of normal control values

**Antithyroid antibodies, serum**
Normal titer <1:100

**Arginine test**
- Human growth hormone levels
- Males: increase to >10 ng/ml (SI, >10 µg/L)
- Females: increase to >15 ng/ml (SI, >15 µg/L)
- Children: increase to >48 ng/ml (SI, >48 µg/L)

**Arterial blood gases**
- pH: 7.35 to 7.45 (SI, 7.35 to 7.45)
- $PaO_2$: 80 to 100 mm Hg (SI, 10.6 to 13.3 kPa)
- $PaCO_2$: 35 to 45 mm Hg (SI, 4.7 to 5.3 kPa)
- $O_2$ CT: 15% to 23% (SI, 0.15 to 0.23)
- $SaO_2$: 94% to 100% (SI, 0.94 to 1.00)
- $HCO_3^-$: 22 to 25 mEq/L (SI, 22 to 25 mmol/L)

**Arylsufatase A, urine**
- Random: 16 to 42 mcg/g creatinine
- 24-hour: 0.37 to 3.60 mcg/day creatinine
- 1-hour test: 2 to 19 mcg/1 hour (SI, 2 to 19 µ/h)
- 2-hour test: 4 to 37 mcg/2 hours (SI, 4 to 37 µ/h)
- 24-hour test: 170 to 2,000 mcg/24 hours (SI, 2.89 to 34.0 µkat/L)

**Aspartate aminotransferase**
12 to 31 U/L (SI, 0.21 to 0.53 µkat/L)

**Aspergillosis antibody, serum**
Normal titer <1:8

**Atrial natriuretic factor, plasma**
20 to 77 pg/ml

## B

**Bacterial meningitis antigen**
Negative

**Bence Jones protein, urine**
Negative

**Beta-hydroxybutyrate**
<0.4 mmol/L (SI, 0.4 mmol/L)

**Bilirubin, amniotic fluid**
- Early: <0.075 mg/dl (SI, <1.3 µmol/L)
- Term: <0.025 mg/dl (SI, <0.41 µmol/L)

**Bilirubin, serum**
- Adults
- Direct: <0.5 mg/dl (SI, <6.8 µmol/L)
- Indirect: 1.1 mg/dl (SI, 19 µmol/L)
- Neonates
- Total: 1 to 12 mg/dl (SI, 34 to 205 µmol/L)

**Bilirubin, urine**
Negative

**Blastomycosis antibody, serum**
Normal titer <1:8

**Bleeding time**
- Template: 3 to 6 minutes (SI, 3 to 6 m)
- Ivy: 3 to 6 minutes (SI, 3 to 6 m)
- Duke: 1 to 3 minutes (SI, 1 to 3 m)

**Blood urea nitrogen**
8 to 20 mg/dl (SI, 2.9 to 7.5 mmol/L)

**B-lymphocyte count**
270 to 640/µl

## C

**Calcitonin, plasma**
- Baseline
- Males: < 16 pg/ml (SI, < 16 ng/L)
- Females: < 8 pg/ml (SI, < 8 ng/L)

**Calcium, serum**
- Adults: 8.2 to 10.2 mg/dl (SI, 2.05 to 2.54 mmol/L)
- Children: 8.6 to 11.2 mg/dl (SI, 2.15 to 2.79 mmol/L)
- Ionized: 4.65 to 5.28 mg/dl (SI, 1.1 to 1.25 mmol/L)

**Calcium, urine**
100 to 300 mg/24 hours (SI, 2.50 to 7.50 mmol/d)

**Candida antibodies, serum**
Negative

### Capillary fragility

| Petechiae per 5 cm: | Score: |
|---|---|
| 11 to 20 | 2+ |
| 21 to 50 | 3+ |
| over 50 | 4+ |

### Carbon dioxide, total, blood
22 to 26 mEq/L (SI, 22 to 26 mmol/L)

### Carcinoembryonic antigen, serum
<5 ng/ml (SI, <5 mg/L)

### Catecholamines, plasma
- Supine
- Epinephrine: undetectable to 110 pg/ml (SI, undetectable to 600 pmol/L)
- Norepinephrine: 70 to 750 pg/ml (SI, 413 to 4,432 pmol/L)
- Standing
- epinephrine: undetectable to 140 pg/ml (SI, undetectable to 764 pmol/L)
- norepinephrine: 200 to 1,700 pg/ml (SI, 1,182 to 10,047 pmol/L)

### Catecholamines, urine
- Epinephrine: 0 to 20 mcg/24 hours (SI, 0 to 109 nmol/24 h)
- Norepinephrine: 15 to 80 mcg/24 hours (SI, 89 to 473 nmol/24 h)
- Dopamine: 65 to 400 mcg/24 hours (SI, 425 to 2,610 nmol/24 h)

### Cerebrospinal fluid
- Pressure: 50 to 180 mm $H_2O$
- Appearance: clear, colorless
- Gram stain: no organisms

### Ceruloplasmin, serum
22.9 to 43.1 mg/dl (SI, 0.22 to 0.43 g/L)

### Chloride, cerebrospinal fluid
118 to 130 mEq/L (SI, 118 to 130 mmol/L)

### Chloride, serum
100 to 108 mEq/L (SI, 100 to 108 mmol/L)

### Chloride, urine
- Adults: 110 to 250 mmol/24 hours (SI, 110 to 250 mmol/d)
- Children: 15 to 40 mmol/24 hours (SI, 15 to 40 mmol/d)
- Infants: 2 to 10 mmol/24 hours (SI, 2 to 10 mmol/d)

### Cholinesterase (pseudocholinesterase)
204 to 532 IU/dl (SI, 2.04 to 5.32 kU/L)

### Coccidioidomycosis antibody, serum
Normal titer <1:2

### Cold agglutinins, serum
Normal titer <1:64

### Complement, serum
- Total
- 40 to 90 U/ml (SI, 0.4 to 0.9 g/L)
- C3
- Males: 80 to 180 mg/dl (SI, 0.8 to 1.8 g/L)
- Females: 76 to 120 mg/dl (SI, 0.76 to 1.2 g/L)
- C4
- Males: 15 to 60 mg/dl (SI, 0.15 to 0.6 g/L)
- Females: 15 to 52 mg/dl (SI, 0.15 to 0.52 g/L)

### Copper, urine
3 to 35 mcg/24 hours (SI, 0.05 to 0.55 µmol/d)

### Cortisol, free, urine
<50 µg/24 hours (SI, <138 nmol/d)

### Cortisol, plasma
- Morning: 7 to 25 mcg/dl (SI, 0.2 to 0.7 µmol/L)
- Afternoon: 2 to 14 mcg/dl (SI, 0.06 to 0.39 µmol/L)

### C-reactive protein, serum
<0.8 mg/dl (SI, <8 mg/L)

### Creatine kinase
Total
- Males: 55 to 170 U/L (SI, 0.94 to 2.89 µkat/L)
- Females: 30 to 135 U/L (SI, 0.51 to 2.3 µkat/L)

### Creatinine clearance
- Males: 94 to 140 ml/min/1.73 m² (SI, 0.91 to 1.35 ml/s/m²)
- Females: 72 to 110 ml/min/1.73 m² (SI, 0.69 to 1.06 ml/s/m²)

### Creatinine, serum
- Males: 0.8 to 1.2 mg/dl (SI, 62 to 115 µmol/L)
- Females: 0.6 to 0.9 mg/dl (SI, 53 to 97 µmol/L)

### Creatinine, urine
- Males: 14 to 26 mg/kg body weight/24 hours (SI, 124 to 230 µmol/kg body weight/d)
- Females: 11 to 20 mg/kg body weight/24 hours (SI, 97 to 177 µmol/kg body weight/d)

### Cryoglobulins, serum
Negative

### Cyclic adenosine monophosphate, urine
- 0.3 to 3.6 mg/day (SI, 100 to 723 µmol/d)
or

- 0.29 to 2.1 mg/g creatinine (SI, 100 to 723 µmol/mol creatinine)

### Cytomegalovirus antibodies, serum
Negative

## D

### D-xylose absorption
- Blood
- Adults: 25 to 40 mg/dl in 2 hours
- Children: >30 mg/dl in 1 hour
- Urine
- Adults: >3.5 g excreted in 5 hours (age 65 of older, >5 g in 24 hours)
- Children: 16% to 33% excreted in 5 hours

## E

### Epstein-Barr virus antibodies
Negative

### Erythrocyte sedimentation rate
- Males: 0 to 10 mm/hour (SI, 0 to 10 mm/h)
- Females: 0 to 20 mm/hour (SI, 0 to 20 mm/h)

### Esophageal acidity
pH >5.0

### Estrogens, serum
- Females
- Menstruating: 26 to 149 pg/ml (SI, 90 to 550 pmol/L)
- Postmenopausal: 0 to 34 pg/ml (SI, 0 to 125 pmol/L)
- Males
- 12 to 34 pg/ml (SI, 40 to 125 pmol/L)
- Children
- <6 years: 3 to 10 pg/ml (SI, 10 to 36 pmol/L)

### Euglobulin lysis time
2 to 4 hours (SI, 2 to 4 h)

## F

### Factor assay, one-stage
50% to 150% of normal activity (SI, 0.50 to 1.50)

### Febrile agglutination, serum
- Salmonella antibody: <1:80
- Brucellosis antibody: <1:80
- Tularemia antibody: <1:40
- Rickettsial antibody: <1:40

### Ferritin, serum
- Males
- 20 to 300 ng/ml (SI, 20 to 300 µg/L)
- Females
- 20 to 120 ng/ml (SI, 20 to 120 µg/L)
- Infants
- 1 month: 200 to 600 ng/ml (SI, 200 to 600 µg/L)
- 2 to 5 months: 50 to 200 ng/ml (SI, 50 to 200 µg/L)
- 6 months to 15 years: 7 to 140 ng/ml (SI, 7 to 140 µg/L)
- Neonates
- 25 to 200 ng/ml (SI, 25 to 200 µg/L)

### Fibrinogen, plasma
200 to 400 mg/dl (SI, 2 to 4 g/L)

### Fibrin split products
- Screening assay: <10 mcg/ml (SI, <10 mg/L)
- Quantitative assay: <3 mcg/ml (SI, <3 mg/L)

### Fluorescent treponemal antibody absorption, serum
Negative

### Folic acid, serum
1.8 to 20 ng/ml (SI, 4 to 45.3 nmol/L)

### Follicle-stimulating hormone, serum
- Menstruating females
- Follicular phase: 5 to 20 mIU/ml (SI, 5 to 20 IU/L)
- Ovulatory phase: 15 to 30 mIU/ml (SI, 15 to 30 IU/L)
- Luteal phase: 5 to 15 mIU/ml (SI, 5 to 15 IU/L)
- Menopausal females
- 5 to 100 mIU/ml (SI, 50 to 100 IU/L)
- Males
- 5 to 20 mIU/ml (5 to 20 IU/L)

### Free thyroxine, serum
0.9 to 2.3 ng/dl (SI, 10 to 30 nmol/L)

### Free triiodothyronine
0.2 to 0.6 ng/dl (SI, 0.003 to 0.009 nmol/L)

## G

### Galactose 1-phosphate uridyl transferase
- Qualitative: negative
- Quantitative: 18.5 to 28.5 U/g of hemoglobin

### Gamma-glutamyltransferase
- Males ≥16 years: 6 to 38 U/L (SI, 0.10 to 0.63 µkat/L)

- Females 16 to 45 years: 4 to 27 U/L (SI, 0.08 to 0.46 µkat/L); >45 years: 6 to 38 U/L (SI, 0.10 to 0.63 µkat/L)
- Children: 3 to 30 U/L (SI, 0.05 to 0.51 µkat)

**Gastric acid stimulation**
- Males: 18 to 28 mEq/hour
- Females: 11 to 21 mEq/hour

**Gastric secretion, basal**
- Males: 1 to 5 mEq/hour
- Females: 0.2 to 3.3 mEq/hour

**Gastrin, serum**
50 to 150 pg/ml (SI, 50 to 150 ng/L)

**Globulin, peritoneal fluid**
30% to 45% of total protein

**Glucose, amniotic fluid**
<45 mg/dl (SI, <2.3 mmol/L)

**Glucose, cerebrospinal fluid**
50 to 80 mg/dl (SI, 2.8 to 4.4 mmol/L)

**Glucose, peritoneal fluid**
70 to 100 mg/dl (SI, 3.5 to 5 mmol/L)

**Glucose, plasma, fasting**
70 to 100 mg/dl (SI, 3.9 to 6.1 mmol/L)

**Glucose-6-phosphate dehydrogenase**
4.3 to 11.8 U/g (SI, 0.28 to 0.76 mU/mol) of hemoglobin

**Glucose tolerance, oral**
Peak at 160 to 180 mg/dl (SI, 8.8 to 9.9 mmol/L) 30 to 60 minutes after challenge dose

**Growth hormone suppression**
Undetectable to 3 ng/ml (SI, undetectable to 3 µg/L) after 30 minutes to 2 hours

# H

**Ham test**
Negative

**Haptoglobin, serum**
40 to 180 mg/dl (SI, 0.4 to 1.8 g/L)

**Heinz bodies**
Negative

**Hematocrit**
- Males
- 42% to 52% (SI, 0.42 to 0.52)
- Females

- 36% to 48% (SI, 0.36 to 0.48)
- Children
- 10 years: 36% to 40% (SI, 0.36 to 0.40)
- Infants
- 3 months: 30% to 36% (SI, 0.30 to 0.36)
- 1 year: 29% to 41% (SI, 0.29 to 0.41)
- Neonates
- At birth: 55% to 68% (SI, 0.55 to 0.68)
- 1 week: 47% to 65% (SI, 0.47 to 0.65)
- 1 month: 37% to 49% (SI, 0.37 to 0.49)

**Hemoglobin (Hb) electrophoresis**
- Hb A: 95% (SI, 0.95)
- Hb $A_2$: 1.5% to 3% (SI, 0.015 to 0.03)
- Hb F: <2% (SI, <0.02)

**Hemoglobin, unstable**
- Heat stability: negative
- Isopropanol: stable

**Hemoglobin, urine**
Negative

**Hemosiderin, urine**
Negative

**Hepatitis B surface antigen, serum**
Negative

**Herpes simplex antibodies, serum**
Negative

**Heterophil agglutination, serum**
Normal titer <1:56

**Hexosaminidase A and B, serum**
Total: 5 to 12.9 U/L (hexosaminidase A constitutes 55% to 76% of total)

**Histoplasmosis antibody, serum**
Normal titer <1:8

**Homovanillic acid, urine**
<10 mg/24 hours (SI, <55 µmol/d)

**Human chorionic gonadotropin, serum**
<4 IU/L

**Human chorionic gonadotropin, urine**
- Pregnant women
- First trimester: 500,000 IU/24 hours
- Second trimester: 10,000 to 25,000 IU/24 hours
- Third trimester: 5,000 to 15,000 IU/24 hours

**Human growth hormone, serum**
- Males: undetectable to 5 ng/ml (SI, undetectable to 5 µg/L)

- Females: undetectable to 10 ng/ml (SI, undetectable to 10 µg/L)
- Children: undetectable to 16 ng/ml (SI, undetectable to 16 µg/L)

**Human immunodeficiency virus antibody, serum**
Negative

**Human placental lactogen, serum**
- Males and nonpregnant females: <0.5 µg/ml
- Pregnant females at term: 9 to 11 µg/ml

**17-hydroxycorticosteroids, urine**
- Males
- 4.5 to 12 mg/24 hours (SI, 12.4 to 33.1 µmol/d)
- Females
- 2.5 to 10 mg/24 hours (SI, 6.9 to 27.6 µmol/d)
- Children
- 8 to 12 years: <4.5 mg/24 hours (SI, < 12.4 µmol/d)
- <8 years: <1.5 mg/24 hours (SI, <4.14 µmol/d)

**5-hydroxyindoleacetic acid, urine**
2 to 7 mg/24 hours (SI, 10.4 to 36.6 µmol/d)

**Hydroxyproline, total, urine**
1 to 9 mg/24 hours (SI, 1.0 to 3.4 IU/d)

## I J

**Immune complex, serum**
Negative

**Immunoglobulins (Ig), serum**
- IgG: 800 to 1,800 mg/dl (SI, 8 to 18 g/L)
- IgA: 100 to 400 mg/dl (SI, 1 to 4 g/L)
- IgM: 55 to 150 mg/dl (SI, 0.55 to 1.5 g/L)

**Insulin, serum**
0 to 35 µU/ml (SI, 144 to 243 pmol/L)

**Insulin tolerance test**
10- to 20-ng/dl (SI, 10- to 20-µg/L) increase over baseline levels of human growth hormone and adrenocorticotropic hormone

**Iron, serum**
- Males: 65 to 175 mcg/dl (SI, 11.6 to 31.3 µmol/L)
- Females: 50 to 170 mcg/dl (SI, 9 to 30.4 µmol/L)

**Iron, total binding capacity, serum**
300 to 360 mcg/dl (SI, 54 to 64 µmol/L)

## K

**17-ketogenic steroids, urine**
- Males: 4 to 14 mg/24 hours (SI, 13 to 49 µmol/d)
- Females: 2 to 12 mg/24 hours (SI, 7 to 42 µmol/d)
- Children
- Infants to 11 years: 0.1 to 4 mg/24 hours (SI, 0.3 to 14 µmol/d)
- 11 to 14 years: 2 to 9 mg/24 hours (SI, 7 to 31 µmol/d)

**Ketones, urine**
Negative

**17-ketosteroids, urine**
- Males: 10 to 25 mg/24 hours (SI, 35 to 87 µmol/d)
- Females: 4 to 6 mg/24 hours (SI, 4 to 21 µmol/d)
- Children
- Infants to 10 years: <3 mg/24 hours (SI, < 10 µmol/d)
- 10 to 14 years: 1 to 6 mg/24 hours (SI, 2 to 21 µmol/d)

## L

**Lactate dehydrogenase (LD)**
- Total: 71 to 207 IU/L (SI, 1.2 to 3.52 µkat/L)
- $LD_1$: 14% to 26% (SI, 0.14 to 0.26)
- $LD_2$: 29% to 39% (SI, 0.29 to 0.39)
- $LD_3$: 20% to 26% (SI, 0.20 to 0.26)
- $LD_4$: 8% to 16% (SI, 0.08 to 0.16)
- $LD_5$: 6% to 16% (SI, 0.06 to 0.16)

**Lactic acid, blood**
0.5 to 2.2 mEq/L (SI, 0.5 to 2.2 mmol/L)

**Leucine aminopeptidase**
- Males: 80 to 200 U/ml (SI, 80 to 200 kU/L)
- Females: 75 to 185 U/ml (SI, 75 to 185 kU/L)

**Leukoagglutinins**
Negative

**Lipase, serum**
10 to 73 U/L (SI, 0.17 to 1.24 µkat/L)

**Lipids, fecal**
Constitute <20% of excreted solids; <7 g excreted in 24 hours

### Lipoproteins, serum
- High-density lipoprotein cholesterol
- Males: 37 to 70 mg/dl (SI, 0.96 to 1.8 mmol/L)
- Females: 40 to 85 mg/dl (SI, 1.03 to 2.2 mmol/L)
- Low-density lipoprotein cholesterol:
- In individuals who don't have coronary artery disease: <130 mg/dl (SI, <3.36 mmol/L)

### Long-acting thyroid stimulator, serum
Negative

### Lupus erythematosus cell preparation
Negative

### Luteinizing hormone, serum
- Menstruating women
- Follicular phase: 5 to 15 mIU/ml (SI, 5 to 15 IU/L)
- Ovulatory phase: 30 to 60 mIU/ml (SI, 30 to 60 IU/L)
- Luteal phase: 5 to 15 mIU/ml (SI, 5 to 15 IU/L)
- Postmenopausal women
- 50 to 100 mIU/ml (SI, 50 to 100 IU/L)
- Males
- 5 to 20 mIU/ml (SI, 5 to 20 IU/L)
- Children
- 4 to 20 mIU/ml (SI, 4 to 20 IU/L)

### Lyme disease serology
Nonreactive

### Lysozyme, urine
0 to 3 mg/24 hours

## M

### Magnesium, serum
1.3 to 2.1 mg/dl (SI, 0.65 to 1.05 mmol/L)

### Magnesium, urine
6 to 10 mEq/24 hours (SI, 3 to 5 mmol/d)

### Manganese, serum
0.4 to 1.4 mcg/ml

### Melanin, urine
Negative

### Myoglobin, urine
Negative

## N

### 5'-nucleotidase
2 to 17 U/L (SI, 0.034 to 0.29 μkat/L)

## O

### Occult blood, fecal
<2.5 ml

### Oxalate, urine
≤40 mg/24 hours (SI, ≤ 456 μmol/d)

## PQ

### Parathyroid hormone, serum
- Intact: 10 to 50 pg/ml (SI, 1.1 to 5.3 pmol/L)
- N-terminal fraction: 8 to 24 pg/ml (SI, 0.8 to 2.5 pmol/L)
- C-terminal fraction: 0 to 340 pg/ml (SI, 0 to 35.8 pmol/L)

### Partial thromboplastin time
21 to 35 seconds (SI, 21 to 35 s)

### Pericardial fluid
- Amount: 10 to 50 ml
- Appearance: clear, straw-colored
- White blood cell count: <1,000/μl (SI, <1.0 × 10⁹/L)
- Glucose: approximately whole blood level

### Peritoneal fluid
- Amount: <50 ml
- Appearance: clear, straw-colored

### Phenylalanine, serum
<2 mg/dl (SI, <121 μmol/L)

### Phosphates, serum
- Adults: 2.7 to 4.5 mEq/L (SI, 0.87 to 1.45 mmol/L)
- Children: 4.5 to 6.7 mEq/L (SI, 1.45 to 1.78 mmol/L)

### Phosphates, urine
<1,000 mg/24 hours

### Phospholipids, plasma
180 to 320 mg/dl (SI, 1.80 to 3.20 g/L)

### Phosphate, tubular reabsorption, urine and plasma
80% reabsorption

### Plasma renin activity
- Normal sodium diet: 1.1 to 4.1 ng/ml/hour (SI, 0.30 to 1.14 ng LS)
- Restricted sodium diet: 6.2 to 12.4 ng/ml/hour (SI, 1.72 to 3.44 ng LS)

**Plasminogen, plasma**
80% to 130%

**Platelet aggregation**
3 to 5 minutes (SI, 3 to 5 m)

**Platelet count**
- Adults: 140,000 to 400,000/µl (SI, 140 to 400 × 10⁹/L)
- Children: 150,000 to 450,000/µl (SI, 150 to 450 × 10⁹/L)

**Potassium, serum**
3.5 to 5 mEq/L (SI, 3.5 to 5 mmol/L)

**Potassium, urine**
- Adults: 25 to 125 mmol/24 hours (SI, 25 to 125 mmol/d)
- Children: 22 to 57 mmol/24 hours (SI, 22 to 57 mmol/d)

**Pregnanediol, urine**
- Nonpregnant females
- 0.5 to 1.5 mg/24 hours (during the follicular phase of the menstrual cycle)
- Pregnant females
- First trimester: 10 to 30 mg/24 hours
- Sesscond trimester: 35 to 70 mg/24 hours
- Third trimester: 70 to 100 mg/24 hours
- Postmenopausal females
- 0.2 to 1 mg/24 hours
- Males
- 0 to 1 mg/24 hours

**Pregnanetriol, urine**
- Males ≥16 years: 0.4 to 2.5 mg/24 hours (SI, 1.2 to 7.5 µmol/d)
- Females ≥16 years: 0 to 1.8 mg/ hours (SI, 0.3 to 5.3 µmol/d)

**Progesterone, plasma**
- Menstruating females
- Follicular phase: <150 ng/dl (SI, <5 nmol/L)
- Luteal phase: 300 to 1,200 ng/dl (SI, 10 to 40 nmol/L)
- Pregnant women
- First trimester: 1,500 to 5,000 ng/dl (SI, 50 to 160 nmol/L)
- Second and third trimesters: 8,000 to 20,000 ng/dl (SI, 250 to 650 nmol/L)

**Prolactin, serum**
Undetectable to 23 ng/ml (SI, undetectable to 23 µg/L)

**Prostate-specific antigen**
- 40 to 50 years: 2 to 2.8 ng/ml (SI, 2 to 2.8 µg/L)

- 51 to 60 years: 2.9 to 3.8 ng/ml (SI, 2.9 to 3.8 µg/L)
- 61 to 70 years: 4 to 5.3 ng/ml (SI, 4 to 5.3 µg/L)
- ≥71 years: 5.6 to 7.2 ng/ml (SI, 5.6 to 7.2 µg/L)

**Protein, cerebrospinal fluid**
15 to 50 mg/dl (SI, 0.15 to 0.5 g/L)

**Protein C, plasma**
70% to 140% (SI, 0.70 to 1.40)

**Protein, total, peritoneal fluid**
0.3 to 4.1 g/dl (SI, 3 to 41 g/L)

**Protein, urine**
50 to 80 mg/24 hours (SI, 50 to 80 mg/d)

**Prothrombin time**
10 to 14 seconds (10 to 14 s)

**Pulmonary artery pressures**
- Right atrial: 1 to 6 mm Hg
- Left atrial: approximately 10 mm Hg
- Systolic: 20 to 30 mm Hg
- Systolic right ventricular: 20 to 30 mm Hg
- Diastolic: 10 to 15 mm Hg
- End-diastolic right ventricular: <5 mm Hg
- Mean: <20 mm Hg
- Pulmonary artery wedge pressure: 6 to 12 mm Hg

**Pyruvate kinase**
- Ultraviolet: 9 to 22 U/g of hemoglobin
- Low substrate assay: 1.7 to 6.8 U/g of hemoglobin

**Pyruvic acid, blood**
0.08 to 0.16 mEq/L (SI, 0.08 to 0.16 mmol/L)

# R

**Red blood cell count**
- Males: 4.2 to 5.4 × 10⁶/mm³ (SI, 4.2 to 5.4 × 10¹²/L)
- Females: 3.6 to 5 × 10⁶/mm³ (SI, 3.6 to 5 × 10¹²/L)
- Neonates: 4.4 to 5.8 million/µl (SI, 4.4 to 5.8 × 10¹²/L)
- 2 months: 3 to 3.8 million/µl (SI, 3 to 3.8 × 10¹²/L) (increasing slowly)
- Children: 4.6 to 4.8 million/µl (SI, 4.6 to 4.8 × 10¹²/L)

**Red blood cell survival time**
25 to 35 days

**Red blood cells, urine**
0 to 3 per high-power field

**Red cell indices**
- Mean corpuscular volume: 84 to 99 $\mu m^3$ (SI, 84 to 99 fL)
- Mean corpuscular hemoglobin: 26 to 32 pg/cell (SI, 0.40 to 0.53 fmol/cell)
- Mean corpuscular hemoglobin concentration: 30 to 36 g/dl (SI, 300 to 360 g/L)

**Respiratory syncytial virus antibodies, serum**
Negative

**Reticulocyte count**
- Adults: 0.5% to 2.5% (SI, 0.005 to 0.025)
- Infants (at birth): 2% to 6% (SI, 0.02 to 0.06), decreasing to adult levels in 1 to 2 weeks

**Rheumatoid factor, serum**
Negative or titer <1:20

**Ribonucleoprotein antibodies**
Negative

**Rubella antibodies, serum**
Titer of 1:8 or less indicates little or no immunity; titer more than 1:10 indicates adequate protection against rubella

## S

**Semen analysis**
- Volume: 0.7 to 6.5 ml
- pH: 7.3 to 7.9
- Liquefaction: within 20 minutes
- Sperm count: 20 to 150 million/ml

**Sickle cell test**
Negative

**Sjögren's antibodies**
Negative

**Sodium chloride, urine**
110 to 250 mEq/L (SI, 100 to 250 mmol/d)

**Sodium, serum**
135 to 145 mEq/L (SI, 135 to 145 mmol/L)

**Sodium, urine**
- Adults: 40 to 220 mEq/L/24 hours (SI, 40 to 220 mmol/d)
- Children: 41 to 115 mEq/L/24 hours (SI, 41 to 115 mmol/d)

**Sporotrichosis antibody, serum**
Normal titers <1:40

## T

**Terminal deoxynucleotidyl transferase, serum**
- Bone marrow: <2%
- Blood: undetectable

**Testosterone, plasma or serum**
- Males: 300 to 1,200 ng/dl (SI, 10.4 to 41.6 nmol/L)
- Females: 20 to 80 ng/dl (SI, 0.7 to 2.8 nmol/L)

**Thrombin time, plasma**
10 to 15 seconds (10 to 15 s)

**Thyroid-stimulating hormone, neonatal**
- ≤ 2 days: 25 to 30 µIU/ml (SI, 25 to 30 mU/L)
- >2 days: <25 µIU/ml (SI, <25 mU/L)

**Thyroid-stimulating hormone, serum**
Undetectable to 15 µIU/ml (SI, undetectable to 15 mU/L)

**Thyroid-stimulating immunoglobulin, serum**
Negative

**Thyroxine, total, serum**
5 to 13.5 mcg/dl (SI, 60 to 165 nmol/L)

**T-lymphocyte count**
1,500 to 3,000/µl

**Transferrin, serum**
200 to 400 mg/dl (SI, 2 to 4 g/L)

**Triglycerides, serum**
- Males: 44 to 180 mg/dl (SI, 0.44 to 2.01 mmol/L)
- Females: 11 to 190 mg/dl (SI, 0.11 to 2.21 mmol/L)

**Triiodothyronine, serum**
80 to 200 ng/dl (SI, 1.2 to 3 nmol/L)

## U

**Uric acid, serum**
- Males: 3.4 to 7 mg/dl (SI, 202 to 416 µmol/L)
- Females: 2.3 to 6 mg/dl (SI, 143 to 357 µmol/L)

**Uric acid, urine**
250 to 750 mg/24 hours (SI, 1.48 to
4.43 mmol/d)

**Urinalysis, routine**
- Color: straw to dark yellow
- Appearance: clear
- Specific gravity: 1.005 to 1.035
- pH: 4.5 to 8.0
- Epithelial cells: 0 to 5 per high-power field
- Casts: none, except 1 to 2 hyaline casts per low-power field
- Crystals: present

**Urine osmolality**
- 24-hour urine: 300 to 900 mOsm/kg
- Random urine: 50 to 1,400 mOsm/kg

**Urobilinogen, fecal**
50 to 300 mg/24 hours (SI, 100 to 400 EU/100 g)

**Urobilinogen, urine**
- 0.1 to 0.8 EU/2 hours (SI 0.1 to 0.8 EU/2 h)
or
- 0.5 to 4.0 EU/24 hours (SI, 0.5 to 4.0 EU/d)

**Uroporphyrinogen I synthase**
≥7 nmol/second/L

# V

**Vanillylmandelic acid, urine**
1.4 to 6.5 mg/24 hours (SI, 7 to 33 µmol/day)

**Venereal Disease Research Laboratory test, cerebrospinal fluid**
Negative

**Venereal Disease Research Laboratory test, serum**
Negative

**Vitamin A, serum**
30 to 80 mcg/dl (SI, 1.05 to 2.8 µmol/L)

**Vitamin $B_2$, serum**
3 to 15 mcg/dl

**Vitamin $B_{12}$, serum**
200 to 900 pg/ml (SI, 148 to 664 pmol/L)

**Vitamin C, plasma**
0.2 to 2 mg/dl (SI, 11 to 114 µmol/L)

**Vitamin C, urine**
30 mg/24 hours

**Vitamin $D_3$, serum**
10 to 60 ng/ml (SI, 25 to 150 nmol/L)

# WXY

**White blood cell count, blood**
4,000 to 10,000/µl (SI, 4 to 10 × $10^9$/L)

**White blood cell count, peritoneal fluid**
<300/µl (SI, <300 × $10^9$/L)

**White blood cell count, urine**
0 to 4 per high-power field

**White blood cell differential, blood**
- Adults
  - Neutrophils: 54% to 75% (SI, 0.54 to 0.75)
  - Lymphocytes: 25% to 40% (SI, 0.25 to 0.40)
  - Monocytes: 2% to 8% (SI, 0.02 to 0.08)
  - Eosinophils: 1% to 4% (SI, 0.01 to 0.04)
  - Basophils: 0 to 1% (SI, 0 to 0.01)

# Z

**Zinc, serum**
70 to 120 mcg/dl (SI, 10.7 to 18.4 µmol/L)

# SELECTED REFERENCES

American Cancer Society. Detailed Guide: Can Cervical Cancer Be Prevented? Available at: *www.cancer.org/docroot/CRI/content/CRI_2_4_2X_Can_cervical_cancer_be_prevented_8.asp.*

Anderson, S.C., and Poulsen, K.B. *Anderson's Atlas of Hematology.* Philadelphia: Lippincott Williams & Williams, 2004.

Behrman, R.E., et al., eds. *Nelson Textbook of Pediatrics,* 17th ed. Philadelphia: W.B. Saunders Co., 2004.

Bishop, M.L., et.al. *Clinical Chemistry,* 5th ed. Philadelphia: Lippincott Williams & Wilkins, 2005.

Black, J.M. *Medical-Surgical Nursing,* 7th ed. Philadelphia: W.B. Saunders Co., 2005.

Bradwell, A.R., et al. "Serum Test for Assessment of Patients with Bence-Jones Myeloma," *Lancet* 361(9356):489-91, February 2003.

Bren, L. *Cervical Cancer Screening.* FDA Consumer Magazine. January-February 2004. Available at: *www.fda.gov/fdac/features/2004/104_cancer.html.*

Cavanaugh, B.M. *Nurse's Manual of Laboratory and Diagnostic Tests,* 4th ed. Philadelphia: F.A. Davis Co., 2003.

Clark, P.M. *Ductal Lavage: A New Look Inside the Breast.* Available at: *www.cancernews.com/data/Article/223.asp.*

Cunningham, F.G., et al. *Williams Obstetrics,* 22nd ed. New York: McGraw-Hill Professional, 2005.

DeGroot, L., and Jameson, J.L., eds. *Endocrinology,* 5th ed. Philadelphia: W.B. Saunders Co., 2006.

*Digene's Hypbrid Capture ® 2HPV DNA Test Frequently Asked Questions.* Available at: *www.thehptest.com.*

Fischbach, F.T. *A Manual of Laboratory and Diagnostic Tests,* 7th ed. Philadelphia: Lippincott Williams & Wilkins, 2004.

Food and Drug Administration. *FDA Approves First DNA-Based Test to Detect Cystic Fibrosis.* FDA News. May 9, 2005. Available at: *www.fda.gov/bbs/topics/NEWS/2005/NEW01178.html.*

Forbes, B., et al. *Bailey and Scott's Diagnostic Microbiology,* 11th ed. St. Louis: Mosby–Year Book, Inc., 2002.

Gilkeson, R.C., and Ciancibello, L. "Virtual Bronchoscopy: Technical Features and Clinical Applications," *Applied Radiology* 32(4), May 2003. *www.medscape.com/viewarticle/452491.*

Goldman, L., and Ausiello, D., eds. *Cecil Textbook of Medicine,* 22nd ed. Philadelphia: W.B. Saunders Co., 2004.

Goodin, L.J. *Gastroesophageal Reflux Imaging and Function Study.* Available at: *www3.sympatical.ca/lgoodin/nmgi/reflux/gi_reflx.htm.*

Greenspan, F.S., and Gardner, D.G. *Basic and Clinical Endocrinology,* 7th ed. Stamford, Conn.: Appleton & Lange, 2004.

Gonzalez-Arriaza, H.L., and Bostwick, J.M. "Acute Porphyrias: A Case Report and Review," *American Journal of Psychiatry* 160(3):450-59, March 2003.

Greci, L.S., et al. "Utility of HbA$_{1c}$ Levels for Diabetes Case Finding in Hospitalized Patients with Hyperglycemia," *Diabetes Care* 26(4):1064-68, April 2003.

Guyton, A.C., and Hall, J.E. *Textbook of Medical Physiology,* 12th ed. Philadelphia: W.B. Saunders Co., 2006.

Hanson, K.A. "Diagnostic Tests and Tools in the Evaluation of Urologic Disease: Part

II," *Urologic Nursing* 23(6):405-15, December 2003.

Hanratty, K., et al., eds. *Obstetrics Illustrated,* 6th ed. St. Louis: Mosby–Year Book, Inc., 2003.

Oweala, O. "HIV Diagnostic Tests: An Overview," *Contraception* 70(2): 141-47, August 2004.

Kasper, D., et al., eds. *Harrison's Principles of Internal Medicine,* 16th ed. New York: McGraw-Hill Book Co., 2005.

Kneale, J., et al. *Orthopaedic Nursing: Elective and Emergency Management,* 2nd ed. London: Churchill Livingstone, 2005.

Lynes, D. "An Introduction to Blood Gas Analysis," *Nursing Times* 99(11):54-55, March 2003.

Mensink, R.P., et al. "Effects of Dietary Fatty Acids and Carbohydrates on the Ratio of Serum Total to HDL Cholesterol and on Serum Lipids and Apolipoprotein: A Meta-analysis of 60 Controlled Trials," *American Journal of Clinical Nutrition* 77(5):1146-55, May 2003.

Monsaingeon, M., et al. "Comparative Values of Catecholamines and Metabolites for the Diagnosis of Neuroblastoma," *European Journal of Pediatrics* 162(6):397-402, June 2003.

Nettina, S. *The Lippincott Manual of Nursing Practice,* 8th ed. Philadelphia: Lippincott Williams & Wilkins, 2005.

*Nursing2006 Drug Handbook,* 26th ed. Philadelphia: Lippincott Williams & Wilkins, 2006.

*Nursing Procedures,* 4th ed. Philadelphia: Lippincott Williams & Wilkins, 2004.

Pagana, K.D., and Pagana, T.J. *Mosby's Diagnostic and Laboratory Test Reference,* 7th ed. St. Louis: Mosby–Year Book, Inc., 2005.

Pillitteri, A. *Maternal & Child Health Nursing,* 4th ed. Philadelphia: Lippincott Williams & Wilkins, 2003.

Porth, C. *Pathophysiology: Concepts of Altered Health States,* 7th ed. Philadelphia: Lippincott Williams & Wilkins, 2005.

*Professional Guide to Diseases*, 8th ed. Philadelphia: Lippincott Williams & Wilkins, 2005.

Ryan, K.J., ed. *Sherris Medical Microbiology: An Introduction to Infectious Diseases,* 3rd ed. Stamford, Conn.: Appleton & Lange, 2003.

Sanchez-Carbayo, M. "Recent Advances in Bladder Cancer Diagnostics," *Clinical Biochemistry* 37(7):562-71, July 2004.

Schnell, Z., et al. *Davis's Comprehensive Handbook of Laboratory and Diagnostic Tests with Nursing Implications.* Philadelphia: F.A. Davis Co., 2003.

Scott, J., et al., eds. *Danforth's Obstetrics and Gynecology,* 9th ed. Philadelphia: Lippincott Williams & Wilkins, 2003.

Stonesifer, E. "Common Laboratory and Diagnostic Testing in Patients with Gastrointestinal Disease," *AACN Clinical Issues* 15(4):582-94, October-December 2004.

Turgeon, M. *Clinical Hematology Theory and Procedures,* 4th ed., Philadelphia: Lippincott, Williams and Wilkins, 2005.

Van Le, T.S., et al. "Functional Characterization of the Bladder Cancer Marker, BLCA-4," *Clinical Cancer Research* 10(4):1384-91, February 2004.

Walton, H.G., et al. "Comparison of Blood Gas and Electrolyte Test Results from the Gem-Premier and the ABL-70 Versus a Conventional Laboratory Analyzer," *Journal of Extracorporeal Technology* 35(1):24-27, March 2003.

Wilkins, R.L., and Stoller, J.K. *Egan's Fundamentals of Respiratory Care,* 8th ed. St. Louis: Mosby–Year Book, Inc., 2003.

Wilkinson, T.M., et al. "Airway Bacterial Load and $FEV_1$ Decline in Patients with Chronic Obstructive Pulmonary Disease," *American Journal of Respiratory and Critical Care Medicine* 167(8):1090-95, April 2003.

Williams, P.B., et al. "Are Our Impressions of Allergy Test Performances Correct?" *Annals of Allergy, Asthma, and Immunology* 91(1):26-33, July 2003.

Yarbo, C.H., et al., eds. *Cancer Nursing: Principles and Practice,* 6th ed. Boston: Jones & Bartlett Pubs., Inc., 2005.

# INDEX

i refers to an illustration; t refers to a table.

i refers to an illustration; t refers to a table.

---

i refers to an illustration; t refers to a table.

---

i refers to an illustration; t refers to a table.

---

i refers to an illustration; t refers to a table.

---

i refers to an illustration; t refers to a table.

i refers to an illustration; t refers to a table.

i refers to an illustration; t refers to a table.

i refers to an illustration; t refers to a table.

---

i refers to an illustration; t refers to a table.

Mean corpuscular hemoglobin concentration in anemias, 379t
Mean corpuscular volume in anemias, 379t
Mediastinoscopy, 284-285
Mediastinum, abnormalities of, in chest X-ray films, 97t
Menghini needle, how to use, 319i
Meningioma, intracranial computed tomography in, 245i, 246
Meningitis
 bacterial meningitis antigen in, 44
 cerebrospinal fluid analysis in, 94t
Meniscal disorders
 arthrography in, 36
 arthroscopy in, 38
Menstrual abnormalities
 plasma progesterone in, 346
 urine pregnanediol in, 342
Metabolic acidosis, 32t
 anion gap and, 16
 arterial blood gas analysis in, 32t
 serum chloride in, 100
Metabolic alkalosis, 32t
 arterial blood gas analysis in, 32t
 serum chloride in, 100
Metastatic carcinoma
 serum calcium in, 72
 urine calcium and phosphates in, 72t
Microagglutination assay, 199
Milk-alkali syndrome, urine calcium and phosphates in, 72t
Minute volume measurement, 360t
Mitogen assay, 275
Mitral stenosis
 echocardiography in, 146i, 147, 148i
 pulmonary artery catheterization in, 359
 real-time echocardiogram in, 147, 148i
Mixed lymphocyte culture assay, 275
Modified Thayer-Martin medium, 215i
Monocytes, influence of disease on, 499t
Mononucleosis, infectious
 alanine aminotransferase in, 5
 anti–smooth-muscle antibodies in, 26
 aspartate aminotransferase in, 39
 bone marrow findings in, 62t
 cryoglobulins in, 126t
MonoVacc test, 467-469
Multiple-gated acquisition scanning, 75-76
Multiple myeloma
 Bence Jones protein in, 48
 B-lymphocyte assay in, 441
 cryoglobulins in, 126t
 erythrocyte sedimentation rate in, 170
 protein levels in, 351

Multiple myeloma *(continued)*
 serum calcium in, 72
 serum immunoglobulin levels in, 365t
 urine calcium and phosphates in, 72t
Multiple sclerosis, visual evoked potentials in, 177i
Muscle disorders
 electromyography in, 158-159
 urine myoglobin in, 288
Myasthenia gravis
 electromyography in, 159
 Tensilon test in, 443-444
Myelography, 285-287
Myocardial infarction
 aspartate aminotransferase in, 39
 complement assays in, 110
 gamma glutamyl transferase in, 208
 lactate dehydrogenase in, 254t, 255
 myoglobins in, 288
 technetium pyrophosphate scanning in, 442
 thallium imaging in, 446
 troponin in, 467
Myoglobin
 blood levels of, 288
 urine, 288

# N

Nasopharyngeal culture, 289-290
 obtaining specimen for, 290i
*Neisseria gonorrhoeae*, culturing for, 214-216, 215i
Neonatal thyroid-stimulating hormone, 290-291
Neoplastic disorders
 gallium scanning in, 207
 human placental lactogen in, 238
 paranasal sinus radiography in, 313t
 protein levels in, 351
Nephritis, urine calcium and phosphates in, 72t
Nephrosis, urine calcium and phosphates in, 72t
Nephrotic syndrome, serum immunoglobulin levels in, 365t
Nephrotomography, 291-293
 differential diagnosis in, 293t
Nerve conduction studies, 158
Nervous system abnormalities, evoked potential studies in, 179
Neural tube defects, alpha-fetoprotein in, 10
Neuroblastoma
 plasma catecholamines in, 86
 urine catecholamines in, 87

---

i refers to an illustration; t refers to a table.

---

i refers to an illustration; t refers to a table.

i refers to an illustration; t refers to a table.

i refers to an illustration; t refers to a table.

---

i refers to an illustration; t refers to a table.

---

i refers to an illustration; t refers to a table.

---

i refers to an illustration; t refers to a table.

---

i refers to an illustration; t refers to a table.